Prospects for Schistosomiasis Elimination

Prospects for Schistosomiasis Elimination

Special Issue Editors

Robert Bergquist
Darren Gray

MDPI • Basel • Beijing • Wuhan • Barcelona • Belgrade

Special Issue Editors
Robert Bergquist
Swiss TPH
Switzerland

Darren Gray
ANU College of Health and Medicine
Australia

Editorial Office
MDPI
St. Alban-Anlage 66
4052 Basel, Switzerland

This is a reprint of articles from the Special Issue published online in the open access journal *Tropical Medicine and Infectious Disease* (ISSN 2414-6366) from 2018 to 2019 (available at: https://www.mdpi.com/journal/tropicalmed/special_issues/schistosomiasis)

For citation purposes, cite each article independently as indicated on the article page online and as indicated below:

LastName, A.A.; LastName, B.B.; LastName, C.C. Article Title. *Journal Name* **Year**, *Article Number*, Page Range.

ISBN 978-3-03921-357-3 (Pbk)
ISBN 978-3-03921-358-0 (PDF)

Cover image courtesy of Darren Gray.

Contents

About the Special Issue Editors . . . . **ix**

Preface to "Prospects for Schistosomiasis Elimination" . . . . **xi**

Robert Bergquist and Darren J. Gray
Schistosomiasis Elimination: Beginning of the End or a Continued March on a Trodden Path
Reprinted from: *Trop. Med. Infect. Dis.* **2019**, *4*, 76, doi:10.3390/tropicalmed4020076 . . . . **1**

Jin Chen, Jing Xu, Robert Bergquist, Shi-Zhu Li and Xiao-Nong Zhou
"Farewell to the God of Plague": The Importance of Political Commitment Towards the Elimination of Schistosomiasis
Reprinted from: *Trop. Med. Infect. Dis.* **2018**, *3*, 108, doi:10.3390/tropicalmed3040108 . . . . **10**

W. Evan Secor and Daniel G. Colley
When Should the Emphasis on Schistosomiasis Control Move to Elimination?
Reprinted from: *Trop. Med. Infect. Dis.* **2018**, *3*, 85, doi:10.3390/tropicalmed3030085 . . . . **14**

Callie J. Weber, Joseph Hargan-Calvopiña, Katy M. Graef, Cathyryne K. Manner and Jennifer Dent
WIPO Re:Search—A Platform for Product-Centered Cross-Sector Partnerships for the Elimination of Schistosomiasis
Reprinted from: *Trop. Med. Infect. Dis.* **2019**, *4*, 11, doi:10.3390/tropicalmed4010011 . . . . **23**

Stefanie J. Krauth, Julie Balen, Geoffrey N. Gobert and Poppy H. L. Lamberton
A Call for Systems Epidemiology to Tackle the Complexity of Schistosomiasis, Its Control, and Its Elimination
Reprinted from: *Trop. Med. Infect. Dis.* **2019**, *4*, 21, doi:10.3390/tropicalmed4010021 . . . . **43**

Remigio M. Olveda and Darren J. Gray
Schistosomiasis in the Philippines: Innovative Control Approach is Needed if Elimination is the Goal
Reprinted from: *Trop. Med. Infect. Dis.* **2019**, *4*, 66, doi:10.3390/tropicalmed4020066 . . . . **54**

Catherine A. Gordon, Johanna Kurscheid, Gail M. Williams, Archie C. A. Clements, Yuesheng Li, Xiao-Nong Zhou, Jürg Utzinger, Donald P. McManus and Darren J. Gray
Asian Schistosomiasis: Current Status and Prospects for Control Leading to Elimination
Reprinted from: *Trop. Med. Infect. Dis.* **2019**, *4*, 40, doi:10.3390/tropicalmed4010040 . . . . **59**

Virak Khieu, Somphou Sayasone, Sinuon Muth, Masashi Kirinoki, Sakhone Laymanivong, Hiroshi Ohmae, Rekol Huy, Thipphavanh Chanthapaseuth, Aya Yajima, Rattanaxay Phetsouvanh, Robert Bergquist and Peter Odermatt
Elimination of Schistosomiasis Mekongi from Endemic Areas in Cambodia and the Lao People's Democratic Republic: Current Status and Plans
Reprinted from: *Trop. Med. Infect. Dis.* **2019**, *4*, 30, doi:10.3390/tropicalmed4010030 . . . . **88**

Reynold Hewitt and Arve Lee Willingham
Status of Schistosomiasis Elimination in the Caribbean Region
Reprinted from: *Trop. Med. Infect. Dis.* **2019**, *4*, 24, doi:10.3390/tropicalmed4010024 . . . . **103**

Rodrigue Mintsa Nguema, Jacques F. Mavoungou, Krystina Mengue Me Ngou-Milama, Modeste Mabicka Mamfoumbi, Aubin A. Koumba, Mariama Sani Lamine, Abdoulaye Diarra, Ghislaine Nkone Asseko, Jean R. Mourou, Marielle K. Bouyou Akotet, Hélène Moné, Gabriel Mouahid and Julienne Atsame
Baseline Mapping of Schistosomiasis and Soil Transmitted Helminthiasis in the Northern and Eastern Health Regions of Gabon, Central Africa: Recommendations for Preventive Chemotherapy
Reprinted from: *Trop. Med. Infect. Dis.* **2018**, 3, 119, doi:10.3390/tropicalmed3040119 . . . . **120**

Moses Adriko, Christina L. Faust, Lauren V. Carruthers, Arinaitwe Moses, Edridah M. Tukahebwa and Poppy H. L. Lamberton
Low Praziquantel Treatment Coverage for *Schistosoma mansoni* in Mayuge District, Uganda, Due to the Absence of Treatment Opportunities, Rather Than Systematic Non-Compliance
Reprinted from: *Trop. Med. Infect. Dis.* **2018**, 3, 111, doi:10.3390/tropicalmed3040111 . . . . **142**

Jean T. Coulibaly, Mamadou Ouattara, Beatrice Barda, Jürg Utzinger, Eliézer K. N'Goran and Jennifer Keiser
A Rapid Appraisal of Factors Influencing Praziquantel Treatment Compliance in Two Communities Endemic for Schistosomiasis in Côte d'Ivoire
Reprinted from: *Trop. Med. Infect. Dis.* **2018**, 3, 69, doi:10.3390/tropicalmed3020069 . . . . **155**

Harrison K. Korir, Diana K. Riner, Emmy Kavere, Amos Omondi, Jasmine Landry, Nupur Kittur, Eric M. Ndombi, Bartholomew N. Ondigo, W. Evan Secor, Diana M. S. Karanja and Daniel G. Colley
Young Adults in Endemic Areas: An Untreated Group in Need of School-Based Preventive Chemotherapy for Schistosomiasis Control and Elimination
Reprinted from: *Trop. Med. Infect. Dis.* **2018**, 3, 100, doi:10.3390/tropicalmed3030100 . . . . **166**

Kosala G. Weerakoon, Catherine A. Gordon and Donald P. McManus
DNA Diagnostics for Schistosomiasis Control
Reprinted from: *Trop. Med. Infect. Dis.* **2018**, 3, 81, doi:10.3390/tropicalmed3030081 . . . . **172**

Zhi-Qiang Qin, Jing Xu, Ting Feng, Shan Lv, Ying-Jun Qian, Li-Juan Zhang, Yin-Long Li, Chao Lv, Robert Bergquist, Shi-Zhu Li and Xiao-Nong Zhou
Field Evaluation of a Loop-Mediated Isothermal Amplification (LAMP) Platform for the Detection of *Schistosoma japonicum* Infection in *Oncomelania hupensis* Snails
Reprinted from: *Trop. Med. Infect. Dis.* **2018**, 3, 124, doi:10.3390/tropicalmed3040124 . . . . **192**

Eniola M. Abe, Yun-Hai Guo, Haimo Shen, Masceline J. Mutsaka-Makuvaza, Mohamed R. Habib, Jing-Bo Xue, Nicholas Midzi, Jing Xu, Shi-Zhu Li and Xiao-Nong Zhou
Phylogeography of *Bulinus truncatus* (Audouin, 1827) (Gastropoda: Planorbidae) in Selected African Countries
Reprinted from: *Trop. Med. Infect. Dis.* **2018**, 3, 127, doi:10.3390/tropicalmed3040127 . . . . **202**

Damilare O. Famakinde
Treading the Path towards Genetic Control of Snail Resistance to Schistosome Infection
Reprinted from: *Trop. Med. Infect. Dis.* **2018**, 3, 86, doi:10.3390/tropicalmed3030086 . . . . **213**

Guo-Jing Yang and Robert Bergquist
Potential Impact of Climate Change on Schistosomiasis: A Global Assessment Attempt
Reprinted from: *Trop. Med. Infect. Dis.* **2018**, 3, 117, doi:10.3390/tropicalmed3040117 . . . . **228**

Miriam Tendler, Marília S. Almeida, Monica M. Vilar, Patrícia M. Pinto and Gabriel Limaverde-Sousa
Current Status of the Sm14/GLA-SE Schistosomiasis Vaccine: Overcoming Barriers and Paradigms towards the First Anti-Parasitic Human(itarian) Vaccine
Reprinted from: *Trop. Med. Infect. Dis.* **2018**, *3*, 121, doi:10.3390/tropicalmed3040121 . . . . **239**

Miriam Tendler, Marília S. Almeida, Monica M. Vilar, Patrícia M. Pinto and Gabriel Limaverde-Sousa
Correction: Tendler, M., et al. Current Status of the Sm14/GLA-SE Schistosomiasis Vaccine: Overcoming Barriers and Paradigms towards the First Anti-Parasitic Human(itarian) Vaccine. *Trop. Med. Infect. Dis.* 2018, *3*, 121
Reprinted from: *Trop. Med. Infect. Dis.* **2019**, *4*, 16, doi:10.3390/tropicalmed4010016 . . . . **249**

Hong You, Pengfei Cai, Biniam Mathewos Tebeje, Yuesheng Li and Donald P. McManus
Schistosome Vaccines for Domestic Animals
Reprinted from: *Trop. Med. Infect. Dis.* **2018**, *3*, 68, doi:10.3390/tropicalmed3020068 . . . . **250**

John B. Malone, Robert Bergquist, Moara Martins and Jeffrey C. Luvall
Use of Geospatial Surveillance and Response Systems for Vector-Borne Diseases in the Elimination Phase
Reprinted from: *Trop. Med. Infect. Dis.* **2019**, *4*, 15, doi:10.3390/tropicalmed4010015 . . . . **263**

Robert Bergquist and Hala Elmorshedy
Artemether and Praziquantel: Origin, Mode of Action, Impact, and Suggested Application for Effective Control of Human Schistosomiasis
Reprinted from: *Trop. Med. Infect. Dis.* **2018**, *3*, 125, doi:10.3390/tropicalmed3040125 . . . . **279**

About the Special Issue Editors

Robert Bergquist. After retiring as a medical officer at the UNICEF/UNDP/World Bank/WHO Special Programme for Research and Training in Tropical Diseases (TDR), Geneva, Switzerland, Robert Bergquist became the Editor-in-Chief of the journal *Geospatial Health* and is affiliated to the Swiss Tropical and Public Health Institute (Swiss TPH), Basel, Switzerland. He graduated with an MD, and later a Ph.D., from the Karolinska Institute, Stockholm, Sweden, and is currently the author/coauthor of 250+ scientific communications and textbook chapters. He has been the editor/coeditor of several Special Issues of *Acta Tropica, Advances in Parasitology*, and *Annals of the New York Academy of Sciences.*

Darren Gray is currently the Deputy Director of the Research School of Population Health and Head of its Department of Global Health at the Australian National University. Prof. Gray is an infectious disease epidemiologist and leads a research program that investigates the transmission and control of neglected tropical diseases (including schistosomiasis)—some of the most prevalent and important infections that cause much suffering and economic loss worldwide. He aims to develop new public health interventions against these pathogens that will lead to their sustainable control and eventual elimination. Prof. Gray has worked in global/international health since 2004, particularly focusing on Southeast Asia, and he currently sits on the editorial boards for *Tropical Medicine and Infectious Disease* (MDPI) and *PLoS Neglected Tropical Diseases* (Public Library of Science).

Preface to "Prospects for Schistosomiasis Elimination"

Elimination Becomes a Reality—Preface and a Call to Action

Marcel Tanner
Swiss Tropical and Public Health Institute, Basel, Switzerland
Swiss Academies of Sciences

"It always seems impossible until it's done." (Nelson Mandela)

These papers, compiling global evidence from the past decades, reveal that we are indeed on a path, but surely not on a well-trodden one—and our pace is quickening. The learning from basic parasitology on host–parasite–intermediate host relationships at the genetic, cellular, and population level placed within the different social, cultural, and ecological contexts not only generate the understanding of a given epidemiological context and possible and necessary public health actions, but also stimulate the research and development of control and public health tools for (i) diagnosis and surveillance, (ii) the prediction of risk areas and decision support/decision-making, (iii) the repurposing of existing safe and efficacious drugs and pediatric formulations, (iv) the potential and position of vaccines, and (v) integrated approaches tailored to specific endemic settings in relation to the schistosome species involved. The present Special Issue brings together evidence and experience in a most comprehensive way, providing a cornerstone for any national control program to seriously consider the elimination of schistosomiasis as a very realistic public health goal.

The complexity of the specificity of the host–parasite–intermediate host relationships and the dynamic influence of the socioecological settings are recognized as well as the individual host–parasite interrelations that govern the pathological outcomes. This in turn helps us explain the focality of transmission and the transmission patterns as we observe them in their natural settings. While the great intricacy of basic parasitology and epidemiology makes us initially shy away from the idea of the possible elimination of schistosomiasis, a more cautious look with the currently available scientific evidence and tools in mind makes us realize that the key to elimination lies precisely in this manifold.

With the achievements of control tools, well-reflected in the present series of papers, further activities towards elimination rest mainly on the backbone of effective surveillance–response approaches within the national programs. Detection and interruption of transmission redirects the focus to the peripheral, point-of-care level, making local surveillance the key intervention. Strategies developed towards effective approaches, capable of detecting ongoing, new, or reintroduced transmission foci, can be swiftly followed by integrated public health response packages tailored to any given transmission setting. This tactic is currently also central to the elimination approaches for malaria guided by the Global Technical Strategy (GTS) endorsed by all WHO member countries in 2015. The GTS for malaria consists of three key pillars: (i) ensure universal access to prevention, diagnosis, and treatment; (ii) accelerate efforts towards elimination; and (iii) transform malaria surveillance into a core intervention. Not only through analogy, but also based on the current state of knowledge, evidence, experience, and ongoing R&D activities, we are now in a very comparable situation for schistosomiasis. Indeed, we are in a promising position allowing the formulation of a global technical strategy for both diseases that is even generally applicable for most of the neglected tropical diseases, thus forming a realistic, operational basis to reach the goals of the London Declaration of 2012.

I congratulate the editors and authors for having produced a stimulating text, and I thank all those working towards the veracity of schistosomiasis elimination. This call to action helps in translating science into meaningful public health and development engagement, making schistosomiasis elimination a realistic goal.

Robert Bergquist, Darren Gray
Special Issue Editors

Tropical Medicine and Infectious Disease

MDPI

Editorial

Schistosomiasis Elimination: Beginning of the End or a Continued March on a Trodden Path

Robert Bergquist [1,*] and Darren J. Gray [2]

1 Ingerod, SE-454 94 Brastad, Sweden
2 Research School of Population Health, Australian National University, Canberra, ACT 2601, Australia; darren.gray@anu.edu.au
* Correspondence: robert.bergquist@outlook.com; Tel.: +46-523-43336

Received: 12 April 2019; Accepted: 15 April 2019; Published: 5 May 2019

Abstract: In spite of spectacular progress towards the goal of elimination of schistosomiasis, particularly in China but also in other areas, research gaps and outstanding issues remain. Although expectations of achieving elimination of this disease have never been greater, all constraints have not been swept aside. Indeed, there are some formidable obstacles, such as insufficient amounts of drugs to treat everybody and still limited use of high-sensitive diagnostic techniques, both for the definitive and the intermediate hosts, which indicate that prevalence is considerably underrated in well-controlled areas. Elimination will be difficult to achieve without a broad approach, including a stronger focus on transmission, better diagnostics and the establishment of a reliable survey system activating a rapid response when called for. Importantly, awareness of the crucial importance of transmission has been revived resulting in renewed interest in snail control together with more emphasis on health education and sanitation. The papers collected in this special issue entitled 'Prospects for Schistosomiasis Elimination' reflect these issues and we are particularly pleased to note that some also discuss the crucial question when to declare a country free of schistosomiasis and present techniques that together create an approach that can show unequivocally when interruption of transmission has been achieved.

Keywords: schistosomiasis elimination; snail control; high-sensitivity diagnostics; chemotherapy; vaccine development; health education; sanitation

1. Introduction

Although severe morbidity due to schistosomiasis is disappearing, the distribution of the disease has not changed since the atlas of schistosomiasis distribution was published in 1987 [1]. Considering the population increase since then, the number of humans currently at risk must be well over a billion rather than the commonly cited figure of 800 million. According to latest available information somewhere between 230 and 250 million people are actually infected [2,3]. However, these data must be even more strongly underestimated since they are based on stool examination according to Kato-Katz [4] for intestinal schistosomiasis (basically *Schistosoma mansoni*, *S, japonicum* and *S. mekongi*) and urine filtration for the urogenital form of the disease (*S. haematobium*). Diagnosis based on the schistosome circulating cathodic antigen (CCA) finds up to four times more infected individuals compared to egg detection [5], which is supported by molecular diagnostics, e.g., the quantitative polymerase chain reaction (qPCR), a highly sensitive and specific technique [6,7]. However, the total number of infected people is not necessarily as high as four times more (as indicated by CCA) since the discrepancies reported also depend on the intensity of infection. Nonetheless, even with a multiplicator as low as two, we remain far from elimination of schistosomiasis and one wonders why control efforts for such a widespread infection have been so inadequate that the World Health Organization (WHO) lists the disease among the neglected tropical diseases (NTDs). The funds going into schistosomiasis research, however, tell another story, and we are already starting to benefit from a wide spectrum of new results ranging from improved diagnostics over vaccine development to better satellite-generated ecological data.

Why did schistosomiasis become such a scourge in the first place? A strong reason is the high concentration of people near rivers and lakes harbouring the intermediate snail hosts, while curative measures could not be contemplated until the parasite had been discovered [8] and its life-cycle demonstrated [9]. Although these findings clarified the epidemiology, effective disease prevention would not be available until the introduction of praziquantel in the 1970s [10]. Promoting sanitation and telling people to avoid lakes and streams in rural areas without infrastructures were as unrealistic then as it is today, so early activities relied primarily on snail control through various molluscicides released into water bodies used by people in the endemic areas [11] and environmental management (useful only for the type of snail transmitting *S. japonicum*). After the 1980s, however, mass drug administration (MDA) with praziquantel started to make inroads and although reinfection remained a problem, severe morbidity could now be managed through repeated drug treatments. Indeed, chemotherapy proved so efficient that it soon became the only approach contributing to WHO's 1984 recommendation that morbidity control be the main goal [12], a strategy that is still largely in place.

Different countries need different approaches since large epidemiological differences between them exist, not the least due to the intermediate sail host, which makes it impossible to apply the same approach everywhere. Although the scope for elimination of schistosomiasis is promising in some countries, the People's Republic of China (PR China), Brazil, Egypt, Morocco and Oman among them, the situation is altogether different in sub-Saharan Africa, which currently harbours 92% of all schistosomiasis in the world [13]. Thus, research gaps and outstanding issues still remain, one of which is the highly unsatisfactory situation of depending on a single drug for the control of a major disease, even if there is still no evidence of widespread resistance. Equally disconcerting is the realization that the number of people with schistosomiasis will continue to rise as a reflection of the ongoing population growth, while the proportion of people actually receiving drug treatment lingers far behind that of those requiring it [14].

2. Can Schistosomiasis be Eliminated?

The special issue Prospects for Schistosomiasis Elimination was conceived in response to the need for an all-round view of the present situation with special reference to the tools needed to reach the goal of elimination of one of the worst NTDs that may have caused more human suffering than any other parasitic disease after malaria. Schistosomiasis elimination in PR China has a 60-year history. Repeating this achievement, briefly described in the first paper in this volume [15], in other countries will require long-term governmental support and the incorporation of social and economic approaches boosting local economies and global health development.

Secor and Colley [16] feel that elimination may well be currently feasible in some endemic countries where there have been improvements in sanitation and access to clean water, but point out that sub-Saharan Africa, this strategy switch remains premature. They emphasize the need to develop and evaluate approaches for achieving and validating elimination, as well as defining the level of infection at which a stepped-up approach to interruption of transmission would be feasible. These ideas are echoed by Krauth et al. [17] who discuss possible hidden drivers of transmission that might hamper intervention success and sustainability. They propose a holistic research approach integrating classical epidemiology with modern knowledge of biology, ecology and the social sciences to uncover processes that indirectly influence exposure and transmission. Addressing persisting disease hotspots and neglected population groups could help overcome barriers holding us back from achieving schistosomiasis elimination. An opinion paper by Olveda and Gray [18] emphasizes that the integrated measures pioneered by PR China cannot be duplicated in the Philippines because of the geographical diversity and topography of this country, and the fact that transmission is not seasonal as in PR China. In fact, the situation in the Philippines is more like that of sub-Saharan

Africa plus the added problem of dealing with zoonotic transmission. For that reason, they feel an innovative, multi-component approach is critical for long-term sustainable schistosomiasis control and eventual elimination in the Philippines. The key is to ensure high praziquantel coverage of endemic populations and realize the role of bovines in transmission. The bovine population in the endemic areas must either be rigorously treated, vaccinated or replaced with mechanized tractors (as in PR China). Another, more general, opinion paper by Weber et al. [19] highlights the opportunities for public–private partnerships (PPPs) to play a key role in the elimination of schistosomiasis. They point out the critical need for diversified therapeutics and they note gaps in the vaccine and diagnostic product R&D pipelines.

3. Progress Vis-à-Vis the Distribution of Schistosomiasis

Asian schistosomiasis is zoonotic, which is a cause of concern as successful elimination not only requires management of the human definitive host, but also the animal reservoir hosts. Within Asia, three species affect humans (*S. japonicum*, *S. mekongi* and *S. malayensis*). Most of the published research has focused on *S. japonicum* with comparatively little attention paid to *S. mekongi* and even less to *S. malayensis*. In this special issue, Gordon et al. [20] examined all three species, highlighting the prospects for elimination and current occurrence in their various endemic countries: Cambodia, Lao People's Democratic Republic (Lao PDR), Malaysia, Myanmar, Thailand, Indonesia, PR China and the Philippines. Apart from the spectacular advancements made in PR China, briefly discussed in the paper by Chen et al. [15], progress in areas and countries, such as the Caribbean, Gabon and Lao PDR, are presented in some detail in this special issue. Excellent progress has been reported previously from Morocco, Africa's Mediterranean coast and Oman [13], but is not further discussed here.

Schistosomiasis in Lao PDR was first reported 60 years ago and 10 years later in Cambodia. The infection there is caused by a specific species, *S. mekongi*, which is distributed along a limited part of the Mekong River. Control activities based on mass drug administration resulted in strong advances reducing prevalence to less than 5% according to stool microscopy [21]. Even so, the true number of infected people is probably higher than that reported and further progress will depend on interruption of transmission. Although this type of well-characterized setting offers an exemplary potential for elimination, the local topography, reservoir animals, and a dearth of safe water sources make transmission control a challenge. On the other hand, these limited endemic foci would indeed be excellent testing grounds for what it takes to keep prevalence permanently low.

In the Caribbean, here chronicled by Hewitt and Willingham [22], elimination of schistosomiasis appears achievable in the near term. Transmission has already been eliminated on three islands with six more awaiting official verification. Saint Lucia is now the remaining island with clear evidence of ongoing transmission. Although mass treatment together with snail control using environmental, chemical and biological methods along with public service improvements are important elements in achieving and sustaining elimination, the economic switch from sugarcane and banana production to tourism obviously played a major role.

Mintsa Nguema et al. [23] report the results of mapping the prevalence of schistosomiasis in Gabon (primarily caused by *S. haematobium*), together with the situation with regard to soil transmitted helminthiases (STH) in the northern and eastern regions of the country, which covers 12% of the population. While many STH infections were found to be very common, schistosomiasis prevalence was only 1.7% across the two regions investigated, with no significant difference between them. However, the combined schistosomiasis/STH rate was shown to reach 56.6% and the conclusion was to recommend an integrated approach using praziquantel and mebendazole, supplemented with levamisole due to the high prevalence and intensity of *Trichuris* infections.

4. Risk for Fragmented Treatment Coverage

The world burden of schistosomiasis remains considerable, and factors influencing intervention coverage are important. To cover all needs with respect to chemotherapy in a country or region can be difficult, even if the drug and means for its distribution are available. The papers collected here highlight three such situations, though there may well be others, both different and even perhaps more serious. Coverage of praziquantel is an important research area since breaking the transmission of schistosomiasis may remain unattainable without a thorough understanding of this issue.

Adriko et al. [24] carried out a cross-sectional household surveys in an endemic district in Uganda where half the entire population reported never having taken praziquantel. It was found that odds improving use of the drug includes school enrolment and stable settlement in a village. The most frequent reasons that prevented treatment during the latest MDA for a person was either not being offered the drug even if present (49.2%) or being away when it was offered (21.4%). Contrary to expectations, chronically-untreated individuals were rarely systematic non-compliers but rather people who, for various reasons, had repeatedly not been offered treatment.

Coulibaly et al. [25] studied the reasons for low-treatment coverage rates in two endemic villages in Côte d'Ivoire. Based on a questionnaire survey, they found a considerable inter-village heterogeneity (27.7% versus 52.3%) that turned out to be multifactorial. The main reason was work-related (agricultural activities), but the bitter taste of praziquantel and previous experiences with adverse events also played an important role. More than three-quarters of those interviewed who had taken praziquantel declared that they would not participate in future treatments. Therefore, careful consideration should be given to attitudes and practices.

Students at the college and university level, a group that normally falls outside the common type of surveys, were investigated in Kenya with regard to schistosomiasis and STH infections by Korir et al. [26]. In a sample of close to 300 persons, each tested by three stools/two slides, *S. mansoni* prevalence was found to be 17.8% with 2.5% having heavy *S. mansoni* infections (≥400 eggs/gram faeces). The STH prevalence was much lower. While one wonders why young adults in higher education do not look after themselves better, it is obvious that this group of the population is as approachable for the national schistosomiasis control programmes, as are school children.

5. New Approaches

The special issue includes many papers outlining new thoughts, such as geospatial techniques, alternative treatments, high-definition diagnostics and vaccine development. For example, the launch of the Soil Moisture Active Passive (SMAP) satellite in 2015 and the new ECOSTRESS instrument launched in 2018 permit the collection of data that define the ecosystems that govern vector sustainability considerably better than was previously possible, while the high spatial resolution available opened for studies at very specific areas, such as the sub-village, even household, level [27]. This will help delineation of the exact possible geographical distribution of schistosomiasis, including changes related to climate change, through the ecological niche requirements by its intermediate host.

It is becoming increasingly clear that praziquantel on its own has insufficient activity against transmission since it only affects mature schistosomes Although several doses of praziquantel over a period of 1–2 months would eventually kill all parasites including the initially refractory young ones as they mature during this time. Use of combined artemether/praziquantel, on the other hand, would have an instantaneous effect as artemether would contribute by wiping out the new, still immature generation in the host, as pointed out by Bergquist and Elmorshedy [28]. However, this approach must be limited to areas without malaria co-endemicity to avoid the risk of the development of resistance against artemether, a key drug against malaria.

6. Diagnostics

Low infection intensities are now common thanks to long-term, widespread preventive chemotherapy. Surveillance in this situation requires considerably more sensitive diagnostics than stool microscopy, which is still the standard approach in the endemic areas. Indeed, overlooked low-intensity infections and the fact that praziquantel does not kill all schistosomes in the body, conspire to keep transmission ongoing.

While diagnosis based on the schistosome circulating cathodic antigen (CCA) [5,29] is clearly more sensitive than stool examination, it does not represent the first high-definition diagnostic technique to be applied for schistosomiasis. Molecular approaches, such as the loop-mediated isothermal amplification (LAMP) [30] and the polymerase chain reaction (PCR) [31], have both been used earlier. The detection of schistosome components based on molecular techniques provide high specificity and high sensitivity, as well as detection of pre-patent infections, and are therefore essential at the elimination stage. Weerakoon et al. present all the various diagnostic techniques in great detail in this special issue [32]. While the assays discussed are similar with respect to sensitivity and can be applied to both blood and faeces, the circulating antigens are also excreted with the urine, which is an advantage that should improve compliancy of continued testing over long periods of time.

7. Vaccine Development

Work on schistosomiasis vaccines remains in the doldrums due to the difficulties in convincing donors of the need for a vaccine. The lack of funding for schistosomiasis vaccine development has been debilitating; not that vaccination in itself is a cure-all solution, but even a partially effective vaccine would be a long-term complement to effective chemotherapy. Against all odds, a few candidate molecules for human use have reached the clinical-trials level. One of these is the Sm14/GLA-SE schistosomiasis vaccine, primarily developed against *S. mansoni*, but which cross-reacts with *S. haematobium* and *S. japonicum*, has successfully completed Phase I and Phase IIa clinical trials, with Phase II/III trials underway in Senegal and further trials planned for Brazil. The paper by Tendler et al. [33] in this special issue reviews the development of this vaccine candidate based on the fatty acid-binding protein (FABP) and formulated with the glucopyranosyl lipid A (GLA-SE) adjuvant. The paper follows the development of this product from the initial experiments delivering strongly supportive data to the ongoing Phase II studies.

Studies undertaken in PR China [34] and the Philippines [35] have identified bovines as major reservoir hosts for *S. japonicum*, and so have provided the rationale for a veterinary-based transmission-blocking vaccine targeting bovines in these settings, benefitting animals directly and humans indirectly. The SjCTPI vaccine [36] has shown promise in experimental trials, and field trials have recently been completed in PR China and the Philippines [37,38]. Interestingly, as shown by You et al. [39] in this special issue, this kind of vaccine would also be useful in African countries although not for humans, only for animals. This work covers the whole field of veterinary schistosomiasis vaccines from irradiated larvae to the recombinant DNA technology revolution. Future challenges to be overcome to design and deliver effective anti-schistosome vaccines are summarized. The fact that schistosomiasis can cause significant animal morbidity and mortality, both in Asia and Africa, is an overlooked cause of economic loss. Although schistosome species, such as *S. bovis*, *S. curassoni* and *S. mattheei*, do not infect humans, they do infect a wide range of domestic animals, resulting in low economic output, reduced productivity and poor reproduction [40]. Furthermore, the ability of *S. bovis* to form interspecific hybrids naturally with the human parasite *S. haematobium* which has been observed in West Africa [41] should be noted as it presents the potential for zoonotic transmission also in Africa.

A vaccine complemented by praziquantel would not only reduce morbidity for the long term, but also reduce transmission, something that is notoriously difficult to achieve. While vaccination of cattle and water buffaloes can be successful in reducing the risk for human (and bovine) infection in an zoonotic environment, elimination of schistosomiasis in Africa may never be achievable without a human vaccine. However, even if good protection can be shown, full validation, large-scale production and release of a product for human use is still a long time away.

8. Research on the Snail

Efforts to control schistosomiasis started with molluscicides against the snail host and largely ineffectual medicines with serious side effects, vividly described by Jordan [42]. As mentioned above, once introduced on a large scale in the 1980s, the drug praziquantel was so effective that snail control was abandoned for morbidity control. We are now witnessing the return of snail control, here reflected by the submission of as many as four snail-related papers. Two of them deal with the genetic diversity of snails providing findings on the complex biology of this vector, which can be used to define snail phylogeography [43] or to study the molecular basis of snail susceptibility to schistosome infection [44]. The two other papers have completely different foci, one discusses the potential influence of climate change on the distribution of snails capable of transmitting schistosomiasis [45], while the other deals with highly sensitive schistosome diagnosis of infection with the snail based on loop-mediated isothermal amplification (LAMP) [46]. While the very nature of climate change makes the former paper speculative, the latter presents a validated approach to accreditation of schistosomiasis eradication (see below), something of great practical importance.

9. Accreditation

So far, only two infections, both viral, have successfully been eradicated: smallpox in 1979 [47] and cattle rinderpest in 2010 [48]. Rigorous investigations and specifications were required before these diseases were finally eradicated (the viruses still remain in a few high-security laboratories). However, the discussion before the announcements led to an exact definition of the terms "elimination" and "eradication". The former is defined as the "reduction to zero of the incidence of infection (or to a very low defined target rate) caused by a specified agent in a defined geographical area as a result of deliberate efforts", while the latter is defined as the "permanent reduction to zero of the worldwide incidence of infection caused by a specific agent as a result of deliberate efforts". While elimination requires continued measures to prevent re-establishment of disease transmission, intervention measures are no longer needed in the case of eradication.

The stated aim to eliminate schistosomiasis must rely on considerably more sensitive assays than stool microscopy [4]. It is also important not to forget snail diagnostics. A very important outcome of this special issue is that some of its papers show that we now have the tools needed for the detection of the smallest number of schistosomes in the definitive host (CAA, qPCR or LAMP), as well as in the intermediate snail host, i.e. sporocysts and cercariae (PCR or LAMP). It should, however, be noted that long-term elimination is only possible if neither the intermediate nor the definitive hosts keep the *Schistosoma* life cycle moving as was achieved, and remains the case, in Japan. In addition, regular surveillance would be required, as well as control for potential infections in visiting people.

Funding: This research received no external funding.

Conflicts of Interest: The authors declare no conflict of interest.

References

1. Doumenge, J.P.; Mott, K.E. Global distribution of schistosomiasis: CEGET*-CNRS**/WHO Atlas. *World Health Stat. Q.* **1984**, *37*, 186–199. [PubMed]
2. Vos, T.; Flaxman, A.D.; Naghavi, M.; Lozano, R.; Michaud, C.; Ezzati, M.; Shibuya, K.; Salomon, J.A.; Abdalla, S.; Aboyans, V.; et al. Years lived with disability (YLDs) for 1160 sequelae of 289 diseases and injuries 1990–2010: A systematic analysis for the Global Burden of Disease Study 2010. *Lancet* **2012**, *380*, 2163–2196. [CrossRef]

3. Hotez, P.; Alvarado, M.; Basáñez, M.; Bolliger, I.; Bourne, R.; Boussinesq, M.; Brooker, S.; Brown, A.; Buckle, G.; Budke, C.; et al. (DALYs and HALE Collaborators). The gobal burden of disease study 2010: Interpretation and implications for the neglected tropical diseases. *PLoS Negl. Trop. Dis.* **2014**, *8*, e2865. [CrossRef] [PubMed]
4. Katz, N.; Chaves, A.; Pellegrino, J. A simple device for quantitative stool thick-smear technique in schistosomiasis mansoni. *Rev. Inst. Med. Trop. São Paulo.* **1972**, *14*, 397–400. [PubMed]
5. Colley, D.G.; Binder, S.; Campbell, C.; King, C.H.; Tchuem Tchuenté, L.A.; N'Goran, E.K.; Erko, B.; Karanja, D.M.; Kabatereine, N.B.; van Lieshout, L.; et al. A five-country evaluation of a point-of-care circulating cathodic antigen urine assay for the prevalence of *Schistosoma mansoni*. *Am. J. Trop. Med. Hyg.* **2013**, *88*, 426–432. [CrossRef] [PubMed]
6. He, P.; Gordon, C.A.; Williams, G.M.; Li, Y.; Wang, Y.; Hu, J.; Gray, D.J.; Ross, A.P.; Harn, D.; McManus, D.P. Real-time PCR diagnosis of *Schistosoma japonicum* in low transmission areas of China. *Infect. Dis. Poverty* **2018**, *7*, 8. [CrossRef] [PubMed]
7. Gordon, C.A.; Acosta, L.; Gobert, G.N.; Olveda, R.; Ross, A.G.; Jis, M.; Gray, D.J.; Williams, G.M.; Harn, D.A.; Li, Y.S.; et al. Real-time PCR demonstrates high prevalence of *Schistosoma japonicum* in the Philippines: Implications for surveillance and control. *PLoS Negl. Trop. Dis.* **2014**, *9*, e0003483. [CrossRef]
8. Bilharz, T.M. Fernere Beobachtungen über das die Pfortader des Menschen bewohnende Distomum Haematobium und sein Verhältnis zu gewissen pathologischen Bildungen, von Dr. Th. Bilharz in Cairo (aus brieflichen Mittheilungen an Professor v. Siebold vom 29 März 1852). *Zeitschrift Wissenschaftliche Zoologie* **1853**, *4*, 72–76. (In German)
9. Leiper, R.T. The relation between the terminal spined and lateral-spined eggs of bilharzia. *Br. Med. J.* **1916**, *1*, 411. [CrossRef]
10. Davis, A.; Wegner, D.H. Multicentre trials of praziquantel in human schistosomiasis: Design and techniques. *Bull. World Health Organ.* **1979**, *57*, 767–771. [PubMed]
11. McCullough, F.S.; Gayral, P.; Duncan, J.; Christie, J.D. Molluscicides in schistosomiasis control. *Bull. World Health Organ.* **1980**, *58*, 681–689.
12. WHO Expert Committee on the Control of Schistosomiasis & World Health Organization. *The Control of Schistosomiasis: Report of a WHO Expert Committee [Meeting Held in Geneva from 8 to 13 November 1984]*; World Health Organization: Geneva, Switzerland, 1985. Available online: http://www.who.int/iris/handle/10665/39529 (accessed on 17 February 2019).
13. WHO Fact Sheet (Data from 2017). Available online: https://www.who.int/neglected_diseases/preventive_chemotherapy/sch/en/ (accessed on 17 February 2019).
14. WHO Schistosomiasis Fact Sheet 2018. Available online: http://www.who.int/news-room/fact-sheets/detail/schistosomiasis (accessed on 17 February 2019).
15. Chen, J.; Xu, J.; Bergquist, R.; Li, S.-Z.; Zhou, X.-N. Farewell to the God of Plague: The importance of political commitment towards the elimination of schistosomiasis. *Trop. Med. Infect. Dis.* **2018**, *3*, 108. [CrossRef]
16. Secor, E.S.; Colley, D.G. When should the emphasis on schistosomiasis control move to elimination? *Trop. Med. Infect. Dis.* **2018**, *3*, 85. [CrossRef] [PubMed]
17. Krauth, S.J.; Balen, J.; Gobert, G.N.; Lamberton, P.H.L.A. Call for Systems Epidemiology to Tackle the Complexity Of Schistosomiasis, Its Control, And Its Elimination. *Trop. Med. Infect. Dis.* **2019**, *4*, 21. [CrossRef] [PubMed]
18. Olveda, R.M.; Gray, D.J. Schistosomiasis in the Philippines: Innovative control approach is needed if elimination is the goal. *Trop. Med. Infect. Dis.* **2019**, *4*, 66. [CrossRef]
19. Weber, C.J.; Hargan-Calvopiña, J.; Graef, K.M.; Manner, C.K.; Dent, J. WIPO Research—A platform for product-centered cross-sector partnerships for the elimination of schistosomiasis. *Trop. Med. Infect. Dis.* **2019**, *4*, 11. [CrossRef] [PubMed]
20. Gordon, C.A.; Kurscheid, J.; Williams, G.M.; Clements, A.C.A.; Li, Y.; Zhou, X.N.; Utzinger, J.; McManus, D.P.; Gray, D.J. Asian Schistosomiasis: Current Status and Prospects for Control Leading to Elimination. *Trop. Med. Infect. Dis.* **2019**, *4*, 40. [CrossRef] [PubMed]
21. Khieu, V.; Sayasone, S.; Muth, S.; Kirinoki, M.; Laymanivong, S.; Ohmae, H.; Huy, R.; Chanthapaseuth, T.; Yajima, A.; Phetsouvanh, R.; et al. Elimination of schistosomiasis mekongi from endemic areas in cambodia and the lao people's democratic republic: Current status and plans. *Trop. Med. Infect. Dis.* **2019**, *4*, 30. [CrossRef]

22. Hewitt, H.; Willingham, A.L. Status of Schistosomiasis Elimination in The Caribbean Region. *Trop. Med. Infect. Dis.* **2019**, *4*, 24. [CrossRef]
23. Mintsa Nguema, R.; Mavoungou, J.F.; Mengue Me Ngou-Milama, K.; Mabicka Mamfoumbi, M.; Koumba, A.A.; Sani Lamine, M.; Diarra, A.; Nkone Asseko, G.; Mourou, J.R.; Bouyou Akotet, M.K.; et al. Baseline Mapping of Schistosomiasis and Soil Transmitted Helminthiasis in the Northern and Eastern Health Regions of Gabon, Central Africa: Recommendations for Preventive Chemotherapy. *Trop. Med. Infect. Dis.* **2018**, *3*, 119. [CrossRef]
24. Adriko, M.; Faust, C.L.; Carruthers, L.V.; Moses, A.; Edridah, M.; Tukahebwa, E.M.; Lamberton, P.H.L. Low Praziquantel Treatment Coverage for *Schistosoma mansoni* in Mayuge District, Uganda, Due to the Absence of Treatment Opportunities, Rather Than Systematic Non-Compliance. *Trop. Med. Infect. Dis.* **2018**, *3*, 111. [CrossRef] [PubMed]
25. Coulibaly, J.T.; Ouattara, M.; Barda, B.; Utzinger, J.; N'Goran, E.K.; Keiser, J. A Rapid Appraisal of Factors Influencing Praziquantel Treatment Compliance in Two Communities Endemic for Schistosomiasis in Côte d'Ivoire. *Trop. Med. Infect. Dis.* **2018**, *3*, 69. [CrossRef]
26. Korir, H.K.; Riner, D.K.; Kavere, E.; Omondi, A.; Landry, J.; Kittur, N.; Ndombi, E.M.; Ondigo, B.N.; Secor, W.E.; Karanja, D.M.S.; et al. Young Adults in Endemic Areas: An Untreated Group in Need of School-Based Preventive Chemotherapy for Schistosomiasis Control and Elimination. *Trop. Med. Infect. Dis.* **2018**, *3*, 100. [CrossRef] [PubMed]
27. Malone, J.B.; Bergquist, R.; Martins, M.; Luvall, J.C. Use of geospatial surveillance and response systems for vector-borne diseases in the elimination phase. *Trop. Med. Infect. Dis.* **2019**, *4*, 15. [CrossRef] [PubMed]
28. Bergquist, R.; Elmorshedy, H. Artemether and Praziquantel: Origin, mode of action, impact, and suggested application for effective control of human schistosomiasis. *Trop. Med. Infect. Dis.* **2018**, *3*, 125. [CrossRef] [PubMed]
29. Corstjens, P.L.; De Dood, C.J.; Kornelis, D.; Fat, E.M.; Wilson, R.A.; Kariuki, T.M.; Nyakundi, R.K.; Loverde, P.T.; Abrams, W.R.; Tanke, H.J.; et al. Tools for diagnosis, monitoring and screening of *Schistosoma* infections utilizing lateral-flow based assays and upconverting phosphor labels. *Parasitology* **2014**, *141*, 1841–1855. [CrossRef]
30. Notomi, T.; Okayama, H.; Masubuchi, H.; Yonekawa, T.; Watanabe, K.; Amino, N.; Hase, T. Loop-mediated isothermal amplification of DNA. *Nucleic Acids Res.* **2000**, *28*, E63. [CrossRef] [PubMed]
31. Pontes, L.A.; Oliveira, M.C.; Katz, N.; Dias-Neto, E.; Rabello, A. Comparison of a polymerase chain reaction and the Kato-Katz technique for diagnosing infection with *Schistosoma mansoni*. *Am. J. Trop. Med. Hyg.* **2003**, *68*, 652–656. [CrossRef]
32. Weerakoon, K.G.; Gordon, C.A.; McManus, D.P. DNA diagnostics for schistosomiasis control. *Trop. Med. Infect. Dis.* **2018**, *3*, 81. [CrossRef]
33. Miriam Tendler, M.; Almeida, M.S.; Vilar, M.M.; Pinto, P.M.; Limaverde-Sousa, G. Current status of the Sm14/GLA-SE Schistosomiasis vaccine: Overcoming barriers and paradigms towards the first anti-parasitic human(itarian) vaccine. *Trop. Med. Infect. Dis.* **2018**, *3*, 121. [CrossRef]
34. Gray, D.J.; Williams, G.M.; Li, Y.; Chen, H.; Li, R.S.; Forsyth, S.J.; Barnett, A.G.; Guo, J.; Feng, Z.; McManus, D.P. A cluster-randomized bovine intervention trial against *Schistosoma japonicum* in the People's Republic of China: Design and baseline results. *Am. J. Trop. Med. Hyg.* **2007**, *77*, 866–874. [CrossRef] [PubMed]
35. Gordon, C.A.; Acosta, L.P.; Gray, D.J.; Olveda, R.M.; Jarilla, B.; Gobert, G.N.; Ross, A.G.; McManus, D.P. High prevalence of *Schistosoma japonicum* infection in Carabao from Samar Province, the Philippines: Implications for transmission and control. *PLoS Negl. Trop. Dis.* **2012**, *6*, e1778. [CrossRef]
36. Da'Dara, A.A.; Li, Y.S.; Xiong, T.; Zhou, J.; Williams, G.M.; McManus, D.P.; Feng, Z.; Yu, X.L.; Gray, D.J.; Harn, D.A. DNA-based vaccine protects against zoonotic schistosomiasis in water buffalo. *Vaccine* **2008**, *26*, 3617–3625. [CrossRef]
37. Gray, D.J.; Li, Y.S.; Williams, G.M.; Zhao, Z.Y.; Harn, D.A.; Li, S.M.; Ren, M.Y.; Feng, Z.; Guo, F.Y.; Guo, J.G.; et al. A multi-component integrated approach for the elimination of schistosomiasis in the People's Republic of China: Design and baseline results of a 4-year cluster-randomised intervention trial. *Int. J. Parasitol.* **2014**, *44*, 659–668. [CrossRef]

38. Williams, G.; Li, Y.-S.; Gray, D.J.; Zhao, Z.-Y.; Harn, D.; Shollenberger, L.M.; Li, S.-M.; Yu, X.; Feng, Z.; Guo, J.-G.; et al. Field testing integrated interventions for schistosomiasis elimination in the People's Republic of China: Outcomes of a multifactorial cluster-randomised controlled trial. *Front. Immunol.* **2019**, *10*, 645. [CrossRef] [PubMed]
39. You, H.; Cai, P.; Tebeje, B.M.; Yuesheng Li, Y.-S.; McManus, D.P. Schistosome vaccines for domestic animals. *Trop. Med. Infect. Dis.* **2018**, *3*, 68. [CrossRef]
40. Charlier, J.; van der Voort, M.; Kenyon, F.; Skuce, P.; Vercruysse, J. Chasing helminths and their economic impact on farmed ruminants. *Trends Parasitol.* **2014**, *30*, 361–367. [CrossRef]
41. Oey, H.; Zakrzewski, M.; Gravermann, K.; Young, N.D.; Korhonen, P.K.; Gobert, G.N.; Nawaratna, S.; Hasan, S.; Martínez, D.M.; You, H.; et al. Whole-genome sequence of the bovine blood fluke *Schistosoma bovis* supports interspecific hybridization with *S. haematobium*. *PLoS Pathog.* **2019**, *15*, e1007513. [CrossRef] [PubMed]
42. Jordan, P. From katayama to the Dakhla Oasis: The beginning of epidemiology and control of bilharzia. *Acta Trop.* **2000**, *77*, 9–40. [CrossRef]
43. Abe, E.M.; Guo, Y.-H.; Shen, H.; Mutsaka-Makuvaza, M.J.; Habib, M.R.; Xue, J.-B.; Midzi, N.; Xu, J.; Li, S.-Z.; Zhou, X.-N. Phylogeography of *Bulinus truncatus* (Audouin, 1827) (Gastropoda: Planorbidae) in selected African countries. *Trop. Med. Infect. Dis.* **2018**, *3*, 127. [CrossRef]
44. Famakinde, D.O. treading the path towards genetic control of snail resistance to schistosome infection. *Trop. Med. Infect. Dis.* **2018**, *3*, 86. [CrossRef] [PubMed]
45. Yang, G.-J.; Bergquist, R. Potential impact of climate change on schistosomiasis: A global assessment attempt. *Trop. Med. Infect. Dis.* **2018**, *3*, 117. [CrossRef] [PubMed]
46. Qin, Z.-Q.; Xu, J.; Feng, T.; Lv, S.; Qian, Y.-J.; Zhang, L.-J.; Li, Y.-L.; Lv, C.; Bergquist, R.; Li, S.-Z.; et al. Field Evaluation of a loop-mediated isothermal amplification (LAMP) platform for the detection of *Schistosoma japonicum* infection in *Oncomelania hupensis* snails. *Trop. Med. Infect. Dis.* **2018**, *3*, 124. [CrossRef]
47. Strassburg, M.A. The global eradication of smallpox. *Am. J. Infect. Control* **1982**, *10*, 53–59. [CrossRef]
48. Hamilton, K.; Baron, M.D.; Matsuo, K.; Visser, D. Rinderpest eradication: Challenges for remaining disease free and implications for future eradication efforts. *Rev. Sci. Tech.* **2017**, *36*, 579–588. [CrossRef]

Tropical Medicine and Infectious Disease

MDPI

Editorial

"Farewell to the God of Plague": The Importance of Political Commitment Towards the Elimination of Schistosomiasis

Jin Chen [1], Jing Xu [1], Robert Bergquist [2], Shi-Zhu Li [1] and Xiao-Nong Zhou [1,*]

1 National Institute of Parasitic Diseases, Chinese Center for Disease Control and Prevention; Chinese Center for Tropical Diseases Research; WHO Collaborating Centre for Tropical Diseases; National Center for International Research on Tropical Diseases; Key Laboratory of Parasite and Vector Biology, Ministry of Health, Shanghai 200025, China; jinchen@nipd.chinacdc.cn (J.C.); xujing@nipd.chinacdc.cn (J.X.); stoneli1130@126.com (S-Z.L.)

2 Ingerod, SE-454 94 Brastad, Sweden; robert.bergquist@outlook.com

* Correspondence: ipdzhouxn@sh163.net; Tel.: +86-21-6437-8058; Fax: +86-021-6433-2670

† This editorial constitutes part of a special issue entitled Prospects for Elimination of Schistosomiasis of the journal Tropical Medicine and Infectious Disease and is published for the 60-year commemoration of the first publication of the poem Farewell to the God of Plague.

Received: 25 September 2018; Accepted: 27 September 2018; Published: 3 October 2018

Schistosomiasis control in China has always been conducted with strong political leadership and support at the highest level of government [1]. In the 1950s, massive surveys were conducted. It eventually became clear that a large part of the country was highly endemic for schistosomiasis japonica. An estimated 11 million people were infected, and local infection rates ranged from 10 to 90% [1–4]. Realizing the severity of the situation in as many as 12 provinces along the Yangtze River, Chairman Mao Zedong himself took the reins and launched a call for schistosomiasis to be wiped out.

The Chinese Central Government prioritized control of the disease. Regarding it as a political issue, the mechanism of "political leadership, government support and mass involvement" was established in 1956. The Yujiang County in Jiangxi Province responded rapidly and worked out a multifaceted scheme with the focus on snail control through environmental modification, repeated screening and molluscicide treatment [5,6]. After the implementation of this strategy for two years, the county authorities reported that schistosomiasis had been eliminated in their area. Chairman Mao was jubilant. He would later spoke of jotting down " ... as sunlight falls on my window, I look towards the distant southern sky and in my happiness pen the following lines". What he referred to is the now famous, sonnet-style poem in two parts *Farewell to the God of Plague* that was published in the Chinese newspaper *People's Daily* on 3 October 1958. (Figure 1) The poem eulogizes the remarkable achievement in Yujiang and encourages work towards schistosomiasis elimination in more endemic areas [5,6]. Inspired by these enthusiastic lines, active people in all endemic counties devoted themselves to schistosomiasis control following what became known as the Yujiang Model.

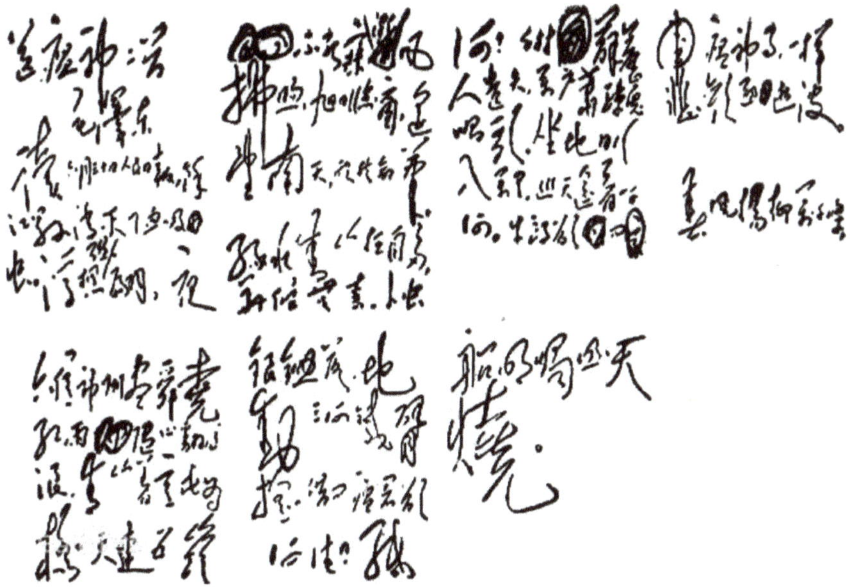

Figure 1. Chairman Mao Zedong's "Farewell to the God of Plague" in his own handwriting.

The year 2018 marks the 60th anniversary of this first step on the road that eventually should lead to the reality of schistosomiasis elimination. This goal has attracted increased support from the Chinese Government, promoting national schistosomiasis epidemiology surveys as well as research, control and prevention. However, political commitment as well as work at the bench and in the field have gone through different stages over the years. After Chairman Mao's passionate approach in 1958, Chairman Jiang Zemin stated 45 years later that the control and elimination of schistosomiasis is the responsibility of the government. This spoken and written declaration promoted schistosomiasis control to a level of priority within the broad range of public health issues. Human, material and financial resources were allocated to the cause and the health sector was strengthened, which eventually led to intersectoral collaboration between several departments of the central government. This proved essential in the fight against the neglected tropical diseases (NTDs), schistosomiasis in particular. At the first stage (1950s–1985), the mass campaigns and vertical control was conducted with an emphasis on snail eradication. This was achieved through environment modification and molluscicide treatment of the snail habitats, together with auxiliary individual protection of the human population. As a result, the snail habitat were reduced by 11 billion m^2 by 1981. Whole provinces met the criteria of schistosomiasis elimination: Guangdong Province and Shanghai Municipality in 1985, Fujian Province in 1987 and Guangxi Zhuang Autonomous Region in 1989 [6]. At the second stage (1986–2003), the chemotherapy-based morbidity control strategy with praziquantel treatment was prioritized through the World Bank Loan Project on schistosomiasis control 1992–2001 [3]. The number of cases and morbidity of the infected residents in the endemic provinces decreased by half [7,8]. During the third stage (2004–2015), the Chinese Government promulgated the Schistosomiasis Prevention and Control Regulation, which accelerated the implementation of an integrated strategy, focusing on controlling all sources of transmission [9,10]. In parallel with continued snail control, the interventions included agricultural mechanization (exchange of water buffaloes for tractors), the construction of lavatories with running water, and the institution of drug treatment and health education [11]. By 2015, all endemic provinces/autonomous regions had achieved control of the infection, i.e., the estimated number of infected people had fallen by a dramatic 91% (from 842,500 to 77,200) [12].

With respect to schistosomiasis, China is now saying 'enough is enough'—this disease must go! According to the latest endemicity report in 2016, five out of 12 endemic provinces have eliminated schistosomiasis; one has reached the stage of transmission control, and six have met the criteria of transmission interruption [13]. Based on the achievement gained, the Chinese Government has issued a decree that schistosomiasis should be eliminated by 2025 [14], which would coincide with reaching United Nations' Sustainable Development Goal: *End the NTDs* [15]. The Healthy China 2030 Plan requests that all counties still endemic for schistosomiasis reach the elimination stage via an integrated strategy and an efficient surveillance and response approach [16,17]. To achieve this ambitious goal, China must interrupt the transmission of schistosomiasis in more than 90% of endemic counties and eliminate the infection in 75% of them by 2020. They must also further achieve transmission interruption in all endemic counties and elimination in 90% of them by 2025 [13].

In parallel with the elimination of schistosomiasis at home, China also assists other endemic countries. This is based on the successful experience mentioned above and then tailored to local settings [18]. The China-Zanzibar-WHO project on schistosomiasis control is a good example of this strategy, adopting the model of high-level governmental communication and technical cooperation. At the 2014 World Health Assembly (WHA) in Geneva, Switzerland, the Government of Zanzibar, the World Health Organization (WHO) and China agreed to jointly work towards the control of schistosomiasis in Zanzibar. With financial support for advisors, health education of local staff and assistance with laboratory renovation from the Chinese Government and China's Ministry of Commerce, a baseline survey and disease control study of urogenital schistosomiasis (due to *Schistosoma haematobium*) was initiated on Pemba Island in 2016. So far, the pilot intervention has completed a baseline survey providing current prevalence rates and the biological situation with regard to the local intermediate snail host *Bulinus globosus*. By systematic disease investigation and snail surveys followed by treatment in cooperation with the local NTD office, the prevalence of schistosomiasis haematobia in Pemba has already showed signs of reduction.

Schistosomiasis elimination in China has a 60-year history. Its early success needed Chairman Mao Zedong's initiative and is now being advanced by long-term political commitment, along with strong developments in society and the economy. Repeating this achievement abroad will only be possible with long-term support from local governments and the incorporation of social and economic approaches. Local import and appreciation of Chinese technologies and products, such as the current Belt and Road Initiative project aimed at boosting local economies with global health development, will be crucially depended on to achieve the ultimate goal of worldwide elimination of the NTDs, including schistosomiasis.

Funding: This research was supported by the National Key Research and Development Program of China (No. 2016YFC1202001), by the International Development Research Center (IDRC), Canada (grant No. 108100-001).

Conflicts of Interest: The authors declare no conflict of interest.

References

1. Berry-Cabán, C.S. Return of the God of Plague: Schistosomiasis in China. *J. Rural Trop. Publ. Health* **2007**, *6*, 45–53.
2. Maegraith, B. Schistosomiasis in China. *Lancet* **1958**, *1*, 208–214. [CrossRef]
3. Utzinger, J.; Zhou, X.N.; Chen, M.G.; Bergquist, R. Conquering schistosomiasis in China: The long march. *Acta Trop.* **2005**, *96*, 69–96. [PubMed]
4. Wang, L.; Utzinger, J.; Zhou, X.N. Schistosomiasis control: Experiences and lessons from China. *Lancet* **2008**, *372*, 1793–1795. [CrossRef]
5. Sandbach, F.R. Farewell to the god of plague–the control of schistosomiasis in China. *Soc. Sci. Med.* **1977**, *11*, 27–33. [CrossRef]
6. Hou, T.C.; Chung, H.L.; Ho, L.Y.; Weng, H.C. Achievements in the fight against parasitic diseases in new China. *Chin. Med. J.* **1959**, *79*, 493–520. [PubMed]

7. Wu, X.H.; Chen, M.G. Zheng, J. Surveillance of schistosomiasis in five provinces of China which have reached the national criteria for elimination of the disease. *Acta Trop.* **2005**, *96*, 276–281. [CrossRef] [PubMed]
8. Zhou, X.N.; Guo, J.G.; Wu, X.H.; Jiang, Q.W.; Zheng, J.; Dang, H.; Wang, X.H.; Xu, J.; Zhu, H.Q.; Wu, G.L.; et al. Epidemiology of schistosomiasis in the People's Republic of China, 2004. *Emerg. Infect. Dis.* **2007**, *13*, 1470–1476. [CrossRef] [PubMed]
9. Collins, C.; Xu, J.; Tang, S. Schistosomiasis control and the health system in P.R. China. *Infect. Dis. Poverty* **2012**, *1*, 8. [CrossRef] [PubMed]
10. Wang, L.D.; Chen, H.G.; Guo, J.G.; Zeng, X.J.; Hong, X.L.; Xiong, J.J.; Wu, X.H.; Wang, X.H.; Wang, L.Y.; Xia, G.; et al. A strategy to control transmission of *Schistosoma japonicum* in China. *N. Engl. J. Med.* **2009**, *360*, 121–128. [CrossRef] [PubMed]
11. Xu, J.; Steinman, P.; Maybe, D.; Zhou, X.N.; Lv, S.; Li, S.Z.; Peeling, R. Evolution of the National Schistosomiasis Control Programmes in The People's Republic of China. *Adv. Parasitol.* **2016**, *92*, 1–38. [PubMed]
12. Lei, Z.L.; Zhang, L.J.; Xu, Z.M.; Dang, H.; Xu, J.; Lv, S.; Cao, C.L.; Li, S.Z.; Zhou, X.N. Endemic status of schistosomiasis in People's Republic of China in 2015. *Zhongguo Xue Xi Chong Bing Fang Zhi Za Zhi* **2016**, *28*, 611–617.
13. Zhang, J.L.; Xu, M.Z.; Qian, J.Y.; Dang, H.; Shan, L.Ü.; Jing, X.U.; Li, Z.S.; Zhou, N.X. Endemic status of schistosomiasis in People's Republic of China in 2016. *Zhongguo Xue Xi Chong Bing Fang Zhi Za Zhi* **2017**, *29*, 669–677.
14. Zhou, X.N. *Tropical Diseases in China: Schistosomiais*; People's Medical Publishing House: Beijing, China, 2018.
15. United Nations Sustainable Development Goals 2015. Available online: https://www.un.org/sustainabledevelopment/health/ (accessed on 28 July 2018).
16. WHO. Healthy China 2030 (from Vision to Action). Available online: http://www.who.int/healthpromotion/conferences/9gchp/healthy-china/en/ (accessed on 20 August 2018).
17. Sun, L.P.; Wang, W.; Zuo, Y.P.; Hong, Q.B.; Du, G.L.; Ma, Y.C.; Wang, J.; Yang, G.J.; Zhu, D.J.; Liang, Y.S. A multidisciplinary, integrated approach for the elimination of schistosomiasis: A longitudinal study in a historically hyper-endemic region in the lower reaches of the Yangtze River, China from 2005 to 2014. *Infect. Dis. Poverty* **2017**, *6*, 56. [CrossRef] [PubMed]
18. Bergquist, R.; Zhou, X.N.; Rollinson, D.; Reinhard-Rupp, J.; Klohe, K. Elimination of schistosomiasis: the tools required. *Infect. Dis. Poverty* **2017**, *6*, 158. [CrossRef] [PubMed]

Tropical Medicine and Infectious Disease

MDPI

Review

When Should the Emphasis on Schistosomiasis Control Move to Elimination?

W. Evan Secor [1] and Daniel G. Colley [2,*]

1 Division of Parasitic Diseases and Malaria, Centers for Disease Control and Prevention, Atlanta, GA 30329, USA; was4@cdc.gov
2 Center for Tropical and Emerging Global Diseases and Department of Microbiology, University of Georgia, Athens, GA 30602, USA
* Correspondence: dcolley@uga.edu; Tel.: +1-706-542-4112

Received: 29 June 2018; Accepted: 10 August 2018; Published: 15 August 2018

Abstract: The stated goal of the World Health Organization's program on schistosomiasis is paraphrased as follows: to control morbidity and eliminate transmission where feasible. Switching from a goal of controlling morbidity to interrupting transmission may well be currently feasible in some countries in the Caribbean, some areas in South America, northern Africa, and selected endemic areas in sub-Saharan Africa where there have been improvements in sanitation and access to clean water. However, in most of sub-Saharan Africa, where programmatic interventions still consist solely of annual mass drug administration, such a switch in strategies remains premature. There is a continued need for operational research on how best to reduce transmission to a point where interruption of transmission may be achievable. The level of infection at which it is feasible to transition from control to elimination must also be defined. In parallel, there is also a need to develop and evaluate approaches for achieving and validating elimination. There are currently neither evidence-based methods nor tools for breaking transmission or verifying that it has been accomplished. The basis for these statements stems from numerous studies that will be reviewed and summarized in this article; many, but not all of which were undertaken as part of SCORE, the Schistosomiasis Consortium for Operational Research and Evaluation.

Keywords: schistosomiasis; control; elimination; Africa; operational research; goals; guidelines

1. Introduction

In 2001, the World Health Assembly (WHA) passed resolution 54.19 that called for regular administration of praziquantel for schistosomiasis (and albendazole or mebendazole for soil-transmitted helminthiasis, STH) to at least 75% of school-aged children at risk of morbidity [1]. The passage of WHA 54.19 helped stimulate governments, pharmaceutical companies, and private donors to provide the resources to allow a considerable expansion of mass drug administration (MDA) for schistosomiasis and STH along with the operational research to inform programs on how to best deliver treatments and monitor impact. Buoyed by this progress, as well as by promising advances towards the elimination of other neglected tropical diseases (NTDs), the WHA passed resolution 65.21 in 2012, which called for interrupting the transmission of schistosomiasis (elimination) where appropriate [2].

The exuberance that led to WHA 65.21 was based on progress towards the WHA 54.19 goals and elimination as a public health problem (<5% prevalence of high-intensity infections in children), success with other NTD elimination programs, and the desire to set program endpoints. However, the critical modifier 'where appropriate' is often overlooked in discussions of schistosomiasis elimination and currently remains undefined. This has led to a certain degree of confusion for programs and dissonance among schistosomiasis stakeholders and the larger NTD community in the development of strategic plans and the allocation of resources.

Schistosomiasis control programs in most endemic countries still consist almost solely of MDA with praziquantel. Considerably less progress has been made towards WHA 54.19's other goals of promoting access to safe water, sanitation, and health education. WHA 65.21 also called for guidance to help countries determine when to switch from control to elimination campaigns, how to implement them, and the process for documenting success. However, these requested guidelines still have not been generated, primarily because the data needed to generate them (i.e., from successful elimination programs) simply do not exist. Thus, one of the most pressing schistosomiasis research needs is to define when it is appropriate to switch from a focus on control to a goal of interrupting transmission.

The few countries that have successfully interrupted the transmission of schistosomiasis have largely been successful when their public health programs were combined with social and economic development. Even for these countries, the process to certify elimination remains unclear. In this review, we detail why we believe that for now an emphasis on interrupting transmission in most of sub-Saharan Africa is overly ambitious. There is no question that elimination remains the laudable and ultimate goal, but, for the immediate future, efforts should be focused on laying the groundwork that will be necessary to accomplish it [3]. Interventions beyond MDA must become widely available, and the evidence regarding when to pursue and how to document elimination must be generated. Clearly, operational research and the development and evaluation of the essential tools needed for elimination and verification should move forward, but we propose that a reasonable balance needs to be struck between the emphases placed upon control and elimination efforts.

2. Once-Annual MDA of School-Aged Children Is Not Enough to Interrupt the Transmission of Schistosomiasis

MDA alone has led to substantial progress towards elimination of several NTDs. For example, MDA for lymphatic filariasis stops or nearly stops transmission, and annual MDA can continue until adult worms die with little risk of new infection. However, with schistosomiasis, given the rapid rates of reinfection that can occur in endemic areas, the incomplete effectiveness of praziquantel, and the considerable amplification of parasite numbers that occurs within the intermediate snail host, MDA alone is unlikely to achieve elimination. Furthermore, if interventions are stopped before bringing prevalence down to the still undefined level at which transmission cannot be sustained, rapid recrudescence is likely.

The Schistosomiasis Consortium for Operational Research and Evaluation (SCORE; https://score.uga.edu/) is an initiative funded by the Bill and Melinda Gates Foundation that has the goal to provide schistosomiasis control program managers the information they need to better do their jobs. The bulk of SCORE-funded operational research has focused on studies to compare different MDA strategies. In western Kenya, when children in primary schools with an initial *Schistosoma mansoni* prevalence of 10–24% were provided school-based treatment (SBT) at high coverage (>90%), one round of treatment was sufficient to drastically reduce prevalence and intensity of infection. However, subsequent rounds, even when provided annually over four years, never brought infection levels below approximately 50% of the baseline prevalence [4]. Thus, even with rigorous implementation in a research setting, MDA alone was not adequate for accomplishing elimination.

3. Modifications to Improve MDA Effectiveness Still Do Not Achieve Elimination

It is possible that community-wide treatment (CWT) in the villages with 10–24% baseline prevalence could have been more effective to achieve the interruption of transmission, especially if there are some adults (e.g., fishermen, sand harvesters, shepherds, or car washers) who have occupations that make them important contributors to transmission in a particular setting. However, in keeping with the current World Health Organization (WHO) guidelines that only recommend CWT when prevalence is greater than 50%, the SCORE studies in areas with 10–24% initial prevalence did not evaluate the impact of CWT. Nevertheless, a SCORE study on Zanzibar (both Pemba and Unguja), which was designed to understand how to achieve elimination in an area that had already received extensive MDA for control of *Schistosoma haematobium* infection for many years, did evaluate CWT [5,6]. This study was part of a major effort called ZEST (Zanzibar Elimination of Schistosomiasis Transmission) involving multiple partners, including a strong commitment by political leaders, to achieve elimination throughout Zanzibar. The SCORE study within ZEST examined three strategies designed to drive schistosomiasis haematobia to elimination. All three strategies utilized twice yearly CWT, either alone, in combination with a community-designed behavioral change intervention, or alongside periodic focal snail control with niclosamide. In areas with low baseline prevalence, it is clear that while schistosomiasis prevalence and infection intensity decreased in most shehias (villages), in some it did not [7]. This variability in response to MDA, resulting in 'persistent hotspots,' has been observed in other SCORE studies [8,9], as well as other tropical disease control programs [10,11]. Persisting hotspots are a reality that must be appreciated, identified, and addressed when contemplating elimination goals. Whether the goal is morbidity control or elimination, both field studies and mathematical modeling suggest that it will be necessary to adapt MDA approaches to address persistent hotspots, including monitoring MDA programs more often than the currently recommended 5–6 years [12,13].

4. Interventions in Addition to MDA Are Needed for Elimination but Are Challenging to Apply

The development and implementation of a community-designed behavioral intervention on Zanzibar required both considerable time and effort [14]. The interventions that the community developed under the guidance of a social scientist and a trained team resulted in the greatly increased involvement of children in activity-based health education about schistosomiasis and the use of participant-designed and -installed concrete washing platforms and clean water to wash clothes. While enabling communities to identify their own problems and solutions is attractive with respect to both self-determination and sustainability, the financial and time investments required are an obstacle to many large control programs.

Adding snail control to MDA also takes some time to be fully implemented due to the training required and the need to identify water-contact sites likely to be important in the transmission of schistosomiasis. On Zanzibar, snail control was implemented focally in identified water-contact sites in which snails were found [5]. This generally occurred 3–4 times per year. Because of the seasonality of the rainy seasons, the sites needing treatment with niclosamide varied at each visit. Thus, as with behavioral change interventions, mollusciciding needs to be tailored to individual sites for effective use and requires considerable training and person-power.

There was a time when snail control was the mainstay of schistosomiasis control. In Africa, the Danish Bilharziasis Laboratory (DBL) and other institutions trained many field personnel in the science and art of snail control. Both molluscicides and environmental interventions designed by water and sanitation engineers were effective snail control measures. In East Asia, both the Chinese and Japanese programs were highly proficient in this practice, and it was effective for reducing schistosomiasis prevalence in humans [3]. However, upon the advent of a safe, generally effective drug, funding for these approaches dwindled to a point where they are now largely non-existent in control programs. It is encouraging that two training workshops for snail control were held in 2017 under the auspices of the WHO/AFRO's Expanded Special Project for the Elimination of NTDs (ESPEN), one on Zanzibar and the other in Burkina Faso, and the WHO has now produced a snail control manual [15]. Nevertheless, the malacology capacity in most of Africa remains very limited, and most ministries have not invested in snail control for their schistosomiasis control programs. This contrasts with programs for vector-borne NTDs, where measures to control mosquitoes, blackflies, tsetse flies, and the like are an integral part of control and elimination efforts. Encouragingly, at least a few environmental engineers are beginning to think about transmission and control of schistosomiasis [16]. Getting more people trained in these areas and getting more NTD programs to acknowledge and utilize these approaches is very likely to be essential for effective elimination within an acceptable timeframe.

As for many other public health issues, the availability of water, sanitation, and hygiene (WASH) in addition to MDA is likely the key intervention for breaking schistosomiasis transmission. For example, schistosomiasis used to be a severe problem in several islands in the Caribbean. In the 1970s and 1980s, Saint Lucia had many residents who suffered from severe hepatosplenic disease as a result of *S. mansoni* infection [17]. After the Rockefeller/Ministry of Health Research and Control project ended in 1981, there was no specific control program for schistosomiasis. However, the economic development that has occurred over the last 30 years has resulted in a vast expansion of WASH throughout most of the island and a concurrent reduction, and possible interruption of transmission, of schistosomiasis. While it may not be possible to completely attribute this change to the greater utilization of WASH (competitor snails were introduced in some areas as part of Research and Control project and some have flourished at the expense of *Biomphalaria glabrata*), the coincident decline in schistosomiasis prevalence is striking. Puerto Rico and the Dominican Republic have similarly experienced great economic development leading to increased WASH and reductions in schistosomiasis prevalence to the point where they are ready for surveys to determine whether elimination has been achieved. The late Professor George Hillyer, who was a leading schistosomiasis researcher in Puerto Rico from the 1970s until his death in 2015, liked to quip that the best control measure for schistosomiasis was concrete. Considering that Puerto Rico at one time had levels of schistosomiasis that rivaled anywhere in Africa and is now ready to verify elimination, even in the absence of large-scale MDA, his point seems prescient.

It is likely that elimination will only be achieved in countries (or areas within countries) with some basal level of a clean water supply and sanitation. However, what that basal level is remains unknown, and there is a clear need for operational research to determine what that level might be. Preliminary results from a follow-on SCORE study in western Kenya designed to identify the factors associated with schistosomiasis persistent hotspots suggest that villages with higher levels of sanitation have greater reductions in prevalence following MDA compared with those that do not [18]. Research to define what level of WASH is needed for effective schistosomiasis control or elimination will require input from behavioral scientists and water and sanitation engineers. Unfortunately, people who have this training and also know or care about schistosomiasis control are in short supply. Nevertheless, schistosomiasis investigators and control advocates, including the WHO, have now begun to cultivate and develop partnerships within the WASH sector [19]. These partnerships need to grow and lead to real WASH implementation to accomplish the sought after goals of both schistosomiasis control and its elimination.

5. What Else Is Needed for Elimination?

Another challenge to achieving elimination is the difficulty of demonstrating significant decreases in infection levels in areas with very low baseline prevalence and intensity. If there is any appreciable variability, such as due to persistent hotspots, demonstrating statistically significant reductions from 2 to 0.5% prevalence requires the evaluation of very large numbers of individuals, which would likely exceed current budgets or implementation abilities of most programs. Proving that prevalence is 0% will require the development of reliable sampling schemes and the wide availability of sensitive tools. Urine filtration is not adequate for monitoring low levels of *S. haematobium* infection, as was made clear when urine specimens collected in Zanzibar were assayed by the highly sensitive and specific up-converting phosphor-circulating anodic antigen (UCP-CAA) assay. Parallel use of these two assays on the same urine specimens yielded considerably higher prevalence estimates with the UCP-CAA assay in most shehias [20]. Schools thought to have low prevalence by urine filtration (mean = 3.4%) had an average prevalence of 17.2% by UCP-CAA assay. These differences could not be explained as false positive results, as latent class analysis estimated that the UCP-CAA assay had 90.1% specificity and 97.0% sensitivity [20]. To implement and validate elimination, surveillance tools more sensitive than parasitologic microscopy will be needed. These tools will also need to be sufficiently cost effective for use on large numbers of individuals and perhaps amenable to pooling schemes [21]. At this time, the UCP-CAA assay is only available in a few specialized laboratories, and the costs are too high for routine use in control programs.

The need for a tool appropriate for validating elimination is shared by efforts to eliminate *S. mansoni*. As with *S. haematobium*, microscopy-based assays fail to detect many light *S. mansoni* infections. SCORE studies in Burundi demonstrated that greater than 85% of schools with 0% prevalence based on stool examination tested positive for schistosomiasis when the commercially available point-of-care/circulating cathodic antigen (POC-CCA) test was used [22]. Thus, many areas that appear to be approaching elimination as measured by parasitologic methods may in fact still have a high prevalence of low intensity schistosomiasis. Unfortunately, the POC-CCA assay is not without certain limitations of its own. In areas that have control programs that have achieved very low levels of prevalence and intensity, such as Egypt, or areas that once had schistosomiasis but appear to have eliminated *S. mansoni* transmission, the use of the POC-CCA assay indicates approximately 5–10% trace positive results. Some of these can be attributable to very, very low-level infections, but many are likely false positives [23]. Thus, the POC-CCA is not an adequate tool for validating elimination of transmission, and additional work is needed to define the sampling strategies, tests, and results to confirm that transmission has been interrupted [24].

Testing for schistosome-specific antibodies may also have some utility. Because individuals remain antibody positive to many if not most schistosome antigens long after they have been cured of infection, the currently available serologic tests are only useful in areas where transmission was likely interrupted a number of years before (e.g., the Caribbean) and when persons younger than the projected transmission interruption date demonstrate negative serology. Serologic tests based on crude antigen mixtures, as well as many purified native antigens, do not distinguish between active and former infections. Work to identify recombinant antigens to which the antibody response is more rapidly lost is ongoing, but as of now, antibody testing is only useful for demonstrating elimination that has occurred in the past, not programs that are actively trying to interrupt transmission.

Through the work with the more sensitive antigen detection assays, another challenge has become apparent. Although praziquantel is still indispensable for MDA programs and thankfully, no widespread clinical resistance has developed, it may not be nearly as effective at killing schistosomes as previously thought. In SCORE studies in western Kenya where children with schistosomiasis were treated with praziquantel and retested with the POC-CCA assay, only about 50% cleared infection after one round of treatment, compared with the 70–90% clearance rates observed when parasitologic methods are used to calculate efficacy [25]. Standard doses of praziquantel are even less effective in very young children [26], which is a further cause for concern even as pediatric formulations of praziquantel are undergoing clinical trials (https://www.pediatricpraziquantelconsortium.org/). As with snail control, much of the investment in identifying additional drugs to treat schistosomiasis disappeared with the availability of praziquantel. There is no mistaking that it is still the most readily available and important component of schistosomiasis control throughout the world, but it is becoming clear that additional research on compounds used either alone or in combination with praziquantel should be pursued in order to realize and sustain elimination, or in the event that stable resistance to praziquantel were to arise in schistosome populations.

A final need is a clear definition of when elimination has been achieved. Single serosurveys of children in Morocco, Saint Lucia, and the Dominican Republic have found no individuals with a positive antibody response. However, a single evaluation is unlikely to provide convincing evidence that transmission has been interrupted. But, how many surveys and of what age groups would suffice? Is it possible to only survey in areas of a country that have historically had schistosomiasis transmission, or is it also necessary to evaluate areas that have never had documented infections? If so, is the same stringency of surveillance needed in both areas? Can demonstration of high-level WASH usage or the absence of appropriate intermediate host snails or xenomonitoring be used to bolster claims that transmission has been interrupted? Is absence of infection in schoolchildren sufficient to prove elimination, or must every adult who may have been infected decades in the past be identified and cured before elimination can be certified? Because there are so few places where transmission has been interrupted and fewer still where it has been verified, developing the schistosomiasis elimination guidelines has the feel of building the airplane while learning to fly it. Modeling of data from field studies in elimination projects, both those that are successful as well as those that are not, will be important to answer these questions.

6. New Challenges

In addition to the obstacles to interrupting transmission detailed above, other recent developments that have come to light from schistosomiasis field studies further complicate the goal of achieving elimination. First, rather than the list of countries endemic for schistosomiasis shrinking in recent years, new foci of schistosomiasis have recently been identified in Corsica and Myanmar [27,28]. How these sites were established is unclear; however, human seeding of intermediate host snails that were already present suggests a role for increased global migration and tourism in establishing new transmission foci [29]. Another factor that may impede elimination efforts is the possible contribution of non-human hosts in maintaining the life cycle. While the zoonotic contribution to *Schistosoma japonica* transmission is widely recognized, its role in maintaining environmental life cycles of *S. mansoni* and *S. haematobium* is less clear [30]. Propagation of the life cycle of these species in reservoir hosts and snails could hinder efforts to interrupt transmission or reinitiate transmission in humans following completion of elimination programs [31]. The identification of hybrid human and animal schistosomes in West Africa further complicates this possibility as hybrid species could possibly have a wider host range and greater vigor, thereby increasing transmission potential through the infection of multiple definitive hosts [32].

7. What Is the Way Forward?

While there are settings where elimination of schistosomiasis transmission have been achieved [33], what is usually not acknowledged is how rarely elimination efforts have succeeded and that this has only occurred in relatively isolated situations. It is also often not appreciated that thus far, elimination has always required both extensive public health measures coupled with infrastructure development and a sustained investment over an extended period of time. In the case of Japan, it required the many decades-long use of a multi-pronged major public health push against helminth diseases [34], and then, as the fight was gaining real traction in terms of control, it was coupled with social and economic development that translated into broad-based water supply and sanitation. Even so, for at least 15 years after the elimination of schistosomiasis japonica, the government of Japan maintained a surveillance system for infected snails and people [35].

We and others maintain that elimination of schistosomiasis in sub-Saharan Africa is an unachievable goal using school-based praziquantel MDA alone, and a better use of current resources there would result in more effective control of schistosomiasis morbidity [36]. Interruption of transmission will only be possible with the introduction of additional control measures. Nevertheless, as this part of the world continues to develop, the schistosomiasis community needs to be planning for the future. By this, we mean thinking ahead about what will be needed to achieve and maintain elimination. Again, Japan provides an example. Anyone who has been so fortunate to have visited Japanese gardens in places like Kyoto, Nara, or Nikko knows that the lovely and tranquil scenes one enjoys, such as through a gracefully arched tree across a lily-dappled pond, did not 'just happen'. It took foresight and work long ahead of when you enjoyed that idyllic botanical scenery as art. That is how schistosomiasis elimination in sub-Saharan Africa should be considered in 2018. There is a need to determine what tools will be needed and how to use them to accomplish and verify elimination and a need to plan how adequate surveillance will be accomplished. Efforts to develop these tools and plans should begin now, not at the expense of much needed control efforts, but in addition to them and alongside them. A haiku at the entrance of such a garden could read as follows:

Seasons of much work
Elimination your goal
Control on your way.

8. Conclusions

Given the obstacles to elimination that we describe, we propose that the major emphasis for schistosomiasis programs in sub-Saharan Africa should still be control of morbidity. Achieving this goal will require better definitions of morbidity due to schistosomiasis and the development of adaptive strategies that are based on more frequent program monitoring and go beyond standard school-based annual MDA. At the same time, we also propose that to be ready to move to a goal of elimination requires a commitment to investments in the basic and operational research needed to develop the tools and strategies that will be essential to achieve and verify elimination. Waiting to do so until countries are ready to move to elimination would be shortsighted and result in continued, long-term control efforts or, in their absence, the inevitable transmission rebound that has been observed following many historical and more recent control efforts.

Author Contributions: Both W.E.S. and D.G.C. contributed equally to the writing of this review.

Funding: The writing of this manuscript and the many of the studies referred to received financial support from the University of Georgia Research Foundation, Inc., which was funded by the Bill & Melinda Gates Foundation for the SCORE project. The funders had no role in the preparation of this manuscript or the studies referred to herein.

Acknowledgments: The findings and conclusions in this report are those of the authors and do not necessarily represent the views of the Centers for Disease Control and Prevention.

Conflicts of Interest: The authors declare no conflicts of interest.

References

1. World Health Organization (WHO). WHA54.19 Schistosomiasis and Soil-Transmitted Helminth Infections. Available online: http://www.who.int/neglected_diseases/mediacentre/WHA_54.19_Eng.pdf?ua=1 (accessed on 20 June 2018).
2. World Health Organization (WHO). Sixty-Fifth World Health Assembly. Available online: http://apps.who.int/gb/DGNP/pdf_files/A65_REC1-en.pdf (accessed on 20 June 2018).
3. Bergquist, R.; Zhou, X.-N.; Rollinson, D.; Reinhard-Rupp, J.; Klohe, K. Elimination of schistosomiasis: The tools required. *Infect. Dis. Poverty* **2017**, *6*, 158. [CrossRef] [PubMed]
4. Karanja, D.M.S.; Awino, E.K.; Wiegand, R.E.; Okoth, E.; Abudho, B.O.; Mwinzi, P.N.M.; Montgomery, S.P.; Secor, W.E. Cluster randomized trial comparing school-based mass drug administration schedules in areas of western Kenya with moderate initial prevalence of *Schistosoma mansoni* infections. *PLoS Negl. Trop. Dis.* **2017**, *11*, e0006033. [CrossRef] [PubMed]
5. Knopp, S.; Mohammed, K.A.; Ali, S.M.; Khamis, I.S.; Ame, S.M.; Albonico, M.; Gouvras, A.; Fenwick, A.; Savioli, L.; Colley, D.G.; et al. Study and implementation of urogenital schistosomiasis elimination in Zanzibar (Unguja and Pemba Islands) using an integrated multidisciplinary approach. *BMC Public Health* **2012**, *12*, 930. [CrossRef] [PubMed]
6. Knopp, S.; Person, B.; Ame, S.M.; Mohammed, K.A.; Ali, S.M.; Khamis, I.S.; Rabone, M.; Allan, F.; Gouvras, A.; Blair, L.; et al. Elimination of schistosomiasis transmission in Zanzibar: Baseline findings before the onset of a randomized intervention trial. *PLoS Negl. Trop. Dis.* **2013**, *7*, e2474. [CrossRef]
7. Pennance, T.; Person, B.; Muhsin, M.A.; Khamis, A.N.; Muhsin, J.; Khamis, I.S.; Mahommed, K.A.; Kabole, F.; Rollinson, D.; Knopp, S. Urogential schistosomiasis transmission on Unguja Island, Zanzibar: Characterisation of persistent hot-spots. *Parasites Vectors* **2016**, *9*, 646. [CrossRef] [PubMed]

8. Wiegand, R.E.; Mwinzi, P.N.M.; Montgomery, S.P.; Chan, Y.L.; Andiego, K.; Omedo, M.; Muchiri, G.; Ogutu, M.O.; Rawago, F.; Odiere, M.R.; et al. A persistent hotspot of *Schistosoma mansoni* infection in a five-year randomized trial of praziquantel preventative chemotherapy strategies. *J. Infect. Dis.* **2017**, *216*, 1425–1433. [CrossRef] [PubMed]
9. Kittur, N.; Binder, S.; Campbell, C.H.; King, C.H.; Kinung'hi, S.; Olsen, A.; Magnussen, P.; Colley, D.G. Defining persistent hotspots: Areas that fail to decrease meaningfully in prevalence after multiple years of mass drug administration with praziquantel for control of schistosomiasis. *Am. J. Trop. Med. Hyg.* **2017**, *97*, 1810–1817. [CrossRef] [PubMed]
10. Lau, C.L.; Sheridan, S.; Ryan, S.; Roineau, M.; Andreosso, A.; Fuimaono, S.; Tufa, J.; Graves, P.M. Detecting and confirming residual hotspots of lymphatic filariasis transmission in American Samoa 8 years after stopping mass drug administration. *PLoS Negl. Trop. Dis.* **2017**, *11*, e0005914. [CrossRef] [PubMed]
11. Mogeni, P.; Williams, T.N.; Omedo, I.; Kimani, D.; Ngoi, J.M.; Mwacharo, J.; Morter, R.; Nyundo, C.; Wambua, J.; Nyangweso, G.; et al. Detecting Malaria Hotspots: A Comparison of Rapid Diagnostic Test, Microscopy, and Polymerase Chain Reaction. *J. Infect. Dis.* **2017**, *216*, 1091–1098. [CrossRef] [PubMed]
12. Toor, J.; Alsallaq, R.; Truscott, J.E.; Turner, H.C.; Werkman, M.; Gurarie, D.; King, C.H.; Anderson, R.M. Are we on our way to achieving the 2020 goals for schistosomiasis morbidity control using current World Health Organization guidelines? *Clin. Inf. Dis.* **2018**, *66*, S245–S252.
13. World Health Organization (WHO). Helminth Control in School Age Children: A Guide for Managers of Control Programmes. Available online: http://www.who.int/neglected_diseases/resources/9789241548267/en/ (accessed on 21 June 2018).
14. Person, B.; Knopp, S.; Ali, S.M.; A'kadir, F.M.; Khamis, A.N.; Ali, J.N.; Lymo, J.H.; Mohammed, K.A.; Rollinson, D. Community co-designed schistosomiasis control interventions for school-aged children in Zanzibar. *J. Biosoc. Sci.* **2016**, *48*, S56–S73. [CrossRef] [PubMed]
15. World Health Organization (WHO). Field Use of Molluscicides in Schistosomiasis Control Programmes: An Operational Manual for Programme Managers. Available online: http://www.who.int/schistosomiasis/resources/9789241511995/en/ (accessed on 20 June 2018).
16. Braun, L.; Grimes, J.E.T.; Templeton, M.R. The effectiveness of water treatment processes against schistosome cercariae: A systematic review. *PLoS Negl. Trop. Dis.* **2018**, *12*, e0006364. [CrossRef] [PubMed]
17. Jordan, P. *Schistosomiasis: The St. Lucia Project*; Cambridge University Press: Cambridge, UK, 1985; ISBN 0 521 30312 5.
18. Musuva, R. (Kenya Medical Research Institute, Center for Global Health Research, Kisumu, Kenya). Personal communication, 2018.
19. World Health Organization (WHO). Water Sanitation and Hygiene for Accelerating and Sustaining Progress on Neglected Tropical Diseases, A Global Strategy 2015–2020. Available online: www.who.int/water_sanitation_health/publications/wash-and-ntd-strategy/en (accessed on 17 June 2018).
20. Knopp, S.; Corstjens, P.L.A.M.; Koukounari, A.; Cercamondi, C.I.; Ame, S.M.; Ali, S.M.; de Dood, C.J.; Mohammed, K.A.; Utzinger, J.; Rollinson, D.; et al. Sensitivity and specificity of a urine circulating anodic antigen test for the diagnosis of *Schistosoma haematobium* in low endemic settings. *PLoS Negl. Trop. Dis.* **2015**, *9*, e0003752. [CrossRef] [PubMed]
21. Lo, N.C.; Bogoch, I.I.; Blackburn, B.G.; Raso, G.; N'Goran, E.K.; Coulibaly, J.T.; Becker, S.L.; Abrams, H.B.; Utzinger, J.; Andrews, J.R. Comparison of community-wide, integrated mass drug administration strategies for schistosomiasis and soil-transmitted helminthiasis: A cost-effectiveness modelling study. *Lancet Glob. Health* **2015**, *3*, e629–e638. [CrossRef]
22. Ortu, G.; Ndayishimiye, O.; Clements, M.; Kayugi, D.; Campbell, C.H.; Lamine, M.S.; Zivieri, A.; Magalhaes, R.S.; Binder, S.; King, C.H.; et al. Countrywide reassessment of *Schistosoma mansoni* infection in Burundi using a urine-circulating cathodic antigen rapid test: Informing the National Control Program. *Am. J. Trop. Med. Hyg.* **2017**, *96*, 664–673. [CrossRef] [PubMed]
23. Clements, M.N.; Corstjens, P.L.A.M.; Binder, S.; Campbell, C.H., Jr.; de Dood, C.J.; Fenwick, A.; Harrison, W.; Kayugi, D.; King, C.H.; Kornelis, D.; et al. Latent class analysis to evaluate performance of point-of-care CCA for low-intensity *Schistosoma mansoni* infections in Burundi. *Parasites Vectors* **2018**, *11*, 111. [CrossRef] [PubMed]

24. Haggag, A.A.; Rabiee, A.; Abd Elaziz, K.M.; Gabrielli, A.F.; Abdel Hay, R.; Ramzy, R.M.R. Mapping of *Schistosoma mansoni* in the Nile Delta, Egypt: Assessment of the prevalence by the circulating cathodic antigen urine assay. *Acta Trop.* **2017**, *167*, 9–17. [CrossRef] [PubMed]
25. Mwinzi, P.N.; Kittur, N.; Ochola, E.; Cooper, P.J.; Campbell, C.H., Jr.; King, C.H.; Colley, D.G. Additional evaluation of the point-of-contact circulating cathodic antigen assay for *Schistosoma mansoni* infection. *Front. Public Health* **2015**, *3*, 48. [CrossRef] [PubMed]
26. Bustinduy, A.L.; Waterhouse, D.; de Sousa-Figueiredo, J.C.; Roberts, S.A.; Atuhaire, A.; van Dam, G.J.; Corstjens, P.L.; Scott, J.T.; Stanton, M.C.; Kabatereine, N.B.; et al. Population pharmacokinetics and pharmacodynamics of praziquantel in Ugandan children with intestinal schistosomiasis: Higher dosages are required for maximal efficacy. *MBio* **2016**, *7*, e00227-16. [CrossRef] [PubMed]
27. Boissier, J.; Grech-Angelini, S.; Webster, B.L.; Allienne, J.F.; Huyse, T.; Mas-Coma, S.; Toulza, E.; Barré-Cardi, H.; Rollinson, D.; Kincaid-Smith, J.; et al. Outbreak of urogenital schistosomiasis in Corsica (France): An epidemiological case study. *Lancet Infect. Dis.* **2016**, *16*, 971–979. [CrossRef]
28. ProMED. Schistosomiasis-Myanmar. Available online: http://www.promedmail.org/post/5921911 (accessed on 31 July 2018).
29. Ramalli, L.; Mulero, S.; Noël, H.; Chiappini, J.D.; Vincent, J.; Barré-Cardi, H.; Malfait, P.; Normand, G.; Busato, F.; Gendrin, V.; et al. Persistence of schistosomal transmission linked to the Cavu River in southern Corsica since 2013. *Eurosurveillance* **2018**, *23*. [CrossRef] [PubMed]
30. Catalano, S.; Sène, M.; Diouf, N.D.; Fall, C.B.; Borlase, A.; Léger, E.; Bâ, K.; Webster, J.A. Rodents as natural hosts of zoonotic *Schistosoma* species and hybrids: An epidemiological and evolutionary perspective from West Africa. *J. Infect. Dis.* **2018**, *218*, 429–433. [CrossRef] [PubMed]
31. Hanelt, B.; Mwangi, I.N.; Kinuthia, J.M.; Maina, G.M.; Agola, L.E.; Mutuku, M.W.; Steinauer, M.L.; Agwanda, B.R.; Kigo, L.; Mungai, B.N.; et al. Schistosomes of small mammals from the Lake Victoria Basin, Kenya: New species, familiar species, and implications for schistosomiasis control. *Parasitology* **2010**, *137*, 1109–1118. [CrossRef] [PubMed]
32. Borlase, A.; Webster, J.P.; Rudge, J.W. Opportunities and challenges for modelling epidemiological and evolutionary dynamics in a multihost, multiparasite system: Zoonotic hybrid schistosomiasis in West Africa. *Evol. Appl.* **2018**, *11*, 501–515. [CrossRef] [PubMed]
33. Rollinson, D.; Knopp, S.; Levitz, S.; Stothard, J.R.; Tchuem Tchuenté, L.-A.; Garba, A.; Mohammed, K.A.; Schur, N.; Person, B.; Colley, D.G.; et al. Time to set the agenda for schistosomiasis elimination. *Acta Trop.* **2013**, *128*, 423–440. [CrossRef] [PubMed]
34. Kajihara, N.; Hirayama, K. The war against a regional disease in Japan: A history of the eradication of schistosomiasis japonica. *Trop. Med. Health* **2011**, *39*, 3–44. [CrossRef] [PubMed]
35. Colley, D.G.; University of Georgia, Athens, Georgia, USA. Personal communication, 2018.
36. French, M.D.; Evans, D.; Fleming, F.M.; Secor, W.E.; Biritwum, N.-K.; Brooker, S.J.; Bustinduy, A.; Gouvras, A.; Kabatereine, N.; King, C.H.; et al. Schistosomiasis in Africa: Improving strategies for long-term and sustainable morbidity control. *PLoS Negl. Trop. Dis.* **2018**, *12*, e0006484. [CrossRef] [PubMed]

Tropical Medicine and Infectious Disease

MDPI

Opinion

WIPO Re:Search—A Platform for Product-Centered Cross-Sector Partnerships for the Elimination of Schistosomiasis

Callie J. Weber, Joseph Hargan-Calvopiña, Katy M. Graef, Cathyryne K. Manner and Jennifer Dent *

BIO Ventures for Global Health, 2101 Fourth Avenue, Suite 1950, Seattle, WA 98121, USA; cweber@bvgh.org (C.J.W.); jhargan@bvgh.org (J.H.-C.); kgraef@bvgh.org (K.M.G.); cmanner@bvgh.org (C.K.M.)
* Correspondence: jdent@bvgh.org

Received: 30 November 2018; Accepted: 2 January 2019; Published: 9 January 2019

Abstract: Schistosomiasis is an acute and chronic disease that affects over 200 million people worldwide, and with over 700 million people estimated to be at risk of contracting this disease, it is a pressing issue in global health. However, research and development (R&D) to develop new approaches to preventing, diagnosing, and treating schistosomiasis has been relatively limited. Praziquantel, a drug developed in the 1970s, is the only agent used in schistosomiasis mass drug administration (MDA) campaigns, indicating a critical need for a diversified therapeutic pipeline. Further, gaps in the vaccine and diagnostic pipelines demonstrate a need for early-stage innovation in all areas of schistosomiasis product R&D. As a platform for public-private partnerships (PPPs), the WIPO Re:Search consortium engages the private sector in early-stage R&D for neglected diseases by forging mutually beneficial collaborations and facilitating the sharing of intellectual property (IP) assets between the for-profit and academic/non-profit sectors. The Consortium connects people, resources, and ideas to fill gaps in neglected disease product development pipelines by leveraging the strengths of these two sectors. Using WIPO Re:Search as an example, this article highlights the opportunities for the PPP model to play a key role in the elimination of schistosomiasis.

Keywords: schistosomiasis; neglected tropical diseases; WIPO Re:Search; BIO Ventures for Global Health; cross-sector collaboration; capacity-building; drug discovery; public-private partnerships

1. The Multifaceted Impact of Schistosomiasis

Schistosomiasis is an acute and chronic disease that affects an estimated 219 million people worldwide [1] and results from infection by parasitic trematode worms of the genus *Schistosoma*. Initial infection occurs when humans come into contact with parasite-infested water sources, and the free-swimming larvae of the parasite, the cercariae, penetrate the skin and migrate into the blood in order to mature. Once inside the circulatory system, these juvenile worms mature into the adult stage [2]. In a study conducted by Warren K.S et al. on Yemeni agricultural workers, it was estimated that in the case of *S. mansoni*, adult worms can have a mean lifespan of five to ten years [3,4] and in some cases have been shown to live as long as 40 years [3,5]. While inside the host, the adult worms are capable of reproducing and laying eggs throughout their lifetimes, leading to a state of chronic infection for the host that, depending on the species, can result in symptoms such as abdominal pain, diarrhea, hepatosplenic inflammation, liver fibrosis, and rectal bleeding (*S. mansoni*, *S. japonicum*, and *S. mekongi*), or obstructive disease in the urinary system, haematuria, chronic fibrosis of the urinary tract, and potentially renal dysfunction (*S. haematobium*). In addition to these species-specific symptoms, all species of *Schistosoma* have been associated with co-morbidities such as anemia [4,6].

Schistosomiasis is endemic in 78 countries, 42 of which are in the World Health Organization (WHO) African Region [7]. It is estimated that over 700 million people are at risk of contracting schistosomiasis worldwide and over 200 million people are currently infected, making this a pressing issue in global health [8]. There are six species of *Schistosoma* that are largely responsible for human infection. *S. japonicum* occurs only in Asia and *S. mansoni* occurs in sub-Saharan Africa, the Middle East, South America, and the Caribbean; these two species are responsible for intestinal schistosomiasis. *S. mekongi* is primarily restricted to Laos and Cambodia [9], whereas *S. haematobium* occurs predominantly in Africa and the Middle East [4] and leads to various urogenital clinical presentations that include urinary tract fibrosis, obstructive renal failure, and squamous cell carcinoma (SCC) of the bladder [10,11]. The less common *S. intercalatum* [12] and *S. guineensis* live in the rectal veins and are also known to cause disease [13].

Due to the disabling systemic morbidities associated with schistosomiasis, such as anemia, malnutrition, and impaired childhood development [14], it is estimated that 18.3 age-standardized disability adjusted life years (DALYs) per 100,000 population were lost to schistosomiasis for both males and females in 2017 [15]. This not only places an enormous burden on healthcare systems in endemic countries, but also interferes with economic productivity due to the reduced ability of the affected population to perform physical activities and participate in the workforce [14,16,17]. In addition to the considerable impact schistosomiasis has on adult and working populations, it is also important to consider its long-term impacts on the next generation. Schistosomiasis has been associated with reduced functional scores and malnutrition [18]. This can severely affect a child's ability [19–21] to become educated [22], lead a productive life [21,22], and break out of the vicious cycle of disease-related poverty.

A growing threat to people living in *S. haematobium*-endemic countries is schistosomiasis-associated SCC of the bladder [23]. This disease is thought to be caused by the inflammatory reaction triggered by schistosomal eggs deposited in the bladder [24]. Eggs are typically excreted through urination but can remain lodged in the patient's bladder. The continued exposure to antigen-releasing eggs during the long lifespan of the adult schistosome [25], and the resulting chronic inflammation and augmented cellular proliferation [4,11,26], increase the likelihood of SCC of the urinary bladder [27], which is estimated to occur at a rate of three to four cases per 100,000 [28]. *S. haematobium* is classified as a carcinogenic agent to humans by the International Agency for Research on Cancer (IARC) [29], and thus it is of high priority to develop more efficacious drugs and better diagnostics to stop acute schistosomiasis from leading to other severe and non-reversible bladder pathologies such as cancer. When treated with praziquantel (PZQ), which is the only approved drug for schistosomiasis, pathological lesions present in the urinary tract are eliminated, indicating that the high cost of caring for patients with schistosomiasis-induced bladder cancer can be avoided by addressing schistosomiasis at an early stage [30]. For the purpose of their studies, Botelho et al. estimated that the current annual treatment cost of PZQ per schistosomiasis patient is $0.16 USD, or approximately $17.92 million USD globally [31]. By not addressing schistosomiasis infection at an early stage, it is estimated that *S. haematobium*-associated bladder cancer results in additional treatment costs of at least $20 million USD per year worldwide [31]. These numbers demonstrate the economic benefits that can result from the development of more efficacious drugs that target this disease.

S. haematobium infection has also been shown to be disproportionately detrimental to women's reproductive and sexual health [32]. Infection-associated genital tract damage can lead to infertility [33], stress incontinence, ectopic pregnancy, increased risk of abortion [4], adverse birth outcomes such as low birth weight, and increased infant and maternal mortality [34]. Further, in multiple population-based studies, *S. haematobium* infection has been linked to an increase in HIV infection in women [35,36], with evidence showing that CD4-positive cells in peripheral blood express increased concentrations of HIV co-receptors [37]. This data implies that cells from patients infected by schistosomiasis may be more susceptible to HIV-1 infection.

Although *S. haematobium* has been known to primarily affect the urinary tract, studies have also shown that in males, *S. haematobium* eggs are found in the seminal vesicles and prostate [38]. In a community-based study of genital schistosomiasis in men from Madagascar, *S. haematobium* eggs were detected in 43% of the semen samples, providing preliminary evidence that male genital organs can also be affected by schistosomiasis [39]. The authors of the study hypothesized that egg deposition in a male's genital organs could potentially lead to an increased accumulation of lymphocytes, eosinophils, and other white cells, which in turn could increase the viral load in semen from males infected with HIV. Along these lines, other population-based studies demonstrated that schistosomiasis has been linked to an increase in HIV infection due to increased concentrations of CD4-positive cells in semen of men with schistosomiasis compared to men who had been cleared of the infection [40]. By successfully detecting and treating schistosomiasis, the global health community is not only removing the burden of this debilitating disease from the population, but also reducing the chances of people suffering from other high-mortality co-morbidities such as HIV.

According to the 5th Progress Report on the London Declaration on Neglected Tropical Diseases (NTDs) [41], the WHO has set a goal of 75% of at-risk populations covered by schistosomiasis control efforts. Regrettably, there has been very little measurable progress made towards elimination [41]. Although strong evidence suggests that PZQ targets schistosome voltage-gated calcium channels, leading to calcium-dependent contraction and paralysis in treated worms [42,43], and the drug has proven to be very useful in controlling morbidity, it is not effective against immature schistosomes [44,45]. Further, it is currently the only drug that is being used in schistosomiasis mass drug administration (MDA) campaigns [46], thus increasing the risk that schistosomes will develop resistance. While it is imperative that new drugs be developed to continue treating infected and at-risk populations, there has not been significant progress in developing alternative treatments since the development of PZQ by Merck KGaA in the 1970s. In fact, due to limited commercial incentives, very little has been done by the for-profit sector in terms of developing new diagnostics, drugs, and vaccines and fueling the early-stage product development pipeline for schistosomiasis. Although these hurdles, among others, currently stand in the way of the elimination of schistosomiasis, the global community is determined to identify solutions through cross-sector partnerships that not only distribute the risk of product development over various stakeholders, but also engage worldwide expertise. While the barriers are high, and the challenge is significant, this article focuses on the incredible efforts being employed in product research and development (R&D) through cross-sector collaborations to make progress toward elimination of schistosomiasis, and the critical roles public-private partnerships (PPPs) play in making that a reality.

2. Limitations of Current Control Efforts and Product Gap Analysis

Current control efforts for schistosomiasis include education programs to promote preventive behavioral and lifestyle changes, such as limiting contact with infected waters, boiling fresh water prior to drinking or bathing, wearing DEET (diethyltoluamide) insect repellent, and implementing vigorous towel drying to prevent parasites from penetrating the skin [47]. However, such preventive strategies focus on decreasing the individual risk of infection, rather than prevention on a large scale. Another approach is to control the host snail population through the administration of effective molluscicides, habitat modification, and biologic control strategies such as introducing competing snail species or natural predators [48]. Despite resulting in high snail mortality, the administration of molluscicides must be replicated twice annually to be effective, and thus is both expensive and (along with habitat modification and biologic control strategies) potentially detrimental to the environment [48]. Concurrent with educational and host snail-targeted interventions, the expansion of the drug, diagnostic, and vaccine development pipelines are crucial to systematically prevent and combat schistosomiasis. These development efforts are the primary focus of this article.

Schistosomiasis is endemic in 78 countries, and mass-scale administration of PZQ is the primary method of both treatment and prevention in all of the affected nations. Since 2012, MDA, or preventive chemotherapy, has been mandated by the governments of 52 endemic countries, covering approximately 250 million people [47].

The MDA movement is rooted in the 2001 World Health Assembly (WHA) resolution calling for the global scale-up of preventive chemotherapy to at-risk population groups for the control of schistosomiasis morbidity [49]. At-risk population groups include school-aged children in endemic areas, adults with occupational risk due to contact with infested waters, and, in many instances, entire communities living in areas with high disease prevalence [47]. In the absence of a preventive vaccine, the annual administration of PZQ is recognized as an accepted schistosomiasis prevention strategy for both children and adults, even during pregnancy and lactation [50]. Further, Merck KGaA and others are reformulating PZQ to develop a pediatric PZQ to expand MDA coverage to include children as young as three to six months old [51]. Efforts to expand the reach of MDA programs to rural communities have received international support, with the objective of reducing schistosomiasis morbidity in school children and funding national control programs that have been widely adopted. For example, in 2012, a five-year grant from the END Fund and Children's Investment Fund Foundation (CIFF) supported the Kenyan government's implementation of a nationwide school-based deworming program that included annual administration of PZQ to all school children in schistosomiasis-endemic areas [52,53]. After just two years, the prevalence of *S. haematobium* fell from 18% to 7.6%, according to a 2014 survey that randomly tested students from 60 schools selected across 16 counties in the Nyanza, Rift Valley, Western, and Coast regions of Kenya [53]. All PZQ distributed through this program was donated by Merck KGaA, which recently committed to donate 250 million tablets of PZQ per year indefinitely to further support global MDA efforts [54,55].

Efforts put forth for MDA programs have not gone unrewarded. In combination with snail-population control efforts, MDA programs have resulted in the WHO declaring that schistosomiasis is no longer a significant public health issue in several countries including Iran, Japan, Jordan, Mauritius, Morocco, Puerto Rico, and Tunisia [47,48].

Despite such successes, MDA programs face significant challenges due to inadequate infrastructure and drug coverage in rural at-risk communities, poor drug compliance, and insufficient monitoring and evaluation [47,56]. A recent WHO publication capturing data from 38 endemic countries reported that 70.9 million school-age children and 18.3 million adults were treated with PZQ for schistosomiasis in 2016, although this only covers 53.7% and 14.3% of at-risk school-age children and adults respectively. The coverage was calculated by dividing the number of children requiring PZQ and treated, by the total number of children in need of PZQ ("WHO 2017 Report on 2016 Treatment of Schistosomiasis") [57].

Even with an unlimited supply, optimal distribution, and high patient compliance in MDA campaigns, PZQ itself has limitations. PZQ was selected as the best treatment option for MDA due to its mild side effects, affordability, single-dose administration, and proven efficacy against every human schistosome species [42,43,58,59]. However, it is important to note that to optimize efficacy, PZQ is recommended to be administered in three 20 mg/kg doses in a single day, but to promote single-dose administration, MDA campaigns supply a single 40 mg/kg daily dose, which contributes to lower treatment efficacy [58]. According to a meta-analysis of 55 published studies, the 40 mg/kg daily dose is justified as a reasonable compromise, although the cure rate varies significantly between species, ranging from 94.7% for *S. japonicum* and 63.5% for mixed *S. haematobium*/*S. mansoni* infections [60]. Multiple field studies over the last two decades have reported cure rates as low as 52% when administering the recommended 40 mg/kg single dose [56,61,62]. Mild side effects, which include dizziness, nausea, headaches, and diarrhea, further hinder patient compliance [47,56]. In a 2014 tolerability study involving 12,435 participants, incidence of adverse events ranged from 2.3% for urticaria to 31.1% for abdominal pain [60]. This is particularly important to note as children carry most of the schistosomiasis burden and PZQ MDA campaigns often target school-aged children [63]. Additionally, PZQ is not effective against juvenile schistosomes. To ensure parasite clearance and to combat reinfection, repeated treatments are common in endemic areas, although lower efficacy of PZQ is observed in subsequent treatments because surviving juvenile schistosomes experience reduced susceptibility to PZQ as adults [42,62].

Despite its drawbacks, PZQ remains the best available option for both prevention and treatment of schistosomiasis, and thus has global support to improve its access and distribution to all endemic populations. However, this complete reliance on a single drug has raised global concerns about the development of PZQ drug resistance [56,64]. The severity of this issue is compounded by the longevity of MDA programs, which may promote the persistence of drug resistance because reductions in PZQ susceptibility are heritable [43,65]. Adult worms with reduced PZQ susceptibility have been found to have higher basal levels of ABC multidrug transporters, suggesting that they remove PZQ along with metabolic toxins by translocating substrates across the cell membrane [43,62,65]. To combat this, studies suggest that co-administration of ABC multidrug transporter inhibitors with PZQ may restore the efficacy of PZQ against adult *S. mansoni* [43,62,65]. To continue to diversify treatment options beyond monotherapy PZQ, the co-administration of PZQ with artemisinin-based derivatives, such as artemether, artesunate, and dihydroartemisinin, are also being explored and have demonstrated higher efficacy than treatment with PZQ alone [66]. For example, a preclinical study in China found that the combined treatment of PZQ and artemether reduced total *S. japonicum* worm burdens by 79–92% compared to a total worm burden reduction of 28–66% when treated with PZQ alone. The study was conducted in rabbits infected with 7- to 12-day-old schistosomula and 42-day-old adult schistosomes [66]. Because PZQ and artemether target different developmental stages of the parasite (PZQ is only effective against adult-stage *Schistosoma* and artemether acts against juvenile worms), their combined administration targets both developmental stages and demonstrates higher efficacy than monotherapies with either drug [42,66]. However, the high inherent fail rate of PZQ (previously cited at 40%) makes it extremely difficult to accurately measure the efficacy of co-administered treatment regimens or the global prevalence of drug resistance.

Despite more than 30 years of scientific and technological advances, the management of schistosomiasis remains unchanged since the development of PZQ in the early 1970s [58]. There is a need to improve current approaches by developing an integrated and intersectional method to sustainably prevent, diagnose, and treat schistosomiasis [56,61]. An antischistosomal vaccine would halt the overuse of PZQ as both a method of prevention and treatment, limit the geographic spread of schistosomiasis, and reduce the high rates of reinfection. Concurrently, the drug development pipeline must be expanded to include a diversified set of compounds that perturb novel molecular targets of PZQ-resistant parasites and that are active against both adult and immature schistosomes. To permit detection of lower-level infections as disease burden and intensity decrease due to successful interventions, highly sensitive, point-of-care (POC) diagnostics are needed. Accurate diagnostics are required for on-site detection of infection before administering treatment, as well as for certification of parasite clearance to avoid unnecessary and prolonged treatment regimens. This two-pronged diagnostic approach will maximize the efficiency of drug administration and distribution.

3. Product Development Pipelines

3.1. Vaccine Development

Despite increased education and MDA efforts, parasite transmission models predict that, based on the current levels of disease prevalence, the WHO's goal to control schistosomiasis morbidity by 2020 will not be attainable through MDA efforts alone [67]. Incidence rates could be significantly reduced by implementing strategies to prevent initial infection and reinfection. Thus, there is a need for a more permanent method of prevention than mass administration of PZQ. In recognition of this high-need, high-impact development gap, there have been increased efforts toward the development of an antischistosomal vaccine over the past two decades. In a 2013 meeting to develop Preferred Product Characteristics (PPC) for a schistosomiasis vaccine held by the National Institute of Allergy and Infectious Diseases (NIAID), it was agreed that a vaccine should reduce the overall worm burden by at least 75% and reduce egg excretion by close to 75% in order to be considered effective [68].

Currently, there are 10 vaccines in the development pipeline: Five in preclinical; three in Phase I; one in Phase II; and one in Phase III (Table 1) [69–71].

Table 1. Vaccines in development (Phase I-III clinical trials).

Product	Antigen	Phase of Clinical Development [1]	Targeted Species
Bilhvax®	*Sh*-GST28	Phase III	*S. haematobium*
Sm-14	*Sm*-14	Phase II	*S. haematobium* *S. mansoni*
Alhydrogel®	*Sm*-TSP-2	Phase Ib	*S. mansoni*
Sm-97 paramyosin	*Sm*-97	Phase I	*S. mansoni*
Calpain®	*Sm*-p80	Phase I	*S. mansoni*

[1] Vaccines in preclinical stages of development are not included.

The French National Institute of Health and Medical Research (INSERM) and Institut Pasteur took Bilhvax® (Sh-GST28; Phase III), a recombinant *S. haematobium* vaccine, through Phase I clinical testing at Lille University Hospital in France and Phase II in Saint-Louis, Senegal [72,73]. Following positive results, Bilhvax® has progressed into Phase III clinical studies, sponsored by INSERM, in the Saint-Louis Region of Senegal as a potential pediatric vaccine candidate against urinary schistosomiasis, with publication of the trial results pending [74].

Sm-14 (Phase II) is being developed in partnership between the Oswaldo Cruz Foundation (FIOCRUZ), the Brazilian governmental financial agency (FINEP), and Alvos Biotecnologia as a vaccine candidate against both *S. mansoni* and *S. haematobium* [72,75]. The Phase I clinical trial was completed in 2014 in Rio de Janeiro, Brazil, and the candidate advanced into Phase II clinical trials in the Saint-Louis Region of Senegal in collaboration with the Infectious Disease Research Institute (IDRI). The Phase II study was completed in June 2017, with publication pending [75,76].

Alhydrogel® (Sm-TSP-2; Phase I), and Sm-97 paramyosin (Phase I), are both recombinant *S. mansoni* vaccines. Alhydrogel® was developed in partnership between the Sabin Vaccine Institute and Texas Children's Hospital Center for Vaccine Development to target intestinal schistosomiasis caused by *S. mansoni* [77,78]. After 18 years of combined efforts, the vaccine is now entering Phase Ib development with continued efforts to be led by the Baylor College of Medicine and Texas Children's Hospital Center for Vaccine Development [77,78]. The ongoing Phase Ib dose-escalating clinical trial, sponsored by the NIAID, is currently in recruitment phase and will be conducted in the *S. mansoni*-endemic area of Americaninhas, Brazil [79].

Calpain® (Sm-p80; Phase I) has been rapidly progressing through the development pipeline due to the targeted efforts of a team of researchers at Texas Tech University, and is poised to enter Phase I clinical trials in 2019 [80]. Sm-p80 is a highly immunodominant antigen in the surface membranes of the worms, and the vaccine works by disrupting the schistosome's mechanisms to evade the host's natural immune response [81]. A recent study demonstrated that Calpain® significantly reduced both the quantity and size of the *S. mansoni* hepatic egg load in vaccinated baboons, and investigators are moving forward to conduct a large-scale double-blinded experiment to validate the vaccine's transmission-blocking potential in baboons [80,81].

Although the vaccine development pipeline is expanding, the established pathway to market is both expensive and time-consuming. At the moment, the majority of pipeline vaccines only target a single species of schistosome (primarily *S. mansoni*). Ideally, the development pipeline would feature a vaccine effective against the infective form of the parasite for all schistosome species found in humans. However, until such a product has been discovered, there is a continued need to expand and diversify the vaccine pipeline to include products targeting immunogenic antigens that are conserved across all species.

3.2. Diagnostic Development

Innovative, effective, and precise diagnostics are particularly important during schistosomiasis elimination, when it is necessary to identify geographic areas where transmission has been interrupted and ensure that the disease is no longer present in the population. Paralleling the vaccine development pipeline, efforts have also been made to improve the accurate diagnosis of schistosomiasis at low levels of infection to best direct and inform key decisions throughout elimination programs: (1) Mapping prevalence—establish a baseline disease prevalence to inform MDA strategy; (2) monitoring the impact of MDA—track disease prevalence; (3) inform reduction/stopping of MDA—determine when morbidity reduction targets have been achieved; (4) post-elimination surveillance—detect the re-emergence of the disease (PATH, Diagnostics for Neglected Tropical Diseases). A single universal diagnostic is unable to inform the entire elimination process, thus there is a need to develop diagnostic tools of varying levels of field implementation and sensitivity to be effectively partnered and applied with each step of schistosome elimination programs (Table 2) [82] (PATH, Diagnostics for Neglected Tropical Diseases).

Table 2. Applications of diagnostic platforms.

Diagnostic Platform	Qualities	Mechanism of Detection	Stage of Elimination Program for Application
Microscopic Detection	Recommended by WHO Low sensitivity: egg shedding is often not observed upon infection or in instances of low infection	Microscopic egg counting from fecal or urine sample	Mapping prevalence
Lateral flow test	Field deployable Minimal training requirements Relatively low cost Incorporating a reader may improve test performance metrics	Antigen detection: indication of active infection	Mapping prevalence Monitoring the impact of MDA Informing reduction/stopping of MDA
		Antibody detection: indication of past or present exposure to disease	Post-elimination surveillance [1]
Molecular Diagnostic Testing	Implementation is limited to a laboratory setting Requires sample preparation Highly sensitive and specific Too expensive for mass distribution Ability for multiplex pathogen detection Rapid turnaround time	Nucleic acid detection: indication of active infection	Informing reduction/stopping of MDA

[1] Antibody-based technology is limited due to its inability to differentiate between ongoing and previous infections, as the detected antibodies remain present even after clearance of parasites. Antibody-based diagnostics have application for post-elimination surveillance by monitoring antibody prevalence in age cohorts that were born after elimination was certified; if antibodies are detected in this youth population, then there has been a re-emergence of the disease [70] (PATH, Diagnostics for Neglected Tropical Diseases).

The below analysis focuses on clinically available diagnostic tests. Currently, the most commonly practiced method of diagnosis for all schistosome species is microscopic evaluation and detection of parasite eggs in human urine or stool, for which WHO recommends a polycarbonate filtration technique or the Kato-Katz (KK) fecal smear, respectively [83–85]. However, the KK technique is not sufficiently sensitive for low-grade infections and has been repeatedly shown to underestimate disease burden in areas where transmission has declined, and egg burdens are low [85]. Further, egg shedding is often not observed during an initial infection or in cases of low-level infection, due to the PZQ-induced sterilization of worm pairs or the survival of single-sex worm populations following PZQ treatment [83]. Following multiple rounds of PZQ MDA, low levels of infection will become more common, and thus new diagnostic tools with higher specificity and sensitivity are needed to ensure the accurate detection of schistosomiasis. For instance, following a very successful MDA program in Morocco, there have been zero reported cases of urogenital schistosomiasis from *S. haematobium* since 2004. However, when testing the efficacy of three newly developed diagnostic methods—two commercially available antibody tests (haemagglutination and enzyme-linked immunosorbent assay [ELISA] formats) and a lateral flow antigen strip—it was found that some citizens remained infected with *S. haematobium* worms that were simply not producing eggs [83]. There is a need to develop and validate monitoring diagnostics to accurately detect the re-emergence of schistosomiasis in areas where previous MDA campaigns have been successful. Moreover, there remains a need for the development of highly sensitive diagnostics to complement MDA programs that often result in lower levels of eggs in order to inform the decisions to stop MDA.

To identify the best technology to fill the need for accurate disease monitoring, recent studies have conducted comparative analyses of available molecular and immunological diagnostic methods that do not rely on egg counting [83,85,86]. ELISAs are able to accurately monitor low-grade infection through the detection of antibodies or antigens and can be adapted for large-scale implementation. Antibody-based technology is limited due to its inability to differentiate between ongoing and previous infections, as the detected antibodies remain present even after the clearance of parasites [86]. However, this may be useful for post-elimination surveillance by monitoring antibody prevalence in age cohorts that were born after elimination was certified; if antibodies are detected in this youth population, then there has been a re-emergence of the disease [82]. An alternative approach is the development of molecular diagnostics to detect *Schistosoma* DNA. Although PCR-based diagnostics have been developed with the ability to detect the four main human *Schistosoma* species with high sensitivity and specificity, PCR technology remains too expensive for mass distribution, and implementation is limited to laboratory settings [86,87]. Although ELISA and PCR technologies have promising features, POC immunodiagnostics have been adopted as the most common alternatives to the KK fecal smear. One of the most promising diagnostics is the POC-CCA developed by Rapid Medical Diagnostics [84]. POC-CCA is a commercially available serological assay that is able to detect *Schistosoma* circulating cathodic antigen (CCA), which is produced by adult schistosomes, in either human blood or urine samples [86]. As CCA is a genus-specific glycan, this method is able to detect active infections caused by the four main species of schistosome that infect humans—excluding urogenital schistosomiasis—and has consistently been identified as a more sensitive substitute for KK when estimating a region's schistosomiasis prevalence [83–86,88]. However, the POC-CCA diagnostic has high rates of false negatives due to frequent trace CCA results on the test strip. In a 2017 comparative study in Brazil, 461 participants donated feces, blood, and urine samples to comparatively map schistosomiasis prevalence using three diagnostic mechanisms, including the KK fecal smear and POC-CCA diagnostic [83]. The POC-CCA method produced the highest proportion of false-negative results and the lowest proportion of true-positive results, thus demonstrating the need for expanding the product development pipeline and continuing sensitivity testing and validation of available immunodiagnostics [83–85].

Through improved access to sequencing technology, the *S. mansoni* genome has been successfully assembled and new secretion proteins from both adult worms and eggs have been identified as new potential diagnostic targets [86]. This presents opportunities for continued development and improvement of multiplex serological assays to simultaneously detect *S. haematobium, S. mansoni*, and *S. japonicum*. Continued development of accurate diagnostics will also improve the detection of reduced drug efficacy and the subsequent monitoring of the development of PZQ resistance. To date, the development of new diagnostics for schistosomiasis has been primarily driven by the academic sector, and there is a need to also engage and incentivize the private sector to drive pipeline expansion and product development.

3.3. Drug Development

Due to the widespread dependence on PZQ to combat schistosomiasis, the therapeutic development pipeline is critically limited (Table 3). The only candidate in clinical trials is Co-Arinate FDC®, an artemisinin-based combination therapy (ACT) consisting of artesunate and sulfamethoxypyrazine/pyrimethamin that was developed by Dafra Pharmaceuticals as an antimalarial drug [89]. Due to the high rates of co-infection of malaria and *S. haematobium*, artemisinins have been observed to have unexpected antischistosomal effects, particularly against juvenile parasites [89]. Thus, Co-Arinate FDC® was tested in a Phase III clinical trial to compare its efficacy to that of PZQ against *S. haematobium* in children [90]. Although it has a strong safety profile, Co-Arinate FDC® has only partial efficacy against *S. haematobium*, with a 43.9% cure rate, which was lower than the 53% cure rate observed in patients receiving PZQ [89]. These findings indicate the need for the further exploration of the efficacy of various ACT formulations against *Schistosoma* species. Alternative preclinical and discovery stage therapeutic programs include the repurposing of miltefosine (MFS), which is currently a widely adopted treatment for leishmaniasis, and evaluating the efficacy of thioredoxin glutathione reductase (TGR) inhibitors through high-throughput screening [91,92]. MFS was reported to have significant activity against various stages of *S. mansoni* in in vitro studies, thus spurring further exploration of repurposing that drug for the treatment of schistosomiasis [91]. A 2015 preclinical study reported that delivering MFS in lipid nanocapsules allowed for single-dose oral delivery in mice [91].

Table 3. Therapeutics in development.

Product	Phase of Development	Targeted Species
Co-Arinate FDC®	Phase III	*S. haematobium*
Pediatric PZQ	Preclinical	*S. haematobium* *S. mansoni* *S. japonicum*
Miltefosine (MFS)	Preclinical	*S. mansoni*

To date, the majority of drug development efforts have focused on developing derivatives of PZQ, including the development of a PZQ pediatric formulation and deuterated PZQ analogs [93]. However, to prepare for the risk of widespread drug resistance, there is a critical need for a diversified therapeutic pipeline with novel drug targets.

3.4. Call to Action: Expanding Product Development Pipelines

To effectively combat schistosomiasis on a population-wide basis, intersectional technological innovations—new drugs with novel molecular targets and activity against immature schistosomes; POC diagnostics to detect low-level infections, assess treatment efficacy, and inform treatment decisions; and effective vaccines to prevent initial infection and reinfection—must be developed and made broadly accessible.

With over 700 million people at risk for infection, there is a clear and pressing need to develop new tools that make schistosomiasis elimination a reality. However, since schistosomiasis largely affects the world's poorest populations, consumers are unable to pay high prices for new products. This has resulted in limited commercial incentives to develop innovative vaccines, diagnostics, and drugs for schistosomiasis and other diseases of poverty. To develop new products, companies must make substantial monetary investments during the discovery, preclinical, and clinical stages of development [94], and must bear the risk that the resulting product may not receive U.S. Food and Drug Administration (FDA) approval and may fail to make it to market. In order for a company to remain profitable, its products must generate a margin of profit that returns the initial investments made during R&D. In comparison to "high-incentive" diseases with profitable markets such as cancer, hypercholesterolemia, and other cardiovascular diseases, the profitability of the schistosomiasis market and the socioeconomic status of its customers do not align particularly well with the business models of most pharmaceutical and biotechnology companies, particularly if the companies are expected to shoulder the financial risk and resource-heavy investment associated with de novo product development. Although schistosomiasis is a high-priority disease to the WHO due to the number of people who are currently infected and are at risk for infection, the commercial incentives to invest resources into product development for this disease are low and not compatible with many business models.

Along these lines, a study that profiled the drug and vaccine landscape for neglected diseases between 2000 and 2011 found that out of 850 new registered products, only 4% were indicated for neglected diseases [95], illustrating the massive gaps in product development for neglected diseases. In order to incentivize the private sector and distribute the financial risk associated with bringing a healthcare product to the market for high-priority, low-incentive indications, new product development models have emerged. One such model is the PPP, in which the strengths of the public and private sectors are combined and leveraged to develop breakthrough products while simultaneously redistributing the financial risk involved with product development [96]. An example of a PPP focused on schistosomiasis is the Pediatric Praziquantel Consortium, which is working to develop a pediatric formulation of PZQ for preschool-aged children. The Pediatric Praziquantel Consortium was launched in 2012 by Astellas Pharma, Merck KGaA, the Swiss Tropical and Public Health Institute (TPH), and Lygature. Armed with funding from the Bill & Melinda Gates Foundation and the Global Health Innovative Technology Fund (GHIT), the Consortium identified promising candidates and is currently optimizing its formulation before moving into clinical trials [97]. Having the capabilities for a Phase I-III clinical development program that includes FDA recommendations for pediatric development, the Consortium aims to have its pediatric-specific product available by 2020 [97]. With approximately 25 million preschool-aged children requiring treatment for schistosomiasis [97], the need for a pediatric formulation of PZQ is pressing, but not highly profitable. Through the Pediatric Praziquantel Consortium, the private and public sectors are working together to fill this high-priority product development gap by contributing specific know-how. Merck KGaA is the sponsor of the clinical trials and will be providing support and resources in the areas of preclinical, clinical, manufacturing, regulatory, and access, while Astellas provides advice on clinical development and pharmacokinetic modeling. Scientists from Swiss TPH, as well as other academic institutions, will contribute extensive experience in helminth biological and pharmacological research; epidemiology; and clinical research in endemic regions. Further, by pivoting from the current donation-based PZQ-MDA model towards a more sustainable pricing model, the Pediatric Praziquantel Consortium plans to make the product available on a not-for-profit basis. The Pediatric Praziquantel Consortium is exploring alternative business models and will work with relevant stakeholders to examine ways of providing access to its novel formulation in an affordable manner. This type of partnership demonstrates that, through the sharing of resources and expertise between the private and public sectors, it is possible to develop products for a market that historically has not been highly profitable.

Another type of collaborative model that fits under the umbrella of a PPP is the not-for-profit product development partnership (PDP). PDPs focus on product development and uncoupling the cost of R&D from the price of medicines, thereby resulting in a more affordable product [98]. Many PDPs are also PPPs, as they work with the pharmaceutical industry, academic research institutions, and other not-for-profit organizations. PDPs such as the Drugs for Neglected Diseases *initiative* (DND*i*), PATH, Medicines for Malaria Venture (MMV), Global Alliance for Tuberculosis Drug Development (TB Alliance), and the Foundation for Innovative New Diagnostics (FIND) tackle the traditionally high cost of R&D and work to bring new NTD, malaria, and tuberculosis products to the market at affordable prices. In contrast to private industry, which funds its R&D through revenues from marketed products as well as investors, PDPs are supported through various mechanisms that include public funding and philanthropy. This funding mechanism allows PDPs to decouple the price of medicines developed from the cost of R&D. Pharmaceutical companies generally employ cost-based pricing to cover the costs of R&D and to generate a profit. Not only do PDPs keep their costs low through efficient collaborations, and smaller clinical trials [98], but once a product is developed, PDPs are not under pressure to generate high-margin profits to cover development costs. Consequently, PDPs can price products in a manner that can be afforded by those in need. In addition to this, by establishing strong partnerships with private industry, PDPs benefit from access to resources such as compound libraries and the pharmaceutical industry's expertise in getting a product to market. Through this collaborative model, it has been possible to reduce development costs and set prices that can be afforded by low- and middle- income countries (LMICs), thus demonstrating that alternative models for neglected disease R&D are possible [98].

By leveraging world-class infectious disease and biological expertise as well as innovative thinking from various research institutions, and by maximizing the use of the material assets and product development know-how of global pharmaceutical and biotechnology companies, PDPs have made it possible to streamline drug discovery to target diseases of poverty in a coordinated and efficient manner. Not only does this incentivize the sharing of ideas and resources across various sectors as outlined in United Nations Sustainable Development Goal (SDG) 3, but it also successfully addresses SDG 17 by directly engaging the private and public sectors in global partnerships and cooperation. However, due to the limited resources available to support product development for neglected diseases, additional collaborative efforts are needed to fill R&D gaps. Although the Pediatric Praziquantel Consortium is working towards a new pediatric formulation of PZQ, there are currently no PDPs focused on novel schistosomiasis drug discovery, thus necessitating other collaborative models. It is such collaborative agreements and cross-sector-inspired business models that will create a sustainable framework for product development in schistosomiasis and other diseases of poverty.

4. WIPO Re:Search as a Platform for Cross-Sector Collaborations That Accelerate Drug Discovery

New and creative collaborative approaches involving both the for-profit and academic/non-profit sectors are required to catalyze product development for schistosomiasis and other high-priority, low-incentive medical needs. Although many pharmaceutical companies have demonstrated commitment to corporate social responsibility (CSR) through drug donation programs for schistosomiasis and other diseases of poverty, as well as through participation in PDPs and PPPs, additional models that complement those efforts and have a longer-term and more sustainable impact on affected populations are needed. Such models need to not only put in place access plans, so that the resulting products are available to the world's poorest populations (as is done with PDPs), but also continue to drive innovation and product development through alternative frameworks that build the capacity for researchers in endemic countries to jumpstart their own R&D efforts.

One such collaborative model, WIPO Re:Search, was established in 2011 by the World Intellectual Property Organization (WIPO) and BIO Ventures for Global Health (BVGH), and is supported by eight pharmaceutical companies (Eisai Co., Ltd., GlaxoSmithKline, Johnson & Johnson, Merck KGaA, Merck Sharp & Dohme [MSD; known as Merck & Co., Inc. in the U.S. and Canada], Novartis, Pfizer, and Takeda Pharmaceutical Company, Ltd.). WIPO Re:Search is a global initiative that connects people, resources, and ideas across biotechnology and pharmaceutical companies, governments, and non-profits to accelerate drug, diagnostic, and vaccine development for schistosomiasis, other NTDs, malaria, and tuberculosis [99]. WIPO Re:Search operations are supported by the financial contributions of the eight participating companies. While the companies may have internal R&D programs focused on neglected diseases, they have also made commitments to sharing their intellectual property (IP) assets with WIPO Re:Search investigators all over the world, to accelerate the development of novel products that can one day play a critical role in eliminating diseases of poverty. To date, WIPO Re:Search has 140 members in 40 countries across six continents, and has established 140 collaborations, with 14 of them focused on schistosomiasis.

The WIPO Re:Search consortium is a global PPP platform, which, through BVGH's targeted partnering approach, catalyzes product development for neglected diseases. BVGH recruits targeted member organizations based on strategic considerations, which may include the need for additional corporate engagement, specialized subject matter expertise, or other resources such as specific screening assays or animal models. Once an academic/non-profit institution joins the Consortium, BVGH reviews its assets, and identifies and connects with researchers who work on neglected diseases.

The researchers share their partnering interests with BVGH during introductory calls, enabling the identification of potential collaborators with aligned interests. Once mutual interest in collaborating is established, BVGH introduces the parties to each other and coordinates communications between partners to solidify collaboration details, roles, and responsibilities. Once milestones, timelines, deliverables, and action items are developed and agreed upon, the participating organizations execute material transfer agreements (MTAs) or other legal agreements to begin the collaboration. Once an agreement is in place, BVGH provides partnership support and alliance management to help ensure project success.

WIPO Re:Search uses IP sharing to incentivize and promote innovative product development and access in areas that have traditionally yielded low profitability, such as neglected diseases. It is through the sharing of IP assets for neglected disease R&D at no cost to the user organization, and by having members agree to the WIPO Re:Search Guiding Principles (detailed below) [100], that the Consortium promotes the accessibility of the resulting products to populations that are disproportionately affected by those diseases. Each legal agreement is executed in accordance with the Guiding Principles, which state that IP is to be shared on a royalty-free basis for R&D of products, technologies, and services to address public health needs for neglected diseases in least developed countries (LDCs), which are low-income countries currently confronting severe structural impediments to sustainable development that are also highly vulnerable to economic and environmental shocks [101]. Further, the Guiding Principles state that, for any products resulting from WIPO Re:Search collaborations, IP owners agree to provide royalty-free licenses for their use and sale in LDCs. IP owners also agree to consider in good faith the issue of product access for all developing countries. Finally, the institution that is using the shared IP is allowed to retain ownership of any new IP that results from WIPO Re:Search collaborations and is encouraged to share those assets with other members of the Consortium.

Through WIPO Re:Search, the most commonly shared IP assets are pharmaceutical company compounds (both targeted libraries and diversity sets) that have the potential to be repurposed as new drugs for schistosomiasis and other neglected diseases. Compounds provided by pharmaceutical companies may have already undergone preclinical or early-stage clinical testing, thereby reducing the number of experiments that need to be conducted to validate the compounds' safety or metabolic properties. This adds value, as it allows scientists to prioritize compounds with good metabolic and safety data that are more likely to move forward through the drug development pipeline. Alternatively, if a compound has a poor toxicity/safety profile, investigators can save valuable time and resources by focusing their efforts on compounds with better profiles. Further, during the drug development process, pharmaceutical companies synthesize large sets of compounds and structurally similar analogs as inhibitors of human target proteins. Like humans, *Schistosoma* are eukaryotes and thus have similar, yet distinct, cellular targets. Thus, compounds targeting human molecules with weak affinity/activity may have the potential to bind to and inhibit homologous proteins found in parasites such as *Schistosoma*. Such large target-specific compound libraries can be repurposed for schistosomiasis as well as many other diseases. Given that the average time required for a drug to reach the market is 12 years [102], it is important to not only identify ways to reduce the time it takes for that drug to get to market (and potentially the cost of the final product), but also reposition important resources such as compounds, technology platforms, and funding in a way that maximizes the strengths of industry and academic/non-profit scientists.

Since companies are likely to have invested significant time and money in developing compounds that target proteins that are dysregulated in non-communicable diseases such as cancer and hypercholesterolemia, targeting the parasitic homologs of those human proteins can be especially promising for neglected disease drug discovery. The key is to identify homologous target proteins that are essential to the survival of the parasite, and pharmaceutical compounds with biological activity against those homologous targets. One of the earliest schistosomiasis-related collaborations established through WIPO Re:Search began in 2013. Through phenotypic whole-organism screens of various compounds, Dr. Conor Caffrey, then at the University of California, San Francisco (UCSF), found that commercial anti-hypercholesterolemia statin drugs were potent schistosomicidal compounds [103]. The statins had been initially developed to treat patients who suffered from elevated cholesterol levels, but as inhibitors of HMG-CoA reductase (3-hydroxy-3-methyl-glutaryl-CoA reductase or HMGR), they also had the potential to be repurposed to inhibit HMG-CoA reductase activity in other organisms. In particular, *S. mansoni's* survival and egg-producing abilities had been shown to be dependent on schistosomal HMG-CoA reductase (SmHMGR) activity both in vivo and in vitro [104], and Dr. Caffrey was looking to exploit that vulnerability with inhibitors that specifically targeted this protein.

In order to screen chemical analogs that could prove to be even more potent against SmHMGR and develop a drug discovery program around this promising validated target, BVGH connected Dr. Caffrey with MSD. As a successful manufacturer of statin drugs, MSD was able to provide a select set of statin analogs to support Dr. Caffrey's efforts. BVGH also connected Dr. Caffrey with investigators from the Center for Infectious Disease Research (CIDR), and the NIAID-funded Seattle Structural Genomics Center for Infectious Disease (SSGCID) to solve the crystal structure for SmHMGR. In addition, MSD scientists provided scientific input on optimized SmHMGR gene expression methodologies that are being used to express the SmHMGR protein so that the crystal structure can be elucidated. With the crystal structure, Dr. Caffrey, now at the Center for Discovery and Innovation in Parasitic Diseases (CDIPD) at the University of California, San Diego (UCSD), and his collaborators will have the option to optimize the hit compounds utilizing a structure-guided medicinal chemistry approach.

Based on the model of directing drug discovery efforts by using validated targets essential to parasite survival, BVGH has continued to establish fruitful collaborations that involve the sharing of targeted compounds from WIPO Re:Search company members. Eisai Co., Ltd. has also become involved in schistosomiasis R&D by agreeing to provide an investigator with a calcium channel antagonist, as it has been shown that this type of inhibitor has activity against schistosomula and is capable of significantly reducing the viability of adult worms, alone or in combination with PZQ [105]. Further, in line with the hypothesis that polo-like kinases play an important role in *S. mansoni* gametogenesis [106], Takeda Pharmaceutical Company, Ltd., agreed to support efforts surrounding this target by providing a selective polo-like kinase inhibitor that was originally developed to treat solid tumors. By sharing compounds that have selective activity against a verified target, companies are not only providing chemical analogs that researchers would typically have difficulty accessing, they are also directly accelerating the drug discovery process by avoiding the use of compounds with unknown activities, properties, and targets. The use of natural products is also an area that is quite active for drug discovery. Due to the need for novel drugs against schistosomiasis, screening natural products for schistosomicidal activity could potentially lead to the identification of interesting starting points for further drug development, such as novel chemistry or mechanisms of action. For this reason, BVGH connected a researcher at Swiss TPH with the Griffith Institute for Drug Discovery (GRIDD) to gain access to GRIDD's Nature Bank [107] and screen natural product extracts for activity against *S. mansoni*.

Although repurposing pharmaceutical compounds is an important strategy for developing novel therapeutics in a cost-effective way, the value of the WIPO Re:Search IP-sharing model in advancing R&D for schistosomiasis and other diseases of poverty goes beyond compounds. The model also involves the sharing of knowledge and expertise. Such sharing is especially impactful when it involves scientists from LMICs, as it not only incentivizes innovation in neglected disease-endemic countries, but it also promotes R&D capacity building. This type of capacity building plays an essential role in changing the global development landscape from donation-based programs to long-term sustainable R&D models in countries that currently lack the necessary resources to successfully jumpstart their own product development efforts. Many LMIC researchers focus their efforts on diseases that affect their countries, but they may not have the product development know-how or infrastructure to advance those efforts to the clinic. WIPO Re:Search provides LMIC scientists with a platform that reduces the access barrier to industry and academic/non-profit IP assets and facilitates the necessary knowledge transfer that will eventually empower and strengthen the scientists' ability to contribute to product development for diseases that challenge their populations.

WIPO Re:Search collaborations are enabling knowledge and technology transfer between high-income country organizations and LMIC institutions to bolster schistosomiasis R&D capacity in the latter. In one instance, an investigator from Ghana's Kwame Nkrumah University of Science and Technology (KNUST) was interested in receiving training in *S. mansoni* cultivation and maintenance and screening of Ghanaian medicinal plants for antiparasitic activity, to enhance KNUST's research and education programs. BVGH connected the researcher with a faculty member who was at UCSF at the time, and the visiting scientist was able to receive the desired training from a world-renowned schistosomiasis researcher. The collaborative work between these two investigators resulted in a *Journal of Parasitology Research* publication [108]. Other WIPO Re:Search collaborations involve the sharing of reagents critical to LMIC investigators' work plans. For example, Dr. Floriano Paes Silva Junior, an investigator at FIOCRUZ (Brazil), was interested in validating a group of genes as essential to *S. mansoni* through RNA interference (RNAi) and determining whether those proteins could be potential drug discovery targets. BVGH connected the researcher to Alnylam, a pharmaceutical company focused on RNAi therapeutics. Alnylam agreed to design and synthesize optimized siRNAs that would enable the FIOCRUZ team to knock down the genes and determine whether their loss affects parasite viability. An additional example involved the sharing of a recombinant schistosome protein that Dr. Moustapha Mbow at Cheikh Anta Diop University (Senegal) was interested in using to assess in vitro immune responses to the protein. BVGH connected Dr. Mbow to Dr. Michael Hsieh at the Biomedical Research Institute (BRI), who expressed, purified, and shared the protein. This collaboration has led to a joint grant submission.

5. Conclusions

To boost the number of quality novel candidates that enter clinical-stage development, the schistosomiasis product development pipeline needs to be continuously fueled by early-stage research. It is during this stage of the product development process that WIPO Re:Search can have the greatest impact by establishing collaborations between for-profit and academic/non-profit institutions. The pharmaceutical industry not only engages in global health initiatives through its drug donation programs, but it also plays an important role in driving R&D for diseases of poverty. However, many academic/non-profit researchers remain unaware of the partnership opportunities that are available to them to drive their own research forward. The WIPO Re:Search consortium can bridge the gap between academic/non-profit and industry scientists to reduce duplicative efforts and encourage synergy to develop vaccines, diagnostics, and drugs for schistosomiasis and other neglected diseases. Furthermore, through the capacity building activities of WIPO Re:Search, LMIC scientists are not only able to gain valuable expertise, but also to use that expertise to develop new skills, accelerate their research, and advance their careers. The expertise gained through such collaborations provides scientists with a distinct advantage that can result in additional funding to reach important milestones. It is through the mutually beneficial model of WIPO Re:Search, where product development risk and cost are distributed among various key stakeholders, that a tangible and significant impact can be made to eliminate schistosomiasis and other diseases of poverty.

As the fight against schistosomiasis continues, the involvement of private industry and their critical contributions of assets and expertise should be causes for optimism. While promising industry collaborations continue to advance towards novel products and tools that will play a key role in the elimination of schistosomiasis, it is important to remember that this task is too great to be overcome by a single sector. As pharmaceutical companies continue to invest resources and funding to combat schistosomiasis, it is important for these efforts to receive the support of various stakeholders such as governments and international funding agencies. Through a concerted effort that distributes risk, and leverages the strengths and resources of the private and public sectors, every day brings us closer to winning the fight against schistosomiasis.

Author Contributions: C.J.W. and J.H.-C. wrote the manuscript. K.M.G. and C.K.M. reviewed the manuscript and provided valuable feedback. J.D. oversaw operations.

Funding: Jennifer Dent, Katy M. Graef, Joseph Hargan-Calvopiña, Cathyryne K. Manner, and Callie J. Weber are employees of BIO Ventures for Global Health (BVGH). BVGH receives WIPO Re:Search sponsorship funding from Eisai Co., Ltd., GlaxoSmithKline, Johnson & Johnson, MSD, Merck KGaA, Novartis, Pfizer, and Takeda Pharmaceutical Company, Ltd.

Acknowledgments: The authors thank Alnylam, Biomedical Research Institute, Center for Infectious Disease Research, Cheikh Anta Diop University, Eisai Co., Ltd., Griffith Institute for Drug Discovery, Oswaldo Cruz Foundation, Kwame Nkrumah University of Science and Technology, MSD, Swiss TPH, Takeda Pharmaceutical Company, Ltd., and University of California, San Diego for their review and helpful suggestions.

Conflicts of Interest: The authors have no other relevant affiliations or financial involvement with any organization or entity with a financial interest in or financial conflict with the subject matter or materials discussed in the manuscript, apart from those disclosed.

References

1. World Health Organization. Schistosomiasis and soil-transmitted helminthiases: Number of people treated in 2017. *WHO Wkly. Epidemiological Rec.* **2018**, *93*, 681–692.
2. Nour, N.M. Schistosomiasis: Health Effects on Women. *Rev. Obsterics Gynecol.* **2010**, *3*, 28–32.
3. Warren, K.S.; Mahmoud, A.A.; Cummings, P.; Murphy, D.J.; Houser, H.B. Schistosomiasis mansoni in Yemeni in California: Duration of infection, presence of disease, therapeutic management. *Am. J. Trop. Med. Hyg.* **1974**, *23*, 902–909. [CrossRef] [PubMed]
4. Colley, D.G.; Bustinduy, A.L.; Secor, W.E.; King, C.H. Human schistosomiasis. *Lancet* **2014**, *383*, 2253–2264. [CrossRef]
5. Chabasse, D.; Bertrand, G.; Leroux, J.P.; Gauthey, N.; Hocquet, P. Developmental bilharziasis caused by Schistosoma mansoni discovered 37 years after infestation. *Bull. Soc. Pathol. Exot.* **1985**, *78*, 643–647.
6. Gryseels, B.; Polman, K.; Clerinx, J.; Kestens, L. Human Schistosomiasis. *Lancet* **2006**, *368*, 23–29. [CrossRef]
7. World Health Organization. *Schistosomiasis: Progress Report 2001–2011, Strategic Plan 2012–2020*; World Health Organization: Geneva, Switzerland, 2013.
8. Steinmann, P.; Keiser, J.; Bos, R.; Tanner, M.; Utzinger, J. Schistosomiasis and water resources development: Systematic review, meta-analysis, and estimates of people at risk. *Lancet Infect. Dis.* **2006**, *6*, 411–425. [CrossRef]
9. Elbaz, T.; Esmat, G. Hepatic and intestinal schistosomiasis: Review. *J. Adv. Res.* **2013**, *4*, 445–452. [CrossRef]
10. Rambau, P.F.; Chalya, P.L.; Jackson, K. Schistosomiasis and urinary bladder cancer in North Western Tanzania: A retrospective review of 185 patients. *Infect. Agents Cancer* **2013**, *8*, 1–6. [CrossRef]
11. Ray, D.; Nelson, T.A.; Fu, C.L.; Patel, S.; Gong, D.N.; Odegaard, J.I.; Hsieh, M.H. Transcriptional profiling of the bladder in urogenital schistosomiasis reveals pathways of inflammatory fibrosis and urothelial compromise. *PLoS Negl. Trop. Dis.* **2012**, *6*, e1912. [CrossRef] [PubMed]
12. Center For Disease Control and Prevention/Schistosomiasis FAQ. Available online: https://www.cdc.gov/parasites/schistosomiasis/gen_info/faqs.html (accessed on 17 September 2018).
13. Moné, H.; Minguez, S.; Ibikounlé, M.; Allienne, J.F.; Massougbodji, A.; Mouahid, G. Natural Interactions between *S. haematobium* and *S. guineensis* in the Republic of Benin. *Sci. World J.* **2012**, *2012*. [CrossRef] [PubMed]
14. King, C.H.; Dangerfield-Cha, M. The unacknowledged impact of chronic schistosomiasis. *Chronic Illn* **2008**, *4*, 65–79. [CrossRef] [PubMed]
15. GBD 2017 DALYs and HALE Collaborators. Global, regional, and national disability-adjusted life-years (DALYs) for 359 diseases and injuries and healthy life expectancy (HALE) for 195 countries and territories, 1990–2017: A systematic analysis for the Global Burden of Disease Study 2017. *Lancelet* **2018**, *392*, 859–922.
16. King, C.H. Parasites and poverty: The case of schistosomiasis. *Acta Trop.* **2010**, *113*, 95–104. [CrossRef] [PubMed]
17. Ndamba, J.; Makaza, N.; Munjoma, M.; Gomo, E.; Kaondera, K.C. The physical fitness and work performance of agricultural workers infected with Schistosoma mansoni in Zimbabwe. *Anal. Trop. Med. Parasitol.* **1993**, *87*, 553–561. [CrossRef]

18. Friedman, J.F.; Kanzaria, H.K.; Acosta, L.P.; Langdon, G.C.; Manalo, D.L.; Wu, H.; Olveda, R.M.; McGarvey, S.T.; Kurtis, J.D. Relationship between Schistosoma japonicum and nutritional status among children and young adults in Leyte, the Philippines. *Am. J. Trop. Med. Hyg.* **2005**, *72*, 527–533. [CrossRef] [PubMed]
19. McDonald, E.A.; Cheng, L.; Jarilla, B.; Sagliba, M.J.; Gonzal, A.; Amoylen, A.J.; Olveda, R.; Acosta, L.; Baylink, D.; White, E.S.; et al. Maternal infection with Schistosoma japonicum induces a profibrotic response in neonates. *Infect. Immun.* **2014**, *82*, 350–355. [CrossRef]
20. Kurtis, J.D.; Higashi, A.; Wu, H.W.; Gundogan, F.; McDonald, E.A.; Sharma, S.; PondTor, S.; Jarilla, B.; Sagliba, M.J.; Gonzal, A.; et al. Maternal Schistosomiasis japonica is associated with maternal, placental, and fetal inflammation. *Infect. Immun.* **2011**, *79*, 1254–1261. [CrossRef]
21. Sacko, M.; Magnussen, P.; Keita, A.D.; Traore, M.S.; Landoure, A.; Doucoure, A.; Madsen, H.; Vennervald, B.J. Impact of Schistosoma haematobium infection on urinary tract pathology, nutritional status and anaemia in school-aged children in two different endemic areas of the Niger River Basin, Mali. *Acta Trop.* **2011**, *120* (Suppl. 1), S142–S150. [CrossRef]
22. Stothard, J.R.; Sousa-Figueiredo, J.C.; Betson, M.; Bustinduy, A.; Reinhard-Rupp, J. Schistosomiasis in African infants and preschool children: Let them now be treated! *Trends Parasitol.* **2013**, *29*, 197–205. [CrossRef]
23. Mostafa, M.H.; Sheweita, S.A.; O'Connor, P.J. Relationship between Schistosomiasis and Bladder Cancer. *Clin. Microbiol. Rev.* **1999**, *12*, 97–111. [CrossRef] [PubMed]
24. Parkin, D.M. The global health burden of infection-associated cancers in the year 2002. *Int. J. Cancer* **2006**, *118*, 3030–3044. [CrossRef] [PubMed]
25. Adenowo, A.F.; Oyinloye, B.E.; Ogunyinka, B.I.; Kappo, A.P. Impact of human schistosomiasis in sub-Saharan Africa. *Braz. J. Infect. Dis.* **2015**, *19*, 196–205. [CrossRef] [PubMed]
26. Dematei, A.; Fernandes, R.; Soares, R.; Alves, H.; Richter, J.; Botelho, M.C. Angiogenesis in Schistosoma haematobium-associated urinary bladder cancer. *APMIS* **2017**, *125*, 1056–1062. [CrossRef]
27. Rosin, M.P.; Zaki, S.S.E.D.; Ward, A.J.; Anwar, W.A. Involvement of inflammatory reactions and elevated cell proliferation in the development of bladder cancer in schistosomiasis patients. *Mut. Res.* **1994**, *305*, 283–292. [CrossRef]
28. Shiff, C.; Veltri, R.; Naples, J.; Quartey, J.; Otchere, J.; Anyan, W.; Marlow, C.; Wiredu, E.; Adjei, A.; Brakohiapa, E.; et al. Ultrasound verification of bladder damage is associated with known biomarkers of bladder cancer in adults chronically infected with Schistosoma haematobium in Ghana. *Trans. R. Soc. Trop. Med. Hyg.* **2006**, *100*, 847–854. [CrossRef]
29. International Agency for Research on Cancer. Biological Agents. Volume 100B. A Review of Human Carcinogenesis. *IARC Monogr. Evalutation Carcinogenic Risks Hum.* **2012**, *100*, 1–441.
30. Doehring, E.; Ehrich, J.H.; Bremer, H.J. Reversibility of urinary tract abnormalities due to Schistosoma haematobium infection. *Kidney Int.* **1986**, *30*, 582–585. [CrossRef]
31. Botelho, M.C.; Alves, H.; Richter, J. Halting Schistosoma haematobium—Associated bladder cancer. *Int. J. Cancer Manag.* **2017**, *10*, e9430. [CrossRef]
32. Kjetland, E.F.; Leutscher, P.D.; Ndhlovu, P.D. A Review of Female Genital Schistosomiasis. *Trends Parasitol.* **2012**, *28*, 58–65. [CrossRef]
33. Santos, J.; Gouveia, M.J.; Vale, N.; Delgado Mde, L.; Goncalves, A.; da Silva, J.M.; Oliveira, C.; Xavier, P.; Gomes, P.; Santos, L.L.; et al. Urinary Estrogen Metabolites and Self-Reported Infertility in Women Infected With Schistosoma Haematobium. *PLoS ONE* **2014**, *9*, e96774. [CrossRef] [PubMed]
34. Friedman, J.; Mital, P.; Kanzaria, H.K.; Olds, G.R.; Kurtis, J.D. Schistosomiasis and pregnancy. *Trends Parasitol.* **2007**, *23*, 159–164. [CrossRef] [PubMed]
35. Kjetland, E.F.; Ndhlovu, P.D.; Gomo, E.; Mduluza, T.; Midzi, N.; Gwanzura, L.; Mason, P.R.; Sandvik, L.; Friis, H.; Gundersen, S.G. Association between genital schistosomiasis and HIV in rural Zimbabwean women. *AIDS* **2006**, *20*, 593–600. [CrossRef] [PubMed]
36. Brodish, P.H.; Singh, K. Association Between Schistosoma haematobium Exposure and Human Immunodeficiency Virus Infection Among Females in Mozambique. *Am. J. Trop. Med. Hyg.* **2016**, *94*, 1040–1044. [CrossRef] [PubMed]

37. Secor, W.E.; Shah, A.; Mwinzi, P.M.N.; Ndenga, B.A.; Watta, C.O.; Karanja, D.M.S. Increased Density of Human Immunodeficiency Virus Type 1 Coreceptors CCR5 and CXCR4 on the Surfaces of CD4+ T Cells and Monocytes of Patients with Schistosoma mansoni Infection. *Infect. Immun.* **2003**, *71*, 6668–6671. [CrossRef] [PubMed]
38. Gelfand, M.; Ross, C.M.; Blair, D.M.; Castle, W.M.; Weber, M.C. Schistosomiasis of the male pelvic organs. Severity of infection determined by digestion of tissue and histologic methods in 300 cadavers. *Am. J. Trop. Med. Hyg.* **1970**, *19*, 779–784. [CrossRef] [PubMed]
39. Leutscher, P.; Ramarokoto, C.E.; Reimert, C.; Feldmeier, H.; Esterre, P.; Vennervald, B.J. Community-based study of genital schistosomiasis in men from Madagascar. *Lancet* **2000**, *355*, 117–118. [CrossRef]
40. Leutscher, P.D.; Pedersen, M.; Raharisolo, C.; Jensen, J.S.; Hoffmann, S.; Lisse, I.; Ostrowski, S.R.; Reimert, C.M.; Mauclere, P.; Ullum, H. Increased prevalence of leukocytes and elevated cytokine levels in semen from Schistosoma haematobium-infected individuals. *J. Infect. Dis.* **2005**, *191*, 1639–1647. [CrossRef]
41. Reaching a Billion. Fifth Progress Report on the London Declaration on NTDs. 2017. Available online: https://unitingtocombatntds.org/reports/5th-report/ (accessed on 7 January 2019).
42. Greenberg, R.M. New approaches for understanding mechanisms of drug resistance in schistosomes. *Parasitology* **2013**, *140*, 1534–1546. [CrossRef]
43. Greenberg, R.M. ABC multidrug transporters in schistosomes and other parasitic flatworms. *Parasitol. Int.* **2013**, *62*, 647–653. [CrossRef]
44. Cioli, D.; Pica-Mattoccia, L.; Basso, A.; Guidi, A. Schistosomiasis control: Praziquantel forever? *Mol. Biochem. Parasitol.* **2014**, *195*, 23–29. [CrossRef] [PubMed]
45. Caffrey, C.R. Chemotherapy of schistosomiasis: Present and future. *Curr. Opin. Chem. Biol.* **2007**, *11*, 433–439. [CrossRef] [PubMed]
46. World Health Organization: Schistosomiasis Strategy. Available online: http://www.who.int/schistosomiasis/strategy/en/ (accessed on 14 September 2018).
47. Inobaya, M.T.; Olveda, R.M.; Chau, T.N.; Olveda, D.U.; Ross, A.G. Prevention and control of schistosomiasis: A current perspective. *Res. Rep. Trop. Med.* **2014**, *2014*, 65–75.
48. Sokolow, S.H.; Wood, C.L.; Jones, I.J.; Lafferty, K.D.; Kuris, A.M.; Hsieh, M.H.; De Leo, G.A. To Reduce the Global Burden of Human Schistosomiasis, Use 'Old Fashioned' Snail Control. *Trends Parasitol.* **2018**, *34*, 23–40. [CrossRef] [PubMed]
49. Lo, N.C.; Addiss, D.G.; Hotez, P.J.; King, C.H.; Stothard, J.R.; Evans, D.S.; Colley, D.G.; Lin, W.; Coulibaly, J.T.; Bustinduy, A.L.; et al. A call to strengthen the global strategy against schistosomiasis and soil-transmitted helminthiasis: The time is now. *Lancet Infect. Dis.* **2017**, *17*, e64–e69. [CrossRef]
50. Olds, G.R. Administration of Praziquantel to pregnant and lactating women. *Acta Trop.* **2003**, *86*, 185–195. [CrossRef]
51. Reinhard-Rupp, J.; Klohe, K. Developing a comprehensive response for treatment of children under 6 years of age with schistosomiasis: Research and development of a pediatric formulation of praziquantel. *Infect. Dis. Poverty* **2017**, *6*, 122. [CrossRef] [PubMed]
52. Abudho, B.O.; Ndombi, E.M.; Guya, B.; Carter, J.M.; Riner, D.K.; Kittur, N.; Karanja, D.M.S.; Secor, W.E.; Colley, D.G. Impact of Four Years of Annual Mass Drug Administration on Prevalence and Intensity of Schistosomiasis among Primary and High School Children in Western Kenya: A Repeated Cross-Sectional Study. *Am. J. Trop. Med. Hyg.* **2018**, *98*, 1397–1402. [CrossRef]
53. Kenya National School-Based Deworming Programme: Year 2 Report (April 2013–March 2014). Available online: https://ciff.org/documents/16/Kenya_National_SchoolBased_Deworming_Programme_Year2_evaluation.pdf (accessed on 6 January 2019).
54. Savioli, L.; Albonico, M.; Colley, D.G.; Correa-Oliveira, R.; Fenwick, A.; Green, W.; Kabatereine, N.; Kabore, A.; Katz, N.; Klohe, K.; et al. Building a global schistosomiasis alliance: An opportunity to join forces to fight inequality and rural poverty. *Infect. Dis. Poverty* **2017**, *6*, 65. [CrossRef]
55. World Health Organization. *Crossing the Billion. Lymphatic Filariasis, Onchocerciasis, Schistosomiasis, Soil-Transmitted Helminthiases and Trachoma: Preventive Chemotherapy for Neglected Tropical Diseases*; World Health Organization: Geneva, Switzerland, 2017.
56. Ross, A.G.; Chau, T.N.; Inobaya, M.T.; Olveda, R.M.; Li, Y.; Harn, D.A. A new global strategy for the elimination of schistosomiasis. *Int. J. Infect. Dis.* **2017**, *54*, 130–137. [CrossRef]

57. World Health Organization. Schistosomiasis and soil-transmitted helminthiases: Number of people treated in 2016. *WHO Wkly. Epidemiological Rec.* **2017**, *92*, 749–760.
58. Caffrey, C.R. Schistosomiasis and its treatment. *Future Med. Chem.* **2015**, *7*, 675–676. [CrossRef] [PubMed]
59. Doenhoff, M.J.; Hagan, P.; Cioli, D.; Southgate, V.; Pica-Mattoccia, L.; Botros, S.; Coles, G.; Tchuem Tchuente, L.A.; Mbaye, A.; Engels, D. Praziquantel: Its use in control of schistosomiasis in sub-Saharan Africa and current research needs. *Parasitology* **2009**, *136*, 1825–1835. [CrossRef] [PubMed]
60. Zwang, J.; Olliaro, P.L. Clinical efficacy and tolerability of praziquantel for intestinal and urinary schistosomiasis-a meta-analysis of comparative and non-comparative clinical trials. *PLoS Negl. Trop. Dis.* **2014**, *8*, e3286. [CrossRef] [PubMed]
61. Liu, R.; Dong, H.F.; Guo, Y.; Zhao, Q.P.; Jiang, M.S. Efficacy of praziquantel and artemisinin derivatives for the treatment and prevention of human schistosomiasis: A systematic review and meta-analysis. *Parasit Vectors* **2011**, *4*, 201. [CrossRef] [PubMed]
62. Kasinathan, R.S.; Sharma, L.K.; Cunningham, C.; Webb, T.R.; Greenberg, R.M. Inhibition or knockdown of ABC transporters enhances susceptibility of adult and juvenile schistosomes to Praziquantel. *PLoS Negl. Trop. Dis.* **2014**, *8*, e3265. [CrossRef] [PubMed]
63. Zwang, J.; Olliaro, P. Efficacy and safety of praziquantel 40 mg/kg in preschool-aged and school-aged children: A meta-analysis. *Parasit Vectors* **2017**, *10*, 47. [CrossRef]
64. Doenhoff, M.J.; Cioli, D.; Utzinger, J. Praziquantel: Mechanisms of action, resistance and new derivatives for schistosomiasis. *Curr. Opin. Infect. Dis.* **2008**, *21*, 659–667. [CrossRef]
65. Pinto-Almeida, A.; Mendes, T.; Armada, A.; Belo, S.; Carrilho, E.; Viveiros, M.; Afonso, A. The Role of Efflux Pumps in Schistosoma mansoni Praziquantel Resistant Phenotype. *PLoS ONE* **2015**, *10*, e0140147. [CrossRef]
66. Liu, Y.X.; Wu, W.; Liang, Y.J.; Jie, Z.L.; Wang, H.; Wang, W.; Huang, Y.X. New uses for old drugs: The tale of artemisinin derivatives in the elimination of schistosomiasis japonica in China. *Molecules* **2014**, *19*, 15058–15074. [CrossRef]
67. Toor, J.; Alsallaq, R.; Truscott, J.E.; Turner, H.C.; Werkman, M.; Gurarie, D.; King, C.H.; Anderson, R.M. Are We on Our Way to Achieving the 2020 Goals for Schistosomiasis Morbidity Control Using Current World Health Organization Guidelines? *Clin. Infect. Dis.* **2018**, *66*, S245–S252. [PubMed]
68. Mo, A.X.; Colley, D.G. Workshop report: Schistosomiasis vaccine clinical development and product characteristics. *Vaccine* **2016**, *34*, 995–1001. [CrossRef] [PubMed]
69. Policy Cures Research. Neglected Disease R&D Product Pipeline. Available online: https://www.pipeline.policycuresresearch.org/august2017 (accessed on 14 September 2018).
70. Hotez, P.J. The global fight to develop antipoverty vaccines in the anti-vaccine era. *Hum. Vaccin. Immunother.* **2018**, 1–4. [CrossRef] [PubMed]
71. Tendler, M.; Almeida, M.; Simpson, A. Development of the Brazilian Anti Schistosomiasis Vaccine Based on the Recombinant Fatty Acid Binding Protein Sm14 Plus GLA-SE Adjuvant. *Front. Immunol.* **2015**, *6*, 218. [CrossRef] [PubMed]
72. Ricciardi, A.; Ndao, M. Still hope for schistosomiasis vaccine. *Hum. Vaccin. Immunother.* **2015**, *11*, 2504–2508. [CrossRef] [PubMed]
73. Riveau, G.; Deplanque, D.; Remoue, F.; Schacht, A.M.; Vodougnon, H.; Capron, M.; Thiry, M.; Martial, J.; Libersa, C.; Capron, A. Safety and immunogenicity of rSh28GST antigen in humans: Phase 1 randomized clinical study of a vaccine candidate against urinary schistosomiasis. *PLoS Negl. Trop. Dis.* **2012**, *6*, e1704. [CrossRef]
74. Efficacy of Bilhvax in Association With Praziquantel for Prevention of Clinical Recurrences of Schistosoma Haematobium (Bilhvax3). Available online: https://clinicaltrials.gov/ct2/show/NCT00870649?term=Bilhvax&rank=2 (accessed on 14 September 2018).
75. Study of Safety and Immune Response of the Sm14 Vaccine in Adults of Endemic Regions. Available online: https://clinicaltrials.gov/ct2/show/NCT03041766?term=sm-14&cond=Schistosomiasis&rank=2 (accessed on 14 September 2018).
76. Santini-Oliveira, M.; Coler, R.N.; Parra, J.; Veloso, V.; Jayashankar, L.; Pinto, P.M.; Ciol, M.A.; Bergquist, R.; Reed, S.G.; Tendler, M. Schistosomiasis vaccine candidate Sm14/GLA-SE: Phase 1 safety and immunogenicity clinical trial in healthy, male adults. *Vaccine* **2016**, *34*, 586–594. [CrossRef]
77. Merrifield, M.; Hotez, P.J.; Beaumier, C.M.; Gillespie, P.; Strych, U.; Hayward, T.; Bottazzi, M.E. Advancing a vaccine to prevent human schistosomiasis. *Vaccine* **2016**, *34*, 2988–2991. [CrossRef]

78. Sabin Vaccine Institute. Available online: https://www.sabin.org/programs/schistosomiasis (accessed on 14 September 2018).
79. A Phase Ib Study of the Safety, Reactogenicity, and Immunogenicity of Sm-TSP-2/Alhydrogel)(R) with or without AP 10-701 for Intestinal Schistosomiasis in Healthy Exposed Adults. Available online: https://clinicaltrials.gov/ct2/show/NCT03110757?term=Alhydrogel&rank=8 (accessed on 14 September 2018).
80. Le, L.; Molehin, A.J.; Nash, S.; Sennoune, S.R.; Ahmad, G.; Torben, W.; Zhang, W.; Siddiqui, A.A. Schistosoma egg-induced liver pathology resolution by Sm-p80-based schistosomiasis vaccine in baboons. *Pathology* **2018**, *50*, 442–449. [CrossRef]
81. Siddiqui, A.A.; Siddiqui, S.Z. Sm-p80-Based Schistosomiasis Vaccine: Preparation for Human Clinical Trials. *Trends Parasitol.* **2017**, *33*, 194–201. [CrossRef]
82. Faulx, D.; Storey, H.L.; Murray, M.A.; Cantera, J.L.; Hawkins, K.R.; Leader, B.T.; Gallo, K.L.; de los Santntos, T. PATH. Diagnostics for Neglected Tropical Diseases: Defining the Best Tools through Target Product Profiles. 2015. Available online: https://www.finddx.org/wp-content/uploads/2016/03/PATH-2015_Dx-for-NTDs-Target-Products-Profile-report.pdf (accessed on 8 January 2019).
83. Balahbib, A.; Amarir, F.; Corstjens, P.L.; de Dood, C.J.; van Dam, G.J.; Hajli, A.; Belhaddad, M.; El Mansouri, B.; Sadak, A.; Rhajaoui, M.; et al. Selecting accurate post-elimination monitoring tools to prevent reemergence of urogenital schistosomiasis in Morocco: A pilot study. *Infect. Dis. Poverty* **2017**, *6*, 75. [CrossRef] [PubMed]
84. Foo, K.T.; Blackstock, A.J.; Ochola, E.A.; Matete, D.O.; Mwinzi, P.N.; Montgomery, S.P.; Karanja, D.M.; Secor, W.E. Evaluation of point-of-contact circulating cathodic antigen assays for the detection of Schistosoma mansoni infection in low-, moderate-, and high-prevalence schools in western Kenya. *Am. J. Trop. Med. Hyg.* **2015**, *92*, 1227–1232. [CrossRef] [PubMed]
85. Lindholz, C.G.; Favero, V.; Verissimo, C.M.; Candido, R.R.F.; de Souza, R.P.; Dos Santos, R.R.; Morassutti, A.L.; Bittencourt, H.R.; Jones, M.K.; St Pierre, T.G.; et al. Study of diagnostic accuracy of Helmintex, Kato-Katz, and POC-CCA methods for diagnosing intestinal schistosomiasis in Candeal, a low intensity transmission area in northeastern Brazil. *PLoS Negl. Trop. Dis.* **2018**, *12*, e0006274. [CrossRef] [PubMed]
86. Ogongo, P.; Kariuki, T.M.; Wilson, R.A. Diagnosis of schistosomiasis mansoni: An evaluation of existing methods and research towards single worm pair detection. *Parasitology* **2018**, *145*, 1355–1366. [CrossRef] [PubMed]
87. Sandoval, N.; Siles-Lucas, M.; Perez-Arellano, J.L.; Carranza, C.; Puente, S.; Lopez-Aban, J.; Muro, A. A new PCR-based approach for the specific amplification of DNA from different Schistosoma species applicable to human urine samples. *Parasitology* **2006**, *133*, 581–587. [CrossRef] [PubMed]
88. Field Evaluations of the Point-of-Care (POC) Circulating Cathodic Antigen (CCA) Urine Assay for Detection of *S. mansoni* infection. Available online: https://score.uga.edu/projects/poc-cca/ (accessed on 14 September 2018).
89. Sissoko, M.S.; Dabo, A.; Traore, H.; Diallo, M.; Traore, B.; Konate, D.; Niare, B.; Diakite, M.; Kamate, B.; Traore, A.; et al. Efficacy of artesunate + sulfamethoxypyrazine/pyrimethamine versus praziquantel in the treatment of Schistosoma haematobium in children. *PLoS ONE* **2009**, *4*, e6732. [CrossRef]
90. Comparing Praziquantel Versus Artesunate + Sulfamethoxypyrazine/Pyrimethamine for Treating Schistosomiasis. Available online: https://clinicaltrials.gov/ct2/show/NCT00510159?term=Co-Arinate&cond=schistosomiasis&rank=1 (accessed on 14 September 2018).
91. Eissa, M.M.; El-Moslemany, R.M.; Ramadan, A.A.; Amer, E.I.; El-Azzouni, M.Z.; El-Khordagui, L.K. Miltefosine Lipid Nanocapsules for Single Dose Oral Treatment of Schistosomiasis Mansoni: A Preclinical Study. *PLoS ONE* **2015**, *10*, e0141788. [CrossRef] [PubMed]
92. Simeonov, A.; Jadhav, A.; Sayed, A.A.; Wang, Y.; Nelson, M.E.; Thomas, C.J.; Inglese, J.; Williams, D.L.; Austin, C.P. Quantitative high-throughput screen identifies inhibitors of the Schistosoma mansoni redox cascade. *PLoS Negl. Trop. Dis.* **2008**, *2*, e127. [CrossRef]
93. TI Pharma Pediatric Praziquantel Consortium. Available online: https://www.tipharma.com/pharmaceutical-research-projects/neglected-diseases/pediatric-praziquantel-consortium/ (accessed on 14 September 2018).
94. The Truly Staggering Cost of Inventing New Drugs. Available online: https://www.forbes.com/sites/matthewherper/2012/02/22/the-truly-staggering-cost-of-inventing-new-drugs-the-print-version/#6a1435725f81 (accessed on 19 September 2018).

95. Pedrique, B.; Strub-Wourgaft, N.; Some, C.; Olliaro, P.; Trouiller, P.; Ford, N.; Pécoul, B.; Bradol, J.-H. The drug and vaccine landscape for neglected diseases (2000–2011): A systematic assessment. *Lancet Glob. Health* **2013**, *1*, e371–e379. [CrossRef]
96. Goldman, M.; Compton, C.; Mittleman, B.B. Public-private partnerships as driving forces in the quest for innovative medicines. *Clin. Transl. Med.* **2013**, *2*, 2. [CrossRef]
97. Pediatric Praziquantel Consortium. Available online: https://www.pediatricpraziquantelconsortium.org/ (accessed on 14 September 2018).
98. Maxmen, A. Big Pharma's Cost Cutting Challenger. *Nature* **2016**, *536*, 388–390. [CrossRef] [PubMed]
99. Dent, J.; Ramamoorthi, R.; Graef, K.; Nelson, L.M.; Wichard, J.C. WIPO Re:Search: A consortium catalyzing research and product development for neglected tropical diseases. *Pharm. Patent Anal.* **2013**, *2*, 591–596. [CrossRef] [PubMed]
100. WIPO Re:Search Guiding Principles. Available online: http://www.wipo.int/export/sites/www/research/docs/guiding_principles.pdf (accessed on 18 September 2018).
101. Economic Analysis and Policy Division, United Nations. Available online: https://www.un.org/development/desa/dpad/least-developed-country-category.html (accessed on 18 September 2018).
102. Van Norman, G.A. Drugs, Devices, and the FDA: Part 1: An Overview of Approval Processes for Drugs. *JACC Basic Transl. Sci.* **2016**, *1*, 170–179. [CrossRef] [PubMed]
103. Rojo-Arreola, L.; Long, T.; Asarnow, D.; Suzuki, B.M.; Singh, R.; Caffrey, C.R. Chemical and genetic validation of the statin drug target to treat the helminth disease, schistosomiasis. *PLoS ONE* **2014**, *9*, e87594. [CrossRef] [PubMed]
104. Chen, G.Z.; Foster, L.; Bennett, J.L. Antischistosomal action of mevinolin: Evidence that 3-hydroxy-methylglutaryl-coenzyme a reductase activity in Schistosoma mansoni is vital for parasite survival. *N-S Arch. Pharmacol.* **1990**, *324*, 477–482. [CrossRef]
105. Silva-Moraes, V.; Couto, F.F.B.; Vasconcelos, M.M.; Araújo, N.; Coelho, P.M.Z.; Katz, N.; Grenfell, R.F.Q. Antischistosomal activity of a calcium channel antagonist on schistosomula and adult Schistosoma mansoni worms. *Mem. Inst. Oswaldo Cruz* **2013**, *108*, 600–604. [CrossRef] [PubMed]
106. Dissous, C.; Grevelding, C.; Long, T. Schistosoma mansoni Polo-like kinases and their function in control of mitosis and parasite reproduction. *An. Acad. Brasil. Cienc.* **2011**, *83*, 627–635. [CrossRef]
107. Camp, D.; Newman, S.; B Pham, N.; J Quinn, R. Nature Bank and the Queensland Compound Library: Unique international resources at the Eskitis Institute for Drug Discovery. *Comb. Chem. High Throughput Screen.* **2014**, *17*, 201–209. [CrossRef]
108. Kyere-Davies, G.; Agyare, C.; Boakye, Y.D.; Suzuki, B.M.; Caffrey, C.R. Effect of Phenotypic Screening of Extracts and Fractions of Erythrophleum ivorense Leaf and Stem Bark on Immature and Adult Stages of Schistosoma mansoni. *J. Parasitol. Res.* **2018**, *2018*, 1–7. [CrossRef]

Tropical Medicine and Infectious Disease

MDPI

Concept Paper

A Call for Systems Epidemiology to Tackle the Complexity of Schistosomiasis, Its Control, and Its Elimination

Stefanie J. Krauth [1,*], Julie Balen [2], Geoffrey N. Gobert [3] and Poppy H. L. Lamberton [1,4,*]

1. Institute for Biodiversity, Animal Health and Comparative Medicine, University of Glasgow, Glasgow G12 8QQ, UK
2. School of Health and Related Research, University of Sheffield, Sheffield S1 4DA, UK; j.balen@sheffield.ac.uk
3. School of Biological Sciences, Queen's University Belfast, Belfast BT9 7BL, UK; G.Gobert@qub.ac.uk
4. Wellcome Centre for Molecular Parasitology, University of Glasgow, Glasgow G12 8QQ, UK

* Correspondence: Stefanie.Krauth@glasgow.ac.uk (S.J.K.); Poppy.Lamberton@glasgow.ac.uk (P.H.L.L.)

Received: 18 October 2018; Accepted: 24 January 2019; Published: 29 January 2019

Abstract: Ever since the first known written report of schistosomiasis in the mid-19th century, researchers have aimed to increase knowledge of the parasites, their hosts, and the mechanisms contributing to infection and disease. This knowledge generation has been paramount for the development of improved intervention strategies. Yet, despite a broad knowledge base of direct risk factors for schistosomiasis, there remains a paucity of information related to more complex, interconnected, and often hidden drivers of transmission that hamper intervention successes and sustainability. Such complex, multidirectional, non-linear, and synergistic interdependencies are best understood by looking at the integrated system as a whole. A research approach able to address this complexity and find previously neglected causal mechanisms for transmission, which include a wide variety of influencing factors, is needed. Systems epidemiology, as a holistic research approach, can integrate knowledge from classical epidemiology, with that of biology, ecology, social sciences, and other disciplines, and link this with informal, tacit knowledge from experts and affected populations. It can help to uncover wider-reaching but difficult-to-identify processes that directly or indirectly influence exposure, infection, transmission, and disease development, as well as how these interrelate and impact one another. Drawing on systems epidemiology to address persisting disease hotspots, failed intervention programmes, and systematically neglected population groups in mass drug administration programmes and research studies, can help overcome barriers in the progress towards schistosomiasis elimination. Generating a comprehensive view of the schistosomiasis system as a whole should thus be a priority research agenda towards the strategic goal of morbidity control and transmission elimination.

Keywords: schistosomiasis; systems epidemiology; systems thinking; complexity; neglected tropical diseases; interdisciplinarity

---

1. A Brief History of the Discovery, Research, and Control of Schistosomiasis

The parasites now classified as *Schistosoma* spp. were first described in 1851 in Egypt by Theodor Bilharz [1]. Within a year, the involvement of these pathogens in the then-termed "endemic haematuria of warm climates" and the "dysenterische Veränderung des Dickdarms" (dysenteric pathology of the colon) became evident [1,2]. With estimated local prevalence ranging from 50–90% [3,4], and deaths from infections not uncommon, the disease initially named Bilharzia was recognised as a serious public health concern [3,4]. The parasite Bilharz first described as *Distomum haematobium* [1] was later renamed *Bilharzia haematobium* [3] and finally re-classified as *Schistosoma haematobium* [5].

Ever since Bilharz's description, researchers have worked to understand the parasite's developmental biology and identify strategies to help prevent infection, interrupt transmission, and reduce disease burden worldwide.

Bilharzia parasites were described in 1882 as "without question, the most dangerous [of human] parasite[s]" [3]. It was argued that, although other, more serious parasites existed, these were less common and therefore schistosomiasis should be considered the "schlimmerer Feind der Menschheit" ("worse enemy of humankind") [4]. Attempts to control the disease were rolled out soon after its discovery and efforts have increased over the last two decades [6]. For example, one of the first schistosomiasis health education interventions was implemented in 1882. After recognising that infection takes place at water points, a printed memorandum was sent to employees of the British Eastern Telegraph company stationed in Egypt, and later made public [3]. In seeking to prevent human infection, a comprehensive understanding of the life cycle and mode of infection became important research priorities. Observations and experiments in the late 19th century led to hypotheses on how the parasite enters the human body, a point of biology debated in the literature of the time [3,4,7,8]. The most popular theory at the time suggested that ingestion of unclean water was the mode of infection [3,4], but skin penetration was also hypothesised early on and, although at first discounted, led to the policy of forbidding people to bathe in open waters [7,8]. Concurrently, efforts searching for an insect or mollusc intermediate host were ongoing due to analogies drawn from *Distoma* species [4].

Much progress has been made in the understanding of schistosomiasis since these early days. The biology of the parasites is now well described, intermediate host snails identified, and an effective antischistosomal drug—praziquantel—was developed in the 1970s, capable of treating infections caused by all species [9–13]. Nevertheless, Fritsch's 1887 quote, "Even when we understand the life history [of Bilharzia] completely, we might not be able to sufficiently protect ourselves against this malicious foe" (translated from German) [4], remains true today, with over 200 million people still infected and over half of those demonstrating detectable symptoms [14].

Current international strategic goals, as outlined by the World Health Organisation (WHO), aim for morbidity control, and once this is reached for the elimination of schistosomiasis as a public health problem "where appropriate" by 2020 [6,15,16]. With such ambitious goals, it is important to consider how severe historical levels of schistosomiasis once were. If existing interventions were to be discontinued, interrupted, or otherwise unsuccessful, schistosomiasis prevalence, intensity, and associated morbidity could be at risk of returning to former historical levels [17,18].

Despite major research advances, many aspects of the biological, ecological, socio-cultural, economic, and political drivers of schistosomiasis are yet to be elucidated. To identify improved control measures, reduce disease transmission, and achieve elimination in the future, it is key to understand which factors and/or processes directly and indirectly influence exposure, infection, transmission, and disease development, as well as how these are interrelated. One priority area for research should therefore be to better understand, and engage with, the schistosomiasis "system" as a whole.

2. Systems Epidemiology: Systems Thinking for Epidemiology

To overcome current shortcomings of control efforts and move towards schistosomiasis elimination, there is a need to improve intervention strategies. It is well understood that health and disease are affected by multiple, diverse, and complex influences ranging from host immunology and parasite biology through to exposure, social environment, ecology, climate, and access to preventative and curative services [19–23]. Control strategies need to be designed around an improved understanding of the comprehensive range of broader factors influencing disease transmission and intervention successes. Their complex interrelationships, emergent properties, and non-linear feedback-loops all need to be considered. Such interdependencies in a system cannot be identified by considering each of the factors individually. These relationships are best understood by looking at the system as a whole [20,23,24]. Traditional epidemiological approaches, largely reductionist in nature, deal with a limited number of directly related factors, narrowing down causal mechanisms to smaller components that enable us to draw generalisable conclusions [25,26]. This approach has been paramount to uncover many risk factors of *Schistosoma* transmission. However, the direct and indirect interrelated causal mechanisms of the disease are hard to integrate using standard epidemiological approaches. In contrast to reductionist approaches, systems sciences address system-wide behaviours and collective effects. In systems thinking, a system is understood as consisting of many components that, through their interactions with each other, form a complex whole with system-wide properties that can give rise to emergent behaviour, adaptations, and feedback loops [27].

The application of general systems thinking to epidemiology and health research as a tool to integrate knowledge from different areas of research has long been proposed for several diseases [19,28–30]. However, to our knowledge this is the first time it has been proposed specifically for schistosomiasis or any neglected tropical disease (NTD). Systems thinking has well-defined advantages over reductionist approaches. A good example of a health issue of which we now have a system-wide understanding is obesity [24,28,29]. A system influence diagram created by Shiftn (2008) illustrates the complex interrelationships of multiple factors influencing obesity [28]. Such "influence models" can be used to formulate appropriate research hypotheses and address the multiple factors across levels of influence and across disciplines [23,26,29]. With influence diagrams, the whole-disease system can be effectively visualised and analysed for underlying causal mechanisms driving changes in infections and intervention successes/failures. This type of analysis can provide the starting point for more in-depth studies on the dynamics of human–parasite systems as well as for more contextually-relevant intervention/implementation research. Co-creating and discussing influence diagrams can, in turn, enhance stakeholders' understanding of underlying behaviours of a specific system [24].

In their thematic series, "Advancing the application of systems thinking in health" Adam (2014) and colleagues discussed how the application of various systems methods has helped authors uncover reasons for poor health outcomes, such as systems-wide impacts on neonatal health in Uganda and has gone on to identify high leverage points [30]. Other authors linked a range of factors including government opposition, alternative medicine, and strong media coverage to changes in vaccination rates [31]. Adam (2014) emphasised the importance of including evidence beyond traditional epidemiology and economic analysis into the design and evaluation of public health interventions and discussed the usefulness of visual representations for the analysis and interpretation of a system [30]. We build on these ideas by proposing the integration of systems science tools and systems modelling into the field of epidemiology for schistosomiasis and other NTDs. This approach, described as "systems epidemiology", will more effectively integrate knowledge to better understand and control schistosomiasis, as well as focus on contextually relevant factors.

The central goal of a systems epidemiologist would be to uncover principles governing the behaviour and outputs of the entire system, not limited to the behaviour of its individual parts. Working together in a trans-disciplinary manner, researchers, policymakers, health providers, and the affected population could generate much-needed insights into the drivers of persisting *Schistosoma* transmission.

3. Systems Epidemiology as Described in Broader Existing Literatures

Systems epidemiology has, to the best of our knowledge, not yet been applied in the form we propose here. However, the term has been used several times in recent publications across a range of scopes and other topics [19,32–34]. In the majority of these studies, systems epidemiology refers to integrating systems biology tools, such as high-throughput molecular analysis of biomarkers, with epidemiological research questions. For example, the integration of genomics, transcriptomics, proteomics, and metabolomics with epidemiological research was conducted to clarify underlying mechanisms of the effects of food on human health [32]. In addition, a multi-omic approach was employed to understand human pathophysiology in cardiovascular disease and cancer [33,34]. Including multi-omic measurements to analyse complex biological data is an important strategy to uncover the exact mechanisms involved in exposure through to disease development. However, systems biology comprises only the micro-system that influences disease development; i.e., mechanisms only taking place after host exposure to the parasite. In contrast, systems epidemiology can be defined in a wider context, whereby mechanisms related to environmental, social, and demographic aspects of disease are needed to complement the systems biology data, as previously proposed for the control of tuberculosis [19].

We therefore argue that systems epidemiology needs to move beyond the application of systems biology, towards a more holistic understanding of health. Systems epidemiology should combine classical epidemiology with social sciences, natural sciences (including systems biology), ecology, economics, health policy and systems research, and other relevant disciplines and sub-disciplines. This would more effectively characterise the relevant physical and socio-political environments of endemic regions, and access (or lack of) to relevant services, as well as the biology and the co-evolution of the hosts and the pathogen. We argue that applying a systems epidemiology approach to schistosomiasis research is imperative for assessing factors that contribute to persistent disease hotspots, failed intervention programmes, and systematically missed population groups in mass drug administration (MDA) campaigns and/or research studies. Findings from such an approach, we believe, can help overcome current barriers in the progress towards schistosomiasis elimination.

4. The Call for Systems Epidemiology Approaches in Schistosomiasis Control

Over the last two decades, the global agendas outlined in the Millennium and Sustainable Development Goals (MDGs and SDGs, respectively) have raised the profile of schistosomiasis and other poverty-related diseases which had, in the post-colonial era, received reduced attention by international and national governmental agencies [35]. The WHO recommends repeated MDA with praziquantel to reduce schistosomiasis intensity and associated morbidity [14]. In certain areas where the elimination of schistosomiasis as a public health problem, or the interruption of schistosomiasis transmission, are deemed possible, the WHO recommends MDA plus complementary public health interventions [14]. MDA reduces the number of *Schistosoma* eggs released into the environment, thus reducing human to snail transmission and potentially lowering transmission back into humans [14,36,37]. MDA campaigns have made substantial reductions in morbidity rates and have improved public health overall [37]. These successes sparked an increased push towards disease elimination [6,15,16]. However, MDA success varies considerably, with greater reductions in infection intensities and prevalence in areas which were initially classified as low endemicity (<10% of school-aged children infected), but with often disappointing effects in many moderate and high endemicity areas [21,38]. Despite increased funding, extensive praziquantel donations and national control programmes running for over a decade in several countries, hotspots of high transmission and severe morbidity remain [21,38,39].

While the benefits of MDA to schistosomiasis morbidity reductions are well established, it is now evident that MDA alone is unlikely to achieve elimination [21,36,37,40,41]. Many authors have discussed reasons for MDA programme failures, including treatment compliance, inadequate coverage, treatment efficacy, open defecation/urination behaviours, water contact behaviours, snail density, available infrastructure, and many more [21,36,40,42–47]. Because schistosomiasis is so deeply embedded in broader physical, social, political, and economic systems, the factors influencing intervention successes (or failures) also span these systems [40,42,45]. Several integrated control measures have been proposed to overcome currently identified shortcomings of MDA-only strategies. These propose the inclusion of health education, agricultural policy interventions, sanitation improvements, water supply improvements, engineering interventions, snail control, and behavioural interventions, etc. [48–53]. Extending control measures in this way aims to target both the transmission of schistosomiasis from snails to humans and from humans to snails. Most of these measures aim to increase treatment compliance, provide physical barriers around urine or faeces, and/or decrease snail density. The proposed measures in these studies are based on factors known to contribute to transmission and disease burden. However, a comprehensive summary of all prevailing factors influencing the disease and its transmission in specific settings, and how changing one aspect impacts another aspect as well as the overall system, has, to date, not been generated. Due to the complexity of the issues, it is unfeasible to identify, measure, and include all factors in a single study and researchers often need to focus on a subset of relevant factors that are measurable and feasible for analysis. A research approach and associated toolkit able to deal with this complexity, including a variety of influencing factors, is urgently needed if WHO goals are to be met.

5. How to Apply Systems Epidemiology Approaches to Schistosomiasis Control

To exemplify the complexity of the schistosomiasis system, Figures 1 and 2 illustrate a preliminary interrelationship diagram of empirically tested or hypothesised interactions from a large body of literature and expert knowledge. These figures represent a first "brainstormed" draft of the broader interaction network for schistosomiasis that could be created using systems epidemiology tools. Detailing the complete nature and direction of these interactions would take considerable future research. Nevertheless, already from this crude diagram, interesting observations emerge. For example, factors from the social environment are especially well-connected to other factors in the system (Figure 3). While social environment factors rarely directly interact with infection mechanisms, they are connected with other factors which, in turn, influence exposure and/or treatment coverage and thereby infection rates of a community. These factors affect, e.g., the likelihood of having high-risk water contact, access to treatment, and treatment compliance—which are all well-documented MDA programmatic issues [21,47,54]. Social environment factors vary between communities and settings, since social and cultural norms vary between groups [55–57]. Additionally, social environment factors are not easily quantifiable and often need qualitative research approaches to elucidate them. However qualitative research remains neglected and still occasionally overlooked or misunderstood. This is perhaps best exemplified in the 2016 systematic review on treatment compliance in NTD control programmes, in which qualitative findings were discussed in half a sentence noting: "Other studies provided only qualitative or anecdotal data or reasons for low or non-compliance" [47]. Qualitative research is especially valuable and urgently needed when assessing treatment uptake in order to find missing factors to explain low compliance. Complete whole-system diagrams could further be compared with other, more commonly used methods, such as Bayesian networks [58], to compare combined qualitative and quantitative approaches.

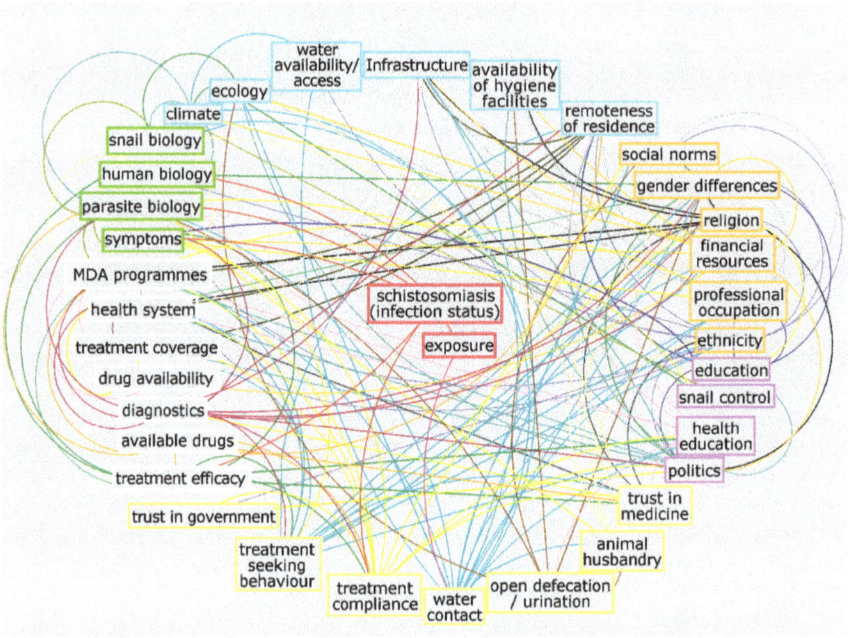

Figure 1. Potential network of factors influencing schistosomiasis infection and disease created with Vensim [59] and GIMP [60]. Connections are a collection of empirically tested or hypothesised relationships. Colours are for illustrative purposes only. This diagram resulted from ongoing brainstorming of connections from a large body of literature and expert knowledge. The diagram aims to exemplify the complexity of the schistosomiasis system without claims of completeness and without detailing the exact nature and direction of interactions. It is meant solely for the purpose of an example of what a systems diagram for schistosomiasis could provide. The full diagram(s) would need to be developed through extensive empirical and theoretical research.

Understanding schistosomiasis control as a systems issue requires a strong interdisciplinary and transdisciplinary approach. Strategies are needed to enable researchers and programme managers to adequately assess and integrate issues across disciplines and in different settings. Creating an empirically based system for understanding interrelationships between relevant issues in schistosomiasis transmission and intervention successes/failures is needed. A comprehensive interrelationship diagram, detailing the nature and direction of the system-wide connections would need to be based on the integration of published knowledge from researchers, with informal knowledge from experts and local populations. Methods to collect and analyse data would include repeated modelling sessions and participatory workshops with stakeholders from a range of backgrounds. This would be the first step towards establishing a systems epidemiology research approach for the control and elimination of schistosomiasis and other NTDs.

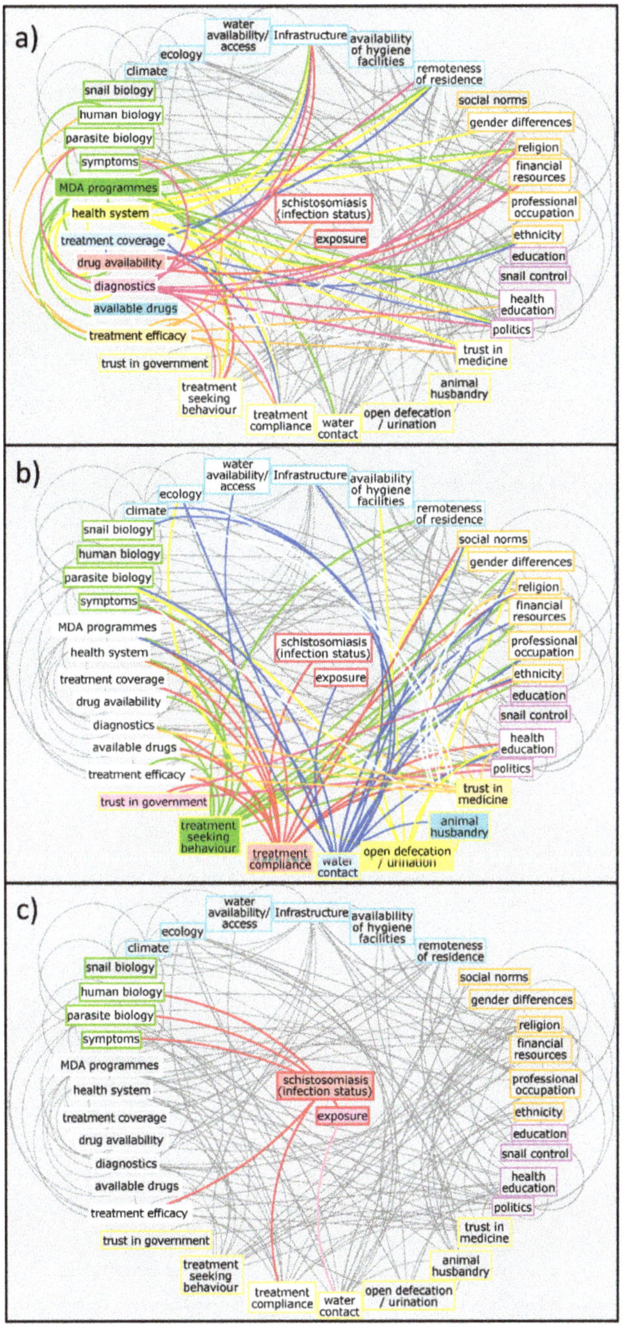

Figure 2. Potential network of factors influencing schistosomiasis infection and disease with individual connections highlighted for (**a**) clinical, (**b**) behavioural, and (**c**) exposure and infection aspects. Colours are for illustrative purposes only; white boxes indicate where the highlighted variables connect to. Different clusters are highlighted by coloured outlines: green: biological aspects; white: clinical aspects; yellow: behavioural aspects; orange: social aspects; purple: politics, policy, and services aspects; turquoise: physical environment; red: exposure and infection.

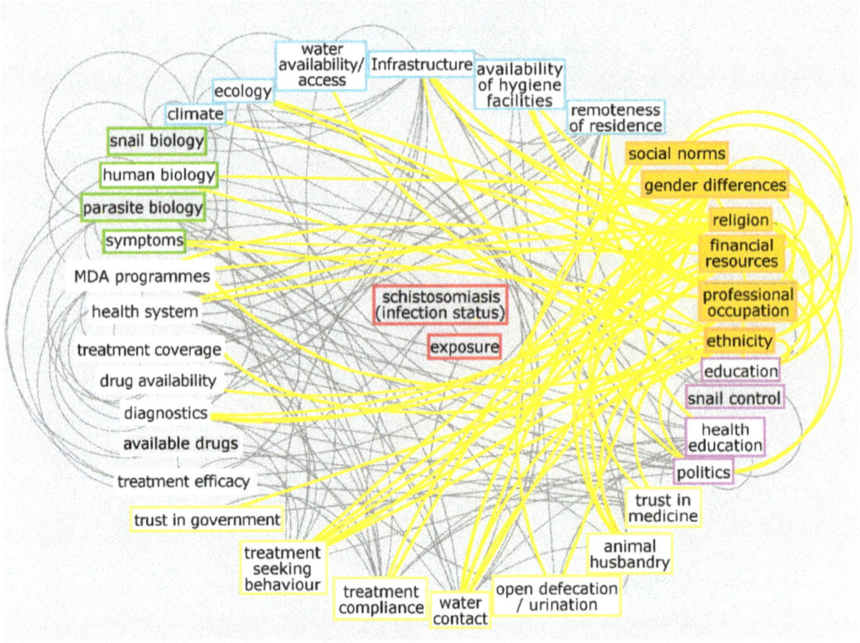

Figure 3. Interconnectedness of social factors with other aspects of the schistosomiasis. White boxes indicate where the highlighted variables connect to. Social aspects illustrated: social norms, gender differences, religion, financial resources, professional occupation, and ethnicity. Although they do not interact directly with infection status or exposure, social aspects underlie and influence many other factors that are, in turn, connected to exposure and infection.

6. Conclusions

Understanding the broader systems-relations and influences of a disease, as well as how best to address these factors with limited resources, is an important challenge. The overall goal is to establish sustainable, contextually relevant, and cost-effective approaches to tackle persistent hotspots of disease transmission. Moving beyond current research and implementation practice, towards complex system analyses and interventions for a disease such as schistosomiasis will help research and policy communities identify how best to achieve WHO goals along the road to elimination. Using a systems thinking toolset, we can connect and integrate knowledge from across a range of disciplines including classical epidemiology, molecular parasitology, ecology, medical anthropology, social and political sciences, and health policy and systems research to identify multiple target points for future schistosomiasis control programmes. This would remove or minimise elusive barriers to success, enabling the global health community to move a step closer towards the elimination of schistosomiasis worldwide.

Author Contributions: Conceptualization, S.J.K. and P.H.L.L.; literature review, S.J.K.; writing—original draft preparation, S.J.K.; writing—review and editing, P.H.L., J.B., G.N.G. visualization, S.J.K.

Funding: This research received no external funding. P.H.L.L. is funded by a European Research Council Starting Grant (SCHISTO_PERSIST_680088), a Medical Research Council Global Challenges Research Fund Foundation Award (MR/P025447/1), and an Engineering and Physical Sciences Research Council Global Challenges Research Fund Grant (EP/R01437X/1). J.B. is core-funded by The University of Sheffield, UK.

Acknowledgments: We would like to thank Axel Hochstetter for his help with the extensive figure editing.

Conflicts of Interest: The authors declare no conflict of interest.

References

1. Bilharz, T.; Siebold, C.T.E. Ein beitrag zur helminthographia humana. *Z. Wiss. Zool. Abt. A* **1852**, *4*, 53–76.
2. Bilharz, T. Fernere mittheilungen über *Distomum haematobium*. *Z. Wiss. Zool. Abt. A* **1852**, *4*, 454–456.
3. Cobbold, T.S. Remarks on injurious parasites of Egypt in relation to water-drinking. *Br. Med. J.* **1882**, *2*, 503–504. [CrossRef]
4. Fritsch, G. Zur anatomie der *Bilharzia haematobia* (cobbold). *Arch. Mikrosk. Anat.* **1887**, *31*, 192–223. [CrossRef]
5. Hemming, F. Opinions and declarations rendered by the international commission on zoological nomenclature. Opinion 147. *Bull. Zool. Nomencl.* **1943**, *2*, 123–132.
6. Rollinson, D.; Knopp, S.; Levitz, S.; Stothard, J.R.; Tchuem Tchuente, L.A.; Garba, A.; Mohammed, K.A.; Schur, N.; Person, B.; Colley, D.G.; et al. Time to set the agenda for schistosomiasis elimination. *Acta Trop.* **2013**, *128*, 423–440. [CrossRef] [PubMed]
7. Kartulis, S. Weitere beiträge zur pathologischen anatomie der bilharzia (*Distomum haematobium*, cobbold). *Arch. Pathol. Anat. Physiol. Klin. Med.* **1898**, *152*, 474–486. [CrossRef]
8. Looss, A. Zur anatomie und histologie der *Bilharzia haematobia* (cobbold). *Arch. Mikrosk. Anat.* **1895**, *46*, 1–108. [CrossRef]
9. Gordon, R.M.; Davey, T.H.; Peaston, H. The transmission of human bilharziasis in Sierra Leone, with an account of the life-cycle of the schistosomes concerned, *S. mansoni* and *S. haematobium*. *Ann. Trop. Med. Parasitol.* **1934**, *28*, 323–418. [CrossRef]
10. King, C.H. The evolving schistosomiasis agenda 2007–2017—Why we are moving beyond morbidity control toward elimination of transmission. *PLoS Negl. Trop. Dis.* **2017**, *11*, e0005517. [CrossRef]
11. Lampe, P. The development of *Schistosoma mansoni*. *Proc. R. Soc. Med.* **1927**, *1510*, 56–62.
12. Leiper, R.T.; Atkinson, E.L. Observations on the spread of Asiatic schistosomiasis. *Br. Med. J.* **1915**, *1*, 201–203. [CrossRef]
13. Machemer, L.; Lorke, D. Mutagenicity studies with praziquantel, a new anthelmintic drug, in mammalian systems. *Arch. Toxicol.* **1978**, *39*, 187–197. [CrossRef] [PubMed]
14. World Health Organization. *Schistosomiasis, W. Progress Report 2001–2011 and Strategic Plan 2012–2020*; World Health Organization: Geneva, Switzerland, 2013.
15. World Health Organization. *Elimination of Schistosomiasis. 65th World Health Assembly, Resolution WHA65*; World Health Organization: Geneva, Switzerland, 2012.
16. Toor, J.; Alsallaq, R.; Truscott, J.E.; Turner, H.C.; Werkman, M.; Gurarie, D.; King, C.H.; Anderson, R.M. Are we on our way to achieving the 2020 goals for schistosomiasis morbidity control using current world health organization guidelines? *Clin. Infect. Dis.* **2018**, *66*, S245–S252.
17. Gurarie, D.; Yoon, N.; Li, E.; Ndeffo-Mbah, M.; Durham, D.; Phillips, A.E.; Aurelio, H.O.; Ferro, J.; Galvani, A.P.; King, C.H. Modelling control of Schistosoma haematobium infection: Predictions of the long-term impact of mass drug administration in Africa. *Parasites Vectors* **2015**, *8*, 529. [CrossRef]
18. Mitchell, K.M.; Mutapi, F.; Mduluza, T.; Midzi, N.; Savill, N.J.; Woolhouse, M.E.J. Predicted impact of mass drug administration on the development of protective immunity against *Schistosoma haematobium*. *PLoS Negl. Tropl. Dis.* **2014**, *8*, e3059. [CrossRef]
19. Comas, I.; Gagneux, S. The past and future of tuberculosis research. *PLoS Pathog.* **2009**, *5*, e1000600. [CrossRef]
20. El-Sayed, A.M.; Galea, S. *Systems Science and Population Health*; Oxford University Press: Oxford, UK, 2017.
21. Kittur, N.; Binder, S.; Campbell, C.H.; King, C.H.; Kinung'hi, S.; Olsen, A.; Magnussen, P.; Colley, D.G. Defining persistent hotspots: Areas that fail to decrease meaningfully in prevalence after multiple years of mass drug administration with praziquantel for control of schistosomiasis. *Am. J. Trop. Med. Hyg.* **2017**, *97*, 1810–1817. [CrossRef]
22. Nithiuthai, S.; Anantaphruti, M.T.; Waikagul, J.; Gajadhar, A. Waterborne zoonotic helminthiases. *Vet. Parasitol.* **2004**, *126*, 167–193. [CrossRef]
23. Sturmberg, J.P. *The Value of Systems and Complexity Sciences for Healthcare*; Springer Publishing: Berlin, Germany, 2016.
24. Newell, B.; Proust, K.; Dyball, R.; McManus, P. Seeing obesity as a systems problem. *N. S. W. Public Health Bull.* **2008**, *18*, 214–218. [CrossRef]

25. Epstein, P.R.; Ferber, D. *Changing Planet, Changing Health: How the Climate Crisis Threatens Our Health and What We Can Do about It*; University of California Press: Berkeley, CA, USA, 2011.
26. Joffe, M.; Gambhir, M.; Chadeau-Hyam, M.; Vineis, P. Causal diagrams in systems epidemiology. *Emerg. Themes Epidemiol.* **2012**, *9*, 1. [CrossRef] [PubMed]
27. Bar-Yam, Y. *General Features of Complex Systems*; Encyclopedia of Life Support Systems (EOLSS), UNESCO, EOLSS Publishers: Oxford, UK, 2002.
28. Shift cvba. Shift Obesity System Influence Diagram. Available online: http://www.shiftn.com/obesity/Full-Map.html (accessed on 6 December 2018).
29. Huang, T.T.; Drewnowski, A.; Kumanyika, S.K.; Glass, T.A. A systems-oriented multilevel framework for addressing obesity in the 21st century. *Prev. Chronic Dis.* **2009**, *6*, A82. [PubMed]
30. Adam, T. Advancing the application of systems thinking in health. *Health Res. Policy Syst.* **2014**, *12*, 50. [CrossRef] [PubMed]
31. Varghese, J.; Kutty, V.R.; Paina, L.; Adam, T. Advancing the application of systems thinking in health: Understanding the growing complexity governing immunization services in Kerala, India. *Health Res. Policy Syst.* **2014**, *12*, 47. [CrossRef]
32. Cornelis, M.C.; Hu, F.B. Systems epidemiology: A new direction in nutrition and metabolic disease research. *Curr. Nutr. Rep.* **2013**, *2*, 225–235. [CrossRef] [PubMed]
33. Haring, R.; Wallaschofski, H. Diving through the "-omics": The case for deep phenotyping and systems epidemiology. *OMICS* **2012**, *16*, 231–234. [CrossRef] [PubMed]
34. Lund, E.; Dumeaux, V. Systems epidemiology in cancer. *Cancer Epidemiol. Biomarkers Prev.* **2008**, *17*, 2954–2957. [CrossRef]
35. Israelian, N. A brief history of neglected tropical diseases. *Immpress Magazine*, 17 October 2016. Available online: http://www.immpressmagazine.com/a-brief-history-of-neglected-tropical-diseases/ (accessed on 6 December 2018).
36. Gurarie, D.; Lo, N.C.; Ndeffo-Mbah, M.L.; Durham, D.P.; King, C.H. The human-snail transmission environment shapes long term schistosomiasis control outcomes: Implications for improving the accuracy of predictive modeling. *PLoS Negl. Trop. Dis.* **2018**, *12*, e0006514. [CrossRef]
37. Webster, J.P.; Molyneux, D.H.; Hotez, P.J.; Fenwick, A. The contribution of mass drug administration to global health: Past, present and future. *Philos. Trans. R. Soc. Lond. Ser. B Biol. Sci.* **2014**, *369*, 20130434. [CrossRef]
38. Crellen, T.; Walker, M.; Lamberton, P.H.L.; Kabatereine, N.B.; Tukahebwa, E.M.; Cotton, J.A.; Webster, J.P. Reduced efficacy of praziquantel against *Schistosoma mansoni* is associated with multiple rounds of mass drug administration. *Clin. Infect. Dis.* **2016**, *63*, 1151–1159.
39. Lo, N.C.; Addiss, D.G.; Hotez, P.J.; King, C.H.; Stothard, J.R.; Evans, D.S.; Colley, D.G.; Lin, W.; Coulibaly, J.T.; Bustinduy, A.L.; et al. A call to strengthen the global strategy against schistosomiasis and soil-transmitted helminthiasis: The time is now. *Lancet Infect. Dis.* **2017**, *17*, E64–E69. [CrossRef]
40. Allen, T.; Parker, M. Deworming delusions? Mass drug administration in east African schools. *J. Biosoc. Sci.* **2016**, *48* (Suppl. 1), S116–S147. [CrossRef] [PubMed]
41. Sokolow, S.H.; Wood, C.L.; Jones, I.J.; Swartz, S.J.; Lopez, M.; Hsieh, M.H.; Lafferty, K.D.; Kuris, A.M.; Rickards, C.; De Leo, G.A. Global assessment of schistosomiasis control over the past century shows targeting the snail intermediate host works best. *PLoS Negl. Trop. Dis.* **2016**, *10*, e0004794. [CrossRef] [PubMed]
42. Chami, G.F.; Kontoleon, A.A.; Bulte, E.; Fenwick, A.; Kabatereine, N.B.; Tukahebwa, E.M.; Dunne, D.W. Profiling nonrecipients of mass drug administration for schistosomiasis and hookworm infections: A comprehensive analysis of praziquantel and albendazole coverage in community-directed treatment in Uganda. *Clin. Infect. Dis.* **2016**, *62*, 200–207. [CrossRef] [PubMed]
43. Dyson, L.; Stolk, W.A.; Farrell, S.H.; Hollingsworth, T.D. Measuring and modelling the effects of systematic non-adherence to mass drug administration. *Epidemics* **2017**, *18*, 56–66. [CrossRef]
44. Hastings, J. Rumours, riots and the rejection of mass drug administration for the treatment of schistosomiasis in Morogoro, Tanzania. *J. Biosoc. Sci.* **2016**, *48*, S16–S39. [CrossRef] [PubMed]
45. Person, B.; Knopp, S.; Ali, S.M.; A'Kadir, F.M.; Khamis, A.N.; Ali, J.N.; Lymo, J.H.; Mohammed, K.A.; Rollinson, D. Community co-designed schistosomiasis control interventions for school-aged children in Zanzibar. *J. Biosoc. Sci.* **2016**, *48* (Suppl. 1), S56–S73. [CrossRef] [PubMed]

46. Riccardi, N.; Nosenzo, F.; Peraldo, F.; Sarocchi, F.; Taramasso, L.; Traverso, P.; Viscoli, C.; Di Biagio, A.; Derchi, L.E.; De Maria, A. Increasing prevalence of genitourinary schistosomiasis in Europe in the migrant era: Neglected no more? *PLoS Negl. Trop. Dis.* **2017**, *11*, e0005237. [CrossRef]
47. Shuford, K.V.; Turner, H.C.; Anderson, R.M. Compliance with anthelmintic treatment in the neglected tropical diseases control programmes: A systematic review. *Parasites Vectors.* **2016**, *9*, 29. [CrossRef]
48. Knopp, S.; Mohammed, K.A.; Ali, S.M.; Khamis, I.S.; Ame, S.M.; Albonico, M.; Gouvras, A.; Fenwick, A.; Savioli, L.; Colley, D.G.; et al. Study and implementation of urogenital schistosomiasis elimination in Zanzibar (Unguja and Pemba islands) using an integrated multidisciplinary approach. *BMC Public Health* **2012**, *12*, 930. [CrossRef]
49. Lee, Y.H.; Jeong, H.G.; Kong, W.H.; Lee, S.H.; Cho, H.I.; Nam, H.S.; Ismail, H.A.H.A.; Alla, G.N.A.; Oh, C.H.; Hong, S.T. Reduction of urogenital schistosomiasis with an integrated control project in Sudan. *PLoS Negl. Trop. Dis.* **2015**, *9*, e3423. [CrossRef] [PubMed]
50. Raso, G.; Esse, C.; Dongo, K.; Ouattara, M.; Zouzou, F.; Hurlimann, E.; Koffi, V.A.; Coulibaly, G.; Mahan, V.; Yapi, R.B.; et al. An integrated approach to control soil-transmitted helminthiasis, schistosomiasis, intestinal protozoa infection, and diarrhea: Protocol for a cluster randomized trial. *JMIR Res. Protoc.* **2018**, *7*, e145. [CrossRef] [PubMed]
51. Tian-Bi, Y.N.T.; Ouattara, M.; Knopp, S.; Coulibaly, J.T.; Hurlimann, E.; Webster, B.; Allan, F.; Rollinson, D.; Meite, A.; Diakite, N.R.; et al. Interrupting seasonal transmission of *Schistosoma haematobium* and control of soil-transmitted helminthiasis in northern and central Côte d'Ivoire: A score study protocol. *BMC Public Health* **2018**, *18*, 186. [CrossRef] [PubMed]
52. Xu, J.; Xu, J.F.; Li, S.Z.; Zhang, L.J.; Wang, Q.; Zhu, H.H.; Zhou, X.N. Integrated control programmes for schistosomiasis and other helminth infections in P.R. China. *Acta Trop.* **2015**, *141*, 332–341. [CrossRef] [PubMed]
53. Yang, Y.; Zhou, Y.B.; Song, X.X.; Li, S.Z.; Zhong, B.; Wang, T.P.; Bergquist, R.; Zhou, X.N.; Jiang, Q.W. Integrated control strategy of schistosomiasis in the People's Republic of China: Projects involving agriculture, water conservancy, forestry, sanitation and environmental modification. *Adv. Parasitol.* **2016**, *92*, 237–268. [PubMed]
54. Ross, A.G.P.; Chau, T.N.; Inobaya, M.T.; Olveda, R.M.; Li, Y.S.; Harn, D.A. A new global strategy for the elimination of schistosomiasis. *Int. J. Infect. Dis.* **2017**, *54*, 130–137. [CrossRef]
55. Henrich, J.; Boyd, R. The evolution of conformist transmission and the emergence of between-group differences. *Evol. Hum. Behav.* **1998**, *19*, 215–241. [CrossRef]
56. Schultz, P.W.; Nolan, J.M.; Cialdini, R.B.; Goldstein, N.J.; Griskevicius, V. The constructive, destructive, and reconstructive power of social norms. *Psychol. Sci.* **2007**, *18*, 429–434. [CrossRef] [PubMed]
57. Sherif, M. *The Psychology of Social Norms*; Harper and Brothers Publishing: New York, NY, USA, 1936.
58. Ghahramani, Z. Learning dynamic Bayesian networks. In *Adaptive Processing of Sequences and DATA Structures*; Giles, C.L., Gori, M., Eds.; Springer: New York, NY, USA, 1998; pp. 168–197.
59. Ventana Systems Inc. *Vensim*; Ventana Systems Inc.: Harvard, MA, USA, 2015.
60. GIMP.org. Available online: https://www.gimp.org/ (accessed on 29 January 2019).

Tropical Medicine and Infectious Disease

MDPI

Opinion

Schistosomiasis in the Philippines: Innovative Control Approach is Needed if Elimination is the Goal

Remigio M. Olveda [1,*] and Darren J. Gray [2]

[1] Research Institute for Tropical Medicine, Manila 1781, Philippines
[2] Research School of Population Health, Australian National University, Canberra 2601, Australia; darren.gray@anu.edu.au
* Correspondence: rolvedamd_ritm_doh@yahoo.com; Tel.: +632-772-2975

Received: 8 January 2019; Accepted: 4 April 2019; Published: 13 April 2019

Abstract: In 1996, schistosomiasis due to *Schistosoma japonicum* was declared eradicated in Japan. In the People's Republic of China, *S. japonicum* transmission has been interrupted in the major endemic areas in the coastal plains but the disease persists in the lake and marshland regions south of the Yangtze River. The disease remains a public health problem in endemic areas in the Philippines and in isolated areas in Indonesia. Comprehensive multidisciplinary campaigns had led to eradication of schistosomiasis in Japan and have been successful in the interruption of disease transmission in the major endemic regions of the People's Republic of China. Unfortunately, the integrated measures cannot be duplicated in schistosomiasis endemic areas in the Philippines because of limited resources. The problem is also more complicated due to the topography in the Philippines and transmission is not seasonal as in China. An innovative approach is needed in the Philippines if schistosomiasis elimination is the goal.

Keywords: Schistosomiasis; Philippines; schistosomiasis elimination; *S. japonicum* zoonosis; bovines

1. Endemic Areas and Transmission of *Schistosoma japonicum* in the Philippines

Schistosomiasis remains a public health problem in endemic areas in the Philippines with approximately 12 million people residing in 28 endemic provinces located across 12 different geographical zones at risk of *S. japonicum* infection [1–5]. A total of 190 municipalities and 1212 barangays (villages) are currently endemic, based on surveys conducted over the past decade. Two new endemic foci reported in the northern (Gonzaga, Cagayan) and central (Calatrava, Negros Occidental) parts of the country were confirmed in 2004 and 2006, respectively [6]. Just like in China, bovines, water buffaloes (carabaos) in particular, play a major role in the transmission of schistosomiasis in the Philippines with infection prevalence close to 90% in some endemic barrangays. A 2011 study carried out in the municipality of Palapag, Northern Samar showed the *S. japonicum* prevalence in cattle to be 87.5% and 77.1% via real-time PCR (qPCR) and the formalin-ethyl acetate sedimentation (FEA-SD), respectively. In carabao, the *S. japonicum* prevalence was 79.1% and 55.2% by qCPR and FEA-SD, respectively [7]. The same study computed the Bovine Contamination Index (BCI) using the FEA-SD technique and gave an average of 195,000 eggs per bovine per day [7]. A recent study in Leyte Province showed a 97% prevalence via perfusion, 67.7% via qPCR and 34.3% by FEA-SD [8].

2. Effect of Long-term Infection with *Schistosoma japonicum*

Prolonged and repeated infection with *S. japonicum* cause two types of morbidities in schistosomiasis japonica: those with clear end-organ complications and those with subtle manifestations. Clear end-organ complications are due to granuloma and fibrosis formed around the parasite eggs trapped in the host tissues. The sequelae can be categorized into hepatosplenic, hepatointestinal, pulmonary, cerebral, and ectopic forms [9,10] Cardiac and renal localization of lesions are rarely encountered. Those with subtle manifestations are due to inflammatory cytokines induced by eggs or worm products of the parasite. Anaemia, growth retardation, malnutrition and impaired cognitive functions have been documented in children with *S. japonicum* infection [11–14]. Maternal schistosomiasis japonica has been shown to exert a negative impact on pregnancy outcomes. Babies born from mothers infected with *S. japonicum* have markedly decreased birth weight. Circulating mediators of inflammation are elevated in the peripheral blood, placental blood, and placental tissues of *S. japonicum* infected pregnant women. Placental TFN-α has also been associated with both *S. japonicum* infection and markedly decreased birth weight [15]. *S. japonicum* infection in pregnant women also result in up-regulation of fibrosis-associated proteins in the cord blood of the neonate. These fibrosis-associated molecules are associated with adverse birth outcomes such as low birth weight (LBW), small for gestational age and prematurity [16]. In addition, endotoxin levels in both maternal and placental compartments in pregnant women with schistosomiasis are 1.3- and 2.4-folds higher, respectively, compared to uninfected women. This higher concentration of endotoxin in placental blood is associated with preterm birth, acute chorioamnionitis, and elevated proinflammatory cytokines [17].

3. Control of Schistosomiasis in the Philippines

In the 1980s, when the highly effective anti-schistosome drug praziquantel (PZQ) was introduced in the Philippines, the schistosomiasis control program rolled out a large-scale community-based chemotherapy approach to eliminate the risk of parasite-associated morbidity – this approach became the backbone of schistosomiasis control in the Philippines [18]. Other control measures to prevent transmission from snail intermediate hosts to humans like health education, behavioural modification, improved sanitation and snail control were continued but not sustained and only on a limited scale. After more than three decades of community-based chemotherapy with PZQ, challenges with this approach have surfaced [18]. Extensive community-based campaigns including mass drug administration (MDA) in the last 10 years has reduced the parasite-associated clinically apparent morbidities, although the hepato-splenic form of schistosomiasis japonica persists in hard to reach endemic zones. Subtle or subclinical morbidities like growth retardation and anaemia in schistosome infected children and poor outcomes of pregnancy in infected women still persist in endemic areas [18,19]. Community-based chemotherapy also failed to interrupt parasite transmission [18,19].

4. Innovative Approach towards Elimination of Schistosomiasis in the Philippines

Despite the limitations of current control measures, it is certain that drug delivery through MDA will be continued for an indefinite period for the control of schistosomiasis in the country. Relaxation of the MDA program or development of parasite resistance to PZQ will result in rebound of schistosome-induced infection and disease [20]. However, while PZQ remains highly effective, additional control measures should be added to augment the community-based chemotherapy control program and move beyond just morbidity control [21]. The next step is elimination of reinfection to prevent all forms of schistosome-induced morbidities. This step will require a comprehensive and more effective phase of disease control and will require incremental expense, but these would ultimately be offset by the greater health benefits achieved with complete elimination of parasite transmission.

Two measures can markedly improve the control program for schistosomiasis in the Philippines. These measures include: (1) Improving delivery or coverage of PZQ to 85% through an intensive MDA program and yearly treatment of 85% of the bovines [22]. Increasing compliance to MDA in humans from less than 50% to 85% is doable. However, yearly treatment of bovines will be very difficult to sustain. (2) MDA (85% coverage) plus removal of water buffaloes (carabaos) from endemic areas and replacing these animals with mechanized tractors. Mechanized farming will prevent exposure of the farmers to the parasite during the tilling of the rice field and planting and harvesting of rice. This approach has proven successful in China where removing buffalos in endemic areas can profoundly reduce the transmission of *S. japonicum* to humans by 75 to >90% [23]. In the

Philippines, recent consultations with the Local Government Unit (LGU) in the Municipality of Javier, a schistosomiasis-endemic area in the Province of Leyte, demonstrated the willingness of the farmers to replace the carabaos with mechanized tractors. In their experience replacing of carabaos by tractors will improve the income of the people in the endemic areas because the cost of labour for rice farming will be markedly reduced and the frequency and volume of rice harvest per year will increase. In addition, they also noted that if they plant hybrid instead of inbred rice the volume of rice recovered per harvest would be significantly increased. Disease transmission from cattle that are also in the endemic areas can be prevented by treating the animals with PZQ—this is would be more sustainable than treating all bovines due to the reduced numbers. This strategy should also include other measures that are doable in the endemic villages like health education and behavioural modification. Recently, mechanization of rice farming is being implemented at pilot scale by a private company in the town of Alang Alang, a schistosomiasis endemic village in the Province of Leyte. In this project it has been demonstrated that the income of farmers can be increased up to ten times compared to their income using the traditional rice farming method [24]. However, the success of this project needs validation in typical endemic areas where resources are limited. It is also important to know by regular monitoring by the Department Health whether the outcome in terms of reduction of *S. japonicum* infection in humans will be significant and sustainable.

Vaccines may also play a crucial role in the elimination of schistosomiasis in the Philippines. No human vaccine is currently available but some veterinary-based transmission blocking vaccines targeting bovines do show some promise and are undergoing field trials [25,26] An alternative elimination strategy would therefore combine human treatment (85% coverage) and treatment of bovines (85% coverage), followed by immunization of these animals with a transmission blocking anti-schistosome vaccine.

5. Conclusions

A multi-component integrated approach towards the control of *S. japonicum* in the Philippines is critical for long-term sustainable control and eventual elimination. Key to such an approach is ensuring high PZQ coverage in endemic populations and the targeting of bovines (carabaos) through either their removal and replacement with mechanized tractors in endemic areas or vaccination.

Author Contributions: R.M.O. & D.J.G. conceived the idea; R.M.O. & D.J.G. drafted and edited the manuscript.

Funding: This research received no external funding

Conflicts of Interest: The authors declare no conflict of interest.

References

1. Tanaka, H.; Tsuji, M. From discovery to eradication of schistosomiasis in Japan: 1847–1996. *Int. J. Parasitol* **1997**, *27*, 1465–1480. [CrossRef]
2. Sleigh, A.; Li, X.; Jackson, S.; Huang, K. Eradication of schistosomiasis in Guangxi, China. Part 1: Setting, strategies, operations, and outcomes, 1953-92. *Bull. World Health Organ.* **1998**, *76*, 361–372.
3. Yuan, H.; Jiagang, G.; Bergquist, R.; Tanner, M.; Xianyi, C.; Huanzeng, W. The 1992-1999 World Bank Schistosomiasis Research Initiative in China: outcome and perspectives. *Parasitol. Int.* **2000**, *49*, 195–207. [CrossRef]
4. Izhar, A.; Sinaga, R.M.; Sudomo, M.; Wardiyo, N.D. Recent situation of schistosomiasis in Indonesia. *Acta Trop.* **2002**, *82*, 283–288. [CrossRef]
5. Blas, B.L.; Rosales, M.I.; Lipayon, I.L.; Yasuraoka, K.; Matsuda, H.; Hayashi, M. The schistosomiasis problem in the Philippines: A review. *Parasitol. Int.* **2004**, *53*, 127–134.
6. Leonardo, L.; Rivera, P.; Saniel, O.; Antonio Solon, J.; Chigusa, Y.; Villacorte, E.; Christoper Chua, J.; Moendeg, K.; Manalo, D.; Crisostomo, B.; et al. New endemic foci of schistosomiasis infections in the Philippines. *Acta Trop.* **2015**, *141*, 354–360. [CrossRef]

7. Gordon, C.A.; Acosta, L.P.; Gobert, G.N.; Jiz, M.; Olveda, R.M.; Ross, A.G.; Gray, D.J.; Williams, G.M.; Harn, D.; Li, Y.; et al. High prevalence of Schistosoma japonicum and Fasciola gigantica in bovines from Northern Samar, the Philippines. *PLoS Negl. Trop. Dis.* **2015**, *9*, e0003108. [CrossRef]
8. Jiz, M.; Mingala, C.; Adriatico, M.; Jarilla, B.; Manalo, D.; Lu, K.; Fu, Z.; Wu, H.; Kurtis, J. High schistosomiasis infection rate among water buffalos living in an endemic area for 10 months in the Philippines. Presented at the 2014 Annual Meeting of the American Soc of Trop Med and Hygiene, New Orleans, LA, USA, 2–6 November 2014.
9. Olveda, R.; Icatlo, F., Jr.; Domingo, E. Clinical aspects of schistosomiasis japonica: A review. *Philipp. J. Int. Med.* **1986**, *24*, 147–150.
10. Weinberg, H.B.; Tillinghast, A.J. The pulmonary manifestations of schistosomiasis caused by Schistosoma japonicum. *Am. J. Trop Med. Hyg.* **1946**, *26*, 801–809. [CrossRef]
11. McGarvey, S.T.; Aligui, G.; Daniel, B.L.; Peters, P.; Olveda, R.; Olds, G.R. Child growth and schistosomiasis japonica in northeastern Leyte, the Philippines: cross-sectional results. *Am. J. Trop. Med. Hyg.* **1992**, *46*, 571–581. [CrossRef] [PubMed]
12. Leenstra, T.; Acosta, L.P.; Langdon, G.C.; Manalo, D.L.; Su, L.; Olveda, R.M.; McGarvey, S.T.; Kurtis, J.D.; Friedman, J.F. Schistosomiasis japonica, anemia, and iron status in children, adolescents, and young adults in Leyte, Philippines 1. *Am. J. Clin. Nutr.* **2006**, *83*, 371–379. [CrossRef] [PubMed]
13. Ezeamama, A.E.; Friedman, J.F.; Acosta, L.P.; Bellinger, D.C.; Langdon, G.C.; Manalo, D.L.; Olveda, R.M.; Kurtis, J.D.; McGarvey, S.T. Helminth infection and cognitive impairment among Filipino children. *Am. J. Trop. Med. Hyg.* **2005**, *72*, 540–548. [CrossRef]
14. Ezeamama, A.E.; McGarvey, S.T.; Hogan, J.; Lapane, K.L.; Bellinger, D.C.; Acosta, L.P.; Leenstra, T.; Olveda, R.M.; Kurtis, J.D.; Friedman, J.F. Treatment for Schistosoma japonicum, reduction of intestinal parasite load, and cognitive test score improvements in school-aged children. *PLoS Negl. Trop. Dis.* **2012**, *6*, e1634. [CrossRef] [PubMed]
15. Kurtis, J.D.; Higashi, A.; Wu, H.W.; Gundogan, F.; McDonald, E.A.; Sharma, S.; PondTor, S.; Jarilla, B.; Sagliba, M.J.; Gonzal, A.; et al. Maternal Schistosomiasis japonica is associated with maternal, placental, and fetal inflammation. *Infect. Immun.* **2011**, *79*, 1254–1261. [PubMed]
16. McDonald, E.A.; Cheng, L.; Jarilla, B.; Sagliba, M.J.; Gonzal, A.; Amoylen, A.J.; Olveda, R.; Acosta, L.; Baylink, D.; White, E.S.; et al. Maternal infection with Schistosoma japonicum induces a profibrotic response in neonates. *Infect. Immun.* **2014**, *82*, 350–355. [CrossRef]
17. McDonald, E.A.; Pond-Tor, S.; Jarilla, B.; Sagliba, M.J.; Gonzal, A.; Amoylen, A.J.; Olveda, R.; Acosta, L.; Gundogan, F.; Ganley-Leal, L.M.; et al. Schistosomiasis japonica during pregnancy is associated with elevated endotoxin levels in maternal and placental compartments. *J. Infect. Dis.* **2014**, *209*, 468–472. [CrossRef]
18. Olveda, R.M.; Tallo, V.; Olveda, D.U.; Inobaya, M.T.; Chau, T.N.; Ross, A.G. National survey data for zoonotic schistosomiasis in the Philippines grossly underestimates the true burden of disease within endemic zones: implications for future control. *Int. J. Infect. Dis.* **2016**, *45*, 13–17. [CrossRef]
19. Mcgarvey, S.T.; Daniel, B.L.; Tso, M.; Wu, G.; Zhong, S.; Olveda, R.; Wiest, P.M.; Olds, G.R. Child growth and schistosomiasis japonica in the Philippines and China. *Clin. Res.* **1990**, *38*, 382.
20. Olveda, R.M.; Daniel, B.L.; Ramirez, B.D.; Aligui, G.D.; Acosta, L.P.; Fevidal, P.; Tiu, E.; de Veyra, F.; Peters, P.A.; Romulo, R.; et al. Schistosomiasis japonica in the Philippines: the long-term impact of population-based chemotherapy on infection, transmission, and morbidity. *J. Infect. Dis.* **1996**, *174*, 163–172. [CrossRef]
21. Gray, D.J.; McManus, D.P.; Li, Y.S.; Williams, G.M.; Bergquist, R.; Ross, A.G. Schistosomiasis elimination: Lessons from the past guide the future. *Lancet Infect. Dis.* **2010**, *10*, 733–736. [CrossRef]
22. Gray, D.J.; Williams, G.M.; Li, Y.S.; Chen, H.G.; Forsyth, S.J.; Li, R.S.; Barnett, A.G.; Guo, J.G.; Ross, A.G.; Feng, Z.; et al. A cluster-randomised intervention trial against *S. japonicum* in the Peoples' Republic of China: Bovine and human transmission. *PLoS ONE* **2009**, *4*, e5900. [CrossRef] [PubMed]
23. Wang, L.-D.; Chen, H.-G.; Guo, J.-G.; Zeng, X.-J.; Hong, X.-L.; Xiong, J.-J.; Wu, X.-H.; Wang, X.-H.; Wang, L.-Y.; Xia, G.; et al. A Strategy to Control Transmission of Schistosoma japonicum in China. *N. Engl. J. Med.* **2009**, *360*, 121–128. [CrossRef] [PubMed]
24. Renucci, P. Challengies in the establishment of mechanized rice farming in schistosomiasis endemic area: Experience in the town of Alang Alang, Province of Leyte. Presented at the International Schistosomiasis Reserch Forum, Crimson Hotel, Alabang, Muntinlupa, Philippines, 12–13 March 2017.

25. Da'dara, A.A.; Li, Y.S.; Xiong, T.; Zhou, J.; Williams, G.M.; McManus, D.P.; Feng, Z.; Yu, X.L.; Gray, D.J.; Harn, D.A. DNA-based vaccines protect against zoonotic schistosomiasis in water buffalo. *Vaccine* **2008**, *26*, 3617–3625. [CrossRef] [PubMed]
26. Jiz, M.; Friedman, J.F.; Leenstra, T.; Jarilla, B.; Pablo, A.; Langdon, G.; Pond-Tor, S.; Wu, H.W.; Manalo, D.; Olveda, R.; et al. Immunoglobulin E (IgE) responses to paramyosin predict resistance to reinfection with Schistosoma japonicum and are attenuated by IgG4. *Infect. Immun.* **2009**, *77*, 2051–2058. [CrossRef] [PubMed]

Tropical Medicine and Infectious Disease

MDPI

Review

Asian Schistosomiasis: Current Status and Prospects for Control Leading to Elimination

Catherine A. Gordon [1,†], Johanna Kurscheid [2,†], Gail M. Williams [3], Archie C. A. Clements [4,5], Yuesheng Li [1], Xiao-Nong Zhou [6], Jürg Utzinger [7,8], Donald P. McManus [1] and Darren J. Gray [2,*]

1 QIMR Berghofer Medical Research Institute, Herston, QLD 4006, Australia; Catherine.Gordon@qimrberghofer.edu.au (C.A.G.); Yuesheng.Li@qimrberghofer.edu.au (Y.L.); Don.McManus@qimrberghofer.edu.au (D.P.M.)
2 Department of Global Health, Research School of Population Health, Australian National University, Acton, ACT 2601, Australia; Johanna.Kurscheid@anu.edu.au
3 School of Public Health, University of Queensland, Herston, QLD 4006, Australia; g.williams@sph.uq.edu.au
4 Faculty of Health Sciences, Curtin University, Bentley, WA 6102, Australia; archie.clements@curtin.edu.au
5 Telethon Kids Institute, Nedlands, WA 6009, Australia
6 Center for Disease Control and Prevention, National Institute for Parasitic Diseases, Shanghai 200025, China; zhouxn1@chinacdc.cn
7 Swiss Tropical and Public Health Institute, CH-4002 Basel, Switzerland; juerg.utzinger@swisstph.ch
8 University of Basel, CH-4003 Basel, Switzerland
* Correspondence: darren.gray@anu.edu.au; Tel.: +61-2-61258595
† Joint first authors.

Received: 14 January 2019; Accepted: 12 February 2019; Published: 26 February 2019

Abstract: Schistosomiasis is an infectious disease caused by helminth parasites of the genus *Schistosoma*. Worldwide, an estimated 250 million people are infected with these parasites with the majority of cases occurring in sub-Saharan Africa. Within Asia, three species of *Schistosoma* cause disease. *Schistosoma japonicum* is the most prevalent, followed by *S. mekongi* and *S. malayensis*. All three species are zoonotic, which causes concern for their control, as successful elimination not only requires management of the human definitive host, but also the animal reservoir hosts. With regard to Asian schistosomiasis, most of the published research has focused on *S. japonicum* with comparatively little attention paid to *S. mekongi* and even less focus on *S. malayensis*. In this review, we examine the three Asian schistosomes and their current status in their endemic countries: Cambodia, Lao People's Democratic Republic, Myanmar, and Thailand (*S. mekongi*); Malaysia (*S. malayensis*); and Indonesia, People's Republic of China, and the Philippines (*S. japonicum*). Prospects for control that could potentially lead to elimination are highlighted as these can inform researchers and disease control managers in other schistosomiasis-endemic areas, particularly in Africa and the Americas.

Keywords: Asia; control; elimination; epidemiology; *Schistosoma japonicum*; *Schistosoma malayensis*; *Schistosoma mekongi*; schistosomiasis

---

1. Introduction

Schistosomiasis is a parasitic disease caused by blood flukes of the genus *Schistosoma*. Six species of schistosomes infect humans: *Schistosoma mansoni* (occurring in Africa, South America, the Caribbean, and the Middle East), *S. haematobium* (mainly occurring in Africa and the Middle East, with recent autochthonous transmission observed in Corsica, France), *S. intercalatum* and *S. guineensis* (two rare species confined to a few countries in Central Africa), *S. japonicum* (Asia), and *S. mekongi* (Mekong Delta including Cambodia, Lao People's Democratic Republic (Lao PDR), and previously Thailand whose current status is transmission interruption) [1–3]. A seventh species, *S. malayensis*, which is thought to be closely related to *S. mekongi*, is endemic in Malaysia [4]. In this review, we focus on only those species currently occurring in Asia: *S. japonicum*, *S. mekongi*, and *S. malayensis*, which cause intestinal schistosomiasis. The three Asian schistosomes are all zoonotic, whereas the remaining species infecting humans are generally considered human-only parasites, with some notable exceptions [5–10].

Schistosomiasis has a long history in Asia with the first descriptions and reports of the disease in modern times appearing in the early 1900s, although it is thought to have been endemic for at least 400 years earlier in Japan, and at least 2200 years ago in the People's Republic of China (P.R. China) after the discovery of *S. japonicum* eggs in a mummy [11–14]. To date, Japan is the only country in Asia to have eliminated schistosomiasis, while Thailand is awaiting verification of transmission interruption by the World Health Organization (WHO) [15]. Currently, schistosomiasis is endemic in six Asian countries: P.R. China, the Philippines, Indonesia, Lao PDR, Cambodia, and Malaysia, and is emerging in a seventh—Myanmar (Figure 1) [16]. Considerable progress in control has been made in recent decades, largely through praziquantel-based preventive chemotherapy (i.e., periodic administration of praziquantel to entire at-risk populations without prior diagnosis). However, preventive chemotherapy alone is insufficient to break the transmission cycle. Lack of safe water, poor sanitation, inadequate hygiene practices, limited health education, and the presence of animal reservoirs are known barriers to the elimination of schistosomiasis from a region [17]. Old challenges remain while new ones emerge, requiring a comprehensive, multi-sectoral, and multifaceted approach across the region to control this disease, and to reach the desired goal of elimination by 2030 [17].

The aim of this review is to provide an overview of the current status of schistosomiasis in Asia, with a particular focus on endemic countries in the region and the unique challenges they face. Our review also aimed to identify current knowledge gaps and future research needs as the affected countries move toward the ultimate goal of control and elimination of this persistent and debilitating disease.

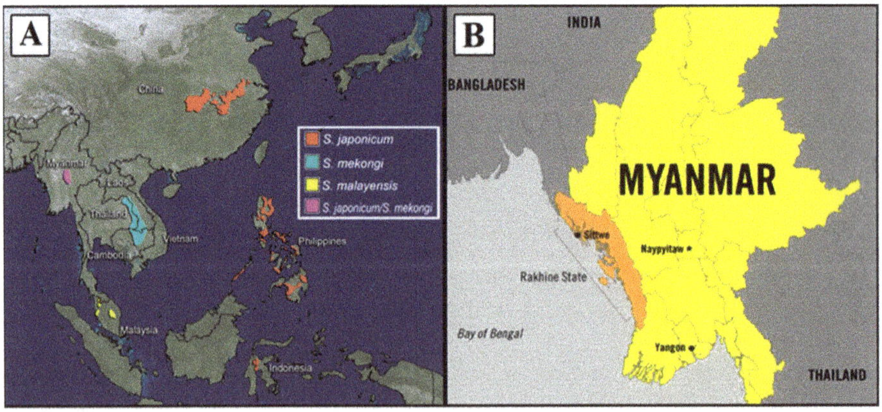

Figure 1. (**A**) Map of Southeast Asia showing the location of endemic areas for schistosomiasis, including a focus in central Myanmar. (**B**) Map of Myanmar highlighting the state of Rakhine.

2. Parasite Features

The genus *Schistosoma* is a group of parasitic blood flukes, or flatworms, of the class Trematoda. Unique amongst the trematode class, schistosomes have separate sexes as adults, whereas all other trematodes are hermaphrodites. The Asian schistosomes discussed in this review are considered zoonotic, unlike schistosome species occurring elsewhere, which are largely human-only excepting some hybrid forms in Africa [5,6,9,10,18], and cases of *S. mansoni* infecting non-human primates in Africa and the Caribbean, and rats in Guadeloupe and Brazil [7,8]. *S. japonicum* is the most cosmopolitan, with 46 mammalian definitive hosts identified thus far, whereas *S. mekongi* has been found in dogs, and *S. malayensis* in rodents, specifically *Rattus muelleri* [19–22] (Table 1). Pigs have been experimentally infected with *S. mekongi*, but, to date, no natural infections have been identified in these hosts [23]. Morphologically, the eggs and adults of the three species are very similar; the eggs are ovoid with a small 'nubby' lateral spine (Table 1) [24].

Table 1. A comparison of features of the three Asian schistosome species that can infect humans [4,25,26].

	Geographic Distribution	Animal Definitive Hosts	Intermediate Hosts	Eggs
S. japonicum	Indonesia, the Philippines, P. R. China	46 known mammalian hosts including water buffalo and cattle, dogs, pigs, and rodents	*Oncomelania* spp. 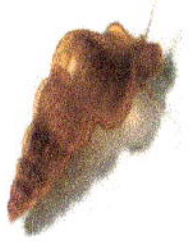	70–100 × 55–64 µm 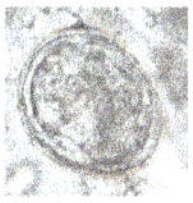
S. mekongi	Cambodia, Lao PDR, Thailand	Dogs and pigs	*Neotricula* spp. 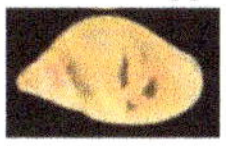	50–80 × 40–65 µm 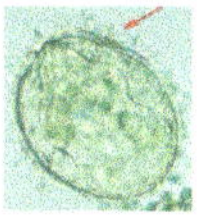
S. malayensis	Malaysia	Rodents	*Robertsiella* spp. 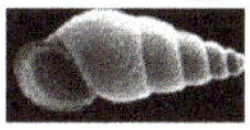	53–90 × 33–62 µm 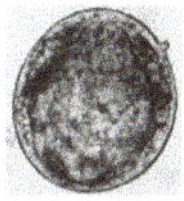

2.1. Lifecycle

The schistosome lifecycle is complex with an intermediate molluscan host, definitive host, and seven lifecycle stages involving both asexual and sexual reproductive phases (Figure 2). An in-depth understanding of social-ecological systems is required to grasp the spatial focality of schistosomiasis distributions [27].

2.1.1. *S. japonicum*

S. japonicum is the most prevalent of the Asian schistosomes. It is endemic in P.R. China, the Philippines, and small foci occur in Indonesia. There are 46 known mammalian definitive hosts of *S. japonicum*, although water buffalo and cattle have previously been shown to be the major reservoirs of infection [19,28,29]. *S. japonicum* was first identified in Japan in 1901, whereas the last new human case was recorded there in 1977. *S. japonicum* parasites in P.R. China and the Philippines have distinct genetic differences, resulting from geographic isolation over time. In general, the strain of *S. japonicum* in P.R. China is more virulent than the parasite in the Philippines; additional genetically variant geographic isolates are known to be present in both countries [30–32].

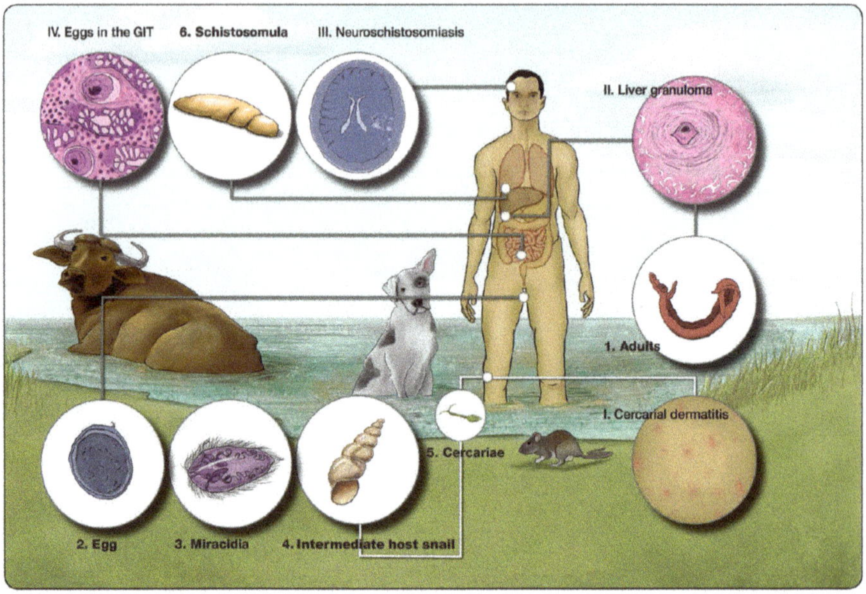

Figure 2. Schistosome lifecycle. Adult worms (**1**) reproduce sexually in the mesenteric veins surrounding the small intestine of the definitive mammalian host. Female worms deposit eggs (**2**), which are excreted in the feces. Upon contact with freshwater, the eggs hatch miracidia (**3**), which penetrate a snail intermediate host (**4**) and undergo asexual reproduction; this includes development of mother and daughter sporocysts, which produce cercariae (**5**). Cercariae exit the snail and swim around until they penetrate the skin of the mammalian definitive host, potentially causing cercarial dermatitis (**I**), shed their tail and become schistosomula (**6**). The schistosomula migrate through the body to the lungs before migrating and maturing to adult worms in the mesenteric veins. Chronic schistosomiasis occurs as the result of an immune reaction to the eggs resulting in granuloma formation in tissues where eggs are lodged. This most commonly occurs in the liver and spleen (**II**), which can result in hepatosplenomegaly and portal hypertension; in the walls of the intestine (**IV**) as eggs pass from the blood into the intestine; and less commonly in the brain (**III**), causing neuroschistosomiasis, characterized by a range of neurological symptoms. (Abbreviation: GIT, gastrointestinal tract).

2.1.2. *S. mekongi*

S. mekongi was first identified in 1857 [33]. While morphologically very similar to *S. japonicum*, *S. mekongi* differs in a number of characteristics that indicate it is a distinct species. These differences include the morphology of the testis and ovary in adult worms [34] and the eggs of *S. mekongi* are smaller and more round than those of *S. japonicum* (Table 1) [35]. Morphological differences in the miracidial stage of the two species are also apparent [35]. Early genetic studies showing electrophoretic enzyme variation indicated sequence differences between *S. japonicum* and *S. mekongi* [36].

Apart from human infection, *S. mekongi* has only been identified naturally in dogs, although there have been successful laboratory infections of pigs. The intermediate host of *S. mekongi* is *Neotricula aperta* (previously *Lithoglyphopsis aperta*), and studies have found *Oncomelania* spp. snails to be refractory to infection with *S. mekongi* [34].

2.1.3. *S. malayensis*

As with the other Asian schistosomes, *S. malayensis* is zoonotic and is primarily a parasite of the rodent *R. muelleri* (Table 1). *S. malayensis* is a sister species to *S. japonicum*, as is *S. mekongi*, to which it is more closely related [24]. Early studies identified the intermediate host of *S. malayensis* as *Robertsiella karporensis* [4,24].

2.2. Clinical Features

There are three clinical stages of schistosome infection. The initial early stage, a second 'silent' phase, also known as Katayama fever (or Katayama syndrome, named after the prefecture in Japan where it was first identified), and the third 'chronic' stage [1,37]. As the average life of an adult schistosome is 10 years and may be as long as 30 years, assuming no treatment, chronic infection can be lifelong [38,39].

The initial disease phase begins as a skin rash caused by an immune reaction to the penetrating cercariae (Figure 2, I). After penetrating the definitive host, the cercariae transform into schistosomula, which migrate to the lungs where they can cause pulmonary schistosomiasis, characterized as small nodules on a chest x-ray and a dry cough in the infected individual. After the lungs, the worms migrate to the venus plexus of the intestine, where they mature and pair up, reproducing sexually (Figure 2, 1). There is little immune response generated against the adult worms; thus, the second silent stage lasts for six to eight weeks post-infection when eggs begin to be produced. At this point, the acute Katayama fever begins, manifesting as fever, cough, rash, abdominal pain, nausea, diarrhea, and eosinophilia. Acute disease is more commonly seen in naïve persons, whereas chronic disease, the third phase, is more likely to occur in individuals resident in schistosome-endemic areas. Chronic disease occurs due to retention of eggs in the liver, spleen, and intestinal walls, and is the result of an immune response generated against the eggs, which causes granuloma formation in the various tissues (Figure 2, II and III). This can result in hepatosplenomegaly, portal hypertension, abdominal pain, and bloody diarrhea. A rarer manifestation of disease is neuroschistosomiasis (Figure 2, IV), which causes neurological symptoms, such as seizures and headaches, due to a granulomatous response against eggs in the brain, appearing as lesions on scans [40–43]. Infection in children is associated with growth stunting and intellectual disability and, in adults, with a reduced ability to work [44,45].

2.3. Diagnostics

A number of diagnostics are available, including coproparasitological examination (CopE), as well as molecular and immunological diagnostics. CopE methods rely on direct detection and visualization of parasite eggs in feces and include the Kato-Katz (KK) thick smear procedure, which is a mainstay of control programs due to the relative ease of performing the test at low cost, although it lacks sensitivity in low-intensity infections [46,47] and FLOTAC [48,49]. Other diagnostic approaches include formal-ethyl acetate sedimentation-digestion (FEA-SD) [50], the Danish Bilharziasis Laboratory (DBL) technique [51,52], and the miracidial hatching technique (MHT) [53,54], which also tests egg viability. Molecular diagnostics rely on detection of parasite DNA in clinical samples, often stool but also in urine, blood, and saliva, and include loop-mediated isothermal amplification (LAMP) [55–58], conventional polymerase chain reaction (cPCR) [59,60], real-time PCR (qPCR) [28,61–64], and digital droplet PCR (ddPCR) [65–67]. Immunological diagnostics rely on detection of circulating parasite antigens or antibodies generated against parasite antigens. Antibody detection might lack specificity and generally does not distinguish between past and current infections. A study by Cai et al., however, suggested that an immunological test combining two antigens (SjSAP4 + Sj23-LHD) may be useful for monitoring schistosomiasis control programs in the Philippines [68]. The main immunological methods include the enzyme-linked immunosorbent assay (ELISA) [69–72] and the rarely used circumoval precipitation test (COPT) [73,74]. Comprehensive reviews of the current diagnostic methods for schistosomiasis were provided by Weerakoon et al. and Utzinger et al. [58,75].

Sensitive and specific diagnostic procedures are required to monitor the success or failure of schistosomiasis control programs as well as to determine whether control efforts have resulted in elimination. However, the most sensitive diagnostics, involving molecular or immunological techniques, can be expensive and require specialized facilities and equipment and trained personnel to perform the procedures [57,76].

2.4. Treatment

Laboratory studies and clinical trials have shown that praziquantel, a pyrazinoisoquinoline derivative, is a safe and highly efficacious oral drug that is active against all schistosome species, although it is less active against juvenile schistosomes compared with adult worms and eggs [77–81]. The effective clinical praziquantel dosage regimen is 60 mg/kg orally in divided doses over one day (3 × 20 mg/kg doses 4-hourly, or 2 × 30 mg/kg either 4- or 6-hourly) for *S. japonicum* and *S. mekongi* [77,78]. Praziquantel is also the mainstay for preventive chemotherapy for morbidity control of schistosomiasis. In the Philippines, the efficacy of a single dose of 40 mg/kg vs. 60 mg/kg was compared; 40 mg/kg was effective and better tolerated and thus 40 mg/kg was adopted for preventive chemotherapy [82]. A single dose is beneficial for large-scale administration as it does not require follow up treatment as occurs with split doses. Despite the reliance on 40 mg/kg for preventive chemotherapy programs, two doses of 60 mg/kg separated by two weeks is recommended by the Philippine government in case finding, i.e., eggs identified in the stool [82].

Treatment with praziquantel does not prevent reinfection [83] and is therefore relatively ineffective at interrupting the transmission cycle. Praziquantel is principally aimed at reducing the prevalence and intensity of infection and to control morbidity over the longer term. Some concern has been expressed that praziquantel-resistant schistosomes may develop, most likely in Africa [84,85], and there is thus a pressing need to develop new anti-schistosomal drugs [86] and other non-pharmaceutical interventions.

3. Epidemiology

Due to the requirement of an intermediate host snail, schistosomiasis is a focal disease, occurring in areas where snail habitats and susceptible transmitting snails are present. This means that village-level prevalence can be very high, whereas country and province prevalence can be low. Demographic factors such as age, sex, and occupation are strongly associated with risk of infection [87,88]. Open defecation remains a common phenomenon in schistosomiasis-endemic countries and is strongly associated with transmission.

Snail habitats generally occur in still or slow moving water bodies such as streams, lakes, dammed waterways, and rice fields. The susceptible snails also have a preference for vegetation and snail control measures can include the removal of this vegetation.

3.1. Mammalian Definitive Hosts

Of the 46 known *S. japonicum* hosts, bovines, particularly water buffalo, are considered the most important for transmission due to the high levels of schistosome eggs they excrete into the environment [89,90] and their predisposition to natural infection. Epidemiological studies conducted in the Poyang and Dongting Lake regions of P.R. China revealed that water buffaloes account for up to 75–80% of *S. japonicum* infections, and hence are considered to be the most important reservoir hosts [29,89–91]. In mountainous and hilly endemic areas, water buffaloes are frequently used for ploughing rice fields and, while rodents have been considered to be important reservoirs, Van Dorssen et al. posited that this may not be the case owing to low levels of egg output and questions around egg viability [92,93]. Other potentially important animal reservoir hosts for *S. japonicum* in P.R. China include goats, pigs, and dogs due to their close contact with humans and water [93,94].

In Indonesia, 13 mammalian species, mostly wild animals (wild rodents, wild pigs, wild deer, wild celedus, and wild civet cats), but also cattle, water buffalo, horses, and dogs, have been identified as susceptible hosts for *S. japonicum* [95]. The prevalence of *S. japonicum* in water buffalo (known also as carabao) in the Philippines has been reported to be as high as 80%, particularly in agricultural areas, and water buffalo are thought to be a major reservoir [96]. In both the Philippines and P.R. China, there are fewer cattle than water buffalo/carabao. Cattle are more susceptible to infection than water buffalo, likely due to their more recent introduction into Asia compared with water buffalo, which have co-evolved with *S. japonicum* for much longer. Although studies suggested that water buffalo exhibit some age-acquired resistance to infection and self-cure [28,97,98], there is still uncertainty regarding this phenomenon [99].

Due to the close genetic relationship between *S. japonicum* and *S. mekongi*, bovines could act as reservoir hosts of *S. mekongi* but, to date, this has not been demonstrated. A range of potential animal hosts have been examined for *S. mekongi*, but currently dogs are the only animal species that have been confirmed as natural hosts of this species [22].

In regards to control, little has been done to target definitive hosts of *S. japonicum*, with the exception of P.R. China, which has practiced both chemotherapy of bovines and removal of the animals, facilitated by mechanization of agriculture (i.e., replacing water buffalo with tractors) [16,29,89,100,101]. Without targeting intermediate host snails, re-infection of humans after treatment can occur almost instantaneously. Animals can also contribute to rebounding infections in areas where humans have been declared free of schistosomiasis [102]. In Lao PDR, chemotherapy of dogs against *S. mekongi* has been highlighted as a priority. This has been proposed as part of community-led initiatives to eliminate schistosomiasis that combine deworming with water, sanitation, and hygiene interventions: community-led school, water, sanitation, and hygiene (CL-SWASH) activities [103].

Animal vaccines against schistosomiasis have been developed and used in controlled trials [104–107]. Whereas none of the currently developed vaccines provide 100% immune protection (0–80% worm reduction in mice and baboons [108]; 41–51% in water buffalo [109]), they do induce a significant reduction in adult worms, decreased egg output, and stunting of adults. A knockdown in adult worm fecundity alone can have a huge impact on transmission. Modeling has shown that an animal vaccine with 75% efficacy will be required to ensure long-term control of schistosomiasis [110].

3.2. Molluscan Intermediate Hosts

The intermediate snail hosts of *S. japonicum* are amphibious and belong to the genus *Oncomelania*, with species dependent on geographical location. Studies investigating the susceptibility of snails from different geographic locations to cercariae from disparate locations have produced mixed results, indicating a certain amount of genetic drift of the parasite [111,112]. Although Japan has successfully eliminated schistosomiasis, the requisite intermediate host snail species, *Oncomelania hupensis nosphora* and *O. hupensis formosana*, are still present [113].

In P.R. China, four sub-species of the intermediate host *Oncomelania hupensis* have been identified based on morphological and molecular characteristics [114–116], each with different growth rates, population genetics, and ecological niches. Control measures have been successful in reducing the populations of *O. h. guangxiensis* and *O. h. tangi* [13] leaving *O. h. hupensis* and *O. h. robertsoni* as the dominant sub-species [114]. Of these, *O. h. hupensis* is the most widely distributed [114]. Few studies have reported *S. japonicum* infection rates in *Oncomelania* snails in endemic regions of P.R. China in the last decade. One study in the marshland regions along the Yangtze River [114] examined more than 70,000 snails over a 15-year period (2001–2015) and found an overall prevalence of 0.05% with no new infections since 2007 [117]. An earlier study reported a decline from 0.88% in 2009 to zero in 2012 in Jiangling county, Hubei province [118]. According to a 2017 WHO meeting report on Asian schistosomiasis, an active sentinel surveillance program, conducted in 2016 in areas where transmission was considered interrupted or under control, also failed to identify infected snails [119]. However, the same report indicated that in two other studies undertaken in 2012 and 2017, in four and seven provinces, respectively, infected snails were found based on LAMP analysis, but no infection was recorded by microscopy, although actual infection rates for the LAMP analysis were not provided [119]. As snail infection rates continue to decline, consistent and highly sensitive diagnostic tests, such as LAMP, will be required to provide accurate information [75,120].

In the Philippines, the sole intermediate host snail for *S. japonicum* is *O. h. quadrasi*. It is amphibious but prefers an aquatic environment, such as wet soil surfaces, swamps, rice fields, ponds, and stream banks, thus making chemical snail control difficult due to the risk of contaminating the water or food source [17]. The current status of *S. japonicum* infection in the snail intermediate hosts in the Philippines is poorly understood. One study, conducted in Samar province, found a mean infection rate of 1.09% across 147 sites with higher infection among snails located in irrigated compared to rain-fed villages [121]. More recent data from 2013 to 2015 indicate infection rates of less than 2% in most endemic provinces, although Northern Samar was found to have a prevalence of above 12% [76].

In Indonesia, the intermediate snail host of *S. japonicum* is *O. h. lindoensis*, which is located focally around Lake Lindu. In 2011, the prevalence of infected *O. h. lindoensis* snails in Lindu Valley was 3.6% and 4.0% in Napu Valley, although the prevalence has fluctuated between 0 and 13.4% in Napu Valley and between 0% and 9.1% in Lindu Valley since 2005 [95]. Prevalence of infected snails in Bada Valley appears to be much lower, with a survey conducted in 2010 identifying a prevalence of only 1% (3 among 299 snails sampled) [122].

The intermediate hosts of *S. mekongi* are *Neotricula* spp., and endemic areas are closely associated with the Mekong Delta where these snails occur. The prevalence of infected snails in Lao PDR was quite low, 0.01% on the Mekong Islands [123] and 0.22% in Khong District, although the snail density was quite high [124]. *Neotricula aperta* snail density in Thailand decreased between 2005 and 2011 in the downstream area of the Nam Theun 2 hydroelectric dam, which began operation in 2010 [125]. A similar decrease in *Oncomelania* snails in low-land areas was initially seen in P.R. China after the building of the Three Gorges Dam [126]. However, snail density began to increase in 2011 after initially decreasing in the years immediately after completion of the dam in 2003. A similar trend may eventually be seen in Thailand with the Nam Theun 2 Dam.

Control of intermediate host snails is an important aspect of schistosomiasis control programs, particularly as the stage of the lifecycle occurring in snails is asexual and involves an exponential increase in parasite numbers. Snail control measures previously implemented in Asia have involved environmental modification and chemical mollusciciding. The snails live in vegetation around rivers and lakes and removal of this vegetation can lead to removal of the snails themselves. This method was used with great success in Japan in combination with mollusciciding. In Japan, the most common method of environmental modification was the use of concreting canals where the snails lived [113]. This method is more difficult to implement in areas where the snail habitats are rice fields or marshland. Early reports from Mindanao in the Philippines showed that the method of farming (weeding and ploughing) practiced in Mindanao reduced snail habitat on the rice fields, and thus snails were primarily found in swampland, at least when intensive farming was practiced [127]. Changing land use in Japan from rice crops to either housing or fruit trees, which did not require flood irrigation and thus no longer provided snail habitats, was an important feature for control.

Mollusciciding has also been used in P.R. China, Indonesia, and the Philippines, although to a limited degree in the latter two countries. Environmental contamination with chemical molluscicides is an important issue, and a number of previously used compounds have been abandoned due to these concerns and as a result of the damage they cause to the environment. In the schistosomiasis foci in Indonesia, the snail habitats occur close to the Lore Lindu National Park, which precludes the use of molluscicides [128] and environmental modification. Early molluscicides included lime, which proved inefficient, calcium cyanamide, and, later, sodium pentachlorohenate (Na-PCP), which was eventually stopped in all countries due to environmental toxicity [129]. In P.R. China, the molluscicide of choice has been niclosamide, used in two different formulations: (1) a 50% niclosamide ethanolamine salt wettable powder and (2) a 4% niclosamide ethanolamine powder [106,130]. Both formulations resulted in substantial, but not 100%, killing of snails, which meant that mollusciciding needed to be performed more than once a year.

Neotricula spp., the intermediate host snails of *S. mekongi*, exhibit a different ecological niche than those transmitting *S. japonicum* in that, rather than being present in marshlands and rice fields, these snails are primarily found in shallow areas of rivers (particularly the Mekong River) and tributaries. Thus, snail control for *S. mekongi* has largely been deemed infeasible [17], although ecological management of snail habitats upstream of human habitation, as occurs in P.R. China, should be explored. Instead, preventive chemotherapy, along with improved WASH is practiced. Lao PDR has previously used niclosamide for snail control, although this did not significantly impact the numbers of snails in the treatment areas [124].

3.3. Environment

The majority of environmental factors associated with *S. japonicum* transmission are related to distance to a snail habitat or those that influence snail habitats, such as the building of dams. The majority of *S. japonicum*-endemic zones are within 1 km of water bodies such as rivers, lakes, or wetlands [131,132]. Environmental factors that influence snail habitat include land cover, particularly the presence of flooded agricultural land [133,134], seasonal land surface temperature (LST), elevation, and rainfall [131].

In P.R. China, endemic areas occupy three different geographical landscapes: (1) marshland and lake areas, (2) mountainous and hilly areas, and (3) water network areas. Of these, marshland and lake areas are characteristic of the major endemic foci for *S. japonicum*, and might account for 95% of the snail habitats [17,87]. *Oncomelania* snails survive best at areas of low elevation—one of the potential environmental factors associated with high prevalence of snails in marshy areas. A study on snail habitats in mountainous and hilly areas identified a maximum elevation of 2300 m above sea level for snail survival [131]. The same study identified an ideal LST of $\geq$22.7 °C and a normalized difference vegetation index (NDVI) of $\geq$0.446 in the mountainous areas. Distance from the nearest stream was also important, as the *Oncomelania* snails are amphibious; yet, require water to survive. A distance of $\leq$1000 m from the nearest stream was found to be ideal for snail habitats [131].

As the marshy and lake areas are categorized by the presence of water bodies, more areas are available for the snails to exist. The area of these landscapes, which cover the four provinces of Hunan, Jiangxi, Anhui, and Hubei, is vast, complicating snail control in these locations [135]. Mountainous and hilly areas, located primarily in the western part of P.R. China in the provinces of Yunnan and Sichuan [131], account for approximately 5% of the remaining snail habitats [17]. The complex environmental conditions present in these areas make it difficult to control snail populations [131]. The third type of landscape are water network areas, mainly located around the Yangtze River, which account for <1% of snail habitats in endemic areas of P.R. China [17].

Local epidemic outbreaks and the geographic distribution of snail hosts are heavily influenced by flooding events caused by the Yangtze River as they facilitate snail dispersion to new localities such as rivers, lakes, and wetlands [136,137]. Large-scale water development projects [138], particularly the aforementioned Three Gorges Dam and the South-North Water Diversion project (SNWD), also influence the transmission and geographic distribution of schistosomiasis [139,140]. The SNWD plans to divert water from the Yangtze River to the North [141]. Climate prediction models have indicated that this project may result in the expansion of viable snail habitats for the main snail intermediate host *O. h. hupensis* as well as *O. h. robertsioni* and *O. h. guangxiensis* [141]. The Three Gorges Dam, begun in 2003 and completed in 2012, was built to decrease flooding events as well as to generate power. As a consequence, it has changed the ecology of the surrounding area and impacted the habitat of *Oncomelania* spp. snails. The decrease in flooding events has decreased the density of snails in some areas, although in others, the density appears unchanged, or is on the increase [126].

In the Philippines, more than 3000 bodies of water are thought to be infested with snails susceptible to *S. japonicum* infection: 80% in Mindanao, 18% in Visayas, and 2% in Luzon [76]. Endemic regions have no distinct dry season and are predominantly comprised of rice fields, where contact between humans and snails is maximized [11,82]. Environmental factors, such as close proximity to large perennial water bodies (PWB), LST, NDVI, and precipitation, influence *S. japonicum* infection prevalence differently in the three main regions of the Philippines [87]. As is the case in P.R. China, the distance from water is an important factor for snail habitats, with the prevalence of schistosomiasis in humans decreasing with distance to PWB [87]. Some differences exist between the three regions, with increased distance to PWB associated with decreased prevalence in Luzon and the Visayas, but not Mindanao, whereas LST increase only significantly associated with decreased prevalence in Luzon. Similarly increased precipitation was associated with higher prevalence in the Visayas but decreased prevalence in Mindanao [87]. A confounding factor may be the differences in average socioeconomic status between the three areas: people in Luzon tend to have higher socioeconomic status compared to schistosomiasis-endemic areas of the Visayas and Mindanao. Natural habitats of *O. h. quadrasi* include flood plains, forests, and swamps, whereas man-made habitats resulting from agricultural development are thought to be important habitats (e.g., drainage channels, roadside ditches, small canals, and drainage canals of irrigation works). These snails are generally found on banks but also occur in shallow water (depth <20 cm) [121]. *O. h. quadrasi* snails prefer areas shaded by vegetation where the temperature is relatively stable and cool.

Endemic regions of Indonesia are located in marshland areas around Lake Lindu and Napu and Bada valleys. Prevalence of *S. japonicum* in snails from this area ranged from 0 to 13.4% in the Lindu Valley and 0 to 9.1% in the Napu Valley, although human prevalence remained <1% as of 2006 [128].

S. mekongi transmission occurs in the Mekong Delta. In Khong and Mounlapamok districts in Lao PDR, 202 villages are situated along the Mekong River with 114 currently or previously endemic for schistosomiasis. The only villages with zero prevalence for *S. mekongi* are in parts of the river where the riverbed is sandy, which is not conducive to the intermediate host snail, or those villages that are more than 6 km away from the river [142].

Limited information is available regarding risk factors and snail intermediate hosts in Myanmar [16]. The current areas where schistosomiasis occurs are around Lake Inlay in Shan State, although a recent outbreak has occurred in Rakhine State on the Coast of the Bay of Bengal [143]. The wet season runs from May to October.

3.4. Transmission and Control

In P.R. China, transmission usually occurs across two distinct seasons [17], coinciding with the natural annual flooding events in the Yangtze River: firstly in April to June/July when flooding is at its peak, and secondly after the waters subside in September/October with transmission continuing until November [140]. Although environmental factors heavily influence the snail intermediate hosts, demographic factors and the presence of host reservoirs play a more significant role in human transmission of *S. japonicum*. Infection with *S. japonicum* is strongly associated with age, sex, and occupational exposure. Males aged 40 years and above who engage in fishing, farming, and herding are at greatest risk of infection [144]. Defecation into lake waters or marshlands by fishermen and grazing water buffalo facilitate the continuance of transmission.

In the Philippines, there is no distinct dry season on the main endemic islands of Leyte and Samar and the province of Mindanao. Hence, transmission is not as variable by season as in P.R. China and occurs all year round [82]. The most common crop in these endemic areas is rice, which provides contact between snails that live in the rice paddies, swamps, and streams, whereas water buffalo and cattle are used to work on the fields (Figure 3). In addition to farming, washing, and recreational use of rivers are associated with higher risk of infection (Figure 4).

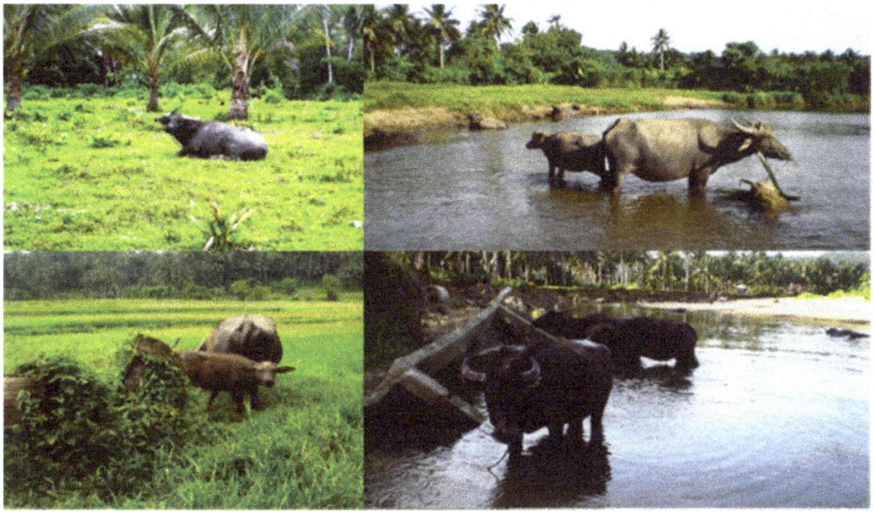

Figure 3. Water buffalo (carabao) in the Philippines are tethered in rivers, rice fields, and wallows—the same areas where the intermediate snail host for *S. japonicum* is also found. (Images from the Philippines, captured by C.A.G.).

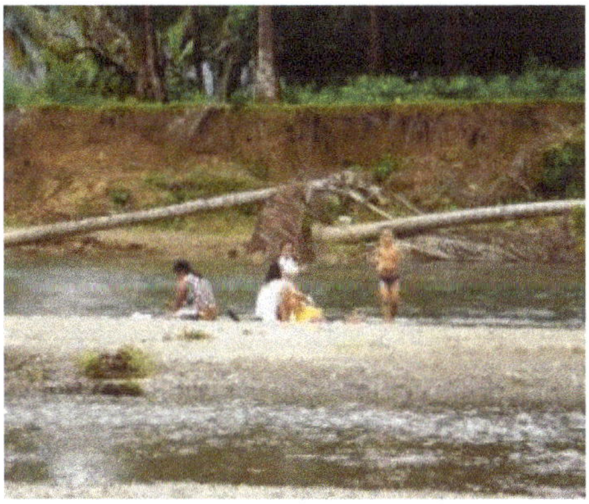

Figure 4. Washing and recreational uses of waterways are risk factors for contracting schistosomiasis. (Image from the Philippines, captured by C.A.G.).

Whereas 13 species of mammalian hosts have been identified in Indonesia, limited research has been undertaken on their involvement in transmission. Rodents of the genus *Rattus* have been suggested as the primary source of transmission, with a peak prevalence of 20% found in one endemic village [128]. Primary species thought to be involved in transmission are *R. exulans*, *R. hoffmani*, *R. chysocomus rallus*, *R. marmosurus*, and *R. celebensis* [128]. Reservations around the role that rodents can play in transmission were addressed earlier [92,93]. As in P.R. China, Indonesia experiences wet and dry seasons; hence, it is likely that schistosome transmission is also seasonal there, with increased transmission occurring in the wet season (November–March).

The transmission season for *S. mekongi* is matched with the lifecycle of the snail. During times of high water levels (2–3 m), the majority of available snails are young, while in times of low water (April–May; 10–60 mm), the snails have matured to adults capable of carrying the infection.

Peak transmission of *S. mekongi* in Cambodia occurs between February and April coinciding with peak water use for fishing [17]; whereas in Lao PDR, the main transmission season occurs in April and May.

In Malaysia, the wet season differs between the southwest where the monsoon season is May–October, and the northeast where the monsoon season runs from November to March, and the typhoon season occurs from April to November. It is therefore difficult in the absence of yearly surveys to pinpoint when transmission in Malaysia might peak, but it is certainly influenced by rainfall brought by the monsoons and typhoons.

Preventive chemotherapy with praziquantel has been the mainstay of schistosomiasis morbidity control and, in addition to targeting mammalian and snail hosts mentioned earlier, efforts to control transmission have also included programs aimed at improving WASH and health education. Until relatively recently, the role of WASH in schistosomiasis control was limited [145–148], despite the strong association of the disease with poverty and poor sanitation. In 2012, the World Health Assembly (WHA) encouraged the incorporation of WASH into control and elimination strategies [149]. Due to the transmission dynamics of schistosomiasis, WASH primarily limits environmental contamination with schistosome eggs and reduces human contact with potentially infested waters [150]. Improvements in sanitation and access to clean water have been shown to reduce the risk of schistosome infection [151], and have the added benefit of reducing infection with other parasites such as soil-transmitted helminths [146]. The impact of WASH is, however, dependent on the setting [151]. For example, access to clean water is not considered to play a significant role in endemic areas where schistosome infections are attributed to occupational or recreational contact with water as opposed to water used for drinking or for everyday activities (e.g., laundry and bathing) [151]. Traditional WASH practices, such as handwashing, have little impact on schistosome infection as the parasite eggs excreted in stools are not infective to human or animal hosts. However, water use practices involving rivers, such as bathing and washing clothes, will increase risk of contact with the infectious cercariae. Hence, much of the WASH emphasis to date has focused on sanitation and sanitary behavior. A number of programs focusing on improving access to clean water and improved sanitation outside of schistosomiasis control are ongoing throughout schistosomiasis-endemic countries in Asia [152–157].

Health education is important not only for educating the public on risk reduction measures and changing behavior, but has also been found to facilitate diagnosis, surveillance, and treatment [157]. Through health education activities and water contact studies, many high-risk behaviors and at-risk populations have been identified [158]. This has enabled health messages to be tailored to specific groups, such as school-age children swimming in freshwater and farmers and fishermen, and has largely been aimed at methods of avoiding water contact and self-protection [158]. However, it can be difficult to change behavior in some groups, such as fishermen or farmers, due to the nature of their occupations [158]. The support of local and national governments, through implementing infrastructure such as public toilets and using sanitary containers for stool on fishing boats, is therefore important in these situations [117,159]. The vehicles used for health education messages are many-fold and include audio-visual (radio, television, film, drama, traditional opera, and exhibits), print media (poems, slogans, posters, magazines, and newspaper), and other daily articles such as printed shirts, towels, fans, and umbrellas, among others [158]. Health information can also be passively disseminated through the community by students, teachers, village leaders, and parents [158]. Although health education is considered an important component of an integrated control program for schistosomiasis [160–163], it needs to be thoroughly planned, targeted, trialed, and evaluated prior to implementation [158], and needs to be sustained over a long period of time in order to maximize effectiveness [164]. To date, health education has been a major focus in P.R. China. Elsewhere, health education has generally been combined with preventive chemotherapy and has played a limited role in schistosomiasis control and elimination programs [82,165].

Research is ongoing for the development of schistosomiasis vaccines targeting humans and, unlike the African schistosomes, the zoonotic nature of the Asian schistosomes allow for the targeting of animal hosts. With bovines, particularly water buffalo/carabao confirmed as the major reservoirs of

S. japonicum, there is the rationale for the development and deployment of a transmission-blocking anti-*S. japonicum* vaccine targeting bovines [29,91,166,167]. The SjCTPI-Hsp70 vaccine is one of the most efficacious to date with an experimental efficacy of ~52% [101] and cluster-randomized controlled trials are currently being finalized to determine efficacy in natural settings. Vaccines may be the key for long-term sustainable control and elimination of schistosomiasis but research needs to be ongoing [167].

4. Current and Historical Status of Schistosomiasis in Asia

Notably, most prevalence estimates reported are based on microscopic detection of schistosome eggs in stool samples, usually using the KK thick smear technique [87,168,169]. However, numerous studies have demonstrated significantly higher prevalence when molecular detection methods have been applied on the same set of samples, with differences of up to 70% reported [28,60,63,170]. Prevalence is also largely influenced by the size of the sampled population. This is particularly relevant to the Philippines and Indonesia where funds are often limited, thus restricting the number of personnel available to interview and process collected samples. Another confounding factor, which is also common in P.R. China, is a fall in participation rates in many endemic areas, often referred to as treatment fatigue. Some communities in highly endemic areas have been participating in surveys for decades; hence, it is not surprising that these villagers have tired of the routine. In areas where prevalence has dropped significantly, the disease is no longer seen as a priority. Based on these factors, it is conceivable that the prevalence of schistosomiasis is considerably underestimated.

4.1. S. japonicum

The first reports of *S. japonicum* in P.R. China and the Philippines occurred around the same time in the early 1900s [171,172] and the epidemiology of the disease is similar in the two countries. The presence of the disease in Indonesia was first reported about three decades later, with an autochthonous infection in a 35-year-old male suffering from chronic schistosomiasis resulting in his death in 1937 [128].

4.1.1. Japan

As indicated in the species name, *S. japonicum* was once found in Japan, the last reported human case was in 1977, and elimination of schistosomiasis was declared in 1996 [17]. There were a number of endemic areas in Japan pre-elimination, including Kofu basin, Fukuoka, and Saga prefectures, which appeared to have had the highest prevalence [173]. Due to a successful control program, transmission of the parasite no longer occurs there, although the requisite intermediate host snail species, *Oncomelania nosphora*, is still present [113]. In addition to the control initiatives implemented, modernization and socioeconomic development had a large impact on elimination of this parasite in Japan. Elimination of schistosomiasis in Japan occurred pre-praziquantel and the available drug at the time, stibnal, caused severe adverse events, which resulted in low treatment compliance. Thus, most control efforts focused on targetting the snail intermediate hosts and preventing transmission to humans.

Environmental modification in the form of concreting canals, where the *Oncomelania* snails bred, began in 1938 and was the primary method used [17]. In addition, the Japanese government purchased and buried snails from people in the endemic areas. Mollusciciding using lime, which proved to be inefficient; calcium cyanamide, which proved to be more efficient; and later Na-PCP were trialed. The use of Na-PCP was eventually stopped after 13 years due to its environmental toxicity. Hot water and flamethrowers were also used to kill snails, and proved effective in small areas. In addition, geese and firefly larvae were released into endemic fields to eat snails, although these measures proved unsuccessful [129]. Land use was changed, with increased urbanization meaning that many paddy fields were converted to housing, and in other areas, crops changed from rice to fruit trees; this precluded the use of flood watering and thus no longer provided areas for snail breeding [17]. Education of farmers to prevent the use of "night soil" as fertilizer was also performed, thus limiting environmental contamination with schistosome eggs from human feces. Bovines were replaced with horses, which can act as reservoir hosts but are less efficient transmitters, and other potential reservoirs such as wild populations of mice and dogs were controlled.

4.1.2. P.R. China

In P.R. China, *S. japonicum* is predominantly found in areas along the middle and upper reaches of the Yangtze River Valley in the southern part of the country where the climate and environment are highly suitable for the propagation of *Oncomelania* snails. Endemic regions are concentrated in the lake regions and in the mountainous region in the western part of the country [131]. Until relatively recently, *S. japonicum* was endemic in 12 provinces, but due to political will and sustained efforts, primarily through snail control and preventive chemotherapy, five provinces have achieved transmission interruption. Of the remaining seven provinces, four (Sichuan, Yunnan, Jiangsu, and Hubei) achieved transmission control (prevalence <5% in humans and animals) by 2014, whereas Anhui, Jiangxi, and Hunan are still in the infection control stage (prevalence <1% in humans and animals) [174,175]. In 2012, an estimated 800,000 people were infected and 65 million people considered at risk [24]. In 2016, the number of reported cases had dropped considerably and was just over 77,000 [17]. Current human prevalence in most endemic villages is between 1% and 3% but among the high-risk population, such as those who have extensive contact with water, infection levels may still exceed 10% [17].

Control approaches in P.R. China have been extensive due to the strong commitment by the national government. Funds from a 10-year World Bank Loan Project (WBLP) implemented in the 1990s [176] were put toward control and prevention strategies for schistosomiasis, including preventive chemotherapy, snail control, and WASH interventions. The mainstay of schistosomiasis control is preventive chemotherapy with praziquantel. In P.R. China, preventive chemotherapy is primarily targeted at fishermen and boat people living within half a kilometer of schistosomiasis-infested water bodies and is administered biannually. Treatment in other high-risk populations is selective, based on the extent of water contact [16]. P.R. China is the only endemic country that also practices mass drug administration for bovines, which are treated annually. The government is replacing animals used for farming with tractors and is removing bovines [16,89,100]. Mollusciciding occurs annually and usually coincides with the onset of the transmission seasons. Ecological methods of snail control have been used in P.R. China, such as changing farming practices, submerging snail habitats, and placing black plastic film over banks post-mollusciciding [17]. P.R. China's efforts to improve WASH began during the third phase of their national schistosomiasis control program (initiated in 2004), which focused on an integrated approach to control transmission [177]. WASH interventions mainly center on fishermen and boatmen [178] in the Poyang and Donting Lake regions and include supplying tap water and stool containers and building latrines close to boat anchoring points [159,179]. Health education has been an integral component of P.R. China's schistosomiasis control program since its inception in the 1950s [164].

4.1.3. Philippines

In the Philippines, *S. japonicum* is distributed throughout all three major island groups (Luzon, Mindanao, and Visayas), although the majority of cases occur in Mindanao and the Visayas [87,180] (Figure 1). Schistosomiasis is currently endemic in 28 of the country's 80 provinces, mostly in Mindanao, with more than 12 million people estimated to be at risk and 2.5 million directly exposed [76]. Distribution of *S. japonicum* is more widespread in the Visayas compared to Luzon and Mindanao, where it is more focal [87]. Among endemic provinces, 10 are considered highly endemic (prevalence >5%), six moderately (1–4.9%), and 12 low or close to elimination levels (<1%) [76]. Prevalence studies conducted since 2000 indicate infection levels vary based on location. In 2000, Acosta et al. reported a prevalence of 60% in adolescent and young adults (aged 15–30 years) in three villages in Leyte [181]. In 2005, a cross-sectional survey in Western Samar Province reported a prevalence range of 0.7% to 47% [182], which is similar to that reported by Ross et al. in 2012 from Northern Samar [96].

A nationwide prevalence study in 2015 identified infection levels >5% in one province, 1–5% in 12 provinces, and less than 1% in 14 provinces [87]. However, a diagnostic study conducted in 2014 in Northern Samar compared the prevalence determined using the gold standard KK method against qPCR results and found a discrepancy of nearly 70% (23% for KK vs. 90% for qPCR) [64], demonstrating the need for more sensitive diagnostic methods to determine true prevalence.

The Philippines experienced a period of success in controlling schistosomiasis after the launch of the Philippines Health Development Project (PHDP) in 1991, which was financially backed by a World Bank loan. The focus shifted to active case finding and mass drug administration with praziquantel; WASH interventions and snail control were included as additional measures. Drug coverage of the target population was reported to be 100% during the 1990s [76]. However, the prevalence of *S. japonicum* increased after the cessation of the program due to a lack of financial support; inadequate resources from the government also led to a diminished capacity to control schistosomiasis in the Philippines compared to P.R. China, where the government has strongly supported control efforts for over 50 years [17,183,184]. Due to insufficient funds to support the continuation of mass examination and treatment of at-risk populations, the Department of Health in the Philippines moved to targeting only high-prevalence endemic areas with mass drug administration [17,183].

In the Philippines, niclosamide has been banned for use in snail control under the Clean Water Act [17]. So, while mollusciciding has been performed in the past, special exemption would be needed for future use. A combination of methods employed in Japan was trialed on Bohol Island in the Philippines, focusing on grass cutting in swamps, followed by mollusciciding. Land reformation from swamps to rice fields, combined with mass drug administration, was effective in reducing prevalence to less than 1% [17]. In general, snail control measures successfully used in P.R. China have not been applicable to the Philippines due to differences in ecology and habitat of the local intermediate host snails [11]. Historically, environmental modification has been used in the Philippines to decrease snail habitats [127,185,186]. This rarely occurs now, and the mainstay of control in the Philippines is preventive chemotherapy with praziquantel [187]; yet, there is low compliance in taking the drug due to a variety of reasons, such as poor community engagement and fear of adverse events, which reduces the effectiveness of this intervention [82,188–191]. A cross-sectional survey undertaken in 2015 in Northern Samar, an area with high prevalence of schistosomiasis, reported treatment coverage of only 27% [28,190].

The success of P.R. China's efforts since after the launch of the WBLP compared to the Philippines is largely attributable to the Chinese targeting both human and animals for chemotherapy as opposed to humans only in the Philippines, which ultimately proved to be far less effective [183]. The Philippines is currently undertaking measures to address the issue of *S. japonicum* infection in animals by strengthening veterinary health teams in priority areas through capacity building and operational research and moving toward implementation of WASH programs, as outlined during the 17th Meeting of the Regional Program Review Group on Neglected Tropical Diseases in the Western Pacific (175). These efforts are laudable and it can be anticipated that WASH will feature more prominently in the Philippines than in the past [187]. Lessons from early efforts (before the advent and wide use of praziquantel) to improve sanitation should be considered [82,96].

4.1.4. Indonesia

In contrast to P.R. China and the Philippines, schistosomiasis in Indonesia is endemic in three comparatively small, isolated highland regions surrounding Lore Lindu National Park in central Sulawesi. These areas include marshes around Lake Lindu, particularly in the villages of Anca, Langko, Tomado, and Puro'o; Napu Valley [11] located 30–50 km southeast of Lake Lindu; and the more recently identified focus of Bada Valley [95]. Although the prevalence of *S. japonicum* has fluctuated over the last decade, prevalence tends to be higher in Napu Valley and overall appears to demonstrate an upward trend. Up to 2005, control efforts had decreased prevalence from 37% to 1% or less in Napu and Lindu valleys, but in the period from 2008 to 2011, prevalence varied between 0.3%

and 4.8% in Napu and 0.8% to 3.2% in Lindu [95]. When Badu was first recognized as a new endemic area in 2008, prevalence was 0.5%, which later increased to 5.9% in 2010 [122].

Schistosomiasis control strategies set by the National Objectives for Health (NOH) directive for 2011–2016 varied based on the degree of endemicity, but overall took a multifaceted approach. Control objectives included mass drug administration coverage of 85% of the entire population in high endemic areas, active selective treatment in moderate endemic areas, and passive selective treatment in low endemic areas. Preventive chemotherapy has been supplemented with strategies that also focused on treating domestic animals, snail control, health education, improving water, and sanitation, and monitoring and evaluation and capacity building [76] in an effort to meet the 2020 elimination goal set by the Indonesian Ministry of Health [192]. Although Indonesia has made great strides in reducing the prevalence of schistosomiasis, control and prevention efforts have been inhibited by a lack of coordination and collaboration between the Ministry of Health and other ministries, as well as insufficient financial and human resources. The lack of funds dedicated to surveillance and control by the Ministry of Health may, in part, be due to the limited area and population affected by the disease or as a result of the decentralized and autonomous government system in Indonesia [193].

4.1.5. Myanmar

Myanmar has been previously thought to be non-endemic for schistosomiasis, although there have been some historical unconfirmed reports of the presence of both *S. japonicum* and *S. mekongi* [16]. Recent studies have indicated that schistosomiasis has been emerging/re-emerging around Lake Inlay in central Myanmar [194]. Serological analysis of patient samples between 2012 and 2013 identified a prevalence of 23.8% (n = 315), whereas 302 cases were identified between 2016 and 2018 [16,195]. The WHO has been involved in supporting efforts to diagnose and treat infections in Myanmar, providing praziquantel, KK thick smear equipment, and urine tests [194]. Recently, molecular diagnostics determined a *S. mekongi* prevalence of 3.9% (n = 205) in the Bago Region of Myanmar [196,197].

A recent schistosomiasis outbreak occurred in Rakhine State with >400 confirmed cases and >800 suspected cases as of August 2018 [143]. Rakhine is the site of unrest due to political strife with Rohingya refugees and is also one of the poorest in terms of socioeconomic status in Myanmar, with a high number of households without access to clean water and proper sanitation [198]. This outbreak is occurring outside the area where schistosomiasis has previously been identified (Figure 1B). A technical team from the WHO and Myanmar Health and Sports Ministry have been to the area and suggested a special control team to carry out activities aimed at treating and preventing infection including health education in schools, diagnostics, treatment, and snail mapping [143]. The schistosome and snail species responsible for this current outbreak have not yet been identified.

It is not immediately clear from published reports if *S. japonicum* has been definitively diagnosed in Myanmar. Until the status of schistosomiasis is further clarified, ideally by molecular methods with which *S. mekongi* has already been confirmed, we rely on early reports that suggest both species are present [196,197].

4.2. *S. mekongi*

4.2.1. Cambodia

The first case of schistosomiasis occurring in Cambodia was identified in 1968 in Eastern Cambodia and was seemingly confined to Vietnamese fishermen living in raft houses. Prevalence among children was higher (14–22%) than in adults (7–10%) [199]. At present, there are an estimated 80,000 people at risk of infection in Cambodia [142].

Control of schistosomiasis in Cambodia has been impacted by political unrest and upheaval through the 1970s and 1980s [200]. It was not until 1993 that control programs targeting schistosomiasis commenced. At the onset of the control program, drug compliance was low due to the treatment not being free. Subsequently, mass drug administration was provided free of charge [200]. This approach has been the mainstay of control in Cambodia for the last 20 years and, in 2016, the schistosome prevalence determined by the KK thick smear technique was 0%. In addition to preventive chemotherapy, CL-WASH programs were implemented in endemic villages in 2016. Facilitators were initially trained in CL-WASH, who then helped lead community-based training when education on schistosomiasis transmission was provided and linked to sanitation and hygiene habitats. In each community, CL-WASH teams, composed of volunteers from each community as well as a facilitator, conducted surveys on village households to determine the provision of sanitation and the level of malnutrition [201]. Initial surveys found that >60% of households did not have toilets and many still practiced open defecation. Survey results were mapped and presented to the community members who discussed how their behaviors led to schistosome infection (and other parasitic worm and intestinal protozoa infections) and how infection could be prevented with the development and implementation of CL-WASH plans. These plans included the building and use of latrines in villages [201]. Elimination was planned for 2017, although this was reliant on more sensitive diagnostic tools being employed, an increase in sentinel site surveillance, and increased use of CL-WASH in endemic areas [202].

4.2.2. Thailand

The first case of *S. mekongi*, described as a *S. japonicum*-like infection, was reported in 1950 in Thailand [199]. This 'patient zero' was a Thai native and thus it is likely this was an autochthonous case. Further investigations identified an endemic region and susceptible intermediate host snail in southern Thailand. In 1964, further cases were identified in northern Thailand. Animals including water buffalo, cattle, dogs, cats, pigs, and rats were also surveyed in the endemic areas but none were positive at that time [199]. Thailand is currently in transmission interruption, waiting on investigation and ratification by the WHO [203].

4.2.3. Lao PDR

Lao PDR followed Thailand in the identification of *S. mekongi* in 1957 in a patient who had been living in Paris for nine years, but had spent the first nine years of life in Lao PDR [34,199]. This observation indicated that the adult worms can live for many years. The patient was admitted with what was thought to be cirrhosis of the liver; a liver biopsy revealed the presence of a *S. japonicum*-like egg. It was not until 1966 that a second case was identified in Lao PDR and, in 1969, an epidemiological survey determined a prevalence of 14.4% (n = 72) on Khong Island. As with *S. japonicum*, hepatosplenomegaly was associated with infection [34,199,204]. On Khong Island, the parasite was first found in animals, specifically in a dog [34].

A study examining the prevalence of a range of parasites in islands of the Mekong in Lao PDR performed in 2011 determined a prevalence of 22.2% (n = 994) in humans and 14.7% (n = 68) in dogs for *S. mekongi* [123]. The infected snail prevalence was very low with 0.01% (n = 29,583) of collected snails being positive [123]. More recent cases have been identified in returning travelers who visited these historically endemic areas, including a Belgian visitor to Khong Island in 2013 and a French woman who was exposed to freshwater habitats in southern Lao PDR [205,206]. These cases indicate that transmission is ongoing.

Mass drug administration in Lao PDR was first carried out yearly from 1989 to 1998. In the first year of the program, only selective chemotherapy was practiced but this was expanded in subsequent years [200]. Before the onset of this preventive chemotherapy-based program, there were an estimated 11,000 cases with a further 60,000 deemed to be at risk of infection. By 1999, the prevalence was significantly reduced, but after cessation of yearly mass drug administration, the prevalence rebounded to pre-intervention levels. Hence, mass drug administration was recommenced in 2007 with financial support from WHO [202]. CL-WASH was implemented in 10 villages in 2016, to be expanded to all endemic villages by 2020 [202].

4.2.4. Myanmar

See Section 4.1.5. for Myanmar under *S. japonicum*.

4.3. *S. malayensis*

Malaysia

Schistosomiasis resembling *S. japonicum* was first identified in Malaysia in 1973 during an autopsy [199]. Previous schistosome infections identified in Malaysia were *S. japonicum* in foreign nationals from P.R. China and Singapore [207]. A review of autopsy materials between 1967 and 1975 uncovered a further nine cases of *S. japonicum*-malaysia (later classified as *S. malayensis* in 1988) [199,207]. No animal infections, snail hosts, or new human cases in the areas that the infected deceased came from could be identified [199]. The strain that caused schistosomiasis in these cases was thought to be different from the Mekong schistosome [199], and likely represents the first case of *S. malayensis*.

Until 1978, all cases of *S. malayensis* were identified in patients who were deceased with schistosomiasis identified in autopsies, although not as the reported cause of death [207,208]. In general, cases of *S. malayensis* have been aboriginal Malaysians (Orang Asli) living in rural areas and patients were either previously or concurrently co-infected with other infectious diseases. The first case identified in a living patient occurred in Selangor State and the patient presented with hepatosplenomegaly [207,208].

In the meantime, *S. malayensis* has only been recorded sporadically in humans, with few recent accounts of infected individuals. The most recent identification of infection in humans was reported in a pathology report of an individual in 2011 [209]. In this case, histology slides of the liver identified liver granulomas, although schistosomiasis had not been diagnosed prior to the death of the patient [209].

5. Concluding Remarks

Multi-component, intersectoral, and integrated control approaches provide a promising path forward for the elimination of schistosomiasis in Asia. Behavioral changes that prevent infection, such as avoiding the practice of open defecation and contact of open freshwater bodies in endemic areas, are necessary. However, without accompanying infrastructure, such as toilets provided in WASH programs, these behaviors will continue. Combined with chemotherapy of both humans and reservoir hosts (e.g., water buffalo), snail control, animal vaccination, health education, and WASH targeting multiple points in the schistosome life cycle will significantly impact the prevalence and re-infection of schistosomiasis. The success achieved in P.R. China in schistosomiasis control and elimination is due to the commitment and support of the Chinese government, including the removal of water buffalo—a major reservoir host in P.R. China—from endemic areas, thus effectively removing them from the transmission cycle. Without such governmental support, sustaining control programs is difficult, particularly those that include more than preventive chemotherapy and require considerable resources to implement, such as required for CL-WASH. There is a niche role for health education that is missing from many schistosomiasis control programs, as knowledge remains limited about the parasite and which behaviors lead to infection in endemic populations.

Limited data are available on prevalence for *S. mekongi*, particularly for *S. malayensis*, the number of human cases, and the role played by animal reservoirs in transmission. Thus, assessing the true importance of schistosomiasis in the countries where these two schistosome species are endemic is difficult.

The true *S. japonicum* prevalence is conceivably underestimated, both in P.R. China and the Philippines, due to the lack of sensitive diagnostics used in control programs. While P.R. China closes in on elimination targets, the use of sensitive diagnostics will be important to determine whether elimination has indeed occurred and to prevent re-bounding infections after treatment and the cessation of the control program. A recent study in P.R. China found a human prevalence <1% by the MHT but 11% by qPCR [63]. Although the majority of the cases detected by qPCR were light-intensity infections, they do present a significant number of individuals who were not identified by widely used diagnostic methods, and who could contribute to resurgence after interventions cease. Limited case finding and prevalence studies have been performed in either country by their national control programs. Another limitation is the lack of snail prevalence surveys performed in many of the schistosome-endemic countries.

Future challenges for schistosomiasis control and elimination include climate change and the potential spread of the disease to new areas [141,210–212]. Europe has, for example, seen a return of autochthonous schistosomiasis cases, although this may initially be due to human migration from endemic areas [213]. Increases in temperature due to climate change will shift the tropical zone, the band in which schistosomiasis currently occurs. In P.R. China, this may lead to a shift in endemic areas further North in the country as the climate changes, and with the implementation of the SNWD project.

Funding: This research received no external funding.

Acknowledgments: The authors would like to thank Andrew Bedford from the Research School of Population Health at the Australian National University, and Tal Bavli and Madeleine Flynn from the Graphics Department at QIMR Berghofer Medical Research Institute for their assistance in producing the figures used in this manuscript.

Conflicts of Interest: The authors declare no conflict of interest.

References

1. McManus, D.P.; Dunne, D.W.; Sacko, M.; Utzinger, J.; Vennervald, B.J.; Zhou, X.N. Schistosomiasis. *Nat. Rev. Dis. Primers* **2018**, *4*, 13. [CrossRef] [PubMed]
2. Boissier, J.; Grech-Angelini, S.; Webster, B.L.; Allienne, J.F.; Huyse, T.; Mas-Coma, S.; Toulza, E.; Barre-Cardi, H.; Rollinson, D.; Kincaid-Smith, J.; et al. Outbreak of urogenital schistosomiasis in Corsica (France): An epidemiological case study. *Lancet Infect. Dis.* **2016**, *16*, 971–979. [CrossRef]
3. Tchuem Tchuente, L.A.; Southgate, V.R.; Jourdane, J.; Webster, B.L.; Vercruysse, J. *Schistosoma intercalatum*: An endangered species in Cameroon? *Trends Parasitol.* **2003**, *19*, 389–393. [CrossRef]
4. Greer, G.J.; Ow-Yang, C.K.; Yong, H.-S. *Schistosoma malayensis* n. sp.: A *Schistosoma japonicum*-complex schistosome from Peninsular Malaysia. *J. Parasitol.* **1988**, *74*, 471–480. [CrossRef] [PubMed]
5. Webster, B.L.; Diaw, O.T.; Seye, M.M.; Webster, J.P.; Rollinson, D. Introgressive hybridization of *Schistosoma haematobium* group species in Senegal: Species barrier break down between ruminant and human schistosomes. *PLoS Negl. Trop. Dis.* **2013**, *7*, e2110. [CrossRef] [PubMed]
6. Leger, E.; Webster, J.P. Hybridizations within the genus *Schistosoma*: Implications for evolution, epidemiology and control. *Parasitology* **2017**, *144*, 65–80. [CrossRef] [PubMed]
7. Kebede, T.; Negash, Y.; Erko, B. *Schistosoma mansoni* infection in human and nonhuman primates in selected areas of Oromia Regional State, Ethiopia. *J. Vector Borne Dis.* **2018**, *55*, 116–121. [CrossRef] [PubMed]
8. Alarcón de Noya, B.; Pointier, J.P.; Colmenares, C.; Théron, A.; Balzan, C.; Cesari, I.M.; González, S.; Noya, O. Natural *Schistosoma mansoni* infection in wild rats from Guadeloupe: Parasitological and immunological aspects. *Acta Trop.* **1997**, *68*, 11–21. [CrossRef]
9. Huyse, T.; Van den Broeck, F.; Hellemans, B.; Volckaert, F.A.M.; Polman, K. Hybridisation between the two major African schistosome species of humans. *Int. J. Parasitol.* **2013**, *43*, 687–689. [CrossRef] [PubMed]
10. Leger, E.; Garba, A.; Hamidou, A.A.; Webster, B.L.; Pennance, T.; Rollinson, D.; Webster, J.P. Introgressed animal schistosomes *Schistosoma curassoni* and *S. bovis* naturally infecting humans. *Emerg. Infect. Dis.* **2016**, *22*, 2212–2214. [CrossRef] [PubMed]
11. Zhou, X.N.; Bergquist, R.; Leonardo, L.; Yang, G.J.; Yang, K.; Sudomo, M.; Olveda, R. Schistosomiasis japonica: Control and research needs. *Adv. Parasitol.* **2010**, *72*, 145–178. [PubMed]
12. Kajihara, N.; Hirayama, K. The war against a regional disease in Japan: A history of the eradication of schistosomiasis japonica. *Trop. Med. Health* **2011**, *39*, 3–44. [PubMed]
13. Ross, A.G.P.; Sleigh, A.C.; Li, Y.; Davis, G.M.; Williams, G.; Jiang, Z.; Feng, Z.; McManus, D.P. Schistosomiasis in the People's Republic of China: Prospects and challenges for the 21st century. *Clin. Microbiol. Rev.* **2001**, *14*, 270–279. [CrossRef] [PubMed]

14. Mao, S.P.; Shao, B.R. Schistosomiasis control in the People's Republic of China. *Am. J. Trop. Med. Hyg.* **1982**, *31*, 92–99. [CrossRef] [PubMed]
15. Rollinson, D.; Knopp, S.; Levitz, S.; Stothard, J.R.; Tchuem Tchuenté, L.-A.; Garba, A.; Mohammed, K.A.; Schur, N.; Person, B.; Colley, D.G.; et al. Time to set the agenda for schistosomiasis elimination. *Acta Trop.* **2013**, *128*, 423–440. [CrossRef] [PubMed]
16. Soe, H.Z.; Oo, C.C.; Myat, T.O.; Maung, N.S. Detection of *Schistosoma* antibodies and exploration of associated factors among local residents around Inlay Lake, Southern Shan State, Myanmar. *Infect. Dis. Poverty* **2017**, *6*, 3. [CrossRef] [PubMed]
17. WHO. Expert consultation to accelerate elimination of Asian schistosomiasis. In *Meeting Report WHO*; WHO: Shanghai, China, 2017.
18. Cameron, T.W.M. A new definitive host for *Schistosoma mansoni*. *J. Helminthol.* **1928**, *6*, 219–222. [CrossRef]
19. He, Y.; Salafsky, B.; Ramaswamy, K. Host-parasite relationships of *Schistosoma japonicum* in mammalian hosts. *Trends Parasitol.* **2001**, *17*, 320–324. [CrossRef]
20. Ho, Y.H.; He, Y.X. On the host specificity of *Schistosoma japonicum*. *Chin. Med. J.* **1963**, *82*, 403–414.
21. Bustinduy, A.L.; King, C.H. 52—Schistosomiasis A2—Farrar, Jeremy. In *Manson's Tropical Infectious Diseases*, 23th ed.; Hotez, P.J., Junghanss, T., Kang, G., Lalloo, D., White, N.J., Eds.; W.B. Saunders: London, UK, 2014.
22. Matsumoto, J.; Muth, S.; Socheat, D.; Matsuda, H. The first reported cases of canine schistosomiasis mekongi in Cambodia. *Southeast Asian J. Trop. Med. Public Health* **2002**, *33*, 458–461. [PubMed]
23. Strandgaard, H.; Johansen, M.V.; Pholsena, K.; Teixayavong, K.; Christensen, N.O. The pig as a host for *Schistosoma mekongi* in Laos. *J. Parasitol.* **2001**, *87*, 708–709. [CrossRef]
24. Blair, D.; van Herwerden, L.; Hirai, H.; Taguchi, T.; Habe, S.; Hirata, M.; Lai, K.; Upatham, S.; Agatsuma, T. Relationships between *Schistosoma malayensis* and other Asian schistosomes deduced from DNA sequences. *Mol. Biochem. Parasitol.* **1997**, *85*, 259–263. [CrossRef]
25. Attwood, S.W.; Cottet, M. Malacological and parasitological surveys along the Xe Bangfai and its tributaries in Khammouane Province, Lao PDR. *Hydroécol. Appl.* **2016**, *19*, 245–270. [CrossRef]
26. CDC. Schistosomiasis Infection. Available online: https://www.cdc.gov/dpdx/schistosomiasis/index.html (accessed on 2 March 2018).
27. Utzinger, J.; N'Goran, E.K.; Caffrey, C.R.; Keiser, J. From innovation to application: Social-ecological context, diagnostics, drugs and integrated control of schistosomiasis. *Acta Trop.* **2011**, *120* (Suppl. 1), S121–S137. [CrossRef] [PubMed]
28. Gordon, C.A.; Acosta, L.P.; Gobert, G.N.; Jiz, M.; Olveda, R.M.; Ross, A.G.; Gray, D.J.; Williams, G.M.; Harn, D.; Yuesheng, L.; et al. High prevalence of *Schistosoma japonicum* and *Fasciola gigantica* in bovines from Northern Samar, the Philippines. *PLoS Negl. Trop. Dis.* **2015**, *9*, e0003108. [CrossRef] [PubMed]
29. Gray, D.J.; Williams, G.M.; Li, Y.; McManus, D.P. Transmission dynamics of *Schistosoma japonicum* in the lakes and marshlands of China. *PLoS ONE* **2008**, *3*, e4058. [CrossRef] [PubMed]
30. Rudge, J.W.; Carabin, H.; Balolong, E.; Tallo, V.; Shrivastava, J.; Lu, D.B.; Basanez, M.G.; Olveda, R.; McGarvey, S.T.; Webster, J.P. Population genetics of *Schistosoma japonicum* within the Philippines suggest high levels of transmission between humans and dogs. *PLoS Negl. Trop. Dis.* **2008**, *2*, e340. [CrossRef] [PubMed]
31. Rudge, J.W.; Lu, D.-B.; Fang, G.-R.; Wang, T.-P.; Basáñez, M.-G.; Webster, J.P. Parasite genetic differentiation by habitat type and host species: Molecular epidemiology of *Schistosoma japonicum* in hilly and marshland areas of Anhui Province, China. *Mol. Ecol.* **2009**, *18*, 2134–2147. [CrossRef] [PubMed]
32. Rudge, J.W.; Webster, J.P.; Lu, D.-B.; Wang, T.-P.; Fang, G.-R.; Basáñez, M.-G. Identifying host species driving transmission of schistosomiasis japonica, a multihost parasite system, in China. *Proc. Natl. Acad. Sci. USA* **2013**, *110*, 11457–11462. [CrossRef] [PubMed]
33. Attwood, S.W.; Fatih, F.A.; Upatham, E.S. DNA-sequence variation among *Schistosoma mekongi* populations and related taxa: Phylogeography and the current distribution of Asian schistosomiasis. *PLoS Negl. Trop. Dis.* **2008**, *2*, e200. [CrossRef] [PubMed]
34. Sornmani, S.; Kitikoon, V.; Thirachantra, S.; Harinasuta, C. Epidemiology of mekong schistosomiasis. *Malacol. Rev.* **1980**, (Suppl. 2), 9–18.
35. Kitikoon, V. Comparison of eggs and miracidia of *Schistosoma mekongi* and *S. japonicum*. *Malacol. Rev.* **1980**, (Suppl. 2), 93–103.
36. Fletcher, M.; Woodruff, D.S.; LoVerde, P.T. Genetic differentiation between *Schistosoma mekongi* and *S. japonicum*: An electrophoretic study. *Malacol. Rev.* **1980**, *2*, 113–122.

37. Ross, A.G.; Vickers, D.; Olds, G.R.; Shah, S.M.; McManus, D.P. Katayama syndrome. *Lancet Infect. Dis.* **2007**, *7*, 218–224. [CrossRef]
38. Gryseels, B. Schistosomiasis. *Infect. Dis. Clin. N. Am.* **2012**, *26*, 383–397. [CrossRef] [PubMed]
39. Gryseels, B.; Polman, K.; Clerinx, J.; Kestens, L. Human schistosomiasis. *Lancet* **2006**, *368*, 1106–1118. [CrossRef]
40. Li, Y.; Ross, A.G.; Hou, X.; Lou, Z.; McManus, D.P. Oriental schistosomiasis with neurological complications: Case report. *Ann. Clin. Microbiol. Antimicrob.* **2011**, *10*, 5. [CrossRef] [PubMed]
41. Kane, C.A.; Most, H. Schistosomiasis of the central nervous system: Experiences in world war II and a review of the literature. *Arch. Neurol. Psychiatry* **1948**, *59*, 141–183. [CrossRef] [PubMed]
42. Ferrari, T.C.A.; Moreira, P.R.R. Neuroschistosomiasis: Clinical symptoms and pathogenesis. *Lancet Neurol.* **2011**, *10*, 853–864. [CrossRef]
43. Liu, H.; Lim, C.C.; Feng, X.; Yao, Z.; Chen, Y.; Sun, H.; Chen, X. MRI in cerebral schistosomiasis: Characteristic nodular enhancement in 33 patients. *Am. J. Roentgenol.* **2008**, *191*, 582–588. [CrossRef] [PubMed]
44. Stecher, C.W.; Sacko, M.; Madsen, H.; Wilson, S.; Wejse, C.; Keita, A.D.; Landoure, A.; Traore, M.S.; Kallestrup, P.; Petersen, E.; et al. Anemia and growth retardation associated with *Schistosoma haematobium* infection in Mali: A possible subtle impact of a neglected tropical disease. *Trans. R. Soc. Trop. Med. Hyg.* **2017**, *111*, 144–153. [CrossRef] [PubMed]
45. WHO. Schistosomiasis: Fact Sheet. Available online: http://www.who.int/mediacentre/factsheets/fs115/en/ (accessed on 20 February 2018).
46. Glinz, D.; Silué, K.D.; Knopp, S.; Lohourignon, L.K.; Yao, K.P.; Steinmann, P.; Rinaldi, L.; Cringoli, G.; N'Goran, E.K.; Utzinger, J. Comparing diagnostic accuracy of Kato-Katz, Koga agar plate, ether-concentration, and FLOTAC for *Schistosoma mansoni* and soil-transmitted helminths. *PLoS Negl. Trop. Dis.* **2010**, *4*, e754. [CrossRef] [PubMed]
47. Habtamu, K.; Degarege, A.; Ye-Ebiyo, Y.; Erko, B. Comparison of the Kato-Katz and FLOTAC techniques for the diagnosis of soil-transmitted helminth infections. *Parasitol. Int.* **2011**, *60*, 398–402. [CrossRef] [PubMed]
48. Cringoli, G. FLOTAC, a novel apparatus for a multivalent faecal egg count technique. *Parassitologica* **2006**, *48*, 381–384.
49. Cringoli, G.; Rinaldi, L.; Maurelli, M.P.; Utzinger, J. FLOTAC: New multivalent techniques for qualitative and quantitative copromicroscopic diagnosis of parasites in animals and humans. *Nat. Protoc.* **2010**, *5*, 503–515. [CrossRef] [PubMed]
50. Xu, B.; Gordon, C.A.; Hu, W.; McManus, D.P.; Chen, H.; Gray, D.J.; Ju, C.; Zeng, X.; Gobert, G.N.; Ge, J.; et al. A novel procedure for precise quantification of *Schistosoma japonicum* eggs in bovine feces. *PLoS Negl. Trop. Dis.* **2012**, *6*, e1885. [CrossRef]
51. Lier, T.; Johansen, M.V.; Hjelmevoll, S.O.; Vennervald, B.J.; Simonsen, G.S. Real-time PCR for detection of low intensity *Schistosoma japonicum* infections in a pig model. *Acta Trop.* **2008**, *105*, 74–80. [CrossRef] [PubMed]
52. Anh, N.T.; Phuong, N.T.; Ha, G.H.; Thu, L.T.; Johansen, M.V.; Murrell, D.K.; Thamsborg, S.M. Evaluation of techniques for detection of small trematode eggs in faeces of domestic animals. *Vet. Parasitol.* **2008**, *156*, 346–349. [CrossRef] [PubMed]
53. Zhu, H.Q.; Xu, J.; Zhu, R.; Cao, C.L.; Bao, Z.P.; Yu, Q.; Zhang, L.J.; Xu, X.L.; Feng, Z.; Guo, J.G. Comparison of the miracidium hatching test and modified Kato-Katz method for detecting *Schistosoma japonicum* in low prevalence areas of China. *Southeast Asian J. Trop. Med. Public Health* **2014**, *45*, 20–25. [PubMed]
54. Jurberg, A.D.; de Oliveira, A.A.; Lenzi, H.L.; Coelho, P.M.Z. A new miracidia hatching device for diagnosing schistosomiasis. *Mem. Inst. Oswaldo Cruz* **2008**, *103*, 112–114. [CrossRef] [PubMed]
55. Xu, J.; Rong, R.; Zhang, H.Q.; Shi, C.J.; Zhu, X.Q.; Xia, C.M. Sensitive and rapid detection of *Schistosoma japonicum* DNA by loop-mediated isothermal amplification (LAMP). *Int. J. Parasitol.* **2010**, *40*, 327–331. [CrossRef] [PubMed]
56. Kumagai, T.; Furushima-Shimogawara, R.; Ohmae, H.; Wang, T.; Lu, S.; Chen, R.; Wen, L.; Ohta, N. Detection of early and single infections of *Schistosoma japonicum* in the intermediate host snail, *Oncomelania hupensis*, by PCR and loop-mediated isothermal amplification (LAMP) assay. *Am. J. Trop. Med. Hyg.* **2010**, *83*, 542–548. [CrossRef] [PubMed]
57. Gordon, C.A.; Gray, D.J.; Gobert, G.N.; McManus, D.P. DNA amplification approaches for the diagnosis of key parasitic helminth infections of humans. *Mol. Cell. Probes* **2011**, *25*, 143–152. [CrossRef] [PubMed]

58. Weerakoon, K.G.; Gobert, G.N.; Cai, P.; McManus, D.P. Advances in the diagnosis of human schistosomiasis. *Clin. Microbiol. Rev.* **2015**, *28*, 939–967. [CrossRef] [PubMed]
59. Gobert, G.N.; Chai, M.; Duke, M.; McManus, D.P. Copro-PCR based detection of *Schistosoma* eggs using mitochondrial DNA markers. *Mol. Cell. Probes* **2005**, *19*, 250–254. [CrossRef] [PubMed]
60. Gordon, C.A.; Acosta, L.P.; Gray, D.J.; Olveda, R.; Jarilla, B.; Gobert, G.N.; Ross, A.G.; McManus, D.P. High prevalence of *Schistosoma japonicum* infection in carabao from Samar province, the Philippines: Implications for transmission and control. *PLoS Negl. Trop. Dis.* **2012**, *6*, e1778. [CrossRef] [PubMed]
61. Lier, T.; Simonsen, G.S.; Haaheim, H.; Hjelmevoll, S.O.; Vennervald, B.J.; Johansen, M.V. Novel real-time PCR for detection of *Schistosoma japonicum* in stool. *Southeast Asian J. Trop. Med. Public Health* **2006**, *37*, 257–264. [PubMed]
62. Lier, T.; Simonsen, G.S.; Wang, T.; Lu, D.; Haukland, H.H.; Vennervald, B.J.; Hegstad, J.; Johansen, M.V. Real-time polymerase chain reaction for detection of low-intensity *Schistosoma japonicum* infections in China. *Am. J. Trop. Med. Hyg.* **2009**, *81*, 428–432. [CrossRef] [PubMed]
63. He, P.; Gordon, C.A.; Williams, G.M.; Yueshang, L.; Wang, Y.; Hu, J.; Gray, D.J.; Ross, A.G.; Harn, D.; McManus, D.P. Real-time PCR diagnosis of *Schistosoma japonicum* in low transmission areas of China. *Infect. Dis. Poverty* **2018**, *7*, 8. [CrossRef] [PubMed]
64. Gordon, C.A.; Acosta, L.P.; Gobert, G.N.; Olveda, R.M.; Ross, A.G.; Williams, G.M.; Gray, D.J.; Harn, D.; Li, Y.; McManus, D.P. Real-time PCR demonstrates high prevalence of *Schistosoma japonicum* in the Philippines: Implications for surveillance and control. *PLoS Negl. Trop. Dis.* **2015**, *9*, e0003483. [CrossRef] [PubMed]
65. Weerakoon, K.G.; Gordon, C.A.; Cai, P.; Gobert, G.N.; Duke, M.; Williams, G.M.; McManus, D.P. A novel duplex ddPCR assay for the diagnosis of schistosomiasis japonica: Proof of concept in an experimental mouse model. *Parasitology* **2017**, *144*, 1005–1015. [CrossRef] [PubMed]
66. Weerakoon, K.G.; Gordon, C.A.; Gobert, G.N.; Cai, P.; McManus, D.P. Optimisation of a droplet digital PCR assay for the diagnosis of *Schistosoma japonicum* infection: A duplex approach with DNA binding dye chemistry. *J. Microbiol. Methods* **2016**, *125*, 19–27. [CrossRef] [PubMed]
67. Weerakoon, K.G.; Gordon, C.A.; Williams, G.M.; Cai, P.; Gobert, G.N.; Olveda, R.M.; Ross, A.G.; Olveda, D.U.; McManus, D.P. Droplet digital PCR diagnosis of human schistosomiasis: Parasite cell-free DNA detection in diverse clinical samples. *J. Infect. Dis.* **2017**, *216*, 1611–1622. [CrossRef] [PubMed]
68. Cai, P.; Weerakoon, K.G.; Mu, Y.; Olveda, D.U.; Piao, X.; Liu, S.; Olveda, R.M.; Chen, Q.; Ross, A.G.; McManus, D.P. A parallel comparison of antigen candidates for development of an optimized serological diagnosis of chistosomiasis japonica in the Philippines. *EBioMedicine* **2017**, *24*, 237–246. [CrossRef] [PubMed]
69. Angeles, J.M.; Goto, Y.; Kirinoki, M.; Asada, M.; Leonardo, L.R.; Rivera, P.T.; Villacorte, E.A.; Inoue, N.; Chigusa, Y.; Kawazu, S. Utilization of ELISA using thioredoxin peroxidase-1 and tandem repeat proteins for diagnosis of *Schistosoma japonicum* infection among water buffaloes. *PLoS Negl. Trop. Dis.* **2012**, *6*, e1800. [CrossRef] [PubMed]
70. Dawson, E.M.; Sousa-Figueiredo, J.C.; Kabatereine, N.B.; Doenhoff, M.J.; Stothard, J.R. Intestinal schistosomiasis in pre school-aged children of Lake Albert, Uganda: Diagnostic accuracy of a rapid test for detection of anti-schistosome antibodies. *Trans. R. Soc. Trop. Med. Hyg.* **2013**, *107*, 639–647. [CrossRef] [PubMed]
71. Lin, D.; Xu, J.; Zhang, Y.; Liu, Y.; Hu, F.; Xu, X.; Li, J.; Gao, Z.; Wu, H.; Kurtis, J.; et al. Evaluation of IgG-ELISA for the diagnosis of *Schistosoma japonicum* in a high prevalence, low intensity endemic area of China. *Acta Trop.* **2008**, *107*, 128–133. [CrossRef] [PubMed]
72. Wang, W.; Li, Y.; Li, H.; Xing, Y.; Qu, G.; Dai, J.; Liang, Y. Immunodiagnostic efficacy of detection of *Schistosoma japonicum* human infections in China: A meta analysis. *Asian Pac. J. Trop. Med.* **2012**, *5*, 15–23. [CrossRef]
73. Hinz, R.; Schwarz, N.G.; Hahn, A.; Frickmann, H. Serological approaches for the diagnosis of schistosomiasis—A review. *Mol. Cell. Probes* **2017**, *31*, 2–21. [CrossRef] [PubMed]
74. Zhou, Y.B.; Zheng, H.M.; Jiang, Q.W. A diagnostic challenge for Schistosomiasis japonica in China: Consequences on praziquantel-based morbidity control. *Parasit. Vectors* **2011**, *4*, 194. [CrossRef] [PubMed]
75. Utzinger, J.; Becker, S.L.; van Lieshout, L.; van Dam, G.J.; Knopp, S. New diagnostic tools in schistosomiasis. *Clin. Microbiol. Infect.* **2015**, *21*, 529–542. [CrossRef] [PubMed]
76. Leonardo, L.; Chigusa, Y.; Kikuchi, M.; Kato-Hayashi, N.; Kawazu, S.I.; Angeles, J.M.; Fontanilla, I.K.; Tabios, I.K.; Moendeg, K.; Goto, Y.; et al. Schistosomiasis in the Philippines: Challenges and some successes in control. *Southeast Asian J. Trop. Med. Public Health* **2016**, *47*, 651–666.

77. Gray, D.J.; Ross, A.G.; Li, Y.; McManus, D.P. Diagnosis and management of schistosomiasis. *Br. Med. J.* **2011**, *342*, d2651. [CrossRef] [PubMed]
78. Utzinger, J.; Keiser, J. Schistosomiasis and soil-transmitted helminthiasis: Common drugs for treatment and control. *Expert Opin. Pharmacother.* **2004**, *5*, 263–285. [CrossRef] [PubMed]
79. Vale, N.; Gouveia, M.J.; Rinaldi, G.; Brindley, P.J.; Gärtner, F.; Correia da Costa, J.M. Praziquantel for schistosomiasis: Single-drug metabolism revisited, mode of action, and resistance. *Antimicrob. Agents Chemother.* **2017**, *61*, e02582-16. [CrossRef] [PubMed]
80. Sabah, A.A.; Fletcher, C.; Webbe, G.; Doenhoff, M.J. *Schistosoma mansoni*: Chemotherapy of infections of different ages. *Exp. Parasitol.* **1986**, *61*, 294–303. [CrossRef]
81. Utzinger, J.; Keiser, J.; Xiao, S.H.; Tanner, M.; Singer, B.H. Combination chemotherapy of schistosomiasis in laboratory studies and clinical trials. *Antimicrob. Agents Chemother.* **2003**, *47*, 1487–1495. [CrossRef] [PubMed]
82. Olveda, D.U.; Li, Y.; Olveda, R.M.; Lam, A.K.; McManus, D.P.; Chau, T.N.; Harn, D.A.; Williams, G.M.; Gray, D.J.; Ross, A.G. Bilharzia in the Philippines: Past, present, and future. *Int. J. Infect. Dis.* **2014**, *18*, 52–56. [CrossRef] [PubMed]
83. Wu, Z.; Shaoji, Z.; Pan, B.; Hu, L.; Wei, R.; Gao, Z.; Li, J.; Uwe, B. Reinfection with *Schistosoma japonicum* after treatment with praziquantel in Poyang Lake Region, China. *Southeast Asian J. Trop. Med. Public Health* **1994**, *25*, 163–169. [PubMed]
84. Wang, W.; Wang, L.; Liang, Y. Susceptibility or resistance of praziquantel in human schistosomiasis: A review. *Parasitol. Res.* **2012**, *111*, 1871–1877. [CrossRef] [PubMed]
85. Cupit, P.M.; Cunningham, C. What is the mechanism of action of praziquantel and how might resistance strike? *Future Med. Chem.* **2015**, *7*, 701–705. [CrossRef] [PubMed]
86. Bergquist, R.; Utzinger, J.; Keiser, J. Controlling schistosomiasis with praziquantel: How much longer without a viable alternative? *Infect. Dis. Poverty* **2017**, *6*, 74. [CrossRef] [PubMed]
87. Soares Magalhães, R.J.; Salamat, M.S.; Leonardo, L.; Gray, D.J.; Carabin, H.; Halton, K.; McManus, D.P.; Williams, G.M.; Rivera, P.; Saniel, O.; et al. Geographical distribution of human *Schistosoma japonicum* infection in The Philippines: Tools to support disease control and further elimination. *Int. J. Parasitol.* **2014**, *44*, 977–984. [CrossRef] [PubMed]
88. Leonardo, L.R.; Rivera, P.; Saniel, O.; Villacorte, E.; Crisostomo, B.; Hernandez, L.; Baquilod, M.; Erce, E.; Martinez, R.; Velayudhan, R. Prevalence survey of schistosomiasis in Mindanao and the Visayas, the Philippines. *Parasitol. Int.* **2008**, *57*, 246–251. [CrossRef] [PubMed]
89. Gray, D.J.; Williams, G.M.; Li, Y.; Chen, H.; Forsyth, S.J.; Li, R.S.; Barnett, A.G.; Guo, J.; Ross, A.G.; Feng, Z.; et al. A cluster-randomised intervention trial against *Schistosoma japonicum* in the People's Republic of China: Bovine and human transmission. *PLoS ONE* **2009**, *4*, e5900. [CrossRef] [PubMed]
90. Gray, D.J.; Williams, G.M.; Li, Y.; Chen, H.; Li, R.S.; Forsyth, S.J.; Barnett, A.G.; Guo, J.; Feng, Z.; McManus, D.P. A cluster-randomized bovine intervention trial against *Schistosoma japonicum* in the People's Republic of China: Design and baseline results. *Am. J. Trop. Med. Hyg.* **2007**, *77*, 866–874. [CrossRef] [PubMed]
91. Gray, D.J.; Williams, G.M.; Li, Y.S.; Chen, H.G.; Forsyth, S.; Li, R.; Barnett, A.; Guo, J.G.; Ross, A.; Feng, Z.; et al. The role of bovines in human *Schistosoma japonicum* infection in the People's Republic China. *Am. J. Trop. Med. Hyg.* **2009**, *81*, 1046.
92. Carlton, E.J.; Bates, M.N.; Zhong, B.; Seto, E.Y.; Spear, R.C. Evaluation of mammalian and intermediate host surveillance methods for detecting schistosomiasis reemergence in southwest China. *PLoS Negl. Trop. Dis.* **2011**, *5*, e987. [CrossRef] [PubMed]
93. Van Dorssen, C.F.; Gordon, C.A.; Li, Y.; Williams, G.M.; Wang, Y.; Luo, Z.; Gobert, G.N.; You, H.; McManus, D.P.; Gray, D.J. Rodents, goats and dogs—Their potential roles in the transmission of schistosomiasis in China. *Parasitology* **2017**, *144*, 1633–1642. [CrossRef] [PubMed]
94. Angeles, J.M.; Leonardo, L.R.; Goto, Y.; Kirinoki, M.; Villacorte, E.A.; Hakimi, H.; Moendeg, K.J.; Lee, S.; Rivera, P.T.; Inoue, N.; et al. Water buffalo as sentinel animals for schistosomiasis surveillance. *Bull. World Health Organ.* **2015**, *93*, 511–512. [CrossRef] [PubMed]
95. Satrija, F.; Ridwan, Y.; Jastal, S.; Rauf, A. Current status of schistosomiasis in Indonesia. *Acta Trop.* **2015**, *141*, 349–353. [CrossRef] [PubMed]
96. Ross, A.G.P.; Olveda, R.M.; Acosta, L.; Harn, D.A.; Chy, D.; Yuesheng, L.; Gray, D.J.; Gordon, C.A.; McManus, D.P.; Williams, G.M. Road to the elimination of schistosomiasis from Asia: The journey is far from over. *Microbes Infect.* **2013**, *15*, 858–865. [CrossRef] [PubMed]

97. Wang, T.; Zhang, S.; Wu, W.; Zhang, G.; Lu, D.; Ørnbjerg, N.; Johansen, M.V. Treatment and reinfection of water buffaloes and cattle infected with *Schistosoma japonicum* in Yangtze river valley, Anhui province, China. *J. Parasitol.* **2006**, *92*, 1088–1091. [CrossRef] [PubMed]
98. Yang, J.; Fu, Z.; Feng, X.; Shi, Y.; Yuan, C.; Liu, J.; Hong, Y.; Li, H.; Lu, K.; Lin, J. Comparison of worm development and host immune responses in natural hosts of *Schistosoma japonicum*, yellow cattle and water buffalo. *BMC Vet. Res.* **2012**, *8*, 25. [CrossRef] [PubMed]
99. Li, Y.-S.; McManus, D.P.; Lin, D.-D.; Williams, G.M.; Harn, D.A.; Ross, A.G.; Feng, Z.; Gray, D.J. The *Schistosoma japonicum* self-cure phenomenon in water buffaloes: Potential impact on the control and elimination of schistosomiasis in China. *Int. J. Parasitol.* **2014**, *44*, 167–171. [CrossRef] [PubMed]
100. Guo, J.; Li, Y.; Gray, D.J.; Hu, G.; Chen, H.; Davis, G.M.; Sleigh, A.C.; Feng, Z.; McManus, D.P.; Williams, G.M. A drug-based intervention study on the importance of buffaloes for human *Schistosoma japonicum* infection around Poyang Lake, People's Republic of China. *Am. J. Trop. Med. Hyg.* **2006**, *74*, 335–341. [CrossRef] [PubMed]
101. Zhou, Y.-B.; Liang, S.; Chen, G.-X.; Rea, C.; He, Z.-G.; Zhang, Z.-J.; Wei, J.-G.; Zhao, G.-M.; Jiang, Q.-W. An integrated strategy for transmission control of *Schistosoma japonicum* in a marshland area of China: Findings from a five-year longitudinal survey and mathematical modeling. *Am. J. Trop. Med. Hyg.* **2011**, *85*, 83–88. [CrossRef] [PubMed]
102. Liang, S.; Yang, C.; Zhong, B.; Qiu, D. Re-emerging schistosomiasis in hilly and mountainous areas of Sichuan, China. *Bull. World Health Organ.* **2006**, *84*, 139–144. [CrossRef] [PubMed]
103. WHO. NTD, WASH, Animal Health, Nutrition and Education Are Joining Forces to Eliminate Schistosomiasis in Mekong Region. Available online: http://www.wpro.who.int/mvp/ntd/ntd_wash/en/ (accessed on 12 September 2018).
104. Chen, S.B.; Ai, L.; Hu, W.; Xu, J.; Bergquist, R.; Qin, Z.Q.; Chen, J.H. New anti-*Schistosoma* approaches in the People's Republic of China: Development of diagnostics, vaccines and other new techniques belonging to the 'omics' group. *Adv. Parasitol.* **2016**, *92*, 385–408. [PubMed]
105. Gray, D.J.; Li, Y.S.; Williams, G.M.; Zhao, Z.Y.; Harn, D.A.; Li, S.M.; Ren, M.Y.; Feng, Z.; Guo, F.Y.; Guo, J.G.; et al. A multi-component integrated approach for the elimination of schistosomiasis in the People's Republic of China: Design and baseline results of a 4-year cluster-randomised intervention trial. *Int. J. Parasitol.* **2014**, *44*, 659–668. [CrossRef] [PubMed]
106. Inobaya, M.T.; Olveda, R.M.; Chau, T.N.P.; Olveda, D.U.; Ross, A.G.P. Prevention and control of schistosomiasis: A current perspective. *Res. Rep. Trop. Med.* **2014**, *2014*, 65–75. [PubMed]
107. McManus, D.P.; Loukas, A. Current status of vaccines for schistosomiasis. *Clin. Microbiol. Rev.* **2008**, *21*, 225–242. [CrossRef] [PubMed]
108. Tebeje, B.M.; Harvie, M.; You, H.; Loukas, A.; McManus, D.P. Schistosomiasis vaccines: Where do we stand? *Parasit. Vectors* **2016**, *9*, 528. [CrossRef] [PubMed]
109. Da'dara, A.A.; Li, Y.S.; Xiong, T.; Zhou, J.; Williams, G.M.; McManus, D.P.; Feng, Z.; Yu, X.L.; Gray, D.J.; Harn, D.A. DNA-based vaccines protect against zoonotic schistosomiasis in water buffalo. *Vaccine* **2008**, *26*, 3617–3625. [CrossRef] [PubMed]
110. Williams, G.; Sleigh, A.C.; Li, Y.; Feng, Z.; Davis, G.M.; Chen, H.; Ross, A.G.P.; Bergquist, R.; McManus, D.P. Mathematical modelling of schistosomiasis japonica: Comparison of control strategies in the People's Republic of China. *Acta Trop.* **2002**, *82*, 253–262. [CrossRef]
111. He, Y.; Guo, Y.; Ni, C.; Xia, F.; Liu, H.; Yu, Q. Compatibility between *Onomelania hupensis* and different isolates of *Schistosoma japonicum* in China. *Southeast Asian J. Trop. Med. Public Health* **1991**, *22*, 245–254. [PubMed]
112. Wang, X.Q.; Mao, S.P. Comparison of morphology, pathogenicity and drug response among three isolates of *Schistosoma japonicum* in the mainland of China. *Ann. Parasitol. Hum. Comp.* **1989**, *64*, 110–119. [CrossRef] [PubMed]
113. Kirinoki, M.; Hu, M.; Yokoi, H.; Kawai, S.; Terrado, R.; Ilagan, E.; Chigusa, Y.; Sasaki, Y.; Matsuda, H. Comparative studies on susceptibilities of two different Japanese isolates of *Oncomelania nosophora* to three strains of *Schistosoma japonicum* originating from Japan, China, and the Philippines. *Parasitology* **2005**, *130*, 531–537. [CrossRef] [PubMed]
114. Zhao, Q.P.; Jiang, M.S.; Littlewood, D.T.; Nie, P. Distinct genetic diversity of *Oncomelania hupensis*, intermediate host of *Schistosoma japonicum* in mainland China as revealed by ITS sequences. *PLoS Negl. Trop. Dis.* **2010**, *4*, e611. [CrossRef] [PubMed]

115. Guan, W.; Li, S.Z.; Abe, E.M.; Webster, B.L.; Rollinson, D.; Zhou, X.N. The genetic diversity and geographical separation study of *Oncomelania hupensis* populations in mainland China using microsatellite loci. *Parasit. Vectors* **2016**, *9*, 28. [CrossRef] [PubMed]
116. Li, S.Z.; Wang, Y.X.; Yang, K.; Liu, Q.; Wang, Q.; Zhang, Y.; Wu, X.H.; Guo, J.G.; Bergquist, R.; Zhou, X.N. Landscape genetics: The correlation of spatial and genetic distances of *Oncomelania hupensis*, the intermediate host snail of *Schistosoma japonicum* in mainland China. *Geospat. Health* **2009**, *3*, 221–231. [CrossRef] [PubMed]
117. Sun, L.P.; Wang, W.; Zuo, Y.P.; Zhang, Z.Q.; Hong, Q.B.; Yang, G.J.; Zhu, H.R.; Liang, Y.S.; Yang, H.T. An integrated environmental improvement of marshlands: Impact on control and elimination of schistosomiasis in marshland regions along the Yangtze River, China. *Infect. Dis. Poverty* **2017**, *6*, 72. [CrossRef] [PubMed]
118. Xia, S.; Xue, J.B.; Zhang, X.; Hu, H.H.; Abe, E.M.; Rollinson, D.; Bergquist, R.; Zhou, Y.; Li, S.Z.; Zhou, X.N. Pattern analysis of schistosomiasis prevalence by exploring predictive modeling in Jiangling County, Hubei Province, P.R. China. *Infect. Dis. Poverty* **2017**, *6*, 91. [CrossRef] [PubMed]
119. WHO. *Expert Consultation to Accelerate Elimination of Asian Schistosomiasis, Shanghai, People's Republic of China, 22–23 May 2017: Meeting Report*; WHO Regional Office for the Western Pacific: Manila, Philippines, 2017; p. 18.
120. Knopp, S.; Corstjens, P.L.; Koukounari, A.; Cercamondi, C.I.; Ame, S.M.; Ali, S.M.; de Dood, C.J.; Mohammed, K.A.; Utzinger, J.; Rollinson, D.; et al. Sensitivity and specificity of a urine circulating anodic antigen test for the diagnosis of *Schistosoma haematobium* in low endemic settings. *PLoS Negl. Trop. Dis.* **2015**, *9*, e0003752. [CrossRef] [PubMed]
121. Madsen, H.; Carabin, H.; Balolong, D.; Tallo, V.L.; Olveda, R.; Yuan, M.; McGarvey, S.T. Prevalence of *Schistosoma japonicum* infection of *Oncomelania quadrasi* snail colonies in 50 irrigated and rain-fed villages of Samar Province, the Philippines. *Acta Trop.* **2008**, *105*, 235–241. [CrossRef] [PubMed]
122. Sumarni, S. The new endemic area of *Schistosoma japonicum* in Bada Highland Western Lore subdistrict, District of Poso, Central Sulawesi Province. *Trop. Med. J.* **2011**, *1*, 1–12.
123. Vonghachack, Y.; Odermatt, P.; Taisayyavong, K.; Phounsavath, S.; Akkhavong, K.; Sayasone, S. Transmission of *Opisthorchis viverrini, Schistosoma mekongi* and soil-transmitted helminthes on the Mekong Islands, Southern Lao PDR. *Infect. Dis. Poverty* **2017**, *6*, 131. [CrossRef] [PubMed]
124. Attwood, S.W. Schistosomiasis in the Mekong Region: Epidemiology and phylogeography. *Adv. Parasitol.* **2001**, *50*, 87–152. [PubMed]
125. Attwood, S.W.; Upatham, E.S. Observations on *Neotricula aperta* (Gastropoda: Pomatiopsidae) population densities in Thailand and central Laos: Implications for the spread of Mekong schistosomiasis. *Parasit. Vectors* **2012**, *5*, 126. [CrossRef] [PubMed]
126. Wu, J.Y.; Zhou, Y.B.; Chen, Y.; Liang, S.; Li, L.H.; Zheng, S.B.; Zhu, S.P.; Ren, G.H.; Song, X.X.; Jiang, Q.W. Three Gorges Dam: Impact of water level changes on the density of schistosome-transmitting snail *Oncomelania hupensis* in Dongting Lake area, China. *PLoS Negl. Trop. Dis.* **2015**, *9*, e0003882. [CrossRef] [PubMed]
127. Pesigan, T.P.; Hairston, N.G.; Jauregui, J.J.; Garcia, E.G.; Santos, A.T.; Santos, B.C.; Besa, A.A. Studies on *Schistosoma japonicum* infection in the Philippines. 2. The molluscan host. *Bull. World Health Organ.* **1958**, *18*, 481–578. [PubMed]
128. Garjito, T.A.; Sudomo, M.; Dahlan, M.; Nurwidayati, A. Schistosomiasis in Indonesia: Past and present. *Parasitol. Int.* **2008**, *57*, 277–280. [CrossRef] [PubMed]
129. Minai, M.; Hosaka, Y.; Ohta, N. Historical view of schistosomiasis japonica in Japan: Implementation and evaluation of disease-control strategies in Yamanashi Prefecture. *Parasitol. Int.* **2003**, *52*, 321–326. [CrossRef]
130. Yang, G.-J.; Li, W.; Sun, L.-P.; Wu, F.; Yang, K.; Huang, Y.-X.; Zhou, X.-N. Molluscicidal efficacies of different formulations of niclosamide: Result of meta-analysis of Chinese literature. *Parasit. Vectors* **2010**, *3*, 84. [CrossRef] [PubMed]
131. Zhu, H.R.; Liu, L.; Zhou, X.N.; Yang, G.J. Ecological model to predict potential habitats of *Oncomelania hupensis*, the intermediate host of *Schistosoma japonicum* in the mountainous regions, China. *PLoS Negl. Trop. Dis.* **2015**, *9*, e0004028. [CrossRef] [PubMed]
132. Chen, Z.; Zhou, X.N.; Yang, K.; Wang, X.H.; Yao, Z.Q.; Wang, T.P.; Yang, G.J.; Yang, Y.J.; Zhang, S.Q.; Wang, J.; et al. Strategy formulation for schistosomiasis japonica control in different environmental settings supported by spatial analysis: A case study from China. *Geospat. Health* **2007**, *1*, 223–231. [CrossRef] [PubMed]

133. Hu, Y.; Zhang, Z.; Chen, Y.; Wang, Z.; Gao, J.; Tao, B.; Jiang, Q.; Jiang, Q. Spatial pattern of schistosomiasis in Xingzi, Jiangxi Province, China: The effects of environmental factors. *Parasit. Vectors* **2013**, *6*, 214. [CrossRef] [PubMed]
134. Hu, Y.; Li, R.; Bergquist, R.; Lynn, H.; Gao, F.; Wang, Q.; Zhang, S.; Sun, L.; Zhang, Z.; Jiang, Q. Spatio-temporal transmission and environmental determinants of schistosomiasis japonica in Anhui Province, China. *PLoS Negl. Trop. Dis.* **2015**, *9*, e0003470. [CrossRef] [PubMed]
135. Li, Y.S.; Sleigh, A.C.; Ross, A.G.P.; Williams, G.; Tanner, M.; McManus, D.P. Epidemiology of *Schistosoma japonicum* in China: Morbidity and strategies for control in the Dongting Lake region. *Int. J. Parasitol.* **2000**, *30*, 273–281. [CrossRef]
136. Yang, K.; Li, L.; Huang, Y.; Zhang, J.; Wu, F.; Hang, D.; Steinmann, P.; Liang, Y. Spatio-temporal analysis to identify determinants of *Oncomelania hupensis* infection with *Schistosoma japonicum* in Jiangsu province, China. *Parasit. Vectors* **2013**, *6*, 138. [CrossRef] [PubMed]
137. Zhou, X.N.; Yang, G.J.; Yang, K.; Wang, X.H.; Hong, Q.B.; Sun, L.P.; Malone, J.B.; Kristensen, T.K.; Bergquist, N.R.; Utzinger, J. Potential impact of climate change on schistosomiasis transmission in China. *Am. J. Trop. Med. Hyg.* **2008**, *78*, 188–194. [CrossRef] [PubMed]
138. Li, Y.S.; Raso, G.; Zhao, Z.Y.; He, Y.K.; Ellis, M.K.; McManus, D.P. Large water management projects and schistosomiasis control, Dongting Lake region, China. *Emerg. Infect. Dis.* **2007**, *13*, 973–979. [CrossRef] [PubMed]
139. Gray, D.J.; Thrift, A.P.; Williams, G.M.; Zheng, F.; Li, Y.-S.; Guo, J.; Chen, H.; Wang, T.; Xu, X.J.; Zhu, R.; et al. Five-year longitudinal assessment of the downstream impact on schistosomiasis transmission following closure of the Three Gorges Dam. *PLoS Negl. Trop. Dis.* **2012**, *6*, e1588. [CrossRef]
140. McManus, D.P.; Gray, D.J.; Li, Y.; Feng, Z.; Williams, G.M.; Stewart, D.; Rey-Ladino, J.; Ross, A.G. Schistosomiasis in the People's Republic of China: The era of the Three Gorges Dam. *Clin. Microbiol. Rev.* **2010**, *23*, 442–466. [CrossRef] [PubMed]
141. Zhu, G.; Fan, J.; Peterson, A.T. *Schistosoma japonicum* transmission risk maps at present and under climate change in mainland China. *PLoS Negl. Trop. Dis.* **2017**, *11*, e0006021. [CrossRef] [PubMed]
142. Zhou, X.; Bergquist, R.; Leonardo, L.R.; Olveda, R. Schistosomiasis: The Disease and Its Control. 2008. Available online: https://www.researchgate.net/publication/242285494_Schistosomiasis_The_Disease_and_its_Control (accessed on 7 January 2019).
143. Nyein, N. WHO's Field Visit Reports over 400 Schistosomiasis Cases in Rakhine State. Available online: http://www.moi.gov.mm/moi:eng/?q=news/14/11/2018/id-14720 (accessed on 7 January 2019).
144. Raso, G.; Li, Y.S.; Zhao, Z.Y.; Balen, J.; Williams, G.M.; McManus, D.P. Spatial distribution of human *Schistosoma japonicum* infections in the Dongting Lake Region, China. *PLoS ONE* **2009**, *4*, e6947. [CrossRef] [PubMed]
145. Ziegelbauer, K.; Speich, B.; Mäusezahl, D.; Bos, R.; Keiser, J.; Utzinger, J. Effect of sanitation on soil-transmitted helminth infection: Systematic review and meta-analysis. *PLoS Med.* **2012**, *9*, e1001162. [CrossRef] [PubMed]
146. Strunz, E.C.; Addiss, D.G.; Stocks, M.E.; Ogden, S.; Utzinger, J.; Freeman, M.C. Water, sanitation, hygiene, and soil-transmitted helminth infection: A systematic review and meta-analysis. *PLoS Med.* **2014**, *11*, e1001620. [CrossRef] [PubMed]
147. Campbell, S.J.; Savage, G.B.; Gray, D.J.; Atkinson, J.M.; Magalhães, R.J.S.; Nery, S.V.; McCarthy, J.S.; Velleman, Y.; Wicken, J.H.; Traub, R.J.; et al. Water, sanitation, and hygiene (WASH): A critical component for sustainable soil-transmitted helminth and schistosomiasis control. *PLoS Negl. Trop. Dis.* **2014**, *8*, e2651. [CrossRef] [PubMed]
148. Campbell, S.J.; Biritwum, N.K.; Woods, G.; Velleman, Y.; Fleming, F.; Stothard, J.R. Tailoring water, sanitation, and hygiene (WASH) targets for soil-transmitted helminthiasis and schistosomiasis control. *Trends Parasitol.* **2018**, *34*, 53–63. [CrossRef] [PubMed]
149. WHO. *Sixty Fifth World Health Assembly: Elimination of Schistosimasis*; WHO: Geneva, Switzerland, 2012.
150. Secor, W.E. Water-based interventions for schistosomiasis control. *Pathog. Glob. Health* **2014**, *108*, 246–254. [CrossRef] [PubMed]
151. Grimes, J.E.T.; Croll, D.; Harrison, W.E.; Utzinger, J.; Freeman, M.C.; Templeton, M.R. The roles of water, sanitation and hygiene in reducing schistosomiasis: A review. *Parasit. Vectors* **2015**, *8*, 156. [CrossRef] [PubMed]

152. WHO. Sanitation, Drinking-Water and Health: Achievements and Challenges Ahead. Available online: http://www.who.int/iris/handle/10665/260222 (accessed on 19 October 2018).
153. USAID. Water, Sanitation and Hygiene in Indonesia. Available online: https://www.usaid.gov/actingonthecall/stories/indonesia-wash (accessed on 19 October 2018).
154. UNICEF. Water, Sanitation and Hygiene: Philippines. Available online: https://www.unicef.org/philippines/wes_21334.html (accessed on 19 October 2018).
155. WGF. Goal Wash Project in the Philippines. Available online: http://www.watergovernance.org/resources/goal-wash-project-philippines/ (accessed on 19 October 2018).
156. UN. *Sanitation, Drinking-Water and Hygiene Status Overview: Indonesia*; UN-Water Global Analysis and Assessment of Sanitation and Drinking-Water: Geneva, Switzerland, 2015.
157. Camon, C.B. *Implementation of Water, Sanitation and Hygiene (WASH) in Public Schools: A Citizen Participatory Audit*; Department of Education: Cagayan de Oro City, Philippines, 2017.
158. Chen, L.; Zhong, B.; Xu, J.; Li, R.Z.; Cao, C.L. Health education as an important component in the national schistosomiasis control programme in the People's Republic of China. *Adv. Parasitol.* **2016**, *92*, 307–339. [PubMed]
159. Wang, L.; Chen, H.; Guo, J.; Zeng, X.; Hong, X.; Xiong, J.; Wu, X.; Wang, X.; Wang, L.; Xia, G.; et al. A strategy to control transmission of *Schistosoma japonicum* in China. *N. Engl. J. Med.* **2009**, *360*, 121–128. [CrossRef] [PubMed]
160. Guo, J.G.; Cao, C.L.; Hu, G.H.; Lin, H.; Li, D.; Zhu, R.; Xu, J. The role of 'passive chemotherapy' plus health education for schistosomiasis control in China during maintenance and consolidation phase. *Acta Trop.* **2005**, *96*, 177–183. [CrossRef] [PubMed]
161. Hu, G.H.; Hu, J.; Song, K.Y.; Lin, D.D.; Zhang, J.; Cao, C.L.; Xu, J.; Li, D.; Jiang, W.S. The role of health education and health promotion in the control of schistosomiasis: Experiences from a 12-year intervention study in the Poyang Lake area. *Acta Trop.* **2005**, *96*, 232–241. [CrossRef] [PubMed]
162. Kloos, H. Human behavior, health education and schistosomiasis control: A review. *Soc. Sci. Med.* **1995**, *40*, 1497–1511. [CrossRef]
163. McManus, D.P.; Bieri, F.A.; Li, Y.S.; Williams, G.M.; Yuan, L.P.; Henglin, Y.; Du, Z.W.; Clements, A.C.A.; Steinmann, P.; Raso, G.; et al. Health education and the control of intestinal worm infections in China: A new vision. *Parasit. Vectors* **2014**, *7*, 344. [CrossRef] [PubMed]
164. Zhou, L.Y.; Deng, Y.; Steinmann, P.; Yang, K. The effects of health education on schistosomiasis japonica prevalence and relevant knowledge in the People's Republic of China: A systematic review and meta-analysis. *Parasitol. Int.* **2013**, *62*, 150–156. [CrossRef] [PubMed]
165. Muth, S.; Sayasone, S.; Odermatt-Biays, S.; Phompida, S.; Duong, S.; Odermatt, P. *Schistosoma mekongi* in Cambodia and Lao People's Democratic Republic. *Adv. Parasitol.* **2010**, *72*, 179–203. [PubMed]
166. McManus, D.P.; Gray, D.J.; Ross, A.G.; Williams, G.M.; He, H.B.; Li, Y.S. Schistosomiasis research in the Dongting Lake region and its impact on local and national treatment and control in China. *PLoS Negl. Trop. Dis.* **2011**, *5*, e1053. [CrossRef] [PubMed]
167. Molehin, A.J.; Rojo, J.U.; Siddiqui, S.Z.; Gray, S.A.; Carter, D.; Siddiqui, A.A. Development of a schistosomiasis vaccine. *Expert Rev. Vac.* **2016**, *15*, 619–627. [CrossRef] [PubMed]
168. Rim, H.-J.; Chai, J.-Y.; Min, D.-Y.; Cho, S.; Eom, K.S.; Hong, S.; Sohn, W.; Yong, T.; Deodato, G.; Standgaard, H.; et al. Prevalence of intestinal parasite infections on a national scale among primary schoolchildren in Laos. *Parasitol. Res.* **2003**, *91*, 267–272. [CrossRef] [PubMed]
169. Hu, Y.; Li, S.; Xia, C.; Chen, Y.; Lynn, H.; Zhang, T.; Xiong, C.; Chen, G.; He, Z.; Zhang, Z. Assessment of the national schistosomiasis control program in a typical region along the Yangtze River, China. *Int. J. Parasitol.* **2017**, *47*, 21–29. [CrossRef] [PubMed]
170. Wu, H.; Qin, Y.; Chu, K.; Meng, R.; Liu, Y.; McGarvey, S.T.; Olveda, R.; Acosta, L.P.; Ji, M.; Fernandez, T.; et al. High prevalence of *Schistosoma japonicum* infection in water buffaloes in the Philippines assessed by real-time polymerase chain reaction. *Am. J. Trop. Med. Hyg.* **2010**, *82*, 646–652. [CrossRef] [PubMed]
171. Logan, O.T. A case of dysentery in Hunan province, caused by the trematode, *Schistosoma japonicum*. *Chin. Med. J.* **1905**, *19*, 243–245.
172. Wooley, P.G. The occurrence of *Schistosoma japonicum* Vel Cattol in the Philippines. *Philipp. J. Sci.* **1906**, *1*, 83–90.

173. Okabe, K. *Progress of Medical Parasitology in Japan*; Meguro Parasitology Museum: Tokyo, Japan, 1964; Volume 1.
174. Lei, Z.L.; Zheng, H.; Zhang, L.J.; Zhu, R.; Xu, Z.M.; Xu, J.; Fu, Q.; Wang, Q.; Li, S.Z.; Zhou, X.N. Endemic status of schistosomiasis in People's Republic of China in 2013. *Chin. J. Schistosomiasis Control* **2014**, *26*, 591–597.
175. WHO. *Elimination of Schistosomiasis from Low-Transmission Areas: Report of a WHO Informal Consultation*; WHO: Geneva, Switzerland, 2008.
176. Yuan, H.; Jiagang, G.; Bergquist, R.; Tanner, M.; Xianyi, C.; Huanzeng, W. The 1992–1999 World Bank Schistosomiasis research initiative in China: Outcome and perspectives. *Parasitol. Int.* **2000**, *49*, 195–207. [CrossRef]
177. Collins, C.; Xu, J.; Tang, S. Schistosomiasis control and the health system in P.R. China. *Infect. Dis. Poverty* **2012**, *1*, 8. [CrossRef] [PubMed]
178. Sun, L.P.; Wang, W.; Hong, Q.B.; Li, S.Z.; Liang, Y.S.; Yang, H.T.; Zhou, X.N. Approaches being used in the national schistosomiasis elimination programme in China: A review. *Infect. Dis. Poverty* **2017**, *6*, 55. [CrossRef] [PubMed]
179. Wang, L.D.; Guo, J.G.; Wu, X.H.; Chen, H.G.; Wang, T.P.; Zhu, S.P.; Zhang, Z.H.; Steinmann, P.; Yang, G.J.; Wang, S.P.; et al. China's new strategy to block *Schistosoma japonicum* transmission: Experiences and impact beyond schistosomiasis. *Trop. Med. Int. Health* **2009**, *14*, 1475–1483. [CrossRef] [PubMed]
180. Leonardo, L.R.; Rivera, P.; Saniel, O.; Villacorte, E.; Labanan, M.A.; Crisostomo, B.; Hernandez, L.; Baquilod, M.; Erce, E.; Martinez, R.; et al. A national baseline prevalence survey of schistosomiasis in the Philippines using stratified two-step systematic cluster sampling design. *J. Trop. Med.* **2012**, *2012*, 936128. [CrossRef] [PubMed]
181. Acosta, L.P.; Aligui, G.D.L.; Tiu, W.U.; McManus, D.P.; Olveda, R.M. Immune correlate study on human *Schistosoma japonicum* in a well-defined population in Leyte, Philippines: I. Assessment of 'resistance' versus 'susceptibility' to *S. japonicum* infection. *Acta Trop.* **2002**, *84*, 127–136. [CrossRef]
182. Tarafder, M.R.; Balolong, E., Jr.; Carabin, H.; Bélisle, P.; Tallo, V.; Joseph, L.; Alday, P.; Gonzales, R.O.; Riley, S.; Olveda, R.; et al. A cross-sectional study of the prevalence of intensity of infection with *Schistosoma japonicum* in 50 irrigated and rain-fed villages in Samar Province, the Philippines. *BMC Public Health* **2006**, *6*, 61. [CrossRef] [PubMed]
183. Inobaya, M.T.; Olveda, R.M.; Tallo, V.; McManus, D.P.; Williams, G.M.; Harn, D.A.; Li, Y.; Chau, T.N.P.; Olveda, D.U.; Ross, A.G. Schistosomiasis mass drug administration in the Philippines: Lessons learnt and the global implications. *Microbes Infect.* **2015**, *17*, 6–15. [CrossRef] [PubMed]
184. Xu, J.; Steinman, P.; Maybe, D.; Zhou, X.N.; Lv, S.; Li, S.Z.; Peeling, R. Evolution of the national schistosomiasis control programmes in the People's Republic of China. *Adv. Parasitol.* **2016**, *92*, 1–38. [PubMed]
185. Pesigan, T.P.; Farooq, M.; Hairston, N.G.; Jauregui, J.J.; Garcia, E.G.; Santos, A.T.; Santos, B.C.; Besa, A.A. Studies on *Schistosoma japonicum* infection in the Philippines: 3. Preliminary control experiments. *Bull. World Health Organ.* **1958**, *19*, 223–261. [PubMed]
186. Pesigan, T.P.; Hairston, N.G. The effect of snail control on the prevalence of *Schistosoma japonicum* infection in the Philippines. *Bull. World Health Organ.* **1961**, *25*, 479–482. [PubMed]
187. DOH. Schistosomiasis Control Program. Available online: http://www.doh.gov.ph/content/schistosomiasis-control-program.html (accessed on 1 September 2014).
188. Leonardo, L.R.; Acosta, L.P.; Olveda, R.M.; Aligui, G.D.L. Difficulties and strategies in the control of schistosomiasis in the Philippines. *Acta Trop.* **2002**, *82*, 295–299. [CrossRef]
189. Tallo, V.L.; Carabian, H.; Alday, P.P.; Balolong, E., Jr.; Olveda, R.M.; McGarvey, S.T. Is mass treatment the appropriate schistosomiasis elimination strategy? *Bull. World Health Organ.* **2008**, *86*, 765–771. [CrossRef] [PubMed]
190. Inobaya, M.T.; Chau, T.N.; Ng, S.-K.; MacDougall, C.; Olveda, R.M.; Tallo, V.L.; Landicho, J.M.; Malacad, C.M.; Aligato, M.F.; Guevarra, J.B.; et al. Mass drug administration and the sustainable control of schistosomiasis: An evaluation of treatment compliance in the rural Philippines. *Parasit. Vectors* **2018**, *11*, 441. [CrossRef] [PubMed]
191. Inobaya, M.T.; Chau, T.N.; Ng, S.K.; MacDougall, C.; Olveda, R.M.; Tallo, V.L.; Landicho, J.M.; Malacad, C.M.; Aligato, M.F.; Guevarra, J.R.; et al. Mass drug administration the sustainable control of schistosomiasis: Community health workers are vital for global elimination efforts. *Int. J. Infect. Dis.* **2018**, *66*, 14–21. [CrossRef] [PubMed]

192. WHO. *Neglected Tropical Diseases in Indonesia: An Integrated Plan of Action 2011–2015*; Ministry of Health Indonesia: Jakarta, Indonesia, 2010.
193. Nasution, A. Government Decentralization Program in Indonesia. Available online: https://www.adb.org/publications/government-decentralization-program-indonesia (accessed on 17 September 2018).
194. WHO. *Schistosomiasis: An Emerging Public Health Problem*; WHO: Geneva, Switzerland, 2018.
195. MoH. Freshwater Snail Parasite that Infects about Schistosomiasis Cases Attended the Professional Union. Available online: http://mohs.gov.mm/ (accessed on 12 December 2018).
196. Han, K.; Wai, K.; Htun, M.W.; Aye, K.; Latt, A.; Chi Aung San, N.; Phyo, A.; Xu, J.; Li, S.-Z.; Zhou, X.-N.; et al. Molecular Verification of Schistosoma mekongi Infection in ShweKyin Township; Myanmar, 2017. In Proceedings of the 16th Annual Workshop of Regional Network on Asian Schistosomiasis and other Zoonotic Helminths (RNAS+), Yangon, Myanmar, 26–28 October 2016.
197. Wai, K.T.; Han, K.T.; Oo, T. Intensifying responsiveness towards neglected intestinal helminth infections in a resource-constrained setting. *Trop. Med. Health* **2017**, *45*, 12. [CrossRef] [PubMed]
198. Gupta, S. *Development in Times of Transition: The Socio-Econommic Status of Rakhine State*; Livelihoods and Food Security Trust (LIFT) Fund: Rakhine, Myanmar, 2018.
199. Harinasuta, C. Introduction: Schistosomiasis in Asia. *Malacol. Rev.* **1980**, *2*, 431–438.
200. Urbani, C.; Sinoun, M.; Socheat, D.; Pholsena, K.; Strandgaard, H.; Odermatt, P.; Hatz, C. Epidemiology and control of mekongi schistosomiasis. *Acta Trop.* **2002**, *82*, 157–168. [CrossRef]
201. WHO. Communities Drive Elimination of Schistosomiasis through Improving Water, Sanitation and Hygiene in Cambodia and the Lao People's Democratic Republic. Available online: http://www.wpro.who.int/mvp/ntd/cl_swash/en/ (accessed on 12 September 2018).
202. WHO. *Seventeenth Meeting of the Regional Programme Review Group on Neglected Tropical Diseases in the Western Pacific*; WHO: Manila, Philippines, 2017.
203. IAMAT. Thailand General Health Risks: Schistosomiasis. Available online: https://www.iamat.org/country/thailand/risk/schistosomiasis (accessed on 29 January 2019).
204. Sornmani, S.; Vivatanasesth, P.; Thirachantra, S. Clinical study of Mekong schistosomiasis at Khong Island, Southern Laos. *Malacol. Rev.* **1980**, *7*, 270–281.
205. Campa, P.; Develoux, M.; Belkadi, G.; Magne, D.; Lame, C.; Carayon, M.-J.; Girard, P.-M. Chronic *Schistosoma mekongi* in a traveler—A case report and review of the literature. *J. Travel Med.* **2014**, *21*, 361–363. [CrossRef] [PubMed]
206. Clerinx, J.; Cnops, L.; Huyse, T.; Tannich, E.; Van Esbroeck, M. Diagnostic issues of acute schistosomiasis with *Schistosoma mekongi* in a traveler: A case report. *J. Travel Med.* **2013**, *20*, 322–325. [CrossRef] [PubMed]
207. Chuah, C.; Gobert, G.N.; Latif, B.; Heo, C.C.; Leow, C.Y. Schistosomiasis in Malaysia: A review. *Acta Trop.* **2019**, *190*, 137–143. [CrossRef] [PubMed]
208. Murugasu, R.; Wang, F.; Dissanaike, A.S. *Schistosoma japonicum*-type infection in Malaysia—Report of the first living case. *Trans. R. Soc. Trop. Med. Hyg.* **1978**, *72*, 389–391. [CrossRef]
209. Latif, B.; Heo, C.C.; Razuin, R.; Shamalaa, D.V.; Tappe, D. Autochthonous human schistosomiasis, Malaysia. *Emerg. Infect. Dis.* **2013**, *19*, 1340–1341. [CrossRef] [PubMed]
210. Gordon, C.A.; McManus, D.P.; Jones, M.K.; Gray, D.J.; Gobert, G.N. The increase of exotic zoonotic helminth infections: The impact of urbanization, climate change and globalization. *Adv. Parasitol.* **2016**, *91*, 311–397. [PubMed]
211. McCreesh, N.; Nikulin, G.; Booth, M. Predicting the effects of climate change on *Schistosoma mansoni* transmission in eastern Africa. *Parasit. Vectors* **2015**, *8*, 4. [CrossRef] [PubMed]
212. Stensgaard, A.S.; Vounatsou, P.; Sengupta, M.E.; Utzinger, J. Schistosomes, snails and climate change: Current trends and future expectations. *Acta Trop.* **2019**, *190*, 257–268. [CrossRef] [PubMed]
213. Boissier, J.; Moné, H.; Mitta, G.; Bargues, M.D.; Molyneux, D.; Mas-Coma, S. Schistosomiasis reaches Europe. *Lancet Infect. Dis.* **2015**, *15*, 757–758. [CrossRef]

Tropical Medicine and Infectious Disease

MDPI

Review

Elimination of Schistosomiasis Mekongi from Endemic Areas in Cambodia and the Lao People's Democratic Republic: Current Status and Plans

Virak Khieu [1,*], Somphou Sayasone [2], Sinuon Muth [1], Masashi Kirinoki [3], Sakhone Laymanivong [4], Hiroshi Ohmae [3], Rekol Huy [1], Thipphavanh Chanthapaseuth [5], Aya Yajima [6], Rattanaxay Phetsouvanh [7], Robert Bergquist [8] and Peter Odermatt [8,9]

1 National Center for Parasitology, Entomology and Malaria Control, Ministry of Health, Phnom Penh 12100, Cambodia; sinuonm@gmail.com (S.M.); kolhuy@gmail.com (R.H.)
2 Lao Tropical and Public Health Institute, Vientiane 01030, Laos; somphou.sayasone@yahoo.com
3 School of Medicine, Dokkyo Medical University, Mibu, Shimotsuga, Tochigi 321-0293, Japan; kirinoki@dokkyomed.ac.jp (M.K.); rsa40370@nifty.com (H.O.)
4 Centre for Malariology, Parasitology and Entomology, Vientiane 01000, Laos; sakhone07@gmail.com
5 World Health Organization, Vientiane Office, Vientiane 01160, Laos; chanthapaseutht@who.int
6 World Health Organization, Western Pacific Regional Office, Manila 1000, Philippines; yajimaa@who.int
7 Department of Communicable Disease Control, Ministry of Health, Vientiane 01130, Laos; rattanaxay@gmail.com
8 Department of Epidemiology and Public Health, Swiss Tropical and Public Health Institute, P.O. Box 4002 Basel, Switzerland; robert.bergquist@yahoo.se (R.B.); peter.odermatt@swisstph.ch (P.O.)
9 University of Basel, P.O. Box 4001 Basel, Switzerland
* Correspondence: virak.khieu@gmail.com; Tel.: +855-12-677-244

Received: 23 December 2018; Accepted: 30 January 2019; Published: 7 February 2019

Abstract: The areas endemic for schistosomiasis in the Lao People's Democratic Republic and in Cambodia were first reported 50 and 60 years ago, respectively. However, the causative parasite *Schistosoma mekongi* was not recognized as a separate species until 1978. The infection is distributed along a limited part of the Mekong River, regulated by the focal distribution of the intermediate snail host *Neotricula aperta*. Although more sensitive diagnostics imply a higher figure, the current use of stool examinations suggests that only about 1500 people are presently infected. This well-characterized setting should offer an exemplary potential for the elimination of the disease from its endemic areas; yet, the local topography, reservoir animals, and a dearth of safe water sources make transmission control a challenge. Control activities based on mass drug administration resulted in strong advances, and prevalence was reduced to less than 5% according to stool microscopy. Even so, transmission continues unabated, and the true number of infected people could be as much as 10 times higher than reported. On-going control activities are discussed together with plans for the future.

Keywords: *Schistosoma mekongi*; *Neotricula aperta*; snail; Cambodia; Lao PDR; elimination

1. Historical Background

The parasitic, trematode genus *Schistosoma* puts more than 800 million people in the world's tropical areas at risk, infecting a third of them [1,2]. Six different species of *Schistosoma* can infect humans, each depending on a specific snail species acting as intermediate host. The various endemic areas for the three main schistosome species have long been well-known, with basically *S. mansoni* in Africa and Latin America, *S. haematobium* in Africa, and *S. japonicum* in China and The Philippines (formerly also in Japan).

The adult schistosomes are miniscule worms with a preference for abdominal capillaries of the definitive human host, where they release a large number of eggs. These are excreted with either urine or feces (which route depends on the schistosome species) and infect the intermediate snail host, which releases many cercariae—a later developmental stage—into the water. The parasite's life cycle is completed when the definitive human host comes into contact with water containing schistosome cercariae that can penetrate the human skin. However, large numbers of parasite eggs fail to be excreted and, instead, cause microscopic lesions due to the host immune reactions in various organs, most often the liver. Generally, this leads to a chronic disease with comparatively low direct mortality. Schistosomiasis as a whole constitutes one of the neglected tropical diseases (NTDs) selected for elimination by the World Health Organization (WHO). Owing to the limited geographical distribution of *Schistosoma mekongi* to endemic areas in Cambodia and the Lao People's Democratic Republic (Lao PDR), strategies aiming at its elimination and eventual eradication can be implemented more effectively than for other, more widespread species.

Before effective chemotherapy became available in the late 1970s, the cornerstone for schistosomiasis control was broad-spectrum molluscicides directed at the intermediate snail host. However, when the drug praziquantel was introduced [3] and started to be used (at 40 mg/kg) for mass drug administration (MDA), it soon replaced most other control activities thanks to safety, high efficacy against the adult parasite worm, and easy administration [1,4]. Praziquantel changed the focus from infection prevention to morbidity reduction, reflected in a decline of the disability-adjusted life years (DALYs) metric for schistosomiasis [5,6]. This decline has, however, been contended since minor, so-called subtle morbidities are not considered by the DALY [5,6].

After schistosomiasis had been discovered in the Mekong River Basin (MRB), first in Lao PDR in 1957 [7] and 10 years later (1968) in Cambodia [8], biological research conducted in the 1970s demonstrated that the eggs from the MRB schistosomes were morphologically different from *S. japonicum* [8]. Furthermore, the former species had a different intermediate snail host [9,10] that could not infect water buffaloes [8] but was found in dogs [11]. By 1978, it became clear that the parasite was sufficiently different from *S. japonicum* to be named a separate species, *S. mekongi* [12]. Schistosomiasis mekongi is only found in specific areas along the MRB as it transverses Lao PDR and Cambodia. Due to the specific environmental variables required by its intermediate host snail, *Neotricula aperta* [9,10,13], transmission of *S. mekongi* is highly focal [14,15]. Compared to other schistosome species, the endemic areas for this kind of schistosomiasis are very limited, and the population at risk is unusually small, comprising only an estimated 150,000 people [14]. However, infection and re-infection sustain the disease, particularly in children, due to their high level of water contact [16,17]. Reservoir hosts, also play a role in maintaining the infection in the environment, although their diversity is not as broad as that seen with *S. japonicum*.

This paper reviews the work carried out after the rediscovery of the *S. mekongi* foci in the early 1990s in Lao PDR and Cambodia. We start with the historical background and continue by summarizing early control activities in each country. Subsequently, we list the achievements and elaborate on the organizational set-up, highlighting most relevant operational research activities. This review also features the more recent switch from morbidity control to elimination, followed by a discussion of the steps to achieve and the challenges involved.

1.1. Lao PDR

The first schistosomiasis mekongi case was diagnosed in Saint Joseph Hospital in Paris in 1957 [7], where an 18-year old Laotian patient was hospitalized, following an episode of severe hematemesis. The patient had advanced hepatosplenic pathology, and the infection was eventually traced back to his first years of life spent on Khong Island, Champasack Province, Lao PDR. Later on, a scientific paper reported on several other schistosomiasis patients originating from the same area [18]. In 1967, a WHO mission was sent to Champasack confirming the infection risk and identifying a transmission focus [19]. High village prevalence rates of schistosomiasis (up to 60%) were observed in certain districts, such as Khong and Mounlapamok in Champasack Province. Severe hepato-biliary morbidity associated with *S. mekongi* infection was frequently seen at the local health facilities. However, further follow-up studies could not be done at this point in time due to war and civil unrest in the 1970s and 1980s. In 1989, the Ministry of Health (MoH) initiated its first chemotherapy-based intervention with support from WHO in all of the endemic communities in Khong and Mounlapamok [14]. It was found that one third of all children tested were positive for *S. mekongi*, leading to the recommendation to implement health information, education, and communication (IEC) in addition to chemotherapy. This type of intervention was performed annually until 1995 and subsequently continued up to 1999 with support from the German Pharma Health Fund. After several annual MDA rounds with praziquantel, the prevalence of schistosomiasis in sentinel villages was as low as 2% [20].

1.2. Cambodia

In the late 1960s, schistosomiasis patients also started to be diagnosed at Phnom Penh's Calmette Hospital in Cambodia [21,22]. All those patients originated from Kratié Province where the presence of a transmission focus was confirmed in primary surveys [23,24]. An extended survey, including the examination of 3, 767 primary school-children in villages along the Mekong River from Strung Treng, towards the Vietnamese border, discovered variable rates of infection with the highest infection (~34%) in Kratié Province, notably lower rates in Stung Treng Province (4%) and no infections in the provinces further downstream [19]. However, intradermal sensitivity tests against *S. japonicum* antigen were positive in some children (<10%) from some downstream villages, and some exposure to the parasite was documented [19].

Early observations on Khong Island in Lao PDR confirmed severe clinical manifestations of the infection [25], such as portal hypertension with dilated superficial abdominal veins or advanced ascites and/or hepatomegaly and/or splenomegaly. Adolescents and young adults were the most heavily affected. Infection rates of 60% and higher were diagnosed with co-infections with *Opisthorchis viverrini* (64%) and hookworm (44%) being very common. However, no mortality was reported [25,26]. In Cambodia, the dramatic, historical events (Cambodian Civil War) that gained momentum in the late 1960s, deterred further studies. Schistosomiasis was only brought back into the national health agenda in 1992, when the non-governmental organization (NGO) 'Action Internationale Contre la Faim' diagnosed marked hepato-splenomegaly in 50% of 120 schoolchildren from Ampil Tuk, a village in Kratié Province [16].

When large-scale monitoring in 1994 resulted in the diagnosis of many severe cases in 20 villages in Kratié Province, the enormity of the schistosomiasis problem in the country became fully recognized [17]. A pilot schistosomiasis control program, mainly based on MDA and IEC, was started in 1995 in Kratié Province [15]. Two years later, the program was scaled up to include all endemic districts in the two hardest hit provinces, Kratié and Stung Treng, bringing the total number of villages to 114 (56 in Kratié and 58 in Stung Treng) with an estimate of 80,000 people at risk [20]. During 1994–1995, several surveys in accessible villages along the Mekong River in Kratié Province showed infection rates between 1% and 68% [17]. Based on the initial epidemiological observations, the Cambodian MoH and the health authorities in Kratié Province, in collaboration with "Médecins sans Frontières", initiated a rehabilitation program at Kratié provincial hospital and the district hospital of Sambo, with integrated community-based and hospital-based schistosomiasis control [15]. In 1996, Hatz et al. [20,27] conducted the first ultrasound profiling of *S. mekongi* infection in the Stung Treng Province in Cambodia, detecting pathological changes in 84% of the 299 participants with periportal thickening in 16% and parenchymal changes in 9% of those investigated.

2. From Morbidity Control to Elimination

2.1. Lao PDR

The first National Policy and Strategy for Control of Helminth Infections was developed and endorsed by the MoH in 2009 [28]. It served as a backbone for the helminth control program, targeting four groups of helminth diseases with public health significance, i.e., lymphatic filariasis (LF), soil-transmitted helminthiasis (STH), food-borne trematodiasis, and schistosomiasis.

2.1.1. Policy, Commitment, and Interdisciplinarity

In 2015, the National Policy and Strategy for Control of Helminth Infections was revised and extended to cover all NTDs with public health significance in Lao PDR, such as leprosy. Following the Policy and Strategy directives, the National Committee for NTD control was established. It included members from the MoH, such as the Department of Communicable Disease Control (CDC), the Lao Tropical and Public Health Institute (Lao TPHI), the National Centre of Malariology, Parasitology and Entomology (CMPE), National Centre for Environmental Health and Water Supply as well as representatives from other administrative authorities, such as the Ministry of Education and Sports, the Ministry of Agriculture and Forestry and the Ministry of Transport and Construction. Chaired by the Deputy Minister of Health, this committee guides, monitors, advocates, and authorizes all NTD control activities in Lao PDR including the MoH budget. It also comprises all activities regarding schistosomiasis control. Its status was updated and its list of members renewed in 2018.

A specific national schistosomiasis elimination action plan for the period 2016–2020 has been developed as a guidance for the National Control Program. This plan is supported by a Technical Taskforce at the central, provincial and district levels, and the taskforce members are experts from the ministries, which are already involved by the National Committee for NTD Control.

2.1.2. Activities after the Millennium Shift

With MDA and IEC discontinued after 1999 due to waning financial support, *S. mekongi* infection prevalence started—unsurprisingly—to rapidly increase. In 2003, a survey was conducted by the MoH, with support from WHO, using the Kato-Katz technique based on a single stool sample. It revealed an overall infection prevalence of 11.0% across the 64 endemic communities in Khong District, varying from 0% to 47.2%. The average infection prevalence in Mounlapamok District was 0.7%, only reaching higher levels (3.5%) in the most highly infected village, and with a majority of villages still completely negative (Figure 1). This re-emergence was later confirmed by a joint Lao–Swiss research project conducted by the Lao TPHI in the period 2005–2006. It showed a *S. mekongi* infection prevalence of 68% and 4% in Khong and Mounlapamok, respectively [29]. These rebounding prevalence rates in the two endemic districts brought infection rates up to the levels common before control was initiated in 1989.

In 2007, the Lao MoH, in collaboration with WHO and other partners, re-established a second chemotherapy-based intervention scheme with the aim to eliminate schistosomiasis as a public health problem by bringing infection intensities below 1% in all areas, using seven specifically defined sentinel villages to monitor the intervention success (MoH, Technical Report on schistosomiasis control program, unpublished). To achieve this goal, WHO recommended maintaining the annual MDA with praziquantel covering at least 75% of each community treated. The high-risk population, namely school-aged children and adults, i.e., people of ages from 5 to 60 years old, were targeted. They conducted ten rounds of MDA, with an average coverage of >80%, which brought the prevalence down to less than 10% in 2016 at all the sentinel sites, with no cases of high-intensity infection (>400 eggs per gram) detected (Figure 2) [30]. In 2017, the infection prevalence was less than 3%, with only 0.1% of them being high-intensity infections. In 2018, less than 6% of villagers at most sentinel sites were infected, with an overall prevalence of 3.2%. No patient with high-intensity infection was diagnosed (Figure 3). In addition, spot-checks were conducted in 20 randomly selected villages with a total of 3,

533 study participants. In 2017, and thus far in 2018, the average infection prevalence reached only 0.7%. No high-intensity infection was diagnosed [31], but continued MDA in the future is planned.

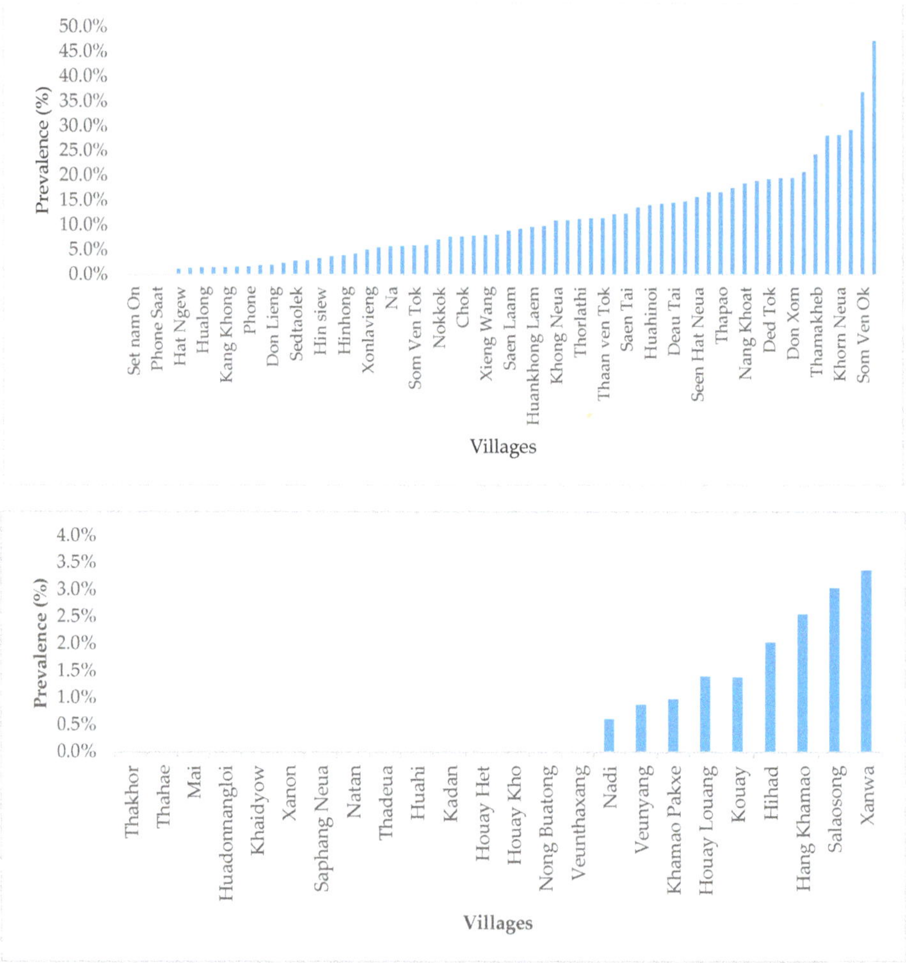

Figure 1. Prevalence of schistosomiasis in Khong (top) and Mounlapamok (bottom), detected by an approach based on a single Kato-Katz smear within the MoH and World Health Organization (WHO) survey in 2003.

With regard to investigating if transmission involving reservoir hosts could become a problem for elimination of schistosomiasis mekongi, Strandgaard et al. [32] conducted a survey focused on domestic pigs in the Khong District. Working with a total number of 98 pigs, detection of *S. mekongi* eggs in the liver, intestines, and stools of 12 (12.2%) of them confirmed this animal as a possible definitive host.

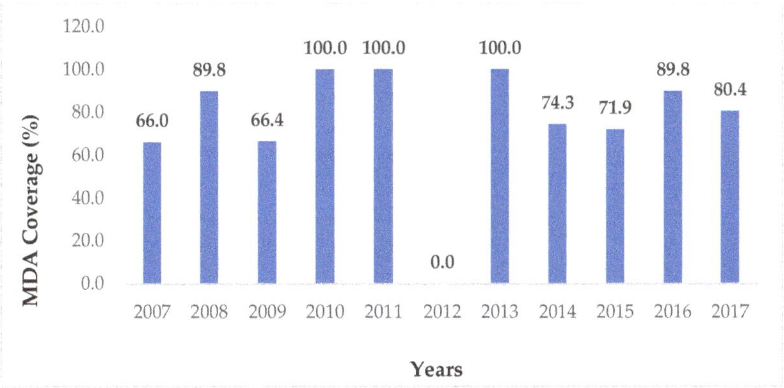

Figure 2. Mass drug administration (MDA) coverage at the *S. mekongi* endemic communities in Lao PDR in the period 2006–2017.

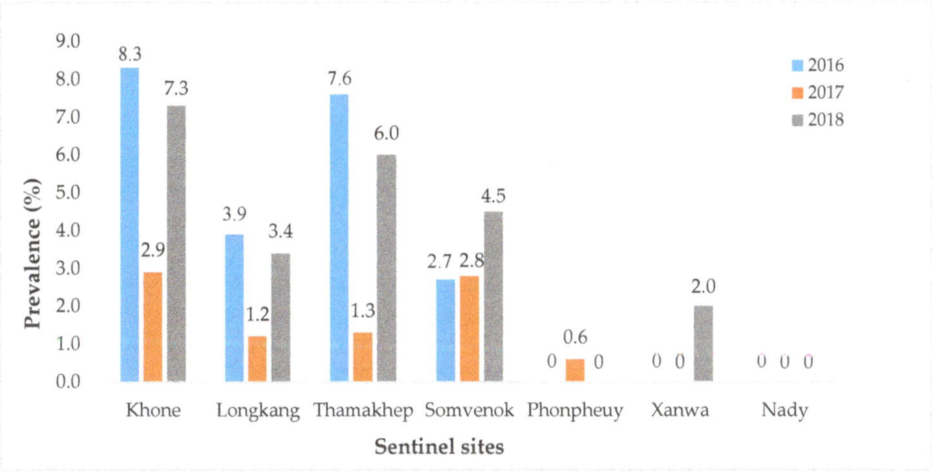

Figure 3. *Schistosoma mekongi* infection prevalence at the seven sentinel sites in the districts Khong and Mounlapamok in the period 2016–2018.

2.2. Cambodia

In collaboration with the MoH National Center for Parasitology, Entomology and Malaria Control (CNM) in Phnom Penh, researchers from Dokkyo Medical University, Mibu, Tochigi, Japan have been conducting epidemiological surveys in Cambodia since 1997. The aim was to elucidate the status of schistosomiasis due to *S. mekongi* [14]. Figure 4 shows the results of a seroepidemiological survey conducted in 1997 and 1998, using the enzyme-linked immunosorbent assay (ELISA) with *S. japonicum* soluble egg antigen (SEA) according to Matsuda et al. [33]. The results were consistent with the stool examinations with regard to the distribution of the infection among the endemic villages [14]. However, egg-positive rates exceeding 50% and ELISA-positive rates higher than 90% were recorded in some villages in the northern part of Kratié Province, while ELISA-positive rates of less than 30% were recorded in some villages in the southern part of the area [14]. None of these parts of Kratié Province had been targeted by surveillance prior to 1997; consequently, no stool examinations had been performed there in the period 1994–1995.

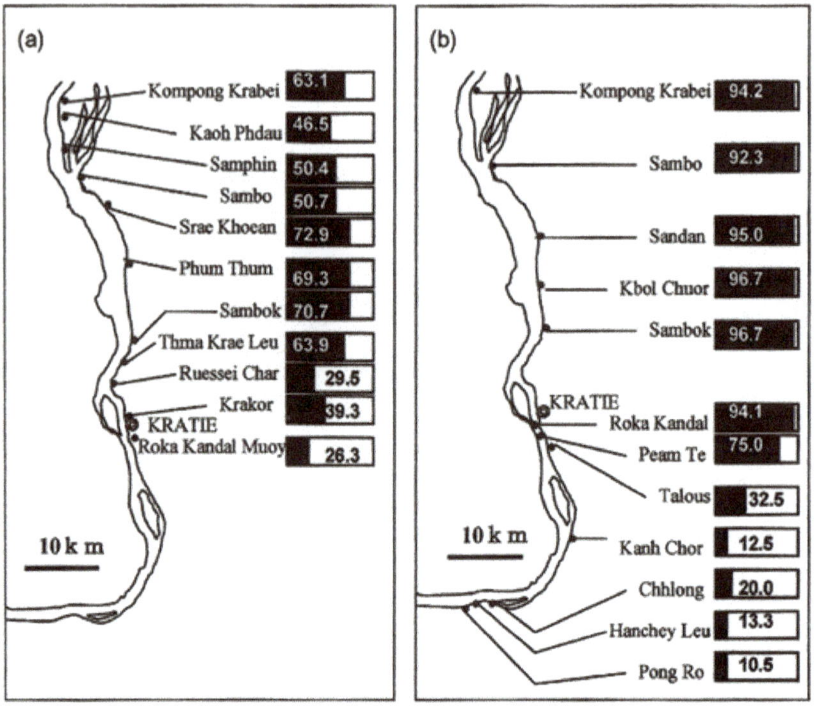

Figure 4. Comparison of results of stool examination and ELISA conducted in villages along the Mekong River in the Kratié Province [14]. Positive ratios (%) are represented by the numbers in the bar charts. (**a**) Prevalence of schistosomiasis mekongi, as determined by stool examination during 1994–1995 [17], and (**b**) prevalence of schistosomiasis mekongi, as determined by ELISA using *S. japonicum* soluble egg antigen (SEA) in the period 1997–1998 [14].

Serology surveys were part of the diagnostic approach, owing to their usefulness for the detection of schistosomiasis risk by village, particularly in low-endemic foci. Since 2003, ELISAs specific for *S. mekongi* were applied, relying on a technique using sodium metaperiodate (SMP) to reduce non-specific cross-reactions via oxidization of polysaccharide residues in the antigen molecules [34]. Ultrasound, a technique showing severe pathological changes in the liver that are often irreversible, was carried out using portable devices. However, this kind of examination can only be used for personal examination as well as for regional risk monitoring and historical evaluation [35]. Such examinations were conducted in 2003 to compare morbidity due to *S. mekongi* infection in villages in Kratié Province characterized by high and low endemicity [36].

Stool examinations were carried out using the Kato-Katz technique [37]. The SMP–ELISA technique was used for surveys in sentinel villages designated by the National Schistosomiasis Control Program (in Achen, Char Thnaol, Srae Kheun and Sambok in Kratié Province as well as several additional spot-check sites). As shown in Figure 5, ELISA-positive rates in sentinel villages and at two additional sites (Roka Kandal and Sambour) dramatically decreased to below 20%, while ELISA-positive rates remained high (>50%) at two spot-check sites (Kampong Krabei and Kbal Chuor).

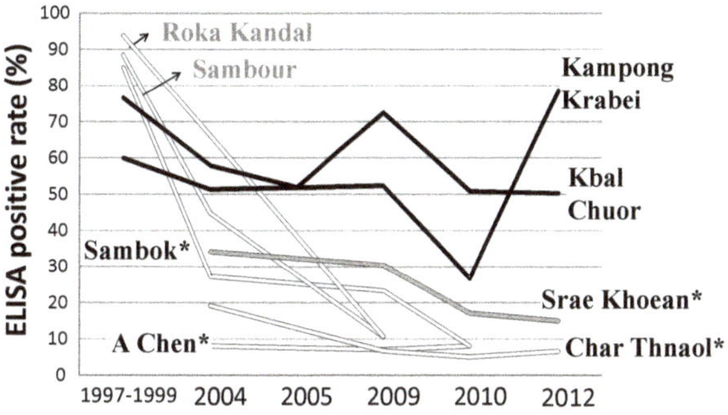

Figure 5. Changes in specific antibody rates in villages in the Kratié Province, Cambodia, during the period 1997–2012. Legend: *Sentinel villages for monitoring, as designated by the National Center for Parasitology, Entomology and Malaria Control (CNM). Black line: high-risk villages (≥50%); grey line: Moderate-risk villages (≥10% and <50%); white line: low-risk village (<10%) SMP–ELISA using *S. mekongi* SEA.

Applying ultrasound examination, dilatation of the portal vein was detected in 139 of 366 participants (38%) in a high-endemic village group and in 10 of the 117 participants (1.2%) in low-endemic villages. The characteristic ultrasound pattern of septum formation in the liver parenchyma producing the fish scale pattern noted in *S. japonicum* infection, was not observed in *S. mekongi* infections. However, in the 1990s, splenomegaly due to *S. mekongi* infection was reported to be more severe than that due to *S. japonicum* infection [38,39].

Various animals have been suspected to act as reservoir infection sources. While pigs have been experimentally shown to be possible natural reservoirs of *S. mekongi* in Lao PDR [32], this finding could only be confirmed for dogs in Cambodia. Natural schistosome infection in dogs in Cambodia was first reported by Matsumoto et al. in 2002 [40]. Schistosome eggs were detected in 1 of the 28 canine stool samples (3.6%) collected from Kbal Chuor village in Kratié Province in 2000 [40]. During a more recent survey in 2010, 15 and 17 canine stool samples were collected from two villages, Kbal Chuor and Kampong Krabei, in Kratié Province; *S. mekongi* eggs were detected in 2 (13.3%) and 1 (5.9%) of the samples from these villages, respectively.

Hisakane et al. [41] constructed a mathematical model for *S. mekongi* transmission in Cambodia, according to which dogs were considered definitive hosts in addition to humans. The simulations indicated that biannual universal and/or targeted treatment could reduce the prevalence to below 5%, within 8 years, based on 85% coverage of the residents [41]. Natural *S. mekongi* infections were not detected in cats, pigs, cows, water buffalos, horses or rats in Cambodia [40]. Rodents have been shown to be susceptible to *S. mekongi* by experimental infection; however, no natural infections have been detected to date. In 2016, ten *S. mekongi* infected *N. aperta* were found in 4840 corrected mollusks (0.2%).

A national task force for the control of STH, schistosomiasis and LF was set up in 2003. The members of the committee were representatives of different departments, ministries, and NGOs. Each department, institution and ministry involved has the responsibility to contribute to specific control/elimination activities. While CNM is responsible for developing the control/elimination strategies of NTDs, including *S. mekongi*, the Department of School Health of the Ministry of Education, Youth and Sports manages health education and support of water, sanitation and hygiene (WASH) approach in schools, the Department of Rural Health of the Ministry of Rural Development (MRD) is in charge of WASH in the communities, and WHO and the United Nations Children's Fund (UNICEF) offer technical and financial support. In 2004, the first National Policy and Guidelines for Helminth Control in Cambodia was established and adopted by the National Task Force for the Control of STH, schistosomiasis and LF [39].

3. Achievements

3.1. Lao PDR

The move from control to elimination is a challenge and recent experience suggests that interruption of MDA without adequate sanitary improvements, would within a few years lead to the parasite reclaiming its previous high endemicity. With this in mind, the MoH has started community-led initiatives to eliminate schistosomiasis by combining MDA with schistosomiasis-adapted Water, Sanitation and Hygiene (WASH) interventions (CL-SWASH) in two pilot villages in 2015, with technical support from WHO and other partners [31,42–44]. CL-SWASH integrates various ongoing MoH components of parasitic infection control with the aim to expand development of Water Safety Plans –a multi-risk management approach ranging from community participation to nationwide activities. Communities will be empowered to self-assess their environmental health risk situation, particularly in relation to schistosomiasis transmission, for instance, by interrupting transmission by eliminating open defecation. CL-SWASH continues to expand and had completed activities in 24 villages by the end of 2018, as well as outlined a plan to cover all 202 endemic villages by 2025. In addition, the MoH national action plan for elimination of schistosomiasis reflects the recommendation by the 'Expert Consultation to Accelerate Elimination of Asian Schistosomiasis' conducted in Shanghai, China under the auspices of the WHO Regional Office for the Western Pacific (WPRO) in May 2017 [45]. The main conclusion was to shift activities from the current chemotherapy-only intervention to an integrated One-Health strategy, aiming to interrupt transmission by 2025 and to achieve certified elimination by 2030 [46].

3.2. Cambodia

Since 1995, the MDA together with the IEC campaigns have been conducted annually in the two provinces endemic for *S. mekongi*. In Kratié Province, four sentinel villages were followed-up annually. Figure 6 shows the rapid decrease in the prevalence of *S. mekongi* infection from 1995 to 2018. The *S. mekongi* prevalence at four sentinel surveillance sites in Kratié Province dropped dramatically from 70% in 1995 to less than 1% in 2018. According to the CNM annual reports no new patients with *S. mekongi* infection were diagnosed in these villages over the last few years, demonstrating the positive impact of the intervention.

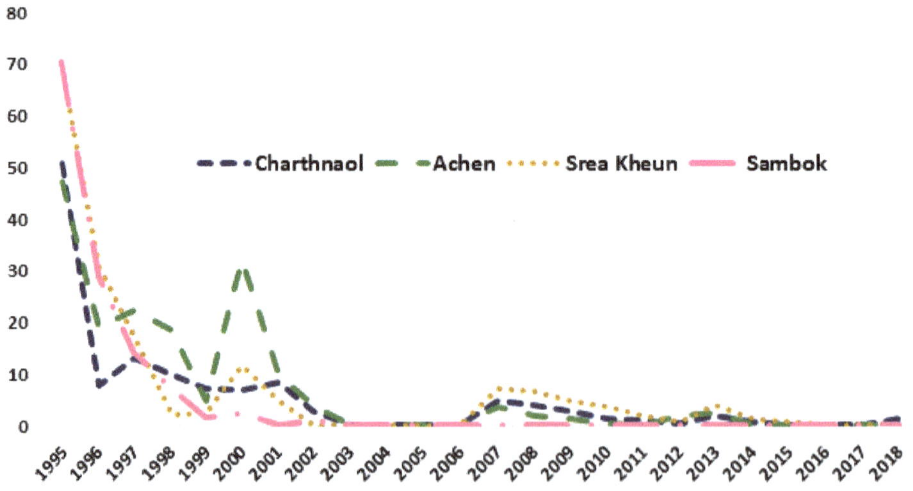

Figure 6. *S. mekongi* prevalence distribution in four sentinel site villages of Kratié, Cambodia 1995–2018.

In 2016, an external evaluation of schistosomiasis control in Cambodia was led by WHO and based on the formalin-detergent diagnostic method [47] proven to have higher sensitivity than the standard Kato-Katz method [37]. The evaluation demonstrated absence of high-intensity infections, both at the sentinel sites and the two additional spot-check sites [48]. Based on this finding, it was concluded that annual rounds of MDA, targeting the entire at-risk population above 5 years of age would be sufficient to achieve elimination of schistosomiasis as a public health problem defined as <1% prevalence of high-intensity infection. This success encouraged the MoH to shift gear from disease control to elimination in alignment with the recommendation of the 2017 WHO Expert Consultation [45]. In 2018, the National Strategic Plan for Elimination of Schistosomiasis (2019–2023) was developed after holding a national consultation workshop with all relevant stakeholders at the national and provincial levels, with input from MoH, MRD, Ministry of Agriculture, Forestry and Fishery, and the Ministry of Education, Youth and Sports. The aim is to interrupt transmission of schistosomiasis by 2025 and validate elimination of schistosomiasis by 2030. Three main elimination strategies were adopted:

1. Universal access to the One-Health intervention package consisting of preventive chemotherapy, CL-SWASH, and treatment of the animal reservoirs;
2. Strengthening community members' health literacy to prevent reinfection and interrupt transmission through a sustained change of sanitation and hygiene behaviour empowering people to act as drivers of schistosomiasis elimination; and
3. Adoption of effective and sustained active and passive surveillance of schistosomiasis in human and reservoirs hosts.

4. Next Steps and Challenges

The prevalence information in Lao PDR and Cambodia discussed here, is based on stool examination by the Kato-Katz technique [49], often based on a single stool sample, which implies that the real prevalence could be considerably higher than that presented. While the use of the Kato-Katz technique is acceptable in areas characterized by high-intensity of infection, the recent reduction of *S. mekongi* intensity of infection, following regular MDA with praziquantel, requires a rapid switch to more sensitive diagnostic techniques [49].

The polymerase chain reaction (PCR) and the loop-mediated isothermal amplification (LAMP) are highly sensitive and specific diagnostic assays that have been validated for schistosomiasis diagnosis [50,51]. The LAMP technique holds the advantage of being applicable in field laboratories, where it has been used to detect *Schistosoma* in the snail host [52,53], an application that should be useful for monitoring transmission. Detecting circulating schistosome antigens (cathodic circulating antigen, CCA or anodic circulating antigen, CAA) in sera from infected humans [54] represents a different approach. An added benefit is that these antigens pass from the blood circulation into the urine, allowing the testing of urine samples rather than blood [54], which should make people more receptive to the recurrent testing that will be needed in the future. A commercial point-of-care (POC-CCA) test for *S. mansoni* has delivered excellent results in Africa [55,56], identifying three to four times more infected individuals compared to the Kato-Katz technique [56]. When POC-CCA and a CAA test were compared with the Kato-Katz stool examination in Lao PDR and Cambodia, the two former assays showed 3- and 6-times better sensitivity, respectively [57]. However, cross-reactivity with other intestinal trematode infections, such as *O. viverrini*, cannot be ruled out, necessitating extended evaluations. Thus, before these tests can become standard assays in control programs, more experience with them are needed. Efforts in this direction are on-going.

The national helminth control programs in Cambodia and Lao PDR implement schistosomiasis control activities independently; however, the two teams regularly visit each other to gain insights into the operational activities and implementation of each program. This is important for sustaining the goals set, and needs now to be complemented by a database encompassing the entire area endemic for *S. mekongi*, distributed to these two countries. The preliminary database, established in Lao PDR to keep track of ongoing control activities and impact measures implemented, has proven useful by contributing to the adoption of standardized measures of infection and morbidity. An online database accessible by all stakeholders would be instrumental for exchange of surveillance data and rapid response action when needed, substantially facilitating the work towards elimination of *S. mekongi* infections. Once a *S. mekongi* database has been established, the information can be leveraged by bundling the data together with cartographic records and remotely sensed data from earth-observing satellites, displaying the information in a geographical information system (GIS) [58,59]. Thanks to the growing accessibility to the Internet and global positioning systems, relevant data can be collected from satellite sensors and analyzed in field settings, or other resource-poor environments, by laptop computers, and even mobile phones.

The multi-sectoral control approach, initiated in pilot villages in both countries, has thus far demonstrated both feasibility and suitability. Nonetheless, scaling up this kind of intervention is a challenge that will require substantial efforts when enlarging activities to cover communities and higher levels. Each endemic village initially requires six provincial-level officials from the different administrative sectors, involved to spend three working days initiating the activities needed. Later all enrolled villages receive follow-up visits to consolidate the various activities started. However, the resources needed, particularly with reference to trained personnel, to implement multi-sectoral activities in all villages endemic for schistosomiasis (114 in Cambodia and 202 in Lao PDR) are currently not available. This notwithstanding, the local health services must become more adapted to surveillance-and-response systems [60]. Today, these services do not have a defined role, neither with respect to diagnosis nor to treatment delivery. Strengthening of the health system has been recognized to be essential for the long-term success of control. Consequently, defining the role of curative and preventive health services in the surveillance and response, and diagnoses and treatment of *S. mekongi* and improving these services accordingly will be indispensable for successful control and future elimination.

In the absence of a schistosomiasis vaccine or alternative drugs, praziquantel has now been used as the mainstay for control, wherever possible complemented by WASH or CL-SWASH. Today, praziquantel treatment through annual MDA is assured as the MoHs in Cambodia and Lao PDR both make substantial efforts to maintain the annual treatment rounds. However, the move towards elimination planned will require transmission control, something which is more difficult in areas endemic for *S. mekongi* than anywhere else. Even if sufficiently sensitive snail diagnostics exist, the collection of specimens for testing is a challenge as the average shell length of *N. aperta* is less than 3 mm [60]. Further, the snails are restricted to shallow areas with water moving fast over wood or stone surfaces. As such conditions only exist during the dry season, the snails mostly originate from eggs laid the previous year [61]. Thus, every year provides new snail populations and they can only be found during a few months in the first half of the year. Transmission control should also involve reservoir host such as dogs and other domestic animals found susceptible for *S. mekongi* infection. The most expedient way of checking these would be serology, even if antibody titers will be less significant than direct tests of circulating or excreted schistosome antigens.

5. Conclusions

Despite the geographically fragmented environment along the Mekong River in Cambodia and Lao PDR, it should be feasible to achieve elimination of *S. mekongi* owing to the confinement of this parasite to extremely restricted areas. In fact, *S. mekongi* has the smallest distribution of any of the schistosome species. However, elimination has proved more difficult than initially thought. Despite strong progress in a large part of the endemic area, thanks to the MDA with praziquantel and the initiation of the multi-sectoral control approach, elimination remains a distant goal. What is needed for improved control are (i) scaling-up of the multi-sectoral control approach; (ii) application of a common database; and (iii), in the longer perspective, local health services to a surveillance-and-response system. A more thorough study of which animals can act as definitive hosts, would also be useful.

These moves, however, will only be bear fruit if a reliable representation of *S. mekongi* prevalence and intensity of infection can be ensured, something that is clearly attainable through the implementation of more sensitive diagnostics, supported by remotely sensed data and GIS technology.

Funding: This research received no external funding

Acknowledgments: We thank Jasmina Saric for her efficient English editing.

Conflicts of Interest: The authors declare no conflict of interest.

References

1. Colley, D.G.; Bustinduy, A.L.; Secor, W.E.; King, C.H. Human schistosomiasis. *Lancet* **2014**, *383*, 2253–2264. [CrossRef]
2. Steinmann, P.; Keiser, J.; Bos, R.; Tanner, M.; Utzinger, J. Schistosomiasis and water resources development: Systematic review, meta-analysis, and estimates of people at risk. *Lancet Infect Dis.* **2006**, *6*, 411–425. [CrossRef]
3. Davis, A.; Wegner, D.H. Multicentre trials of praziquantel in human schistosomiasis: Design and techniques. *Bull. World Health Organ.* **1979**, *57*, 767–771. [PubMed]
4. King, C.H. Parasites and poverty: The case of schistosomiasis. *Acta Trop.* **2010**, *113*, 95–104. [CrossRef] [PubMed]
5. Dalys, G.B.D.; Collaborators, H. Global, regional, and national disability-adjusted life-years (DALYs) for 333 diseases and injuries and healthy life expectancy (HALE) for 195 countries and territories, 1990–2016: A systematic analysis for the Global Burden of Disease Study 2016. *Lancet* **2017**, *390*, 1260–1344. [CrossRef]
6. Murray, C.J.; Vos, T.; Lozano, R.; Naghavi, M.; Flaxman, A.D.; Michaud, C.; Ezzati, M.; Shibuya, K.; Salomon, J.A.; Abdalla, S.; et al. Disability-adjusted life years (DALYs) for 291 diseases and injuries in 21 regions, 1990–2010: A systematic analysis for the Global Burden of Disease Study 2010. *Lancet* **2012**, *380*, 2197–2223. [CrossRef]
7. Vic-Dupont, B.C.; Soubrane, J.; Halle, B.; Richir, C. Bilharziose à *Schistosoma japonicum* à forme hépato-spléenique révélée par une grande hématemese. *Bull. Mem. Soc. Med. Hop. Paris* **1957**, *73*, 933–941.
8. Schneider, C.R.; Kitikoon, V.; Sornmani, S.; Thirachantra, S. Mekong schistosomiasis. III: A parasitological survey of domestic water buffalo (*Bubalus bubalis*) on Khong Island, Laos. *Ann. Trop. Med. Parasitol.* **1975**, *69*, 227–232. [CrossRef] [PubMed]
9. Davis, G.M.; Kitikoon, V.; Temcharoen, P. Monograph on "Lithoglyphopsis" aperta, the snail host of Mekong River schistosomiasis. *Malacologia* **1976**, *15*, 241–287. [PubMed]
10. Kitikoon, V.; Schneider, C.R. Notes on the aquatic ecology of Lithoglyphopsis aperta. *Southeast Asian J. Trop. Med. Public Health* **1976**, *7*, 238–243. [PubMed]
11. Sornmani, S.; Kitikoon, V.; Schneider, C.R.; Harinasuta, C.; Pathammavong, O. Mekong schistosomiasis. 1. Life cycle of *Schistosoma japonicum*, Mekong strain in the laboratory. *Southeast Asian J. Trop. Med. Public Health* **1973**, *4*, 218–225. [PubMed]
12. Voge, M.; Price, Z.; Bruckner, D.A. Changes in tegumental surface of *Schistosoma mekongi* Voge, Bruckner, and Bruce 1978, in the mammalian host. *J. Parasitol.* **1978**, *64*, 944–947. [CrossRef] [PubMed]
13. Attwood, S.W.; Fatih, F.A.; Campbell, I.; Upatham, E.S. The distribution of Mekong schistosomiasis, past and future: Preliminary indications from an analysis of genetic variation in the intermediate host. *Parasitol. Int.* **2008**, *57*, 256–270. [CrossRef] [PubMed]
14. Ohmae, H.; Sinuon, M.; Kirinoki, M.; Matsumoto, J.; Chigusa, Y.; Socheat, D.; Matsuda, H. *Schistosomiasis mekongi*: From discovery to control. *Parasitol. Int.* **2004**, *53*, 135–142. [CrossRef] [PubMed]
15. Sinuon, M.; Tsuyuoka, R.; Socheat, D.; Odermatt, P.; Ohmae, H.; Matsuda, H.; Montresor, A.; Palmer, K. Control of *Schistosoma mekongi* in Cambodia: Results of eight years of control activities in the two endemic provinces. *Trans. R. Soc. Trop. Med. Hyg.* **2007**, *101*, 34–39. [CrossRef] [PubMed]
16. Biays, S.; Stich, A.H.; Odermatt, P.; Long, C.; Yersin, C.; Men, C.; Saem, C.; Lormand, J.D. A foci of *Schistosomiasis mekongi* rediscovered in Northeast Cambodia: Cultural perception of the illness; description and clinical observation of 20 severe cases. *Trop. Med. Int. Health* **1999**, *4*, 662–673. [CrossRef] [PubMed]

17. Stich, A.H.; Biays, S.; Odermatt, P.; Men, C.; Saem, C.; Sokha, K.; Ly, C.S.; Legros, P.; Philips, M.; Lormand, J.D.; et al. Foci of *Schistosomiasis mekongi*, Northern Cambodia: II. Distribution of infection and morbidity. *Trop. Med. Int. Health* **1999**, *4*, 674–685. [CrossRef] [PubMed]
18. Barbier, M. Determination of aocus of arteriovenous bilharziosiin southern Laos (Sithadone Province). *Bull. Soc. Pathol. Exot. Filiales* **1966**, *59*, 4–83. [PubMed]
19. Iijima, T.; Garcia, R.G. *Rapport D'affectation (Enquête Préliminaire sur la Bilharziose au Laos Méridional)*; OMS, Bureau Rég. Pacif. Occid. Doc. WPRO-80, 23 Mai 1967 (11 Pages, 3 Cartes); WPRO: Manila, Philippines, 1967.
20. Urbani, C.; Sinoun, M.; Socheat, D.; Pholsena, K.; Strandgaard, H.; Odermatt, P.; Hatz, C. Epidemiology and control of mekongi schistosomiasis. *Acta Trop.* **2002**, *82*, 157–168. [CrossRef]
21. Audebaud, G.; Tournier-Lasserve, C.; Brumpt, V.; Jolly, M.; Mazaud, R.; Imbert, X.; Bazillio, R. 1st case of human schistosomiasis observed in Cambodia (Kratié area). *Bull. Soc. Pathol. Exot. Filiales* **1968**, *61*, 778–784. [PubMed]
22. Tournier-Lasserve, C.; Audebaud, G.; Brumpt, V.; Jolly, M.; Calvez, F.; Mazaud, R.; Imbert, X.; Bazillio, R. Existence of a focus of human bilharziosis, in Cambodia in the Kratié area. I. Study of the 1st three clinical cases. *Med. Trop. (Mars)* **1970**, *30*, 451–461. [PubMed]
23. Jolly, M.; Bazillio, R.; Audebaud, G.; Brumpt, V.; Sophinn, B. Existence of a focus of human bilharziosis, in Cambodia in Kratié area. II. Epidemiologic survey. Preliminary results. *Med. Trop. (Mars)* **1970**, *30*, 462–471. [PubMed]
24. Jolly, M.; Bazillio, R.; Audebaud, G.; Brumpt, V.; Sophinn, B. First epidemiologic studies on a focus of human biharziasis in Cambodia, in the region of Kratié. *Bull. Soc. Pathol. Exot. Filiales* **1970**, *63*, 476–483. [PubMed]
25. Sornmani, S.; Vivatanasesth, P.; Thirachantra, S. Clinical study of Mekong schistosomiasis at Khong Island, Southern Laos. *Southeast Asian J. Trop. Med. Public Health* **1976**, *7*, 270–281. [PubMed]
26. Sornmani, S. Current status of schistosomiasis in Laos, Thailand and Malaysia. *Southeast Asian J. Trop. Med. Public Health* **1976**, *7*, 149–154. [PubMed]
27. Hatz, C.; Odermatt, P.; Urbani, C. *Preliminary Data on Morbidity Due to Schistosomiasis mekongi Infections among the Population of Sdau Village, Northestern Cambodia*; Médecins Sans Frontières Suisse: Phnom Penh, Cambodia, 1997.
28. MOH. *National Policy and Strategy for Parasite Control 2009, Ministry of Health, Lao People Democratic Republic, Vientiane Lao PDR*; MOH: Long Beach, CA, USA, 2009.
29. Sayasone, S.; Mak, T.K.; Vanmany, M.; Rasphone, O.; Vounatsou, P.; Utzinger, J.; Akkhavong, K.; Odermatt, P. Helminth and intestinal protozoa infections, multiparasitism and risk factors in Champasack province, Lao People's Democratic Republic. *PLoS Negl. Trop. Dis.* **2011**, *5*, e1037. [CrossRef] [PubMed]
30. WHO. Report on Mass Drug Administration to Control of Schistosomiasis in Lao People's Democratic Republic 2018. Available online: https://www.who.int/neglected_diseases/preventive_chemotherapy/sch/en/ (accessed on 19 January 2019).
31. WHO. *Report on Schistosoma mekongi Paratological Surveillance from Village Sentinel Sites (2016–2018)*; WHO: Geneva, Switzerland, 2018.
32. Strandgaard, H.; Johansen, M.V.; Pholsena, K.; Teixayavong, K.; Christensen, N.O. The pig as a host for *Schistosoma mekongi* in Laos. *J. Parasitol.* **2001**, *87*, 708–709. [CrossRef]
33. Matsuda, H.; Tanaka, H.; Blas, B.L.; Nosenas, J.S.; Tokawa, T.; Ohsawa, S. Evaluation of ELISA with ABTS, 2-2′-azino-di-(3-ethylbenzthiazoline sulfonic acid), as the substrate of peroxidase and its application to the diagnosis of schistosomiasis. *Jpn. J. Exp. Med.* **1984**, *54*, 131–138. [PubMed]
34. Kirinoki, M.; Chigusa, Y.; Ohmae, H.; Sinuon, M.; Socheat, D.; Matsumoto, J.; Kitikoon, V.; Matsuda, H. Efficacy of sodium metaperiodate (SMP)-ELISA for the serodiagnosis of schistosomiasis mekongi. *Southeast Asian J. Trop. Med. Public Health* **2011**, *42*, 25–33. [PubMed]
35. Hatz, C.F. The use of ultrasound in schistosomiasis. *Adv. Parasitol.* **2001**, *48*, 225–284. [PubMed]
36. Keang, H.; Odermatt, P.; Odermatt-Biays, S.; Cheam, S.; Degremont, A.; Hatz, C. Liver morbidity due to *Schistosoma mekongi* in Cambodia after seven rounds of mass drug administration. *Trans. R. Soc. Trop. Med. Hyg.* **2007**, *101*, 759–765. [CrossRef] [PubMed]
37. Katz, N.; Chaves, A.; Pellegrino, J. A simple device for quantitative stool thick-smear technique in schistosomiasis mansoni. *Rev. Inst. Med. Trop. São Paulo* **1972**, *14*, 397–400. [PubMed]
38. Chigusa, Y.; Otake, H.; Kirinoki, M.; Ohmae, H.; Socheat, D.; Sinuon, M. Splenomegaly of *Schistosoma mekongi* infection in Kratie province Cambodia. *Clin. Parasitol.* **2001**, *12*, 63–65.

39. CNM. *National Policy and Guideline for Helminth Control in Cambodia by the National Task Force for the Control of Soil-Transmitted Helminthiasis, Schistosomiasis, and for the Elimination of Lymphatic Filariasis*; CNM: Albuquerque, NM, USA, 2004.
40. Matsumoto, J.; Muth, S.; Socheat, D.; Matsuda, H. The first reported cases of canine schistosomiasis mekongi in Cambodia. *Southeast Asian, J. Trop. Med. Public Health* **2002**, *33*, 458–461.
41. Hisakane, N.; Kirinoki, M.; Chigusa, Y.; Sinuon, M.; Socheat, D.; Matsuda, H.; Ishikawa, H. The evaluation of control measures against *Schistosoma mekongi* in Cambodia by a mathematical model. *Parasitol. Int.* **2008**, *57*, 379–385. [CrossRef] [PubMed]
42. WHO. *Report on National Meeting on Neglected Tropical Disease Control Program*; WHO: Geneva, Switzerland, 2018.
43. WHO. *Action Plan for Schistosomiasis Elimination 2016–2020*; WHO: Geneva, Switzerland, 2016.
44. WHO. Water Safety Planning Will Contribute to the Elimination of Schistosomiasis Worms and Improve Nutrition via a Community-Led Approach in the Province of Champassak. 2016. Available online: http://www.wpro.who.int/laos/mediacentre/releases/2016/20160524-lao-cl-swash-water-safety/en/ (accessed on 19 January 2019).
45. WHO. *Expert Consultation to Accelerate Elimination of Asian Schistosomiasis, Shanghai, China, 22–23 May 2017, Meeting Report*; 2017 Report Series; RS/2017/GE/36(CHN); WHO: Geneva, Switzerland, 2017.
46. WHO. *Report on National Policy and Strategies on Neglected Tropical Diseases Prevention and Control, May 2018*; WHO: Geneva, Switzerland, 2018.
47. Elkins, D.B.; Sithithaworn, P.; Haswell-Elkins, M.; Kaewkes, S.; Awacharagan, P.; Wongratanacheewin, S. *Opisthorchis viverrini*: Relationships between egg counts, worms recovered and antibody levels within an endemic community in northeast Thailand. *Parasitology* **1991**, *102*, 283–288. [CrossRef] [PubMed]
48. Kirinoki, M.; Ohmae, H.; Chigusa, Y.; Muth, S.; Khieu, V. *Evaluation of the Status of Schistosomiasis Elimination as a Public Health Problem in Cambodia and Development of Monitoring Protocol and Indicators for Interruption of Transmission of Mekong Schistosomiasis*; Technical Report to WPRO; WHO: Geneva, Switzerland, 2016.
49. Bergquist, R.; Johansen, M.V.; Utzinger, J. Diagnostic dilemmas in helminthology: What tools to use and when? *Trends Parasitol.* **2009**, *25*, 151–156. [CrossRef] [PubMed]
50. Lodh, N.; Mikita, K.; Bosompem, K.M.; Anyan, W.K.; Quartey, J.K.; Otchere, J.; Shiff, C.J. Point of care diagnosis of multiple schistosome parasites: Species-specific DNA detection in urine by loop-mediated isothermal amplification (LAMP). *Acta Trop.* **2017**, *173*, 125–129. [CrossRef] [PubMed]
51. He, P.; Gordon, C.A.; Williams, G.M.; Li, Y.; Wang, Y.; Hu, J. Real-time PCR diagnosis of *Schistosoma japonicum* in low transmission areas of China. *Infect. Dis. Poverty* **2018**, *7*, 8. [CrossRef] [PubMed]
52. Hamburger, J.; Abbasi, I.; Kariuki, C.; Wanjala, A.; Mzungu, E.; Mungai, P. Evaluation of loop-mediated isothermal amplification suitable for molecular monitoring of schistosome-infected snails in field laboratories. *Am. J. Trop. Med. Hyg.* **2013**, *88*, 344–351. [CrossRef] [PubMed]
53. Qin, Z.Q.; Xu, J.; Feng, T.; Lv, S.; Qian, Y.J.; Zhang, L.J.; Li, Y.; Lv, C. Field Evaluation of a Loop-Mediated Isothermal Amplification (LAMP) Platform for the Detection of *Schistosoma japonicum* Infection in *Oncomelania hupensis* Snails. *Trop. Med. Infect. Dis.* **2018**, *3*, 124. [CrossRef] [PubMed]
54. Bergquist, R.; van Dam, G.J.; Xu, J. Diagnostic tests for schistosomiasis. In *Schistosoma: Biology, Pathology and Control*; Jamieson, B.G.M., Ed.; CRC Press: Boca Raton, FL, USA, 2016; pp. 401–439.
55. Colley, D.G.; Binder, S.; Campbell, C.; King, C.H.; Tchuem Tchuente, L.A.; N'Goran, E.K.; Erko, B.; Karanja, D.M.; Kabatereine, N.B.; van Lieshout, L.; et al. A five-country evaluation of a point-of-care circulating cathodic antigen urine assay for the prevalence of *Schistosoma mansoni*. *Am. J. Trop. Med. Hyg.* **2013**, *88*, 426–432. [CrossRef] [PubMed]
56. Kittur, N.; Castleman, J.D.; Campbell, C.H., Jr.; King, C.H.; Colley, D.G. Comparison of *Schistosoma mansoni* Prevalence and Intensity of Infection, as Determined by the Circulating Cathodic Antigen Urine Assay or by the Kato-Katz Fecal Assay: A Systematic Review. *Am. J. Trop. Med. Hyg.* **2016**, *94*, 605–610. [CrossRef] [PubMed]
57. Vonghachack, Y.; Sayasone, S.; Khieu, V.; Bergquist, R.; van Dam, G.J.; Hoekstra, P.T.; Corstjens, P.L.A.M.; Nickel, B.; Marti, H.; Utzinger, J.; et al. Comparison of novel and standard diagnostic tools for the detection of *Schistosoma mekongi* infection in Lao People's Democratic Republic and Cambodia. *Infect. Dis. Poverty* **2017**, *6*, 127. [CrossRef] [PubMed]

58. Malone, J.; Bergquist, R.; Rinaldi, L. Geospatial Surveillance and Repsonse Systems for Schistosomiasis. In *Schistosoma: Biology, Pathology and Control*; Jamieson, B.G.M., Ed.; CRC Press: Boca Raton, FL, USA, 2016; pp. 479–497.
59. Malone, J.B.; Bergquist, R.; Luvall, J.C. Use of Geospatial Surveillance and Response Systems for Vector-borne Diseases in the Elimination Phase. *Trop. Med. Infect. Dis.* **2019**, *18*, 4. [CrossRef] [PubMed]
60. Bergquist, R.; Yang, G.J.; Knopp, S.; Utzinger, J.; Tanner, M. Surveillance and response: Tools and approaches for the elimination stage of neglected tropical diseases. *Acta Trop.* **2015**, *141 Pt B*, 229–234. [CrossRef]
61. Attwood, S.W.; Upatham, E.S. Observations on *Neotricula aperta* (Gastropoda: Pomatiopsidae) population densities in Thailand and central Laos: Implications for the spread of Mekong schistosomiasis. *Parasit. Vectors* **2012**, *5*, 126. [CrossRef] [PubMed]

Tropical Medicine and Infectious Disease

MDPI

Review

Status of Schistosomiasis Elimination in the Caribbean Region

Reynold Hewitt and Arve Lee Willingham *

One Health Center for Zoonoses and Tropical Veterinary Medicine, Ross University School of Veterinary Medicine, Basseterre, Saint Kitts and Nevis; reynoldhewitt@students.rossu.edu

* Correspondence: awillingham@rossvet.edu.kn; Tel.: +1-732-898-0144

Received: 21 December 2018; Accepted: 26 January 2019; Published: 31 January 2019

Abstract: Schistosomiasis elimination status in the Caribbean is reviewed with information on historical disease background, attempts to control it and current situation for each locality in the region where transmission has been eliminated (Sint Maarten, Saint Kitts, Vieques), eliminated but not yet verified (Puerto Rico, Dominican Republic, Antigua, Montserrat, Guadeloupe, Martinique) and still ongoing (Saint Lucia, Suriname). Integrated control initiatives based on selective and mass treatment and snail control using environmental, chemical and biological methods along with public service improvements (housing, safe water, sanitation) and changes in demography (urbanization) and economy (change from sugarcane and banana production to tourism) have resulted in reduction in the burden of schistosomiasis over the past century. Introduction of *Biomphalaria*-competitor snails into the region as a cost-effective, low maintenance control method appears to have had the most sustainable impact on transmission reduction. A regional inventory of *B. glabrata*, other *Biomphalaria* species and *Biomphalaria*-competitor snails as well as investigation of possible animal reservoir hosts in persisting endemic areas would be helpful for control. Elimination of schistosomiasis appears achievable in the Caribbean. However, a regional surveillance and monitoring program is needed to verify elimination in the various localities and identify and monitor areas still endemic or at risk.

Keywords: *Schistosomiasis mansoni*; Caribbean; elimination; snail control; *Biomphalaria glabrata*

1. Introduction

Schistosoma mansoni is the only human-infecting schistosome species that occurs in the Caribbean countries and territories (For the purposes of this article the Caribbean region is considered as all the islands in the Caribbean Sea and those adjoining mainland areas which are politically, historically and culturally associated with the islands (i.e., Belize, Guyana, Suriname, French Guiana) and is thus composed of sovereign states, overseas departments, and dependencies.). The first indication that *S. mansoni* was present in the Caribbean occurred in 1902 when Sir Patrick Manson published a case report [1] regarding the discovery of lateral-spined schistosome ova in the feces of a 38-year-old Caucasian Englishman who had been living in the Caribbean for 15 years at the time of his examination in England. The man had suffered chronic lower back pain and severe headaches over a period of 5 years, which at times had totally incapacitated him, as well as a history of multiple bouts of malaria. He was found to be anemic with eosinophilia and positive for intestinal schistosomiasis. The patient had never been to Africa, only having been in the British and Caribbean Isles during his lifetime. From 1887–1902 the patient had lived in Antigua, Anguilla and St Kitts, paid multiple visits to Nevis and Montserrat and also travelled to St Thomas and Barbados, thus it is difficult to pinpoint the exact island where he had been exposed to schistosomiasis. This first case report from the Caribbean was followed in 1904 by diagnosis of intestinal schistosomiasis in two young boys from the Mayagüez region of Puerto Rico who were found by Doctor I G Martínez to have lateral-spined schistosome ova in their feces [2].

Since the beginning of the 20th century schistosomiasis mansoni has been found endemic in several countries and territories in the Caribbean region, its discontinuous geographic distribution determined to a great extent by the occurrence of its intermediate hosts, freshwater snails of the genus *Biomphalaria* (Preston, 1910) [3]. Phylogenetic studies, supported by the fossil record, suggest that *Biomphalaria* actually originated in the Americas and secondarily colonized Africa within the past 5 million years [4]. Conversely, based on molecular evidence schistosomiasis mansoni in the Americas is considered to have come most likely from West Africa via the slave trade between the 17th to 19th centuries enabling transmission to the *Biomphalaria* snails present and establishing the life cycle of the parasite in the Caribbean and South America [5]. The significance of schistosomiasis mansoni as a zoonosis and the possible role of wild animals maintaining transmission in the Caribbean remains to be clarified with monkeys and rodents found with patent infections in various locations in the region during the past century [6–8].

An overview of the localities with a history of being endemic for schistosomiasis mansoni is provided in Figure 1. Two countries in the Caribbean region, Saint Lucia and Suriname, are still considered endemic for schistosomiasis with possible residual transmission whereas six additional countries and territories of Antigua and Barbuda, Guadeloupe, Martinique, Montserrat, Puerto Rico and Dominican Republic have likely eliminated transmission, but their status needs to be verified by compiling an elimination dossier and/or conducting epidemiological surveys based on WHO recommendations [9]. There are a few islands where schistosomiasis was endemic that became free of the parasite through cessation of transmission. Schistosomiasis cases ceased being detected on the island of Saint Martin/Sint Maarten from 1929 onwards with surveys published in 1980 indicating the absence of snail habitats on the island [3,10]. St Kitts was highly endemic in the early 1900s with more than 25% of the population estimated to be infected in 1932 but by 1959 onwards schistosomiasis was no longer considered a public health problem [11,12]. Schistosomiasis mansoni was eliminated from the small island of Vieques near Puerto Rico in 1962 [13]. Caribbean localities without a history of schistosomiasis include Anguilla, St Barthélemy, Saba, Sint Eustatius, Nevis, Dominica, St Vincent and the Grenadines, Grenada, Barbados, Tobago and Trinidad, Aruba, Bonaire, Curaçao and the British and U.S. Virgin Islands in the Lesser Antilles as well as the Greater Antillean countries/territories of Jamaica, Cuba, Cayman Islands and Haiti, nor in Belize, Guyana or French Guiana which are also included in the Caribbean region [3,14].

Transmission of schistosomiasis in the Caribbean was enhanced through agricultural production, whereby irrigation and drainage systems developed for production of sugarcane, bananas and rice resulted in expansion of habitats for *Biomphalaria* snails and increased exposure of people to water harboring *S. mansoni* cercariae while movement of aquatic plants for ornamental or piscicultural use enabled spread of potential intermediate-host snails between localities in the region [3,14]. Various interventions including hydrological changes, improvement in water and sanitation, targeted chemotherapy, and intermediate-host snail control have been undertaken in the region with varying degrees of success in lowering the burden of schistosomiasis and blocking its transmission. The St Lucia Project undertaken between 1965 and 1981 with support from the Rockefeller Foundation and the local government actually enabled a large-scale, concurrent comparison study of drug-treatment versus intermediate-host snail control versus improvement of water supplies [15,16].

Our aim is to review the schistosomiasis situation in each of the localities of the Caribbean where schistosomiasis mansoni has been and may still be present to better understand the lessons learned and identify continued research and control needs that would help enable elimination of the disease from the entire region.

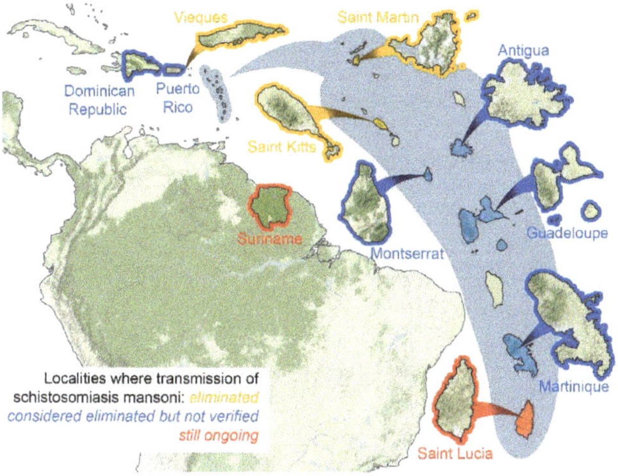

Figure 1. Map of the Caribbean region indicating localities with a history of schistosomiasis mansoni endemicity and their current transmission status.

2. Status of Schistosomiasis in the Caribbean

2.1. Localities Where Transmission of Schistosomiasis Mansoni Eliminated

2.1.1. Saint Martin

In the 1920s over 20 cases of schistosomiasis and multiple snail habitats were detected near a sugar mill in Colombier, considered the wettest valley in the French half of the French/Dutch island of Saint Martin/Sint Maarten [10,11]. No further autochthonous cases have been reported on the island since 1929 [14]. This was attributed to the disappearance of snail habitats as a result of the climate becoming drier and because of extensive deforestation associated with major construction projects resulting in hydrological changes such that surface water from heavy rain drains away quickly [3].

2.1.2. Saint Christopher (Saint Kitts)

The island of St. Kitts was highly endemic for schistosomiasis in the first half of the 20th century with multiple cases reported in 1918 [6] and a 1932 survey based on single saline fecal smears indicating nearly 25% of the island's population infected [11]. Schistosomiasis cases were primarily found in coastal villages bordering the two permanent streams on the island, Wingfield River entering the Caribbean Sea at the village of Old Road and Cayon River entering the Atlantic Ocean at Cayon village, as well as a semi-permanent stream appearing during heavy rainfall which entered the Caribbean Sea at the village of West Farm but during other times only provided piped water to the plantation of West Farm itself. The drinking water at Cayon was piped from a mountain spring free from snails; but the drinking water to Old Road and West Farm, together with the washing/bathing water in all the endemic areas, was not free of snails [17]. Importantly, St Kitts is inhabited by West African Green (Vervet) monkeys (*Chlorocebus aethiops*) and five of seven of these monkeys collected near these streams in 1928 were found infected with schistosomiasis [6].

In the 1940s, a scheme was introduced to secure domestic water supplies by diverting the natural mountain streams such that aquatic snail habitats were destroyed in the low-lying areas as water no longer flowed constantly to those areas [12]. These hydrological changes affected the *B. glabrata* habitats resulting in interruption of schistosomiasis transmission as evidenced by a steep decrease in incidence such that autochthonous clinical cases in St. Kitts have not been detected since 1955 [3]. In 1959 uninfected *B. glabrata* were found to persist in West Farm Gut [3] instigating a randomized survey of

188 randomly selected school children and villagers from the West Farm area with no cases detected [12]. Attempts were made to eliminate *B. glabrata* from the island by applying a molluscicide (Bayluscide) to relevant water bodies in 1965 and 1976 and introducing *Marisa cornuarietis*, the Colombian ramshorn apple snail, as a biological control agent in West Farm Gut [3]. A *B. glabrata* colony was later detected in the isolated Fountains River in the rain forest at an altitude of 450 meters [3]. There is currently no active schistosomiasis surveillance program on the island. Fecal samples collected in 2015 from 94 wild-caught monkeys and subjected to copro-PCR testing at the WHO Collaborating Centre for the Identification and Characterisation of Schistosomes and Snails at the Natural History Museum in London indicated no positives (Jennifer Ketzis, Ross University School of Veterinary Medicine, personal communication).

2.1.3. Vieques

Vieques Island lies off the east coast of Puerto Rico, and as part of the Commonwealth of Puerto Rico is a U.S. territory. In 1954 the prevalence of schistosomiasis in 6-year-old children on the island was 6.7% when a concerted intense control program involving control of snails with molluscicide (sodium pentachlorophenate) and chemotherapy of infected persons (sodium antimony tartrate) was implemented by the Puerto Rico Health Department with technical assistance from the U.S. Public Health Service [13]. By 1958 transmission had stopped among children in schools at high risk, and by 1959 the prevalence was down to zero and has remained there [14]. No autochthonous cases of schistosomiasis have been detected on the island since 1962. Total elimination of *B. glabrata* snails was not achievable; however, the great reduction in their number enabled transmission to be interrupted. The island remains free of schistosomiasis although *B. glabrata* persists.

2.2. Localities Where Schistosomiasis Transmission Considered Eliminated but Not yet Verified

2.2.1. Puerto Rico

Schistosomiasis was first detected on the island of Puerto Rico in1904 when young boys from Mayagüez region were found to have lateral-spined schistosome eggs in their feces and 21 cases of intestinal schistosomiasis were detected by stool survey of 4482 anemic patients from Utuado [2,18]. In 1913, the Institute of Tropical Medicine of Puerto Rico recorded 320 cases of bilharziasis among 10,149 patients [18]. Surveys in the 1930s indicated schistosomiasis cases across the country, with the eastern part of the country having the highest disease prevalence, in particular the heavily irrigated sugarcane-producing region of Guayama-Arroyo-Patillas [19–21]. An island-wide survey in 1943 estimated prevalence at 13.5% while a coprological survey conducted in 1950 on 11,690 schoolchildren between 5 and 18 years of age in 17 municipalities indicated a prevalence of 10% [18]. Schistosomiasis was prevalent along the island's coasts, along lowlands and valleys of the interior where sugarcane is grown and in one mountainous region (Utuado) [18].

In 1943, a national program was instituted to improve availability of water and sanitation through construction of water supply and sewage systems including the channeling of streams through enclosed cement viaducts that likely resulted in reduction of schistosomiasis transmission [20]. A national schistosomiasis control program under the Puerto Rico Health Department was instituted from 1953 to 1980 that emphasized biological, environmental and chemical control of snails as well as health education, improvement of public water supplies, free latrine distribution and limited chemotherapy [20,22,23]. Chemotherapy was initially not widely used due to concerns about dangerous and deadly side effects of available drugs during that time [20]. The control program first used copper sulfate for mollusciciding but soon switched to sodium pentachlorophenate and eventually niclosamide in the 1960s and 1970s [20].

Between 1954 and 1958 the *Biomphalaria*-competitor snails *M. cornuarietis* and *Tarebia granifera* appeared in Puerto Rico and within a decade spread throughout the country effectively displacing the *B. glabrata* populations with profound impact on schistosomiasis transmission [24,25]. In 1956,

M. cornuarietis was intently transferred to 111 irrigation ponds containing *B. glabrata* in the south part of the island and by 1965 was found to have completely displaced the *B. glabrata* populations in 89 of the 97 ponds still in operation [26–28]. In 1997, a national survey of multiple water bodies known to be habitats for *B. glabrata* revealed the presence of *T. granifera* and *M. cornuarietis* but *B. glabrata* had disappeared [24]. Because of the success of competitor snail introductions, biological control was found to be far more cost-effective and sustainable than mollusciciding and thus given priority [29].

An intense control program was undertaken from 1954–1960 in the highly endemic community of Patillas which included health education in primary schools and rural communities, limited chemotherapy, monitoring surveys based on annual fecal testing (formalin-ether concentration) of 1st graders and chemical, environmental and biological control of snails using sodium penta chlorophenate, drainage of habitats and introduction of the predatory *Biomphalaria*-competitor ampullarid snail *M. cornuarietis*, respectively [30]. The program was a joint effort of the Puerto Rico Department of Health and San Juan Laboratories of the Public Health Service, involving biologists, engineers and physicians. At an average annual cost of $8600, the program was effective such that by 1962 prevalence of schistosomiasis among 7-year-old children dropped from 21.5% in 1952 to 0% and the *B. glabrata* snail population no longer existed [30].

The national schistosomiasis control program with its main focus on biological snail control without widespread human treatment showed slow progress initially but had very positive results in the long term. Nationwide prevalence decreased from 15.6% in 1963 to 9% in 1968 [31] to 3.4% in 1975 [32]. By 1976, only 5 of the island's 30 main freshwater reservoirs still harbored *B. glabrata* [33]. Recognizing this progress and facing new challenges the Puerto Rico Department of Health eliminated the schistosomiasis control program in 1980 and transferred its resources to combating dengue virus. There was little in the way of active control efforts in the 1990s however nationwide disease prevalence further decreased to 2% in 1989 [34] and a limited survey in 1997 [19] conducted in previously endemic areas revealed only three positive cases all in older individuals. During this time major demographic changes happened on the island as a result of rapid urbanization with the rural population migrating to cities such that the rural population decreased from 59.5% to 6.4% of the total population between 1950 and 2018 [35,36] greatly reducing the number of persons exposed in rural transmission sites while the island's sanitation and health systems were strengthened. Authorities now consider schistosomiasis transmission interrupted as there are no longer clinical cases and no cases have been detected from coprological or serological surveys in recent years however compilation of an elimination dossier and follow-up studies, per WHO recommendations, are still needed to verify the status [9,18].

2.2.2. Dominican Republic

The first undisputed autochthonous schistosomiasis case in Dominican Republic was reported in 1947 [37]. Historically, active transmission occurs in the eastern part of the country primarily in the provinces of El Siebo, La Altagracia and Hato Mayor, the latter considered the area of highest endemicity [38]. Cases have also been reported further north in Sabana de la Mar and Miches [37]. The area is known for sugarcane and rice production and this has been linked to the high transmission as have the frequent domestic and recreational use of streams and consequent fecal contamination [39]. Infected *B. glabrata* snails were first detected in this area in 1951 [18]. Surveys in the 1960s indicated the geographic range of *B. glabrata* snails to be more extensive than that of schistosomiasis transmission with *B. glabrata* found present in over 1/6th of the country's land area including the capital Santo Domingo [38].

Schistosomiasis control efforts commenced in 1952 initially focused on mollusciciding snail habitats in high transmission areas with sodium pentachlorophenate [40]. In 1970 a Committee to Combat and Control Bilharzia, located in Hato Mayor, was created within the Ministry of Public Health and Social Welfare and a Center for the Eradication of Bilharzia established to serve as a base for implementing and coordinating control efforts [39]. The control program's activities included community education, schistosomiasis surveys involving coprologic detection, environmental control (e.g., draining ponds, filling-in swamps), and snail control based on molluscicide application (Frescon, Bayluscide) as well as biological control using both ampullarid and thiarid competitive snails [39]. In the 1960s and 1970s *M. cornuarietis*, *T. granifera* and *Melinoides tuberculata* were both actively and passively introduced into waterways in the high transmission region all becoming prolific in streams, irrigation canals and drains in rice plantations such that in several locations they completely displaced the *B. glabrata* snails [39]. In 1980 surveillance efforts were taken over by the Bilharzia Institute established through a national resolution under the Autonomous University of Santo Domingo as a public health program to undertake numerous epidemiological and malacological studies until dissolved in 1996 [18].

In 1968, there were an estimated 1000 infected individuals and 6000 at risk nationally [41]. By 1986, these numbers had increased dramatically to 208,000 people infected and an estimated 4.16 million people at risk, with an estimated 5% prevalence [34]. In 2008 estimates indicated 258,000 people to be infected [42] and in 2010 prevalence estimated at 3.0% [43]. Evidence suggests prevalence has decreased significantly in the past few years as a result of urbanization, economic development, improvements in sanitation, and expanding presence of competing snails [39]. In 2013 a serological survey (ELISA and immunoblot) was conducted in the provinces with a history of schistosomiasis transmission with none of 612 samples collected testing positive [18]. The current objective is to update knowledge of the presence and distribution of *Biomphalaria* spp. snails while compiling all of the necessary evidence to verify that transmission has indeed been interrupted through post-elimination surveillance [44].

2.2.3. Antigua

Schistosomiasis cases were first detected on the island of Antigua in 1923 when 18% of persons in St John Parish included in a Rockefeller Foundation hookworm survey were found passing eggs of *S. mansoni* [3]. *Biomphalaria glabrata* snails were found in St John Parish in Bendel's stream in 1928 and later in nearby Body Pond, with these waterbodies continuing to serve as important transmission sites for several decades due to domestic and recreational use [3]. A 1932 report recorded 60% prevalence in a village bordering these water bodies [11]. Official surveillance and control programs were never established in Antigua as transmission was considered low such that malacological and schistosomiasis surveys have been infrequent. A 1977 survey showed *B. glabrata* to be widespread and abundant in pools, dams and canals throughout the island but human contact with them limited [3]. In 1980, the *Biomphalaria*-competitor snail, *T. granifera*, was observed on the island and later *M. tuberculata* also appeared [45].

In the 1980s hydrological changes as a result of several dam projects resulted in the disappearance of any permanent flowing bodies of water as the water was piped to households for domestic use which improved sanitation and also greatly reduced exposure of the population to transmission sites as bathing and washing were increasingly done at home [14]. These water impoundment projects resulting in creation of dams and reservoirs with concomitant improvements in sanitation and protection of water supplies had great impact on the incidence of schistosomiasis [3]. National surveys in 1989, 2000 and 2003, estimated schistosomiasis prevalence at 0.1–0.2% [34,43,46] resulting in the island no longer being considered endemic however compilation of an elimination dossier and snail and schistosomiasis surveys are still needed to verify this status.

2.2.4. Montserrat

Montserrat was reportedly clear of schistosomiasis in the first half of the 20th century with no autochthonous cases reported before 1947 [41]. In 1974, public health officials reported low endemicity of schistosomiasis but provided no data. A 1977 survey indicated the presence of *B. glabrata* snails in the small, sparsely inhabited watersheds of Barzey's Stream where local people washed clothes and bathed and Farms River a local swimming site [3]. In 1978, researchers surveyed schistosomiasis prevalence in the few individuals living close to these two localities finding 14% positive while their survey of 251 school-age children elsewhere on the island did not indicate any positives [47]. In 1989, the WHO estimated that only 145 people out of the island's 11,200 were at risk of contracting schistosomiasis (1.3% at risk) and later removed Montserrat from the list of schistosomiasis endemic countries in 1993 [34,48]. A major volcanic eruption in 1995 buried the two endemic areas of the island thus interrupting schistosomiasis transmission completely. However, due to a lack of data WHO has reinstated the island's place on the list of countries for which the epidemiological status of schistosomiasis remains 'uncertain' [48]. The Thiarid snail *M. tuberculata*, used as a biological competitor to control *B. glabrata* on other islands, was found on Montserrat in 2001 [49].

2.2.5. Guadeloupe

Guadeloupe consists of two islands separated by a narrow strait with the western island, Basse-Terre, being volcanic, mountainous, forested, and containing numerous permanent rivers, streams and canals while the eastern island, Grande-Terre, is low-lying, flat, calcareous, well-drained, and has only temporary streams and natural and artificial ponds and marshes. Cases of schistosomiasis have been reported from the entire island of Grande-Terre, with mangrove swamps important transmission sites. However, more cases were reported from the coastal belt of mountainous Basse-Terre with streams and irrigation canals major sites of transmission [3]. Prevalence of *S. mansoni* peaked in the 1960s and 1970s such that in 1978 human prevalence on the islands was estimated to be 25% [25].

An interesting epidemiological aspect of schistosomiasis on Guadeloupe is the finding of rats serving as definitive hosts of *S. mansoni* with both the black rat, *Rattus rattus*, and brown rat, *Rattus norvegicus*, found naturally infected [8]. At two localities in particular, the mangrove swamps of Grande-Terre and the Grand Etang Lake in the rain forest of south Basse-Terre, rats were found to maintain the life cycle of *S. mansoni* alone in the absence of human infection with both high prevalences and high intensities of infection with some rats harboring more than 500 worms [50]. The *S. mansoni* cercariae in these areas were shown to have a late shedding pattern with an emergence peak adapted to the nocturnal activities of the rodents [51]. Studies indicate that that murine reservoir hosts may not be an important factor in areas where human transmission occurs [52].

In 1978, Guadeloupe established an integrated control program based on treatment of infected persons, environmental management and snail control mainly involving introduction of *Biomphalaria*-competitive snails (*Pomacea glauca* in 1976, *M. cornuarietis* in 1987, *M. tuberculata* in 1985) [25]. Prevalence was reduced to 15% in 1985 [34] and most of the transmission sites were eliminated in the1990s due to the extensive displacement of *B. glabrata* by *M. tuberculata* throughout most of the islands such that prevalence was down to 1% in 2003 [43,53]. *Melanoides tubercalata* was unable to effectively displace but ended up co-existing with *B. glabrata* in the mangrove swamps [54] where murine schistosomiasis was still present in *R. rattus* in 2005 [53]. Authorities consider schistosomiasis transmission on Guadeloupe effectively interrupted however, its status awaits evaluation and verification by the World Health Organization.

2.2.6. Martinique

Biomphalaria glabrata snails were included in an inventory of malacological fauna of Martinique already in 1873 [55] while the first cases of schistosomiasis were detected in 1906 when native persons being treated for dysentery were found passing lateral-spined schistosome eggs in their feces [56]. The prevalence of schistosomiasis was estimated at 6.4% in 1951, 8.4% in 1961 and 12% in 1977 [57]. Important sites of transmission were beds of watercress where people became infected while collecting the vegetation for consumption [58]. These surveys led to recognition of schistosomaisis as a public health problem resulting in establishment in 1978 of a national Department to Combat Intestinal Parasitoses to implement integrated control efforts including sanitation improvements both individually and collectively, health promotion and education, detection and treatment of patients (niridazole from 1978, oxamniquine from 1981, and praziquantel from 1995) and snail control [18].

However, unintended changes in the malacological fauna of the island had profound and sustained impact on schistosomiasis transmission such that the control program eventually became focused on biological control as its long-term strategy.

A 1953 malacological survey of the island reported *B. glabrata* was widespread [59]. During the late 1960s and early 1970s, *Biomphalaria kuhniana* (initially reported as *B. straminea*) entered the island and gradually displaced *B. glabrata* such that *B. kuhniana* rapidly became distributed across the whole hydrogeographic system of the island [60]. Although *B. kuhniana* was compatible as an intermediate-host of *S. mansoni* it was less susceptible to infection than *B. glabrata* which resulted in reducing transmission [61]. In 1979, the *Biomphalaria*-competitor thiarid snail, *M. tuberculata*, which is not susceptible to *S. mansoni*, entered Martinique and rapidly colonized the entire island displacing populations of both *B. glabrata* and *B. kuhniana* as a result reducing the prevalence of schistosomiasis [61].

The success of the accidental introduction of *M. tuberculata* in interrupting schistosomiasis transmission led the Ministry of Health to initiate a biological control program against schistosomiasis, using *M. tuberculata* in 1983 [61]. By 1989, after several intentional introductions of *M. tuberculata* into watercress beds and other transmission sites, the prevalence of *S. mansoni* dropped to 1.33% and by 1990 malacological surveys proved the near total disappearance of both *B. glabrata* and *B. kuhniana* [62]. In the 1990s another thiarid *Biomphalaria*-competitor snail. *T. granifera*, entered Guadeloupe and rapidly spread throughout the island partially displacing *M. tuberculata* [63]. Together the thiarid snails have colonized the whole hydrographic system of the island and maintain dense populations preventing an eventual recolonization by the *Biomphalaria* spp. snails and thus are maintaining sustainable control of schistosomiasis [25]. Disappearance of the intermediate hosts of *S. mansoni* and the absence of any new cases of infection in children under 10 years of age since 1984 support the elimination of schistisomiasis from Martinique. However, this remains to be verified through malacological and human prevalence studies [18].

2.3. Localities Where Schistosomiasis Transmission Still Considered Ongoing

2.3.1. Saint Lucia

Schistosomiasis in St Lucia was first reported in the 1924–1925 period [64]. Although *B. glabrata* were found widespread on the island, schistosomiasis initially remained focal, contained primarily in the southwestern Soufriere Valley until the 1950s when there was a shift in agricultural production from sugarcane to bananas and the *B. glabrata* expanded into the banana root drainage channels in the valleys and the extensive network of associated natural river systems which people used intensively for domestic and recreational use [14,65]. These environmental conditions and socioeconomic determinants including limited water and sanitation services leading to unsafe drinking water, outdoor defecation, and water contact for bathing and washing clothes contributed to transmission [66]. By 1961, the estimated national prevalence based on coprological testing was 17%, and evidence indicated that *S. mansoni* had spread to most parts of the island [15]. By the 1970s schistosomiasis prevalence in many of the endemic communities reached 70% [3].

Between the years 1965 and 1981, the St. Lucia Research and Control Project, a joint effort of the St. Lucia Ministry of Health and the Rockefeller Foundation with financial assistance from the Medical Research Council of the United Kingdom, utilized the natural laboratory setting of an endemic island to conduct research on all facets of schistosomiasis including the biology of *B. glabrata*, treatment of humans and the best methods for controlling transmission [15]. The main focus of the project was on the basic schistosomiasis control methods, namely health education, provision of safe water, chemotherapy and snail control, investigating through a comparative design the impact of these methods separately and in combination in ecologically isolated watersheds throughout the island, referred to as the "experimental valley" approach [4,15]. For chemotherapy those found infected were initially treated with hycanthone in the early 1970s and then with oxamniquine after 1975 [15].

Molluscicidng, using an emulsifiable concentrate of 25% niclosamide, was first applied area-wide and monitored by snail surveillance, then followed up with focal treatment if *B. glabrata* was still found present [65,67,68]. In 1978, the Project intentionally introduced the *Biomphalaria*-competitor snail, *M. tuberculata*, which quickly colonized water bodies on the island resulting in various levels of displacement of *B. glabrata* populations [15]. Surveillance of transmission was achieved using a locally developed sentinel-snail technique [69] and a coprological sedimentation and concentration technique for detecting human infection [70]. Incidence of schistosomiasis was reduced in communities where interventions were implemented compared to control communities [70–74]. When the Project ended in 1981, the risk of disease was considered minimal and prevalence at known endemic areas was less than 2 % [14].

After the joint Ministry of Health–Rockefeller Foundation St. Lucia Research and Control Project ended in 1981 parasite surveillance and control activities were very limited but indicated that schistosomiasis was not totally eliminated from the island [66]. Between 1981–1986 *M. tuberculata* was introduced to the whole hydrographic system of St Lucia. However, in 1993, *B. glabrata* was still found co-existing with *M. tuberculata* in 17 sites and abundantly present in two other sites where *M. tuberculata* was absent, and another *Biomphalaria* species, *B. straminea*, detected on the island [75]. Between 1995 and 2007, 106 schistosomiasis cases were reported mostly through passive surveillance of patients at prenatal health care centers and among food handlers who were routinely tested [66]. A coprological survey of 10,508 people undertaken between 2002–2005 indicated 0.3% prevalence overall with no children under the age of 9 found infected though a prevalence of 0.5% was indicated in children 10–19 [76]. The last data on schistosomiasis in St Lucia came from a limited school-based coprological survey conducted in 2006 of 550 children in three southern, rural villages that detected schistosomiasis in four (0.6%) children between the ages of 5–14 [77] and detection of a case in Babonneau in 2007 [18]. Efforts are currently underway by the St. Lucia Ministry of Health and PAHO to undertake national surveys focusing on children and snails to determine the island's current schistosomiasis status. As a pilot research site, St. Lucia is still considered a model for an integrated approach to schistosomiasis control; however, it also serves as an important example of the long-term needs for surveillance and monitoring and continued application of control measures to achieve complete elimination [43].

2.3.2. Suriname

Biomphalaria glabrata was first reported in Suriname in 1859 while the first schistosomiasis case was detected in 1911 [66,78]. Schistosomiasis is endemic only in the coastal region of the country where the majority of the country's population resides, stretching from the marsh areas north of Wageningen in Nickerie district in the west through the central cultivated areas surrounding Paramaribo to the delta area of Commewijne district in the east [66]. *Biomphalaria glabrata* are found in rice fields, swamps, drainage ditches and canals, their presence and distribution associated with the calcareous sands and alkaline waters of the shell-ridges [79]. Conversion of swamps to rice paddies in the region increased transmission as a major difficulty in control is the lack of proper disposal of feces of people working in rice fields and the irrigation schemes for rice cultivation expanded snail habitats [80,81].

The burden of schistosomiasis in Suriname has been explored through multiple studies. A house-to-house survey in 1956 based on fecal smears of over 10,000 people in multiple coastal plain localities indicated 12.7% excreting *S. mansoni* eggs [79]. A similar survey conducted from 1961–1964 focused on Saramacca district showed 23.1% positive [82] but this number went up to 45% by 1974 [66]. Intermittent national surveys conducted in the period 1986–2008 continually indicated about 3400–4000 people infected nationally [34,46]. A survey of schoolchildren in coastal provinces from 1997 to 2001 found between 0.3% and 4.7% prevalence [83]. Surveys conducted by the Ministry of Health in Commewijne and Saramacca in the period 1997–1998 indicated prevalences of 3.1% and 4.7%, respectively [81]. Countrywide prevalence remained between 0.9% to 1.0% in the period 2003–2010 [43]. High prevalences have been found associated with occupational activities involving water contact such as fishing and agriculture as well as among certain ethnic groups living in rural areas of all the districts of the coastal plain [80]. Studies conducted in the 1990s showed that schistosomiasis was a major cause of morbidity and mortality, with hematemesis, and pulmonary hypertension being the major consequences of infection [81].

Since the 1970s Suriname has implemented schistosomiasis control programs resulting in reduced prevalence of the disease. Initially hycanthone was used effectively to treat schistosomiasis however the drug had significant side effects, afterwards oxamniquine was used until 1983 when it was replaced with praziquantel [84]. The very high schistosomiasis prevalence of 74% detected in Saramacca in 1974 instigated a long-term control project in that district funded by the governments of both Suriname and the Netherlands aimed at reducing prevalence to 5% [85]. Under the project selective chemotherapy was used based on coprological case detection and implementation of other control activities including mollusciciding, mechanizing rice culture, installing pit latrines, draining standing water and swamps, and providing health education regarding schistosomiasis [86]. The first phase of the project was conducted 1974–1983 and then transferred to local authorities and integrated with existing public health programs [85]. National intervention efforts continue including intense information campaigns, detecting and treating infected people through stool sampling and provision of praziquantel, improved sanitation/waste disposal and avoidance of contact with contaminated water. A 2011 survey of six coastal districts and one inland district showed very low prevalence rates, well below the 20% deemed necessary to institute mass drug administration [87].

3. Research and Control Needs

3.1. Updating Epidemiological Surveillance

The 2009 PAHO Resolution CD49.R19 on elimination of neglected diseases and other poverty-related infections noted that in the Caribbean schistosomiasis is still present in Saint Lucia and Suriname and stated the need for studies to confirm its elimination from previously endemic localities, the goal being to reduce prevalence and parasite load in high transmission areas to less than 10% prevalence as measured by quantitative egg counts [91]. In 2012 the World Health Assembly adopted resolution WHA65.21 on elimination of schistosomiasis, calling for increased investment in schistosomiasis control and support for countries to initiate elimination programs [92]. As presented in this review, limited evidence suggests low or no transmission in many localities previously endemic for schistosomiasis including Dominican Republic, Puerto Rico, Antigua, Montserrat, Guadeloupe and Martinique. The epidemiological status of these historically schistosomiasis endemic localities in the Caribbean, in particular the prevalence and intensity of *S. mansoni* infections in children as an indirect indicator, needs to be updated based on WHO guidelines to verify elimination of transmission or, if schistosomiasis is still present, determine the public health interventions needed for control which can lead to elimination [9].

3.2. Regional Snail Inventory

A major component of the effort to combat schistosomiasis in the Caribbean region has been the effective and sustainable control of snails through environmental, chemical and, most importantly, biological interventions resulting in profound reduction or absence of *B. glabrata* populations and consequently *S. mansoni* in many sites. Biological control using the phenomenon of competition by non-medically important snails was found to be a cost-effective, low maintenance, popular way of controlling the disease. Competitive action of the ampullarid snail *M. cornuarietis* through food and predation of eggs and young snails [93] or *B. glabrata*'s avoidance of the prolific and rapidly colonizing parthenogenic thiarid snails *T. granifera* and especially *M. tuberculata* [94] all resulted in varying levels of displacement of *B. glabrata* populations. Biological control does have its limits as shown in St Lucia where *B. glabrata* and *M. tuberculata* were found to co-exist in many habitats [75], and in Guadeloupe the Thiarid snails were unable to displace *B. glabrata* in certain areas where rats served as *S. mansoni* intermediate hosts [54]. In addition, other species of *Biomphalaria* including *B. straminea*, *B. havenensis* and *B. kuhniana* have been found present in the region with varying susceptibility to *S. mansoni* [60,75,78]. With the current aim to eliminate schistosomiasis from the region, it would be worthwhile to now undertake an inventory of *Biomphalaria* spp. as well as *Biomphalaria*-competitor snail species in the Caribbean, to help assess the long-term impact of biological control, determine areas still at risk for schistosomiasis transmission, investigate the potential of other *Biomphalaria* spp. as transmitters of *S. mansoni* and contribute to the verification of schistosomiasis elimination.

3.3. Animal Reservoir Hosts

With the aim to eliminate schistosomiasis from the Americas, the presence and importance of animal reservoir hosts of *S. mansoni* becomes a significant issue for the eventual success of elimination efforts as they could pose a permanent threat of recrudescence of human infection [14]. African Green Monkeys, *Chlorocebus aethiops*, in St Kitts were found infected with *S. mansoni* [6] though apparently dependent on the persistence of human infection as after abatement of schistosomaisis transmission to humans, primate infections were no longer observed [14]. The occurrence of schistosome infections in multiple mammal species in Suriname was considered to have similar incidental status [7,95]. Under the Schistosomiasis Research and Control Project in St Lucia numerous animal species including mammals and birds were tested for infection with none found positive though in many cases the sample sizes were limited (15). The importance of rats as reservoir hosts maintaining transmission of schistosomiasis in Guadeloupe specifically in standing-water habitats where rat-maintained *S. mansoni* populations could persist independent of human intervention has been identified [96,97]. The real significance of murine schistosomiasis in Guadeloupe is not in its current impact on human schistosomiasis transmission but its potential for confounding control and eventual elimination efforts [14]. In areas of the Caribbean region with continued schistosomiasis transmission, e.g., Suriname and St Lucia, the presence and importance of animal reservoir hosts should be investigated to ensure that persistence of the disease is not due to that reason.

4. Conclusions

During the 20th Century schistosomiasis mansoni emerged as an important cause of morbidity and mortality throughout the Caribbean region however, at the beginning of the 21st Century the burden of disease appears dramatically reduced and confined to only a few foci such that its importance as a public health problem has greatly diminished. Integrated control programs based on selective and mass treatment campaigns and snail control through environmental, chemical and biological interventions enabled reductions in prevalence over the decades as evidenced in Puerto Rico and St Lucia. Additionally, the socioeconomic and ecological determinants that enabled schistosomiasis transmission have been impacted dramatically during this time due to demographic changes and improvement in socioeconomic standards resulting in urbanization, improvements in housing, provision of safe water and sanitation and re-focusing of economies from being based on agricultural production (sugarcane, bananas) to tourism that have resulted in reducing both people's exposure to *S. mansoni* as well as outdoor defecation subsequently limiting transmission. One of the most important factors responsible for long-term, sustainable impact on transmission has been the appearance of *Biomphalaria*-competitor snails in the region, both intentional and unintentional, particularly the rapidly colonizing oriental thiarid snail *M. tuberculata*. Based on these factors the elimination of schistosomiasis from the Caribbean region should indeed be achievable (see Table 1). A regional surveillance program is now needed, led by PAHO, CARPHA, CARICOM and local governments to identify in a standardized way remaining endemic foci as well as areas still at risk using the most sensitive methods available.

Table 1. Transmission status of Caribbean localities with a history of schistosomiasis endemicity noting interventions implemented and natural changes affecting transmission as well as presence of animal reservoirs.

Transmission Status.	Locality	Current Population [1]	Interventions/Natural Changes Impacting Transmission	Animal Reservoirs
Eliminated	Saint Martin	32,284 (2018)	Deforestation Hydrological changes Climate change	
	Saint Kitts	34,918 (2011)	Hydrological Changes Water and sanitation improvement Molluscicidng Competitor snails (A) [3]	Monkeys [4]
	Vieques	8669 (2017)	Molluscicidng Chemotherapy	
Considered eliminated but not yet verified	Puerto Rico	3,337,177 (2017) [2]	Water and sanitation improvement Chemotherapy (selective) Molluscicidng Competitor snails (A,B) [3] Health education	
	Dominican Republic	10,649,000 (2016)	Molluscicidng Health education Competitor snails (A,B,C) [3] Environmental management	
	Antigua	90,755 (2015)	Hydrological changes Water and sanitation improvements Competitor snails (B,C) [3]	
	Montserrat	5241 (2015)	Volcanic eruption Competitor snails (C) [3]	
	Guadeloupe	402,119 (2013)	Chemotherapy (selective) Environmental management Competitor snails (A,C,D) [3]	Rats [5]
	Martinique	385,551 (2013)	Water and sanitation improvements Health education Chemotherapy (selective) Competitor snails (B,C) [3]	
Ongoing	Saint Lucia	172,255 (2014)	Health education Water and sanitation improvements Chemotherapy (selective) Molluscicidng Competitor snails (C) [3]	
	Suriname	541,638 (2012)	Chemotherapy (selective) Molluscicidng Environmental management Water and sanitation improvements Agricultural practices Health education	

[1] For Puerto Rico and Vieques: [88]; for Saint Martin: [89] ; for all others: [90]; [2] Puerto Rico population number includes population of Vieques; [3] Competitor snails: A = *Marisa cornuarietis*; B = *Tarebia granifera*; C = *Melanoides tuberculata*; D = *Pomacea glauca*; [4] African Green (Vervet) Monkeys (*Chlorocebus aethiops*); [5] Black and Brown Rats (*Rattus rattus* and *R. norvegicus*)

Author Contributions: R.H. and A.L.W. were both involved in drafting the review, approved the submitted version and are accountable for its contents.

Funding: Funding for this review was provided by the One Health Center for Zoonoses and Tropical Veterinary Medicine, Ross University School of Veterinary Medicine, St Kitts, West Indies.

Acknowledgments: The authors thank Erin Walsh, Postdoctoral Fellow at the Research School of Population Health, ANU College of Health & Medicine, Australian National University, Australia, for designing the map of localities in the Caribbean with a history of schistosomiasis endemicity (Figure 1).

Conflicts of Interest: The authors declare no conflicts of interest.

References

1. Manson, P. Report of a case of bilharzia from the West Indies. *Br. Med. J.* **1902**, *2*, 1894–1895. [CrossRef] [PubMed]
2. Faust, E.C. Studies on Schistosomiasis mansoni in Puerto Rico. I. The history of schistosomiasis in Puerto Rico. *P. R. J. Public Health Trop. Med.* **1933**, *9*, 154–161.
3. Prentice, M.A. Schistosomiasis and its intermediate hosts in the lesser Antillean islands of the Caribbean. *Bull. Pan Am. Health Organ* **1980**, *14*, 258–268. [PubMed]
4. DeJong, R.J.; Morgan, J.A.T.; Paraense, W.L.; Pointier, J.P.; Amarista, M.; Ayeh-Kumi, P.F.K.; Babiker, A.; Barbosa, C.S.; Brémond, P.; Canese, A.P.; et al. Evolutionary relationships and biogeography of *Biomphalaria* (Gastropoda: Planorbidae) with implications regarding its role as host of the human bloodfluke, *Schistosoma mansoni*. *Mol. Biol. Evol.* **2001**, *18*, 2225–2239. [CrossRef] [PubMed]
5. Morgan, J.A.T.; Dejong, R.J.; Adeoye, G.O.; Ansa, E.D.O.; Barbosa, C.S.; Brémond, P.; Cesari, I.M.; Charbonnel, N.; Corrêa, L.R.; Coulibaly, G.; et al. Origin and diversification of the human parasite *Schistosoma mansoni*. *Mol. Ecol.* **2005**, *14*, 3889–3902. [CrossRef] [PubMed]
6. Cameron, T.W.M. A new definitive host for *Schistosoma mansoni*. *J. Helminthol.* **1928**, *6*, 219–222. [CrossRef]
7. Swellengrebel, N.H.; Rijpstra, A.C. Lateral-spined schistosome ova in the intestine of a squirrel monkey from Suriname. *Trop. Geogr. Med.* **1965**, *17*, 80–84. [PubMed]
8. Alarcón de Noya, B.; Pointier, J.P.; Colmenares, C.; Théron, A.; Balzan, C.; Cesari, I.M.; González, S.; Noya, O. Natural *Schistosoma mansoni* infection in wild rats from Guadeloupe: Parasitological and immunological aspects. *Acta Trop.* **1997**, *68*, 11–21. [CrossRef]
9. Zoni, A.C.; Catalá, L.; Ault, S.K. Schistosomiasis prevalence and intensity of infection in Latin America and the Caribbean countries, 1942–2014, A systematic review in the context of a regional elimination goal. *PLoS Negl. Trop. Dis.* **2016**, *10*, e0004493. [CrossRef] [PubMed]
10. Hoffman, W.A. From San Juan to Aruba. *P. R. J. Public Health Trop. Med.* **1929**, *5*, 357–369.
11. Jones, S.B. Intestinal bilharziasis in St. Kitts, British West Indies. *J. Trop. Med.* **1932**, *35*, 129–136.
12. Ferguson, F.F.; Richards, C.S.; Sebastian, S.T.; Buchanan, I.C. Natural abatement of *Schistosoma mansoni* in St. Kitts, British West Indies. *Public Health* **1960**, *74*, 261–265. [CrossRef]
13. Ferguson, F.F.; Palmer, J.R.; Jobin, W.R. Control of schistosomiasis on Vieques Island, Puerto Rico. *Am. J. Trop. Med. Hyg.* **1968**, *17*, 858–863. [CrossRef] [PubMed]
14. Bundy, D.A.P. Caribbean schistosomiasis. *Parasit* **1984**, *89*, 377–406. [CrossRef]
15. Jordan, P. *Schistosomiasis: The St. Lucia Project*; Cambridge University Press: Cambridge, UK, 1985; p. 442.
16. Ivy, J.A.; King, C.H.; Cook, J.A.; Colley, D.G. Historical perspective: Revisiting the St. Lucia Project, a multi-year comparison trial of schistosomiasis control strategies. *PLoS Negl. Trop. Dis.* **2018**, *12*, e0006223. [CrossRef] [PubMed]
17. Cameron, T.W.M. Observations on a parasitological tour of the Lesser Antilles. *Proc. R. Soc. Med.* **1929**, *22*, 37–45.
18. PAHO. *PAHO/WHO Schistosomiasis Regional Meeting: Defining a Road Map toward Verification of Elimination of Schistosomiasis Transmission in Latin America and the Caribbean by 2020*; Pan American Health Organization: Washington, DC, USA, 2014; Available online: https://www.paho.org/hq/dmdocuments/2014/2014-cha-sch-regional-meeting-report.pdf (accessed on 10 December 2018).
19. Giboda, M.; Malek, E.A.; Correa, R. Human schistosomiasis in Puerto Rico: Reduced prevalence rate and absence of *Biomphalaria glabrata*. *Am. J. Trop. Med. Hyg.* **1997**, *57*, 564–568. [CrossRef] [PubMed]
20. Haddock, K.C. Control of schistosomiasis: The Puerto Rican experience. *Soc. Sci. Med. Part D Med. Geogr.* **1981**, *15*, 501–514. [CrossRef]
21. Jobin, W.R. Sugar and snails: The ecology of bilharziasis related to agriculture in Puerto Rico. *Am. J. Trop. Med. Hyg.* **1980**, *29*, 86–94. [CrossRef]
22. Negro-Aponte, H.; Jobin, W.R. Schistosomiasis control in Puerto Rico. Twenty-five years of operational experience. *Am. J. Trop. Med. Hyg.* **1979**, *28*, 515–525. [CrossRef]
23. Hillyer, G.V. The rise and fall of Bilharzia in Puerto Rico: Its centennial 1904–2004. *P. R. Health Sci. J.* **2005**, *24*, 225–235. [PubMed]
24. Harry, H.; Aldrich, D. The ecology of *Australorbis glabratus* in Puerto Rico. *Bull. World Health Organ* **1958**, *18*, 819–832. [PubMed]

25. Pointier, J.P.; Jourdane, J. Biological control of the snail hosts of schistosomiasis in areas of low transmission: The example of the Caribbean area. *Acta Trop.* **2000**, *77*, 53–60. [CrossRef]
26. Pointier, J.P.; David, P.; Jarne, P. The biological control of the snail hosts of schistosomes: The role of competitor snails and biological invasions. In *Biomphalaria Snails and Larval Trematodes*; Toledo, R., Fried, B., Eds.; Springer: New York, NY, USA, 2011; pp. 215–238.
27. Butler, J.M.; Ferguson, F.F.; Palmer, J.R.; Jobin, W.R. Displacement of a colony of *Biomphalaria glabrata* by an invading population of *Tarebia granifera* in a small stream in Puerto Rico. *Caribb. J. Sci.* **1980**, *16*, 73–80.
28. Chaniotis, B.N.; Butler, J.M., Jr.; Ferguson, F.F.; Jobin, W.R. Bionomics of *Tarebia granifera* (Gastropoda: Thiaridae) in Puerto Rico, an Asiatic vector of Paragonimiasis westermani. *Caribb. J. Sci.* **1980**, *16*, 81–90.
29. Jobin, W.R.; Ferguson, F.F.; Palmer, J.R. Control of schistosomiasis in Guayama and Arroyo, Puerto Rico. *Bull. World Health Organ* **1970**, *42*, 151–156. [PubMed]
30. Palmer, J.R.; Colón, A.Z.; Ferguson, F.F.; Jobin, W.R. The control of schistosomiasis in Patillas. *P. R. Public Health Rep.* **1969**, *84*, 1003–1007. [CrossRef]
31. McMullen, D.B. Discussion of the paper by Willard H. Wright: "Schistosomiasis as a world problem". *Bull. N. Y. Acad. Med.* **1968**, *44*, 3–6.
32. Iatroski, L.S.; Davis, A. The schistosomiasis problem in the world: Results of a WHO questionnaire survey. *Bull. World Health Organ* **1981**, *59*, 115–127.
33. Jobin, W.R.; Brown, R.A.; Vélez, S.P.; Ferguson, F.F. Biological control of *Biomphalaria glabrata* in major reservoirs of Puerto Rico. *Am. J. Trop. Med. Hyg.* **1977**, *26*, 1018–1024. [CrossRef]
34. Utroska, J.A.; Chen, M.G.; Dixon, H.; Yoon, S.; Helling-Borda, M.; Hogerzeil, H.V.; Mott, K.E. An Estimate of Global Needs for Praziquantel within Schistosomiasis Control Programmes. Available online: http://whqlibdoc.who.int/HQ/1989/WHO_SCHISTO_89.102_Rev1.pdf (accessed on 15 December 2018).
35. Central Intelligence Organization. *The World Factbook 2017–18*; Washington, DC, USA, 2018. Available online: https://www.cia.gov/library/publications/the-world-factbook/fields/2212.html (accessed on 10 December 2018).
36. U. S. Bureau of the Census. *U.S. Census of Population: 1950, Volume 1 Number of Inhabitants*; U. S. Government Printing Office: Washington, DC, USA, 1952; pp. 53–56. Available online: https://www2.census.gov/prod2/decennial/documents/23761117v1ch12.pdf (accessed on 15 December 2018).
37. Ponce Pinedo, A.M. Schistosomiasis mansoni in the Republic of Santo Domingo with a report of six cases studied. *P. R. J. Public Health Trop. Med.* **1947**, *22*, 308–324.
38. WHO. *Atlas of the Global Distribution of Schistosomiasis—Dominican Republic, Puerto Rico*; World Health Organization: Geneva, Switzerland, 1987.
39. Schneider, C.R.; Hiatt, R.A.; Malek, E.A.; Ruiz-Tiben, E. Assessment of schistosomiasis in the Dominican Republic. *Public Health Rep.* **1985**, *100*, 524–530. [PubMed]
40. Vaughn, C.M.; Olivier, L.; Hendricks, J.R.; Mackie, T.T. Molluscciciding operations in an endemic area of schistosomiasis in the Dominican Republic. *Am. J. Trop. Med. Hyg.* **1952**, *3*, 518–528. [CrossRef]
41. Wright, W.H. Schistosomiasis as a World Problem. *Bull. N. Y. Acad. Med.* **1968**, *44*, 301–312. [PubMed]
42. Hotez, P.J.; Bottazzi, M.E.; Franco-Paredes, C.; Ault, S.K.; Periago, M.R. The neglected tropical diseases of Latin America and the Caribbean: A review of disease burden and distribution and a roadmap for control and elimination. *PLoS Negl. Trop. Dis.* **2008**, *2*, e300. [CrossRef] [PubMed]
43. Rollinson, D.; Knopp, S.; Levitza, S.; Stothard, J.R.; Tchuem Tchuentée, L.A.; Garba, A.; Mohammed, K.A.; Schurb, N.; Person, B.; Colley, D.G.; et al. Time to set the agenda for schistosomiasis elimination. *Acta Trop.* **2013**, *128*, 423–440. [CrossRef] [PubMed]
44. PAHO. *Neglected Infectious Diseases in the Americas: Success Stories and Innovation to Reach the Neediest*; Pan American Health Organization: Washington, DC, USA, 2016; Available online: http://iris.paho.org/xmlui/handle/123456789/31250 (accessed on 15 December 2018).
45. Sodeman, W.A., Jr. Thiara (*Tarebia*) *granifera* (Lamarck): An agent for biological control of *Biomphalaria.* In Aquaculture and Schistosomiasis, Proceedings of the a Network Meeting, Manila, Philippines, 6–10 August 1991; National Research Council, Ed.; National Academy Press: Washington, DC, USA, 1992. Available online: http://www.nzdl.org/gsdlmod?e=d-00000-00---off-0hdl--00-0----0-10-0---0---0direct-10---4-------0-1l--11-en-50---20-about---00-0-1-00-0--4----0-0-11-10-0utfZz-8-00&cl=CL1.1&d=HASHb35dbf907ec64c6abd14b3.6.3.1&gc=0 (accessed on 10 December 2015).

46. Chitsulo, L.; Engels, D.; Montresor, A.; Savioli, L. The global status of schistosomiasis and its control. *Acta Trop.* **2000**, *77*, 41–51. [CrossRef]
47. Tikasingh, E.S.; Wooding, C.D.; Long, E.; Lee, C.P.; Edwards, C. The presence of *Schistosoma mansoni* in Montserrat Leeward Islands. *J. Trop. Med. Hyg.* **1982**, *85*, 41–43.
48. WHO. *WHO Schistosomiasis Progress Report 2001–2011 and Strategic Plan 2012–2020*; World Health Organization: Geneva, Switzerland, 2013.
49. Facon, B.; Pointier, J.P.; Glaubrecht, M.; Poux, C.; Jarne, P.; David, P. A molecular phylogeography approach to biological invasions of the New World by parthenogenetic Thiarid snails. *Mol. Ecol.* **2003**, *12*, 3027–3039. [CrossRef]
50. Théron, A.; Sire, C.; Rognon, A.; Prugnolle, F.; Durand, P. Molecular ecology of *Schistosoma mansoni* transmission inferred from the genetic composition of larval and adult infrapopulations within intermediate and definitive hosts. *Parasit* **2004**, *126*, 1–15. [CrossRef]
51. Théron, A. Early and late shedding patterns of *Schistosoma mansoni* cercariae: Ecological significance in transmission to human and murine hosts. *J. Parasitol.* **1984**, *70*, 652–655.
52. Théron, A.; Pointier, J.P.; Combes, C. Approche écologique du problème de la responsibilité de l'homme et du rat dans le fonctionnement d'un site de transmission à *Schistosoma mansoni* en Guadeloupe. *Ann. Parasitol. Hum. Comp.* **1978**, *53*, 223–234. [CrossRef] [PubMed]
53. Pointier, J.P.; Théron, A. Transmission de la bilharziose intestinale aux Antilles Guyane. *Bull. D'Alerte Surveillance Antilles Guyane* **2006**, *1*, 1–4.
54. Pointier, J.; Théron, A.; Borel, G. Ecology of the introduced snail *Melanoides tuberculata* (Gastropoda; Thiaridae) in relation to *Biomphalaria glabrata* in the marshy forest area of Guadeloupe, French West Indies. *J. Molluscan Stud.* **1993**, *59*, 421–428. [CrossRef]
55. Mazé, H. Catalogue des coquilles terrestres et fluviatiles recueillies à la Martinique en 1873. *J. Conchyliol.* **1874**, *22*, 158–173.
56. Noc, F. La bilharziose á la Martinique. *Bull. Soc. Path Exot.* **1910**, *3*, 26.
57. Guyard, A.; Pointier, J.P. Faune malacologique dulcaquicole et vecteurs de la schistosome en Martinique (Antilles francaises). *Ann. Parasitol. Hum. Comp.* **1979**, *54*, 193–205. [CrossRef]
58. Pointier, J.P.; Guyard, A.; Théron, A.; Dumoutier, A. Le fonctionnement d'un site de transmission à *Schistosoma mansoni* en Martinique (Antilles françaises). *Ann. Parasitol. Hum. Comp.* **1984**, *59*, 589–595. [CrossRef]
59. Dreyfuss, R. Les planorbes de la Martinique. *Bull. Soc. Fr. Hist. Nat. Ant.* **1953**, *2*, 41–45.
60. Guyard, A.; Pointier, J.P.; Théron, A., Gilles, A. Mollusques hotes intermédiaires de la schistosomose intestinale dans les Petites Antilles. Hypothèses sur le rôle de *Biompbalaria glabrata* et *B. straminea* en Martinique. *Malacologia* **1982**, *22*, 103–107.
61. Pointier, J. Invading freshwater snails and biological control in Martinique Island, French West Indies. *Mem. Inst. Oswaldo Cruz* **2001**, *96*, 67–74. [CrossRef] [PubMed]
62. Pointier, J.P.; Guyard, A. Biological control of the snail intermediate hosts of *Schistosoma mansoni* in Martinique, French West Indies. *Trop. Med. Parasitol.* **1992**, *43*, 98–101.
63. Pointier, J.P.; Samadi, S.; Jarne, P.; Delay, B. Introduction and spread of *Thiara granifera* (Lamarck, 1822) in Martinique, French West Indies. *Biodivers. Conserv.* **1998**, *7*, 1277–1290. [CrossRef]
64. Vinter, N.S.B. Schistosomiasis in St. Lucia. *Br. Med. J.* **1964**, *1*, 119. [CrossRef]
65. Sturrock, R.F.; Barnish, G.; Upatham, E.S. Snail findings from an experimental mollusciciding programme to control *Schistosoma mansoni* transmission on St. Lucia. *Int. J. Parasitol.* **1974**, *4*, 231–240. [CrossRef]
66. PAHO. *Schistosomiasis in Suriname. PAHO/WHO Preparatory Meeting on Epidemiological Data Needed to Plan Elimination of Schistosomiasis in the Caribbean*; Pan American Health Organization: Washington, DC, USA, 2007.
67. Sturrock, R.F. Field studies on the transmission of schistosomiasis mansoni and on the bionomics of its intermediate host, *Biomphalaria glabrata,* on St Lucia, West Indies. *Int. J. Parasitol.* **1973**, *3*, 175–194. [CrossRef]
68. Sturrock, R.F. Control of *Schistosoma mansoni* transmission: Strategy for using molluscicides on St Lucia. *Int. J. Parasitol.* **1973**, *3*, 795–801. [CrossRef]
69. Upatham, E.S. Exposure of caged *Biomphalaria glabrata* (Say) to investigate dispersion of miracidia of *Schistosoma mansoni* Sambon in outdoor habitats in St Lucia. *J. Helminthol.* **1972**, *46*, 297–306. [CrossRef]

70. Jordan, P.; Woodstock, L.; Unrau, G.O.; Cook, J.A. Control of *Schistosoma mansoni* transmission by provision of domestic water supplies: A preliminary report of a study in St Lucia. *Bull. World Health Organ* **1975**, *52*, 9–20. [PubMed]
71. Unrau, G.O. Individual household water supplies as a control measure against *Schistosoma mansoni*: A study in rural St Lucia. *Bull. World Health Organ* **1975**, *52*, 1–8.
72. Jordan, P. Schistosomiasis—Research to control. *Am. J. Trop. Med. Hyg.* **1977**, *26*, 877–886. [CrossRef] [PubMed]
73. Jordan, P.; Barnish, G.; Bartholomew, R.K.; Grist, E.; Christie, J.D. Evaluation of an experimental mollusciding programme to control *Schistosoma mansoni* transmission in St Lucia. *Bull. World Health Organ* **1978**, *56*, 139–146. [PubMed]
74. Jordan, P.; Bartholomew, R.K.; Unrau, G.O.; Upatham, E.S.; Grist, E.; Christie, J.D. Further observations from St Lucia on control of *Schistosoma mansoni* transmission by provision of domestic water supplies. *Bull. World Health Organ* **1978**, *56*, 965–973. [PubMed]
75. Pointier, J.P. The introduction of *Melanoides tuberculata* (Mollusca: Thiaridae) to the island of Saint Lucia (West Indies) and its role in the decline of *Biomphalaria glabrata*, the snail intermediate host of *Schistosoma mansoni*. *Acta Trop.* **1993**, *54*, 13–18. [CrossRef]
76. Kurup, R.; Hunjan, G.S. Intestinal parasites in St Lucia: A retrospective, laboratory-based study. *J. Rural Trop. Public Health* **2010**, *9*, 24–30.
77. Kurup, R.; Hunjan, G.S. Epidemiology and control of schistosomiasis and other intestinal parasitic infections among children in three rural villages of south Saint Lucia. *J. Vector Borne Dis.* **2010**, *47*, 228–234. [PubMed]
78. Paraense, W.L. The schistosome vectors in the Americas. *Mem. Inst. Oswaldo Cruz* **2001**, *96*, 7–16. [CrossRef]
79. Van Der Kuyp, E. Schistosomiasis in the Surinam District of Surinam. *Trop. Geogr. Med.* **1961**, *13*, 357–373.
80. PAHO. *Control and Elimination of Five Neglected Diseases in Latin America and the Caribbean, 2010–2015. Analysis of Progress, Priorities and Lines of Action for Lymphatic filariasis, Schistosomiasis, Onchocerciasis, Trachoma and Soil-Transmitted Helminthiases*; Pan American Health Organization: Washington, DC, USA, 2010.
81. Noya, O.; Katz, N.; Pointier, J.P.; Théron, A.; Alarcón de Noya, B. Schistosomiasis in America. In *Neglected Tropical Diseases—Latin America and the Caribbean, Neglected Tropical Diseases*; Franco-Paredes, C., Santos-Preciado, J.I., Eds.; Springer: Vienna, Austria, 2015; pp. 11–43.
82. Van Der Kuyp, E. Schistosomiasis mansoni in the Saramacca District of Surinam. *Trop. Geogr. Med.* **1969**, *21*, 88–92.
83. PAHO. *Epidemiological Profiles of Neglected Diseases and Other Infections Related to Poverty in Latin America and the Caribbean*; Pan American Health Organization: Washington, DC, USA, 2009.
84. Alberda, A.; Weits, J.; Limburg, A.J.; Grond, J.; Ilic, P. Chronic schistosomiasis in Surinam subjects: Symptoms, treatment and course. *Nederlands tijdschrift voor Geneeskunde* **1987**, *131*, 2308–2312.
85. WHO. *WHO Technical Report Series 830, The Control of Schistosomiasis, Second Report of the WHO Expert Committee*; World Health Organization: Geneva, Switzerland, 1993.
86. Locketz, L. Health education in rural Surinam: Use of videotape in a national campaign against schistosomiasis. *Bull. Pan Am. Health Organ* **1976**, *10*, 219–226. [PubMed]
87. Colston, J.; Saboyá, M. Soil-transmitted helminthiasis in Latin America and the Caribbean: Modelling the determinants, prevalence, population at risk and costs of control at sub-national level. *Geospat. Health* **2013**, *7*, 321–340. [CrossRef] [PubMed]
88. U.S. Department of Commerce. United States Census Bureau: Quick Facts Puerto Rico. Available online: https://www.census.gov/quickfacts/fact/table/pr/PST045218 (accessed on 15 January 2019).
89. U.S. Central Intelligence Agency: World Factbook, Saint Martin. Available online: https://www.cia.gov/library/publications/the-world-factbook/geos/print_rn.html (accessed on 15 January 2019).
90. PAHO. Health in the Americas. Available online: https://www.paho.org/salud-en-las-americas-2017/ (accessed on 15 January 2019).
91. PAHO. Resolution CD49.R19 Elimination of Neglected Diseases and Other Poverty-Related Infections. In Proceedings of the 49th Directing Council, 61st Session of the Regional Committee, PAHO, Washington, DC, USA, 28 September–2 October 2009; Available online: http://iris.paho.org/xmlui/bitstream/handle/123456789/399/CD49.R19%20%28Eng.%29.pdf?sequence=1&isAllowed=y (accessed on 15 December 2018).

92. WHO. Resolution WHA65.21 Elimination of Schistosomiasis. Agenda Item 13.11. In Proceedings of the Sixty-fifth World Health Assembly, Geneva, Switzerland, 26 May 2012; Available online: https://www.who.int/neglected_diseases/mediacentre/WHA_65.21_Eng.pdf (accessed on 10 December 2018).
93. Chernin, E.; Michelson, E.H.; Augustine, D.L. Studies on the biological control of schistosome-bearing snails. I. The control of *Australorbis glabratus* populations by the snail, *Marisa cornuarietis*, under laboratory conditions. *Am. J. Trop. Med. Hyg.* **1956**, *5*, 297–307. [CrossRef]
94. Gomez Perez, J.; Vargas, M.; Malek, E.A. Displacement of *Biomphalaria glabrata* by *Thiara granifera* under natural conditions in the Dominican Republic. *Mem. Inst. Oswaldo Cruz* **1991**, *86*, 341–347. [CrossRef] [PubMed]
95. Rijpstra, A.C.; Swellengrebel, N.H. Lateral-spined schistosome ova in a great anteater, *Myrmecophaga tridactyla* L. (Edentata) from Suriname. *Trop. Geogr. Med.* **1962**, *14*, 279–483. [PubMed]
96. Combes, C.; Imbert-Establet, D. Infectivity in rodents of *Schistosoma mansoni* cercariae of human and murine origin. *J. Helminthol.* **1980**, *54*, 167–171. [CrossRef] [PubMed]
97. Combes, C.; Leger, N.; Golvan, Y.J. Rats et Bilharzia en Guadeloupe. *Acta Trop.* **1975**, *32*, 304–308.

Tropical Medicine and Infectious Disease

MDPI

Article

Baseline Mapping of Schistosomiasis and Soil Transmitted Helminthiasis in the Northern and Eastern Health Regions of Gabon, Central Africa: Recommendations for Preventive Chemotherapy

Rodrigue Mintsa Nguema [1,2,3,*], Jacques F. Mavoungou [1], Krystina Mengue Me Ngou-Milama [3,4], Modeste Mabicka Mamfoumbi [2], Aubin A. Koumba [1], Mariama Sani Lamine [5], Abdoulaye Diarra [5,†], Ghislaine Nkone Asseko [5], Jean R. Mourou [2], Marielle K. Bouyou Akotet [2], Hélène Moné [6], Gabriel Mouahid [6] and Julienne Atsame [3]

1. Research Institute in Tropical Ecology, National Center for Scientific and Technological Research, Libreville BP 13354, Gabon; mavoungoujacques@yahoo.fr (J.F.M.); aubinho25@yahoo.fr (A.A.K.)
2. Department of Parasitology-Mycology, Faculty of Medicine, University of Health Sciences of Libreville, Libreville BP 4009, Gabon; mabikmamfoumbi@yahoo.fr (M.M.M.); mangondu20@yahoo.fr (J.R.M.); mariellebouyou@gmail.com (M.K.B.A.)
3. Control Program of Parasitic Diseases, Libreville BP 2434, Gabon; ngoukrystina@yahoo.fr (K.M.M.N.-M.); julienneatsame@yahoo.fr (J.A.)
4. National Laboratory of Public Health, Libreville BP 10736, Gabon
5. Word Health Organization Country Office Gabon, Libreville BP 820, Gabon; salamarine_06@yahoo.fr (M.S.L.); diarraa@who.int (A.D.); nkoneassokog@who.int (G.N.A.)
6. IHPE, Univ Montpellier, CNRS, UM, IFREMER, Univ Perpignan Via Domitia, Perpignan F-66860, France; mone@univ-perp.fr (H.M.); mouahid@univ-perp.fr (G.M.)

* Correspondence: rodriguemintsa@yahoo.fr; Tel.: +241-04-37-61-31

† Current Address: WHO Country Office Union des Comores, P.O. Box 435, Moroni, Union des Comores.

Received: 24 August 2018; Accepted: 7 November 2018; Published: 11 November 2018

Abstract: In order to follow the Preventive Chemotherapy (PC) for the transmission control as recommended by WHO, Gabon initiated in 2014 the mapping of Schistosomiasis and Soil Transmitted Helminthiasis (STH). Here, we report the results of the Northern and Eastern health regions, representing a third of the land area and 12% of its total population. All nine departments of the two regions were surveyed and from each, five schools were examined with 50 schoolchildren per school. The parasitological examinations were realized using the filtration method for urine and the Kato-Katz technique for stool samples. Overall 2245 schoolchildren (1116 girls and 1129 boys), mean aged 11.28 ± 0.04 years, were examined. Combined schistosomiasis and STH affected 1270 (56.6%) with variation between regions, departments, and schools. For schistosomiasis, prevalence were 1.7% across the two regions, with no significant difference ($p > 0.05$) between the Northern (1.5%) and the Eastern (1.9%). Schistosomiasis is mainly caused by *Schistosoma haematobium* with the exception of one respective case of *S. mansoni* and *S. guineensis*. STH are more common than schistosomiasis, with an overall prevalence of 56.1% significantly different between the Northern (58.1%) and Eastern (53.6%) regions ($p = 0.034$). *Trichuris trichiura* is the most abundant infection with a prevalence of 43.7% followed by *Ascaris lumbricoides* 35.6% and hookworms 1.4%. According to these results, an appropriate PC strategy is given. In particular, because of the low efficacy of a single recommended drug on *T. trichiura* and hookworms, it is important to include two drugs for the treatment of STH in Gabon, due to the high prevalence and intensities of *Trichuris* infections.

Keywords: schistosomiasis; soil-transmitted-helminthiasis; mapping; preventive chemotherapy; transmission control; Gabon; Central Africa

1. Introduction

Combined schistosomiasis and Soil Transmitted Helminthiasis (STH) are the most prevalent infectious diseases in the world. They are the cause of serious global public health problems and impose a great burden on poor populations in the developing world [1]. Indeed, with the exclusion of malaria, the World Health Organization (WHO) further estimated that schistosomiasis and STH were responsible for more than 40% of the disease burden due to tropical diseases [2].

Schistosomiasis is acknowledged to be distributed in Africa, Asia, and South America with about 200 million infected people [3]. The WHO regards the disease as a Neglected Tropical Disease (NTD), with an estimated 732 million persons being vulnerable to infection worldwide in renowned transmission areas [4]. The Sub-Sahara African region remains the most affected with still high prevalence with about 192 million people infected [5]. In Gabon, with confirmed occurrence of *Schistosoma guineensis*, formely *S. intercalatum* lower Guinea strain, [6,7] and *S. haematobium*, with some cases of *S. mansoni*, it is estimated that a total of 310,391 people require preventive chemotherapy (PC) [8]. However, these 2010 estimates likely need revising.

Soil Transmitted Helminthiasis corresponds to a group of parasitic diseases that are caused by nematode worms that are transmitted to humans by faecally contaminated soil. The three major human diseases are caused by *Ascaris lumbricoides*, *Trichuris trichiura*, and hookworms (*Necator americanus* and *Ancylostoma duodenale*). The latest estimates indicate that more than two billion people are infected by at least one species worldwide and more frequently in areas where sanitation and water supply are insufficient [9]. STH infections are most common in children and such children have malnutrition, growth stunting, intellectual retardation, and cognitive and educational deficits [10]. It is estimated that over 35.4 million African school-aged children (SAC) are infected by *A. lumbricoides*, 40.1 million with *T. trichiura*, and 41.1 million with hookworms [11]. Since many children have multiple infections, it is estimated that 89.9 million are infected by at least one STH species [11]. In 2009, according to the burden of STH per country in the WHO African Region, 145,518 preschool (1−5 years) and 349,386 SAC (6−14 years), with a need of revising, were requiring PC in Gabon [9]. Indeed, the situation of STH in Gabon remains of concern and the latest local studies that were carried out showed that the prevalence is low in the sub-urban area (Melen, Libreville) and moderate in the rural area (Ekouk, 80 km of Libreville) [12].

Despite the burden that they cause in world public health, schistosomiasis and STH are considered as NTD's. Since the World Health Assembly in 2001, access to essential medicines for schistosomiasis and STH in endemic areas for the treatment of both clinical cases and groups at high risk for morbidity was recommended and endorsed by World Health Assembly resolution WHA54.19. The resolution urges member states to ensure access to essential drugs against schistosomiasis and STH in all health services in endemic areas for the treatment of clinical cases and groups at high risk of morbidity such as women and children. The declared that the aim of this resolution was to achieve at least the 75% coverage target of regular administration of anthelminthic drugs and up to 100% of all SAC at risk of morbidity by 2010 [13]. The strategy that was adopted by WHO since 2006 advocates integrated PC using a school-based approach with the concept of coordinated use of anthelminthic medicines against schistosomiasis and STH given the consideration that the diseases are largely co-endemic and that these medicines can safely be co-administered [14]. The 2010 target was not achieved, only 200 million SAC of the 600 million in need received treatment in 2010 [9]. The current goal is to revitalize the control strategy for achieving the 75% coverage target by 2020. PC for the populations at-risk in endemic areas was adopted once or twice a year, depending on risk levels, over a five-year period. Preschool and SAC in endemic areas were the primary target of PC interventions. Therefore, the target population was expanded to include all adults in high-risk areas. Communities can be classified into low-risk (<10% for schistosomiasis and <20% for STH), moderate-risk (≥10% for schistosomiasis and ≥20% for STH but <50% for both), and high-risk (≥50% for both) areas. These prevalence based on the SAC sampling are essential to adapt the frequency of PC (including SAC and at risk adults in the whole communities) according to the WHO disease specific thresholds [15].

Thus, the first step for establishing the PC strategy for schistosomiasis and STH is the knowledge of the geographic distribution of prevalence and the degree of overlap of the diseases in endemic areas [16]. The distribution of schistosomiasis and STH is particularly sensitive to environmental changes whose heterogeneity reflects numerous human and ecological factors, including changes of human origin and focal transmission [17]. For these purposes, there is a need to identify restricted areas where infection remains a public health problem for an integrated control identifying the broad scale patterns. A successful role for GIS applications in investigating the spatial epidemiology of the major human helminths was well recognized and helping to this purpose [18]. In 2009, 20 of the 32 African endemic countries had initiated the mapping of schistosomiasis and STH in order to implement the PC interventions [9]. In Gabon, schistosomiasis and STH are known to occur in many areas [8,9]; however, there has not been any sustained effort to control the diseases, apart from the establishment of the National Program for Control of Parasitic Disease in 1999, and to date, no major action had been taken at the national level by this program.

Until early 2014, PC interventions for schistosomiasis and STH had not been started in Gabon. To be in line of the WHO's target for the control of schistosomiasis and STH, Gabon initiated, in April 2014, the evaluation of the prevalence levels of schistosomiasis and STH throughout its territory. The aim was to report the outcome of schistosomiasis and STH at several levels in order to provide recommendations that are related to the implementation of PC interventions according to the WHO requirement. The present paper publishes the results regarding the Northern and Eastern health regions of Gabon.

2. Materials and Methods

2.1. Authorization and Ethical Assessment

Gabon aligns with the NTD coordinated mapping guidelines of WHO [15]. The implementation of the present study will enable the rapid scaling up of national mass treatment interventions and achieve the WHO targets that are set for 2020. An agreement was obtained for the implementation of this study as a public health exercise assumed for the Ministry of Health. Surveys were conducted in schools with the approval of the Ministry of National Education, school inspectors, directors, and teachers. Informed written consent was sought from the directors of selected schools as the legal guardian of all study schoolchildren. The school director receives prior verbal consent of the parents or guardians of schoolchildren after having explained to them the study and its objectives, with a translation in local language when necessary. Each individual that was involved in the study was registered in a data file and assigned to an anonymous identification number. At the end of the trial, infected persons were provided with appropriate chemotherapy, before the beginning of PC interventions, according to the WHO recommendations.

2.2. Study Area

Gabon is part of Central Africa. The Ministry of Public Health divides the country into 10 health regions and 52 departments. The health regions analyzed in this paper represent a third of the land of Gabon and include nine health departments, with five (Woleu, Ntem, Haut-Ntem, Haut-Okano and Okano) in the North region and four (Ivindo, Lopé and Mvoung and Zadié) in the East region (Figure 1). The General Direction for Statistic (GDS) estimated the total Gabonese population at 1,811,079 inhabitants, of which 34.7% were pre and SAC, and an urbanization rate of 87% [19]. However, predominantly urban population live in only 1% of the total space of the country, whereas the majority of territory (99% of superficies) is rural and hosts only 13% of population of the county. The study area comprises a total population of 218,279 inhabitants (154,986 and 63,293 in the North and East health regions, respectively).

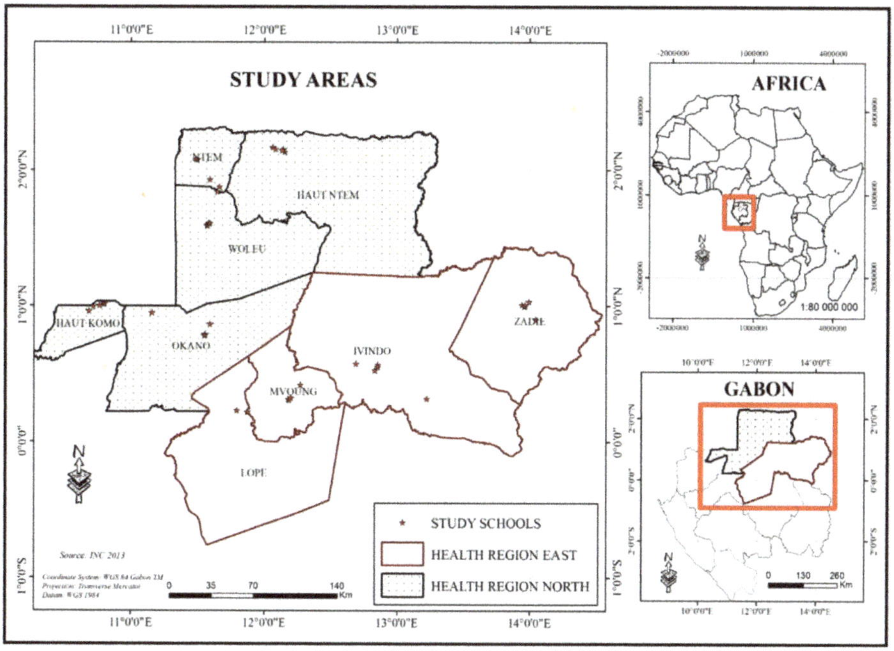

Figure 1. Study area showing the nine health departments surveyed: in the Northen region (gray): Woleu, Ntem, Haut-Ntem, Haut-Okano, Okano and in the Eastern region (white): Ivindo, Lopé, Mvoung, and Zadié.

2.3. Study Type, Period and Population

A cross-sectional prospective study was carried out from January to February 2015. It included both male and female schoolchildren aged 10 to 14 years in priority (where the infection rates will be the highest and where WHO base their guidelines from) in the selected schools. Each included schoolchild must have provided both stool and urine, otherwise they were excluded from the survey.

2.4. Selection and Location of Schools

Each health department was considered as an ecologically homogeneous area. Five schools were selected randomly among those available for each department. Schools were either urban or rural and either public or private. The geographical coordinates of each school were recorded while using a Garmin GPS (Global Positioning System) (Table S1).

2.5. Schoolchildren Sampling

In each school, select 50 schoolchildren (25 girls and 25 boys) aged 10 to 14 years from the upper class, for a total of 250 schoolchildren in each health department. For the sampling, align all schoolchildren in the age group of interest from the upper class in two rows according to their gender (girl and boy). In each row (gender), select 25 schoolchildren.

If the row contains more than 25 schoolchildren, then a systematic random sampling method is used. For example, say there are 100 schoolchildren in the row, divide the total number of schoolchildren (100) by the number of schoolchildren you want in the sample (25), the answer is 4. This means that you are going to select every fourth schoolchildren from the row. Choose randomly a number between 1 and 4. This is your random starting point. Say your random starting point is

"3", this means you select schoolchild 3 in the row as your first schoolchild, and then every fourth schoolchild down the row (3, 7, 11, 15, 19, etc.) until you have 25 schoolchildren.

If the row contains exactly 25 schoolchildren, no random sampling is necessary; all 25 schoolchildren are directly selected.

If the row contain less than 25 schoolchildren, select them and complete the sample with schoolchildren in the age group of interest from the next upper class using a random sampling method, as described above.

2.6. Sample Collection and Parasitological Examination

Stool and urine samples of each individual were collected from 9.00 to 11.00 h am in a 100 and 50 mL of plastic screw-cap vial respectively and forwarded for examination in the laboratories equipped for the circumstance at the department level. Small cakes have been distributed to encourage them. Those who did not provide both samples despite any efforts were replaced according to the schoolchildren sampling protocol. For schools with fewer than 50 schoolchildren, enrollment is completed among the other schools that were selected in the same district. For each selected schoolchild, the urine and stool samples were collected, along with information on gender and age.

Urine was analyzed for the presence and the number of *S. haematobium* eggs, using a slightly modified Nucleopore syringe urine filtration method [20], filtering a 10 mL unique aliquot from each urine sample [21]. When the volume of the sample was less than 10 mL, it was measured before filtration and the number of eggs per 10 mL was estimated. Intensity of *S. haematobium* infection was expressed as the number of eggs per 10 mL of urine (eggs/10 mL). Stool samples were examined for the presence and the number of both STH and intestinal *Schistosoma* (*S. mansoni* and *S. guineensis*) eggs while using the Kato-Katz technique [22]. A single thick smear equivalent to 41.7 mg of stool was analyzed for each stool sample. The method used is that described in the Kato-Katz kit (VESTERGAARD FRANDSEN). Eggs were immediately examined and counted by microscopy to avoid egg lysis of hookworm eggs. Individual intensity of infection was expressed as eggs per gram of feces (epg).

2.7. Data Analysis

All the collected data: age, gender, and parasitological results, were reported on an Excel sheet. Prevalence of infection (percentage of infected schoolchildren among those examined) was estimated for each parasite, for each parasite group: schistosomiasis and STH and for the combined schistosomiasis and STH, at the overall, regional, departmental, school, school category (public/private), school location (urban/rural), and gender levels. The 95% confidence intervals (CI) for prevalence were calculated using the exact method in the software R version 3.2.2. Arithmetic mean intensities of infection (number of egg per infested schoolchild) with standard deviations (SD) for each parasite species were estimated, including only the positives schoolchildren [23]. The Chi squared or Fisher exact tests were used to compare the prevalence differences in relation to the region, gender, school category (private/public), and school area (urban/rural), while the non-parametric Wilcoxon or Mann-Whitney rank sum test were used to compare differences in mean intensities of infection using R version 3.2.2 or SPSS 10.0 for Windows software. The significance of tests was defined at $p < 0.05$. Prevalence generated in each department were used to produce the prevalence maps of distribution for each species using software ArcGis version 10.1.

3. Results

3.1. Characteristics of Sampling

A total of 45 schools were examined, 25 for North and 20 for East region, 27 for urban versus 18 for rural area and 27 for public versus 18 for private category. A total of 2245 schoolchildren (1116 girls and 1129 boys) and the mean number of schoolchildren per school was 49.9 ± 3.9. The number of examined schoolchildren is 1236 (632 girls and 604 boys) in the North region and 1009 (484 girls and 525 boys) in the East region. 1754 schoolchildren were from urban versus 491 from rural area and 1420 public versus 825 private. Age of schoolchildren ranged from 4 to 17 years with median age of 11 years. The total average ages of examined schoolchildren were 11.28 ± 0.04; 11.39 ± 0.05 in the Northern and 11.26 ± 0.09 in the Eastern region.

3.2. Prevalence

3.2.1. Combined Schistosomiasis and Soil Transmitted Helminthiasis

Of the 2245 schoolchildren surveyed, 1270 (56.57%; 95% CI 54.49–58.63%) were affected by schistosomiasis (at least one species) and/or STH (at least one species) (Table 1). Schoolchildren from the North region: 723 (58.50%; 95% CI 55.3–60.9%) were significantly more infected than those from the East region: 548 (54.31%; 95% CI 50.5–56.7%), (X-squared=4.5129, df = 1; $p = 0.04169$). At the department level, prevalence was from 44.4% (WLE department) to 73.6% (HKO department) in the Northern region and from 46.56% (LPE department) to 67.45% (ZAD department) in the Eastern. Prevalence was significantly different between departments (X-squared = 84.672, df = 8, $p < 0.0001$). All of the schools were infected with prevalence ranging from 28.6% at school 3 of WLE to 92.9% at school 3 of NTM in the North region and from 8.3% at school 4 of MVG department to 88.2% at school 4 of IVD in the East region (Table S2). There were significant differences between schools (X-squared = 325.31, df = 44, $p < 0.0001$). Gender and school category had no influence on prevalence of the combined schistosomiasis and/or STH ($p > 0.05$), while STH infections in rural schoolchildren (72.10%; 95% CI 67.90–76.02%) were significantly more prevalent than the urbans (51.60; 95% CI 49.23–53.96%), (X-squared = 64.633, df = 1, $p < 0.00001$).

Of the total 1270 affected schoolchildren, 718 had one species, 537 two species, 15 three species, and no schoolchild had four, five, six or more parasites concomitantly. For those affected with schistosomiasis only one had two species, and for those with STH, 528 had two species, eight had three species, and the rest had one species (Table 2).

Table 1. Percentage of infected schoolchildren (prevalence) [95% confidence intervals], at overall level, at regional level, according to gender, school area, and school category.

	N	Schistosomiasis			Soil Transmitted Helminthiasis			SCH	STH	SCH-STH
		S. haematobium	*S. mansoni*	*S. guineensis*	*A. lumbricoides*	*T. trichiura*	Hookworms			
Overall	2245	1.65 [1.16–2.27]	0.04 [0.0–0.25]	0.04 [0.0–0.25]	35.59 [33.61–37.59]	43.74 [41.68–45.82]	1.43 [0.98–2.01]	1.69 [1.2–2.32]	56.08 [54.0–58.15]	56.57 [54.49–58.63]
By region										
Northern	1236	1.46 [0.87–2.29]	0.08 [0.0–0.45]	0.08 [0.0–0.45]	29.13 * [26.60–31.75]	52.83 * [50.0–55.65]	1.62 [0.99–2.49]	1.54 [0.93–2.39]	58.09 * [55.29–60.86]	58.5 * [55.69–61.26]
Eastern	1009	1.88 [1.14–2.93]	0.00 [0.0–0.37]	0.00 [0.0–0.37]	43.51 [40.42–46.63]	32.61 [29.72–35.60]	1.19 [0.62–2.07]	1.88 [1.14–2.93]	53.62 [50.48–56.73]	54.2 [51.08–57.32]
By gender										
Girl	1116	1.25 [0.69–2.1]	0.00 [0.0–0.33]	0.09 [0.0–0.5]	34.14 [31.36–37.01]	42.47 [39.55–45.43]	0.81 [0.37–1.53]	1.34 [0.75–2.2]	54.84 [51.87–57.79]	55.11 [52.13–58.05]
Boy	1129	2.04 [1.30–3.04]	0.09 [0.0–0.49]	0.00 [0.0–0.49]	37.02 [34.20–39.92]	45.00 [42.07–47.95]	2.04 * [1.30–3.04]	2.04 [1.30–3.04]	57.31 [54.36–60.21]	58.02 [55.08–60.91]
By school area										
urban	1754	1.48 [0.97–2.16]	0.06 [0.0–0.32]	0.06 [0.0–0.32]	30.84 [28.69–33.06] *	40.59 [38.28–42.93] *	1.37 [0.88–2.03]	1.54 [1.02–2.23]	51.60 [49.23–53.96] *	52.17 [49.80–54.48] *
rural	491	2.24 [1.12–3.97]	0.00 [0.0–0.75]	0.00 [0.0–0.75]	52.55 [48.02–57.04]	54.99 [50.47–59.45]	1.63 [0.71–3.19]	2.24 [11.24–3.97]	72.10 [67.90–76.02]	72.51 [68.33–76.41]
By school category										
Public	1420	1.97 [1.31–2.84]	0.07 [0.0–0.39]	0.07 [0.0–0.39]	36.76 [34.25–39.33]	45.35 [43.74–47.98] *	1.62 [1.03–2.42]	2.04 [1.37–2.92]	57.61 [54.99–60.19]	58.24 [55.62–60.82] *
Private	825	1.09 [0.50–2.06]	0.00 [0.0–0.45]	0.00 [0.0–0.45]	33.58 [30.36–36.91]	40.97 [37.59–44.41]	1.09 [0.50–2.06]	1.09 [0.50–2.06]	53.46 [49.98–56.90]	53.82 [50.35–57.26]

* $p < 0.05$ (Chi squared test), SCH = combined Schistosomiasis (together *S. haematobium*, *S. mansoni* and *S. guineensis*); STH = combined soil transmitted helminthiasis (together *A. lumbricoides*, *T. trichiura* and Hookworms). SCH-STH = presence at least one schistosomiasis and/or soil transmitted helminthiasis.

Table 2. Proportion of polyparasitism for schistosomiaisis, soil transmitted helminthiasis (STH) and combined (schistosomiais-STH). N is the total number of examined schoolchildren.

Number of Species	N	Schistosomiasis	STH	Schistosomiasis-STH
1	2245	37	723	718 *
2		1	528	537
3		0	8	15
4		0	0	0
5		0	0	0
6		0	0	0
>6		0	0	0
Negative		2207	986	975

* In the STH column some of those also have schistosomiasis, so this decreases the number with 1 species in the SCH-STH column.

3.2.2. Combined Schistosomiasis

Including all three species, overall 38 cases (1.7%) were positive for schistosomiasis in 21 schools of the 45 surveyed, with no significant difference ($p > 0.05$) between the North, 19 cases (1.5%; 95% CI 0.9–2.4%), and the East region, 19 cases (1.88%; 95% CI 1.1–2.9%), (Table 1). Gender, school area and school category had no influence on prevalence of the combined schistosomiasis ($p > 0.05$). At the department level, prevalence was all <10%. It varied from 0.8% at WLE to 2.6% at HKO department in the North region ($p > 0.05$) and from 0.0% at ZAD to 4.4% at MVG department in the East region (X-squared = 22.032, df = 8, $p = 0.004857$). At the school level, prevalence was all < 10% (0% in 25 schools), with the exception of school 5 in MVG department, it was 15.8% (X-squared = 84.762, df = 44, $p = 0.0002171$).

3.2.3. Schistosomiasis Haematobium

It is the most frequent schistosomiasis that was found to be prevalent in 20 schools from the 45 studied (Table S2). Overall, *S. haematobium* affected 37 (1.45%; 95% CI 1.16–2.27%) schoolchildren with 18 (1.46%. 95% CI 0.87–2.29%) in the North and 19 (1.88%; 95% CI 1.14–2.93%) in the East region ($p > 0.05$). Gender, school area, and school category had no influence on prevalence of *S. haematobium* ($p > 0.05$). At the department level (Figure 2), the prevalence of *S. haematobium* was all <10%, from 0.8% (HNT department) to 2.4% (NTM department) in the North region and from 0% (ZAD department) to 4.36% (MVG department) in the East region, (X-squared = 21.741, df = 8, $p = 0.00542$). At the school level, prevalence varied from 0 (in 25 schools) to15.8% (six cases in school 5 in the MVG department) (X-squared = 85.959, df = 44, $p = 0.0001583$).

3.2.4. Other Schistosomiasis

S. guineensis and *S. mansoni* are very unusual, only one case of each respectively was listed in the North region. The *S. mansoni* case was encountered in school 4 of NTM department, while the *S. guineensis* case was in school 1 of HKO department (Table S2). All the distribution maps of schistosomiasis are presented in the Figure 2.

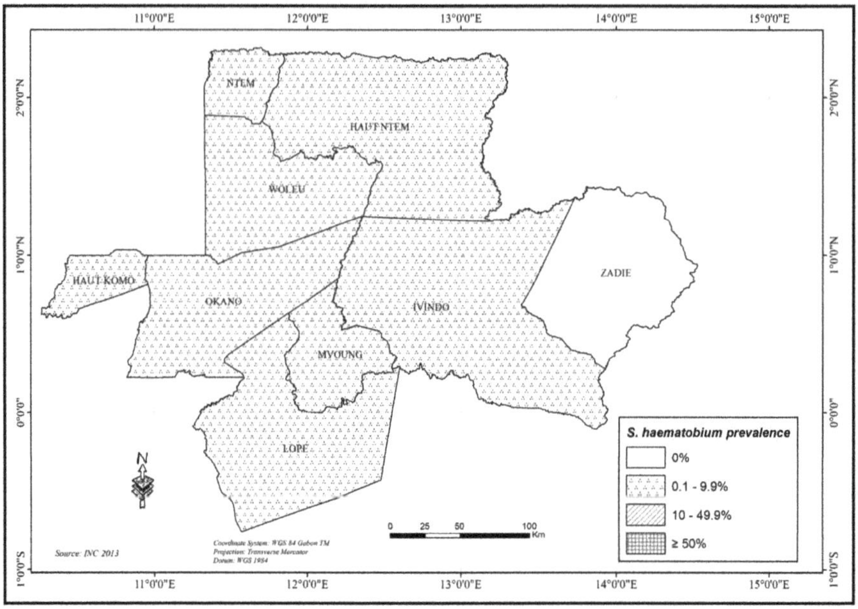

(A)

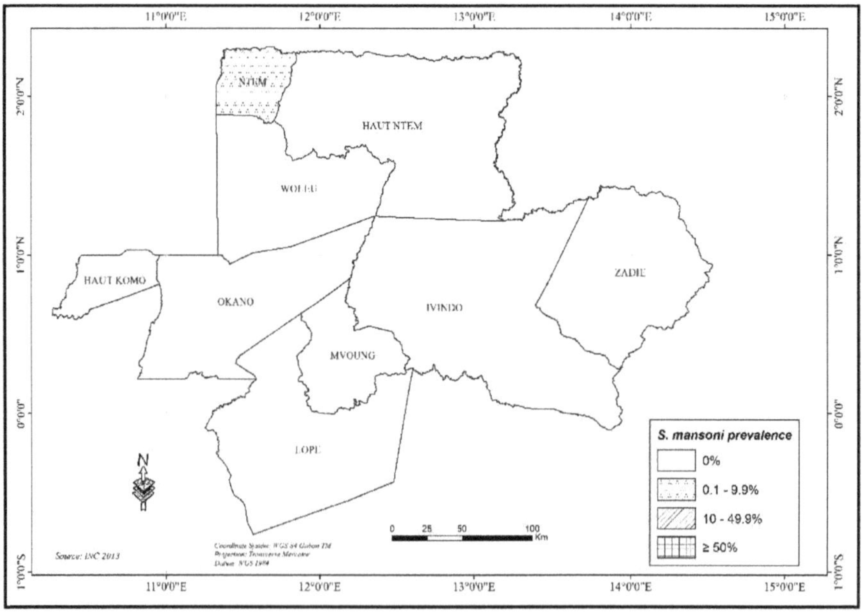

(B)

Figure 2. *Cont.*

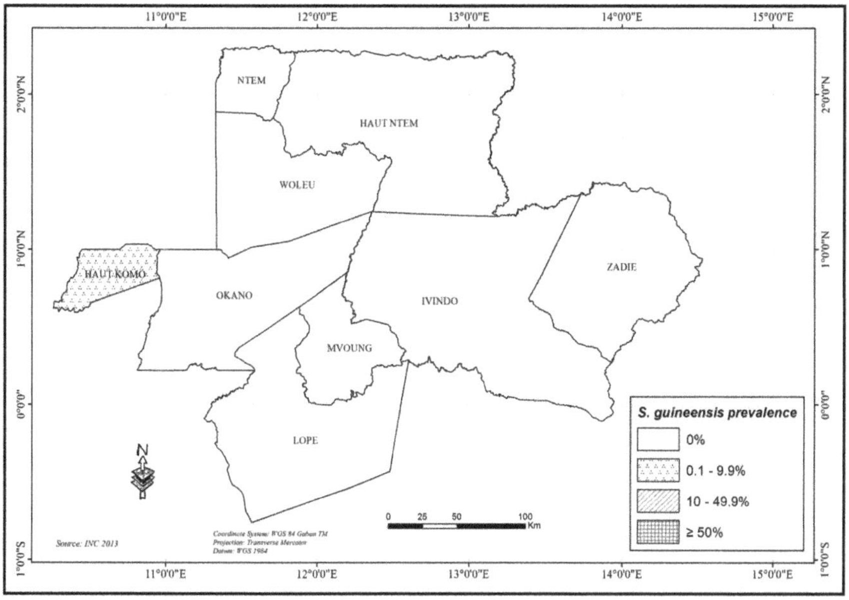

(C)

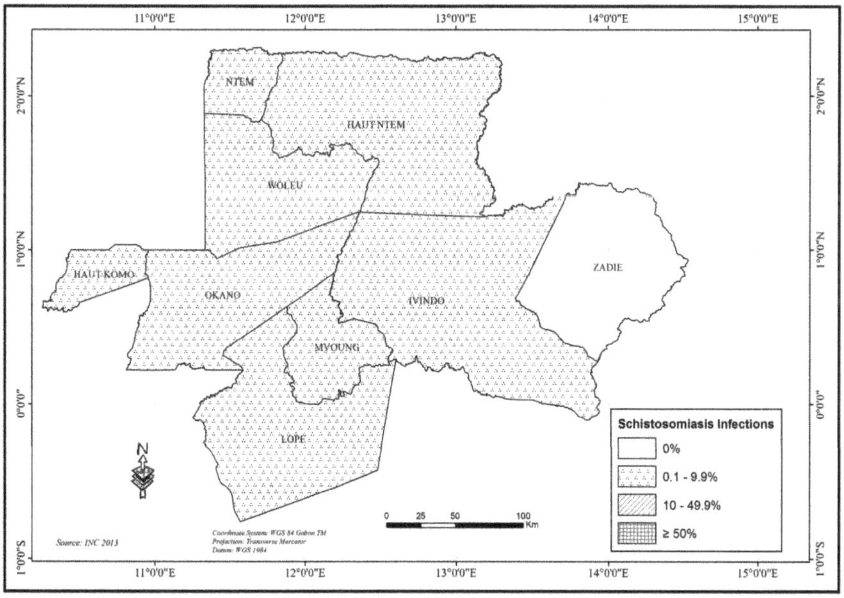

(D)

Figure 2. Map of prevalence levels for Schistosomiasis at department scale: (**A**) *Schistosoma haematobium*; (**B**) *S. mansoni*; (**C**) *S. guineensis*; and, (**D**) Combined schistosomiasis.

3.2.5. Combined Soil Transmitted Helminthiasis (STH)

Including all the STH, a total of 1259 (56.08%; 95% CI 54.0–58.15%) schoolchildren were affected by STH (Table 1). At the regional level, the North health region (58.09%; 95% CI 55.29–60.86%) was more affected than Eastern (53.62%; 95% CI 50.48–56.73%), (X-squared = 4.3331, df = 1, p = 0.03738). At the department level, significant differences were found (X-squared = 85.435, df = 8, $p < 0.0001$). Prevalence varied from 44.736% (WLE department) to 73.16% (HKO department) in the North and from 46.56% (LPE department) to 67.45% (LPE department) in the East region. At the school level, there were heterogeneity between schools (X-squared = 326.25, df = 44, $p < 0.00001$). One school had a prevalence of STH < 20%, 14 schools had a prevalence ≥20%, but <50% and 29 had a prevalence ≥50% (Table S2). Gender and school category had no influence on overall prevalence of STH ($p > 0.05$) while according to school area: schoolchildren of rural schools (72.1% [67.90–76.02]) had significantly higher prevalence than those of urban schools (51.6%; 95% CI 49.23–53.96%), X-squared = 64.633, df = 1, $p < 0.0001$.

3.2.6. *Ascaris lumbricoides*

A. lumbricoides was identified in 44 of the 45 schools studied for a total of 799 (35.59% (95% CI 33.61–37.59%)) schoolchildren affected (Table 1). According to the health region, East (43.51% (95% CI 40.42–46.63%)) was more affected than North (29.13% (95% CI 26.60–31.75%)), (X-squared = 50.126, df = 1, $p < 0.0001$). Gender and school category had no influence on overall prevalence of *A. lumbricoides* ($p > 0.05$) while rural schools (52.55% (95% CI 48.02–57.04%)) were more affected by *A. lumbricoides* than urban schools (30.84% (95% CI 28.69–33.06%)), (X-squared = 77.872, df = 1, $p < 0.0001$). At the department level (Figure 3), prevalence ranged from 12.9% in the WLE department to 58.04% in ZAD, (X-squared = 160.82, df = 8, $p < 0.0001$). Significant heterogeneity (X-squared = 382.81, df = 44, $p < 0.0001$) existed between schools: one is non-infected (0%), nine schools had a low prevalence (<20%), 19 had a moderate prevalence (≥20% but <50%), and 16 had a high prevalence (≥50%) (Table S2).

3.2.7. *Trichuris trichiura*

T. trichiura was prevalent in all schools surveyed and it was the more frequently found species with a total of 982 (43.7% (95% CI 41.68–45.8%)) infected schoolchildren. According to health region, a higher prevalence was found in the North (52.8% (95% CI 50–55.7%)) as compared to the East (32.6% (95% CI 29.7–35.6%)), (X-squared = 91.521, df = 1, $p < 0.0001$). There was a significant difference between rural (55%; 95% CI 50.5–59.5%) and urban schools (40.6%; 95% CI 38.3–42.9%), (X-squared = 31.729, df = 1, $p < 0.0001$)); and, between public (45.4%; 95% CI 43.7–48%) and private schools (41%; 95% CI 37.6–44.4%), (X-squared = 3.8965, df = 1, $p < 0.0001$) for the overall prevalence of *T. trichiura*. There was no significant difference of overall prevalence of *T. trichiura* according to gender ($p > 0.05$). At the department level, (Figure 3) the prevalence of *T. trichiura* varied from 27.13% in LPE to 67.53% in HKO department with significant heterogeneity (X-squared = 142.85, df = 8, $p < 0.0001$). At the school level, six schools had a prevalence of *T. trichiura* <20%, 21 schools had a prevalence ≤20% but <50%, and 18 had a prevalence ≥50% (Table S2). There was a significant difference in the distribution of *T. trichiura* among schools (X-squared = 340.14, df = 44, $p < 0.0001$).

3.2.8. Hookworms

Hookworms were present in 12 of the 45 studied schools with an overall prevalence of 1.43% (95% CI 1–2%): 1.6% (95% CI 0.99–2.49%) in the North region, 1.2% (95% CI 0.6–2.1%) in the East region. There was no significance difference between regions, school areas, and school categories (p>0.05), while there was a significant difference in overall prevalence of hookworm between girls (1.3%; 95% CI: 0.8–2.2%) and boys (2%; 95% CI: 1.3–3%) (X-squared = 5.2061, df = 1, p = 0.02251). At the department level (Figure 3), the prevalence was from 0 (for three departments) to a maximum of 6% in the WLE department with significant difference between departments (X-squared = 53.552, df = 8, $p < 0.0001$). Prevalence of hookworm in schools ranged from 0% (33 of the 45 schools surveyed) to 14.3% (Table S2). There were significant differences between schools (X-squared = 159.25, df = 44, $p < 0.0001$). Geographical distribution of the STH is presented in Figure 3.

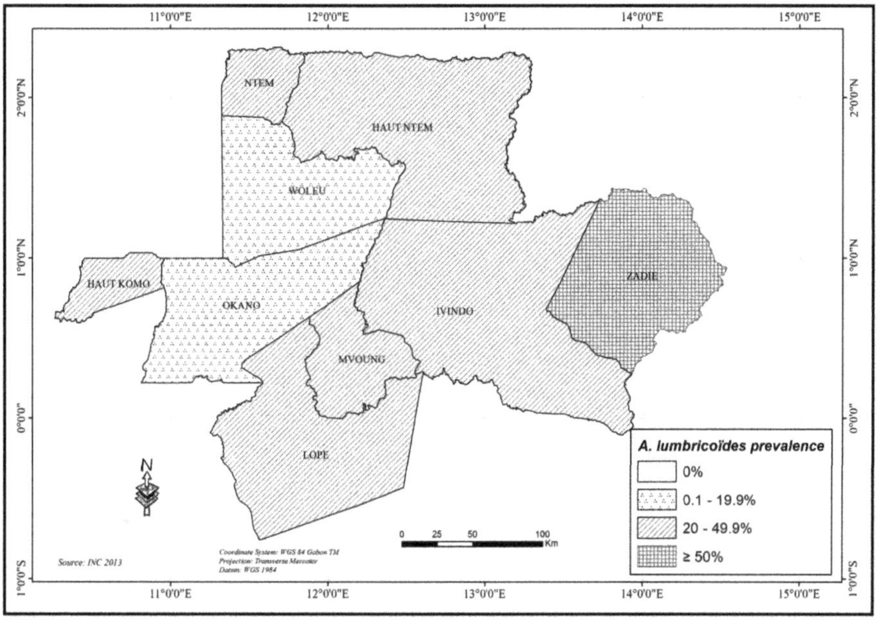

(**A**)

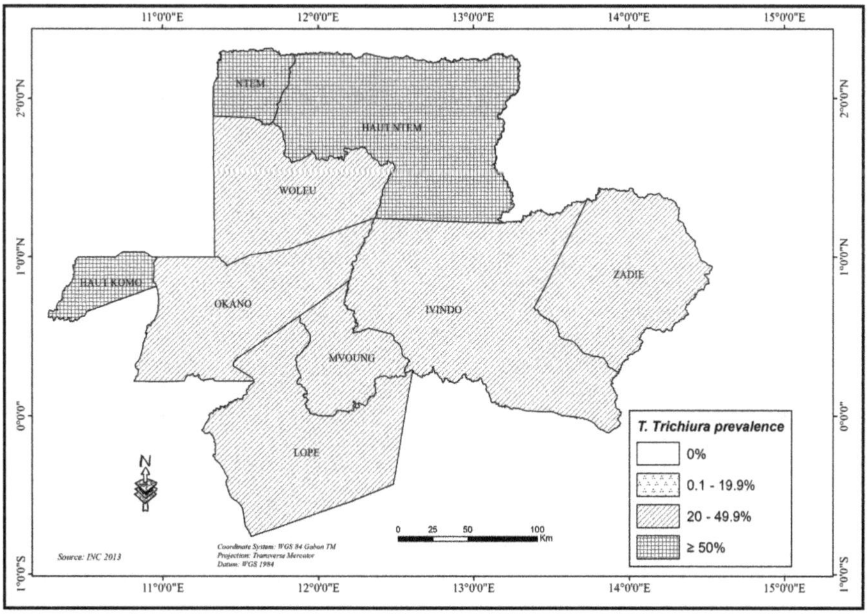

(**B**)

Figure 3. *Cont.*

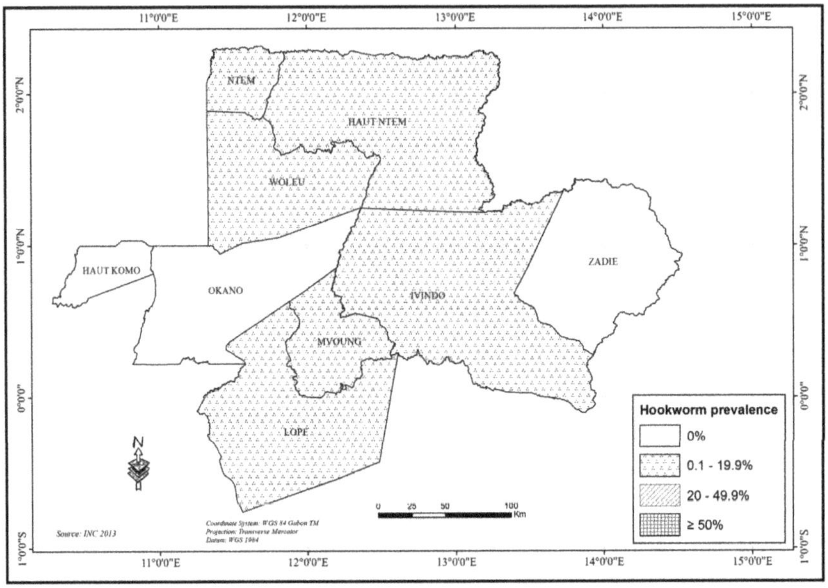

(C)

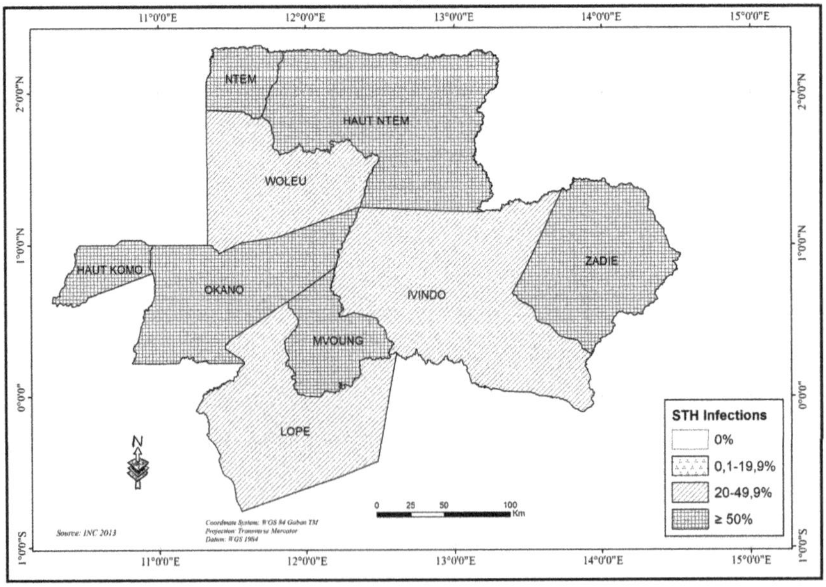

(D)

Figure 3. Map of prevalence levels for Soil Transmitted Helminthiasis at the department scale: (**A**) *Ascaris lumbricoides*; (**B**) *Trichurus trichuira*; (**C**) Hookworm; and, (**D**) Combined STH.

3.3. Intensity of Infection

3.3.1. Schistosomiasis

For the 37 schoolchildren that were infected with *S. haematobium*, the mean intensity of infections was 101.9 ± 41.1 eggs per 10 mL of urine with a significant difference between the North (18.3 ± 8.2 epg) and the East region (181.1 ± 85.6 epg), (W = 246, $p = 0.02176$) (Table 3). On the 20 schools prevalent with *S. haematobium*, light-intensity infections (<50 eggs/10 mL) occurred in 12 schools (11 in the North region and one in the East Region) and heavy-intensity infections (≥50 eggs/10 mL) occurred in eight schools (one in the North region and seven in the East Region) (Table S3). The maximum individual egg counts was 1534 eggs/10 mL of urine; 73% of infected schoolchildren had low-intensity infections and 27% had heavy-intensity infections. Overall, there is no significant difference between the genders, the school areas, and the school categories ($p > 0.05$).

Intensity of infections was 72 epg for the only case of *S. mansoni* and 240 epg for the only case of *S. guineensis* (Table 3).

3.3.2. *Ascaris lumbricoides*

Overall mean intensity of infection was moderate: 9586.6 ± 618.3 epg and significantly different between the two regions: 11,433.6 ± 1061.7 epg for the North and 8071.9 ± 707.3 epg for the East region (W = 69,804, $p = 0.004523$) (Table 3). Of the 44 schools prevalent with *A. lumbricoides*, light-intensity infections (1–4999 epg) occurred in 10 schools (four in the North region and six in the East region), moderate-intensity infections (5000–49,999 epg) occurred in 33 schools (20 in the North region and 13 in the East region), and heavy-intensity infections (≥50,000 epg) occurred in one school (in the North region) (Table S3). The maximum individual egg counts was 176,640, whereas 59.1% of infected schoolchildren had low-intensity infections, 37.5% with moderate-intensity infection, and 3.4% with heavy-intensity infections. Overall, gender, school area, and school category had no influence on the *A. lumbricoides* intensity of infection ($p > 0.05$).

3.3.3. *Trichuris trichiura*

The overall mean intensity of infection was moderate: 1143.2 ± 97 with a significant difference between the North (1395.2 ± 126.6 epg) and the East region (642.9 ± 140.2 epg), (W = 76,502, $p = 1.551 \times 10^{-13}$) (Table 3). Intensities of infection were classified in the light-intensity infections class (1–999 epg) for 30 schools (13 in the North region and 17 in the East region), in the moderate-intensity infections class (1000–9999) for 15 schools (12 in the North region and three in the East region). No school had the heavy intensity infections (≥10,000 epg) (Table S3). The maximum individual egg count was 37,440; 77.8% of the infected schoolchildren had low-intensity infections, 20.1% moderate-intensity infections, and 2.1% heavy-intensity infections. Overall, gender and school area had no influence on the *T. trichiura* intensity of infection ($p > 0.05$), while intensities of infection were higher in public schools (1193.5 ± 113.1 epg) than in private schools (1047.3 ± 182.1 epg) (W = 98,024, p-value = 0.01032) in the same class of intensity.

3.3.4. Hookworm

The overall mean intensity of infection was light: 618.0 ± 499.6 epg; 130.8 ± 31.1 epg in the North region and 1430.0 ± 1369.1 epg in the East region (Table 3). No significant difference was found between regions, gender, school areas, and school categories. The maximum individual egg count was 15,840 eggs and 96.9% of the schoolchildren had light-intensity infections (Table S3).

Table 3. Mean intensity of infection ± standard deviation at overall, by region, gender, school area, and school category. (N).

	Schistosomiasis			Soil Transmittted Helminthiasis		
	S. haematobium	***S. mansoni***	***S. guineensis***	***A. lumbricoides***	***T. trichiura***	**Hookworms**
Overall	101.9 ± 45.1 (37)	72 (1)	240 (1)	9586.6 ± 618.3 (799)	1143.2 ± 97.0 (982)	618.0 ± 499.6 (32)
By region						
North	18.3 ± 8.2 (18)	72 (1)	240 (1)	11433.6 ± 1061.7 (360)	1395.2 ± 126.6 (653)	130.8 ± 31.1 (20)
East	181.1 ± 85.6 (19)	-	-	8071.9 ± 707.3 (439)	642.9 ± 140.2 (329)	1430.0 ± 1369.1 (12)
By gender						
Girl	65.3 ± 32.4 (14)	-	240 (1)	10131.3 ± 1053.6 (381)	1152.6 ± 147.4 (474)	1861.3 ± 1853.7 (9)
Boy	124.2 ± 70.9 (23)	72 (1)	-	9018.1 ± 688.7 (418)	1130.1 ± 127.7 (508)	131.5 ± 35.0 (23)
By school area						
urban	109.5 ± 61.0 (26)	72 (1)	240 (1)	9144.6 ± 665.8 (541)	1139.9 ± 113.9 (712)	791.0 ± 669.2 (24)
rural	174.7 ± 55.3 (11)	-	-	10513.4 ± 1313.1 (258)	1151.7 ± 185.9 (270)	99.0 ± 46.9 (8)
By school category						
Public	73.3 ± 26.3 (28)	72 (1)	240 (1)	8874.4 ± 624.4 (522)	1193.5 ± 113.1 (644)	97.0 ± 18.9 (23)
Private	504.9 ± 178.5 (9)	-	-	10928.7 ± 1340.5 (277)	1047.3 ± 182.1 (338)	1949.3 ± 1843.5 (9)

3.4. Community Diagnosis and Recommended Treatment Strategies

According to our results on the prevalence and the intensity of infection, the recommended treatment strategies by department were summarized in Table 4.

Table 4. Diagnosis of health department and recommended treatment strategies.

Department	Category	MDA Interventions in Schools (Enrolled and Non-Enrolled)	Drug
Schistosomiasis infections			
Woleu Ntem Haut-Ntem Haut-Okano Okano Ivindo Lopé Mvoung	Low prevalence	MDA of SAC twice during primary schooling (once on entry, again on leaving)	Praziquantel
Zadié	Not endemic	No required MDA. Treatment of individual confirmed cases	
Soil Transmitted Helminthiasis infections			
Woleu	Moderate prevalence and moderate intensity	Annual MDA	
Ntem Haut-Ntem Haut-Komo Okano	High prevalence	Biannual MDA	Mebendazole + Levamisole
Ivindo Lopé	Moderate prevalence and moderate intensity	Annual MDA	
Mvoung Zadié	High prevalence	Biannual MDA	

MDA = mass drug administration; SAC = school-aged children.

4. Discussion

Our study showed that schistosomiasis and STH remain common in schoolchildren of both North and East health regions of Gabon with heterogenic proportions. Of the 2245 examined schoolchildren, 1270 (56.6%) were diagnosed by at least one schistosomiasis and/or STH. Infections were more influenced by both regions and school area. Indeed, schoolchildren in the North region (58.5%) were more affected than those in the East region (54.2%) and rural schoolchildren (72.10%) were more affected than urban schoolchildren (51.6%). Gender (girl/boy) and school category (public/private) had no influence on the burden of combined schistosomiasis or combined STH. However, hookworms affect more the boys than the girls and *T. trichiura* affect more the public than the private schoolchildren burden was most supported by STH than by schistosomiasis that is very low.

For schistosomiasis, the present study indicates that the infection is low endemic in the surveyed area, with the prevalence being 1.7% (all three species). Exhaustive results indicate that distribution of schistosomiasis is heterogeneous with an overall low endemicity for all the three species in the whole of the study area. Schistosomiasis haematobium was the most frequent and was diagnosed with at least one case in 20 schools from the 45 studied and from these 20 schools only one school was moderately endemic with a prevalence at 15.8%. Overall infection of *S. haematobium* was low (1.7%) in both the North (1.5%) and the East regions (1.9%). At the departmental level, prevalence was from 0.8% to 2.4% in the North region and from 0 to 4.4% in the Eastern region. Schistosomiasis *mansoni* and *guineensis* were rare in the surveyed areas with only one case of *S. mansoni* and *S. guineensis* respectively from the total schoolchildren examined. Data obtained here contrast with the results available for other areas and for the overall estimations in Gabon. Indeed, Mintsa *et al.* reported prevalence for *S. haematobium* at 17% and 26% in Melen, Libreville and Ekouk (80 km to Libreville), respectively [24], Gabon. Even wider, the estimation of prevalence of schistosomiasis in Gabon was about 45% [3]. Outside Gabon, in Central Africa, prevalence of schistosomiasis is generally high. For instance, in Cameroon, some localities in the East, West, and Central regions had prevalence of between 20 and 50%, and for some of them >50% [25]. In the Littoral, North-West and South-West Cameroon regions [26], prevalence were also much higher than those recorded in our study. This contrast confirms the patching distribution of schistosomiasis. Some parameters can explain the patching distribution of schistosomiasis and they include human and ecological factors [27], temperature, and rainfall [28]. The use of GIS for epidemiological survey in Tanzania showed that schistosomiasis was not endemic in areas where the temperature was below 20 °C [18,29]. By contrast, in Cameroon, prevalence is >10% for the areas where temperature is >40 °C and precipitation <1500 mm [30]. These differences can be attributed to both distribution of the intermediate snail host species in Africa [31] and their optimal conditions for development in West Africa [32]. In our study sites, temperature is >30 °C and precipitation >1000 mm, this should be in favor of high prevalence. Besides temperature and rainfall, relief [33], demography and living conditions [34] can also play a role in the distribution of schistosomiasis. Otherwise, the low presence *S. guineensis* can also be attributed to the possibilities of hybrid species which are mentioned in the country and are very indistinguishable using microscopy [24]. The hypothesis of the hybridization zones between *S. guineensis* and *S. haematobium* has been suggested in two provinces of western Gabon, Moyen-Ogooué [35] and Estuaire [36]. Hydridization between *S. guineensis* and *S. haematobium* led to the extinction of *S. guineensis* in favor of *S. haematobium*, as at Loum in Cameroon [37]. The low prevalence of *S. mansoni* in this study is not surprising because its distribution in the country is uncertain [38].

In addition to the low prevalence recorded in this study, schistosomiasis was characterized by low intensity of infections. Indeed, 73% of schoolchildren that were infected by *S. haematobium* had a light (<50 eggs/10 mL urine) intensity of infection, and 27% a heavy one (≥50 eggs/10 mL urine). These results are lower than those that were recorded at baseline results in the Barombi Kotto focus, Cameroon where the total intensity of infection was 212.1 e/10 mL urine in schoolchildren of ages between 3 and 22 years [23] and in the Sahel region, Burkina Faso [39]. The intensity of infection to *Schistosoma* is often correlated to the morbidity in SAC and other susceptible groups [40,41] and it plays an important role for the estimation of prevalence with consequences for the treatment strategy in PCT [38,42]. Although the microscopic techniques that were used in our study (urine filtration for *S. haematobium* diagnosis and Kato-Katz for *S. mansoni* and *S. guineensis* diagnosis) are the most recommended by WHO [43] and the most widely used diagnostic approaches in epidemiological surveys, their sensitivity is very discussed in foci with low intensity of infection because of day to day egg variations [44]. Hence, multiple Kato-Katz thick smears are required to enhance sensitivity [45], but this poses operational challenges and strains financial resources. As an alternative to these conventional diagnostic methods, novel tools showing a very high diagnostic accuracy have recently been developed. They include the detection of monoclonal antibody-based circulating antigens CCA and CAA [46] and the molecular approaches [47]. For example, it has been shown that estimation of prevalence with Kato-Katz technique underestimates the prevalence of active *S. japonicum* infections in China by a factor of 10 compared with the UCP-LF CAA assay [48]. Similarly, estimation of *S. haematobium* prevalence was several-fold higher with UCP-LF CAA assay than the one detected with a single urine filtration [49]. Since 2008, a more sophisticated Point-Of-Care (POC) test detecting *Schistosoma* CCA in urine has been developed and is now commercially available and is recommended by the authors for *S. mansoni* diagnosis [50,51]. A POC-CCA test revealed higher sensitivity than triplicate Kato-Katz, and it produced similar prevalence as nine Kato-Katz in many field survey evaluations [21,52]. The use of CCAs or CAAs might thereby affect the results and the recommendations for treatment strategies

Our results showed that STH were highly endemic. Overall, 56.1% of the schoolchildren examined were affected by the combined STH (together *A. lumbricoides*, *T. trichiura*, and Hookworms). This confirms the important level of STH in Central Africa, as in Cameroun [53]. Factors that may explain high levels of STH infections include lacks of sanitation and access to drinking water [9]. Our results indicate that the North region (58.1%) was most prevalent that the East (53.1%) and schoolchildren from rural schools (72.1%) were more affected than those from urban schools (51.6%).Various factors, such as genetics, poly-parasitism, demography, and urbanization, may explain these differences [11]. The most common STH was *T. trichiura* (43.7%), followed by *A. lumbricoides* (35.6%), with heterogeneous distributions between departments (Figure 3) and between schools. Indeed, *T. trichiura* and *A. lumbricoides* were moderately prevalent (≥20 and <50%) in 21 and 19 schools, respectively, and both were very highly prevalent (≥50%) in 16 schools. In contrast to the high prevalence of *A. lumbricoides* and *T. trichiura*, the prevalence of hookworm was low, 1.4% at overall, 1.6% in the North, and 1.2% in the East region. These results confirm the well documented observation that the prevalence of *T. trichiura* and *A. lumbricoides* were always higher than prevalence of hookworms [12,25,26]. Besides prevalence, the intensity of infection is a good indicator for epidemiology of STH. Indeed, most of the morbidity is accounted for by infected individuals who are the most heavily infected [54]. Our results showed a moderate-intensity infections for *T. trichiura*. (1143.2 epg overall) and *A. lumbricoides* (overall 9586.6 epg) and light-intensity infection for hookworms (overall 618 epg). However, 2.1% and 3.4% of schoolchildren had heavy-intensity of infections for *T. trichiura* and *A. lumbricoides*, respectively, attesting the burden of these STH in the surveyed foci.

One of the objectives of our study was to address recommendations for SCH and STH preventive chemotherapy in Gabon. Following WHO guidelines, based on prevalence and intensity of infections, the program is classifying communities according to three strategies: (1) a high prevalence (≥50% for both Schistosomiasis and STH) or heavy-intensity infections, schoolchildren are treated every year, and high risk groups, such as fishermen, are treated; (2) a moderate prevalence (≥10% for Schistosomiasis and ≥20% for STH, but <50% for both schistosomiasis and STH) and light-intensity infections, schoolchildren are treated once every two years; and (3) a low prevalence (<10% for Schistosomiasis and <20% for STH) and light-intensity infections, chemotherapy is made available in health facilities for treatment of suspected cases [15]. For schistosomiasis, considering the low prevalence recorded in our study, we recommend PC of SAC twice during primary schooling (once on entry, again on leaving) for eight departments and individual treatment for the confirmed cases in the Zadié department. We also recommend the diagnosis of other communities at high risk (such as pre-schoolchildren, pregnant women, and special occupation groups) and chemotherapy will be made available in health facilities for treatment of suspected cases according to OMS guidelines [15]. WHO recommended the drug Praziquantel (PZQ) with a dosage of 40mg/Kg for the treatment of schistosomiasis in PTC. Impact of treatment varies according to region and treatment strategy. An annual treatment strategy has significantly reduced prevalence of schistosomiasis 1, 2, and 3 years post-treatment in West Africa, i.e., Burkina Faso [38], Niger [55], Ghana [56]; East Africa i.e., Uganda [57], and in Central Africa, i.e., Cameroun [23,26]. For STH, we recommend a biannual PC strategy including pre and SAC, women of child bearing age including pregnant women in the 2nd and 3rd trimesters and lactating women and adults at high risk in certain occupations (e.g. tea-pickers and miners) for the six departments (Ntem, Haut-Ntem, Haut-Komo, Okano, Mvoung and Zadié), where the prevalence was high (≥50%) and an annual PC strategy for the three departments (Woleu, Ivindo, Lopé) with moderate prevalence. Four anthelminthics are currently on the WHO model list of essential medicines for the treatment and control of STH: albendazole, mebendazole, levamisole, and pyrantel-pamoate [15]. Impact of these different drugs on STH are discussed by Keizer and Utzinger [58]. For these authors, oral single-doses of these drugs show high cure rates against *A. lumbricoides*, but not always against *T trichiura* and hookworms. Combination of mebendazole and levamisole shows the best cure rate against STH [59]. Furthermore, considering the total costs per child treated against schistosomiasis and STH, including drug and delivery, US$ 0.32 in Burkina Faso [35], the PC should integrate and progress with both schistosomiasis and STH.

Supplementary Materials: The following are available at http://www.mdpi.com/2414-6366/3/4/119/s1, Table S1: list of schools surveyed per region and department with their respective geographical position. Non-italic = public school; italics = private school. In bold = urban school; normal = rural school, Table S2: Number of infected schoolchildren (prevalence in %) for each parasite according to school and department investigated. N is the number of schoolchildren examined. * $p < 0.05$ (Fisher-Exact-test); * is followed by school number or by department name with a significant difference, Table S3: Intensity of infection (mean ± standard deviation) for each parasite according to school and department investigated. N is the number of schoolchildren examined. * $p < 0.05$ (Mann-Whitney test); * is followed by the school number or department code with significant difference. L, M and H indicate class intensity of infection. L = light-intensity infection, M = moderate-intensity infections, H = heavy-intensity infections according to each species.

Author Contributions: Conceptualization: R.M.N., K.M.M.N.-M., J.A. and M.S.L. Data curation: R.M.N., J.F.M. and K.M.M.N.-M. Formal analysis: R.M.N., J.F.M., A.A.K., H.M. and G.M. Funding acquisition and relevant documents: J.A., A.D., and G.N.A. Investigation: R.M.N., K.M.M.N.-M., J.A. and M.M.M. Methodology: R.M.N., K.M.M.N.-M., M.S.L. and J.A. Project administration: R.M.N., K.M.M.N.-M., A.D., G.N.A. and J.A. Resources: J.A., K.M.M.N.-M., M.M.M., J.R.M. and M.K.B.A. Software: R.M.N., A.A.K., H.M. and G.M. Supervision: J.A., M.S.L., M.M.M. and J.R.M. Validation: M.S.L., G.N.A., M.K.B.A., G.M., H.M. and J.A. Visualization: R.M.N., G.M. and H.M. Original draft preparation: R.M.N. and J.F.M. Review and editing: All the authors.

Funding: This study was entirely funded by WHO delegation office Gabon in Libreville, and with the implementation of the Gabonese Ministry of Public Health through the Control Program of Parasitic Diseases.

Acknowledgments: The authors are grateful to the both Regional Directors of Health: Dr. Guikombi Jean Réné in the North and Ms. Mbeng Mba Félicité in the East for planning and communication work in the field. We want to thank all the participants in this study, particularly the schoolchildren and their parents, the directors and teachers of the schools surveyed. We are very grateful to Lilody Ikoutsi Gertrude, Ollomo Nziengui Fabrice, Oniane Nicole, Emane Alain Georges, Nzamba Boulingui Antoine Chyder, Minko mi Engone Gui, and Inguimba Elvis for the technical supports and assistance.

Conflicts of Interest: The authors declare no conflict of interest. The funders had no role in the design of the study; in the collection, analyses, or interpretation of data; in the writing of the manuscript, or in the decision to publish the results.

References

1. Hotez, P.J.; Kamath, A. Neglected tropical diseases in sub-Saharan Africa: Review of their prevalence, distribution, and disease burden. *PLoS Negl. Trop. Dis.* **2009**, *3*, e412. [CrossRef] [PubMed]
2. World Health Organization. Schistosomiasis and soil-transmitted helminth infections—preliminary estimates of the number of children treated with albendazole or mebendazole. *Wkly. Epidemiol. Rec.* **2006**, *81*, 145–163.
3. Steinmann, P.; Keiser, J.; Bo, R.; Tanner, M.; Utzinger, J. Schistosomiasis and water resources development: Systematic review, meta-analysis, and estimates of people at risk. *Lancet Infect. Dis.* **2006**, *6*, 411–425. [CrossRef]
4. WHO. *World Health Organization Schistosomiasis Fact Sheet*; World Health Organization: Geneva, Switzerland, 2014.
5. Adenowoa, A.F.; Oyinloyea, B.E.; Ogunyinkaa, B.I.; Kappo, A.P. Impact of human schistosomiasis in sub-Saharan Africa. *Braz. J. Infect. Dis.* **2015**, *19*, 196–205. [CrossRef] [PubMed]
6. Kane, R.A.; Southgate, V.R.; Rollinson, D.; Littlewood, D.T.J.; Lockyer, A.E.; Pagès, J.R.; Tchuem Tchuente, L.A.; Jourdane, J. A phylogeny based on three mitochondrial genes supports the division of *Schistosoma intercalatum* into two separate species. *Parasitology* **2003**, *127*, 131–137. [CrossRef] [PubMed]
7. Pagès, J.R.; Jourdane, J.; Southgate, V.R.; Tchuem Tchuente, L.A. Reconnaissance de deux espèces jumelles au sein du taxon *Schistosoma intercalatum* Fisher, 1934, agent de la schistosomose humaine rectale en Afrique. Description de *Schistosoma guineensis* n. sp. In *Taxonomy, Ecology and Evolution of Metazoan Parasites*; tome II; Combes, C., Jourdane, J., Eds.; Presses Universitaire de Perpignan: Perpignan, France, 2003; pp. 139–146.
8. WHO. *Schistosomiasis: Progress Report 2001–2011 and Strategic Plan 2012–2020*; WHO/HTM/NTD/PTC; World Health Organization: Geneva, Switzerland, 2013; p. 2.
9. WHO. *Soil-Transmitted Helminthiases: Eliminating Soil-Transmitted Helminthiases as a Public Health Problem in Children: Progress Report 2001–2010 and Strategic Plan 2011–2020*; WHO/HTM/NTD/PTC; World Health Organization: Geneva, Switzerland, 2012; p. 4.

10. WHO. *Deworming for Health and Development*; Report of the Third Global Meeting of the Partners for Parasite Control; World Health Organization: Geneva, Switzerland, 2005.
11. Brooker, S.; Clements, A.C.A.; Bundy, D.A.P. Global epidemiology, ecology and control of soil-transmitted helminth infections. *Adv. Parasitol.* **2006**, *62*, 221–261. [PubMed]
12. Mabika-Mamfoumbi, M.; Moussavou-Boussougou, M.N.; Nzenze-Afene, S.; Owono-Medang, M.; Bouyou-Okotet, M.; Kendzo, E.; Kombila, M. Prevalence evaluation of intestinal parasites in rural and sub-urban area in Gabon. *Bull. Med. Owendo* **2009**, *12*, 85–88.
13. Schistosomiasis and Soil-Transmitted Helminth Infections. Fifty-fourth World Health Assembly: Resolution WHA54.192001. 2001. Available online: http://apps.who.int/gb/archive/pdf_files/WHA54/ea54r19.pdf (accessed on 12 April 2018).
14. Namwanje, H.; Kabatereine, N.; Olsen, A. A randomised controlled clinical trial on the safety of co-administration of albendazole, ivermectin and praziquantel in infected schoolchildren in Uganda. *Trans. R. Soc. Trop. Med. Hyg.* **2011**, *105*, 181–188. [CrossRef] [PubMed]
15. WHO. *Preventive Chemotherapy in Human Helminthiasis: Coordinated Use of Anthelminthic Drugs in Control Interventions*; World Health Organization: Geneva, Switzerland, 2006.
16. Kolaczinski, J.; Kabatereine, N.B.; Onapa, A.; Ndyomugyengi, R.; Kakmebo, A.S.; Brooker, S. Neglected tropical diseases in Uganda: The prospect and challenge of integrated control. *Trend Parasitol.* **2007**, *23*, 485–493. [CrossRef] [PubMed]
17. Hunter, J.M.; Rey, L.; Chu, K.Y.; Adekolu-John, E.O.; Mott, K.E. *Parasitic Diseases in Water Resources Development: The Need for Intersectoral Collaboration*; World Health Organization: Geneva, Switzerland, 1993.
18. Brooker, S.; Micheal, E. The potential of geographical information systems and remote sensing in the epidemiology and control of human heliminths infections. *Adv. Parasitol.* **2000**, *47*, 246–288.
19. Direction Générale de la Statistique. Résultats globaux du Recensement Général de la Population et des Logements de 2013 du Gabon (RGPL-2013). Libreville, Publication de la Direction Générale de la Statique (DGS). 2015. Available online: https://www.mays-mouissi.com/wp-content/uploads/2016/07/Recensement-general-de-la-population-et-des-logements-de-2013-RGPL.pdf (accessed on 01 December 2017).
20. Peters, P.A.; Mahmoud, A.A.; Warren, K.S.; Ouma, J.H.; Siongok, T.K. Field studies of a rapid, accurate means of quantifying *Schistosoma haematobium* eggs in urine samples. *Bull. World Health Organ.* **1976**, *54*, 159–162. [PubMed]
21. Coulibaly, J.T.; Knopp, S.; N'Guessan, N.A.; Silue, K.D.; Furst, T.; Lohourignon, L.K.; Brou, J.K.; N'Gbesso, Y.K.; Vounatsou, P.; N'Goran, E.K.; et al. Accuracy of Urine Circulating Cathodic Antigen (CCA) Test for *Schistosoma mansoni* diagnosis in different settings of Côte d'Ivoire. *PLoS Negl. Trop. Dis.* **2011**, *5*, e1384. [CrossRef] [PubMed]
22. Katz, N.; Chaves, A.; Pellegrino, J. A simple device for quantitative stool thick-smear technique in *Schistosomiasis mansoni. Rev. Inst. Med. Trop. Sao Paulo* **1972**, *14*, 397–400. [PubMed]
23. Nkengazong, L.; Njiokou, F.; Asonganyi, T. Two years impact of single praziquantel treatment on infection of urinary schistosomiasis in the Barombi Kotto focus, Cameroon. *Int. J. Biosci.* **2013**, *3*, 98–107.
24. Mintsa Nguema, R.; Mengue Ngou-Milama, K.; Kombila, M.; Rechard-Lenoble, D.; Tisseyre, P.; Ibikounlé, M.; Moné, H.; Mouahid, G. Morphometric and molecular characterizations of schistosome populations in Estuaire province Gabon. *J. Helminthol.* **2010**, *84*, 81–85. [CrossRef] [PubMed]
25. Tchuem Tchuenté, L.A.; Kamwa Ngassam, R.I.; Sumo, L.; Ngassam, P.; Dongmo Noumedem, C.; Luogbou Nzu, D.D.; Dankoni, E.; Kenfack, C.M.; Gipwe, N.F.; Akame, J.; et al. Mapping of Schistosomiasis and Soil-Transmitted Helminthiasis in the Regions of Centre, East and West Cameroon. *PLoS Negl. Trop. Dis.* **2012**, *6*, e1553. [CrossRef] [PubMed]
26. Tchuem Tchuenté, L.A.; Dongmo Noumedem, C.; Ngassam, P.; Mérimé Kenfack, C.; Feussom Gipwe, N.; Dankoni, E.; Merrime Kenfack, C.; Feussom Gipwe, N.; Akame, J.; Tarini, A.; et al. Mapping of schistosomiasis and soil transmitted helminthiasis in the regions of Littoral, North-West, South and South-West Cameroon and recommendations for treatment. *BMC Infect. Dis.* **2013**, *13*, 602. [CrossRef] [PubMed]

27. Woolhouse, M.E.J.; Chandiwana, S.K. Spatial and temporal heterogeneity in the population dynamics of *Bulinus globosus* and *Biomphalaria pfeifferi* and in the epidemiology of their infection with Schistosomes. *Parasitology* **1989**, *98*, 21–34. [CrossRef] [PubMed]
28. Brooker, S. Schistosomes, snails and satellites. *Acta Trop.* **2002**, *82*, 207–214. [CrossRef]
29. Brooker, S.; Hay, S.I.; Issae, W.; Hall, A.; Kihamia, C.M.; Lwambo, N.J.S.; Wint, W.; Rogers, D.J.; Bundy, D.A.P. Predicting the distribution of urinary schistosomiasis in Tanzania using satellite sensor data. *Trop. Med. Int. Health* **2001**, *6*, 998–1007. [CrossRef] [PubMed]
30. Brooker, S.; Hay, S.I.; Tchuem Tchuenté, L.A.; Ratard, R. Modelling human helminth distributions for planning disease control in Cameroon. *Photogramm. Eng. Remote Sens.* **2002**, *68*, 175–179.
31. Brown, S.D. *Freshwater Snail of Africa and Their Medical Importance*; Taylor and Francis: London, UK, 1994.
32. Greer, G.J.; Mimpfoundi, R.; Malek, E.A.; Joky, A.; Ngonseu, E.; Ratard, R.C. Human schistosomiasis in Cameroon II. Distribution of the snail hosts. *Am. J. Trop. Med. Hyg.* **1990**, *6*, 573–580. [CrossRef]
33. Kabatereine, N.B.; Brooker, S.; Tukahebwa, E.M.; Kazibwe, F.; Onapa, A. Epidemiology and geography of *Schistosoma mansoni* in Uganda: Implications for planning control. *Trop. Med. Int. Health* **2004**, *9*, 372–380. [CrossRef] [PubMed]
34. WHO. *Report on the WHO Informal Consultation on Schistosomiasis Control*; World Health Organization: Geneva, Switzerland, 1999; p. 2.
35. Burchard, G.D.; Kern, P. Probable hybridization between *S. intercalatum* and *S. haematobium* in Western Gabon. *Trop. Geogr. Med.* **1985**, *37*, 119–123. [PubMed]
36. Richard-Lenoble, D.; Kombila, M.; Duong, T.H.; Gendrel, D. Bilharziose à *Schistosoma intercalatum*, bilharziose récente et oubliée. *Rev. Pratc.* **1993**, *43*, 432–439.
37. Webster, B.L.; Tchuem Tchuenté, L.A.; Jourdane, J.; Southgate, V.R. The interaction of *Schistosoma haematobium* and *S. guineensis* in Cameroon. *J. Helminthol.* **2005**, *79*, 193–197. [CrossRef] [PubMed]
38. Mintsa Nguema, R.; Mve Ondo, B.; Mabika Mamfoumbi, M.; Koumba, A.A.; Bouyou Akotet, M.K.; Kombila, M. Recent Examination for Assessing Epidemiological Status of Schistosoma *Mansoni* in Plaine Orety, Urban Area of Libreville, Gabon, Central Africa. *CAJPH* **2018**, *4*, 81–85. [CrossRef]
39. Toure, S.; Zhang, Y.; Bosque-Oliva, E.; Ky, C.; Ouedraogo, A.; Koukounariet, A.; Gabrielli, A.F.; Sellin, B.; Websterb, J.P.; Fenwickb, A. Two-year impact of single praziquantel treatment on infection in the national control programme on schistosomiasis in Burkina Faso. *Bull. World Health Organ.* **2008**, *86*, 780–787. [CrossRef] [PubMed]
40. Smith, D.H.; Warren, K.S.; Mahmoud, A.A.F. Morbidity in *Schistosomiasis Mansoni* in relation to intensity of infection: Study of a community in Kisumu, Kenya. *Am. J. Trop. Med. Hyg.* **1979**, *28*, 220–229. [PubMed]
41. Genming, Z.; Brinkmann, U.K.; Qingwu, J.; Shaoji, Z.; Zhide, L.; Hongchang, Y. The relationship between morbidity and intensity of *Schistosomiasis japonicum* infection of a community in Jiangxi Province, China. *Southeast. Asian J. Trop. Med. Public Health* **1977**, *28*, 245–250.
42. Utzinger, J.; Becker, S.L.; van Lieshout, L.; van Dam, G.J.; Knopp, S. New diagnostic tools in schistosomiasis. *Clin. Microbiol. Infect.* **2015**, *21*, 529–542. [CrossRef] [PubMed]
43. WHO. *Basic Laboratory Methods in Medical Parasitology*; World Health Organization: Geneva, Switzerland, 1991.
44. Braun-Munzinger, R.A.; Southgate, B.A. Repeatability and reproducibility of egg counts of *Schistosoma haematobium* in urine. *Trop. Med. Parasitol.* **1992**, *43*, 149–154. [PubMed]
45. Lamberton, P.H.L.; Kabatereine, N.B.; Oguttu, D.W.; Fenwick, A.; Webster, J.P. Sensitivity and specificity of multiple Kato-Katz thick smears and a Circulating Cathodic Antigen test for *Schistosoma mansoni* Diagnosis Pre-and Post-repeated-Praziquantel treatment. *PLoS Negl. Trop. Dis.* **2014**, *8*, e3139. [CrossRef] [PubMed]
46. Van Lieshout, L.; Polderman, A.M.; Deelder, A.M. Immunodiagnosis of schistosomiasis by determination of the circulating antigens CAA and CCA, in particular in individuals with recent or light infections. *Acta Trop.* **2000**, *77*, 68–80. [CrossRef]
47. Obeng, B.B.; Aryeetey, Y.A.; de Dood, C.J.; Amoah, A.S.; Larbi, I.A.; Deelder, A.M.; Yazdanbakhsh, M.; Hartgers, F.C.; Boakye, D.A.; Verweij, J.J.; et al. Application of a circulating-cathodic-antigen (CCA) strip test and real-time PCR, in comparison with microscopy, for the detection of *Schistosoma haematobium* in urine samples from Ghana. *Ann. Trop. Med. Parasitol.* **2008**, *102*, 625–633. [CrossRef] [PubMed]

48. Van Dam, G.J.; Xu, J.; Bergquist, R.; de Dood, C.J.; Utzinger, J.; Qin, Z.Q.; Guanb, W.; Fengb, T.; Yug, X.L.; Zhoug, J.; et al. An ultra-sensitive assay targeting the circulating anodic antigen for the diagnosis of *Schistosoma japonicum* in a low-endemic area, People's Republic of China. *Acta Trop.* **2015**, *141*, 190–197. [CrossRef] [PubMed]
49. Knopp, S.; Corstjens, P.L.A.M.; Koukounari, A.; Cercamondi, C.I.; Ame, S.M.; Ali, S.M.; de Dood, C.J.; Mohammed, K.A.; Utzinger, J.; Rollinson, D.; et al. Sensitivity and specificity of a urine circulating anodic antigen test for the diagnosis of *Schistosoma haematobium* in low endemic settings. *PLoS Negl. Trop. Dis.* **2015**, *9*, e0003752. [CrossRef] [PubMed]
50. Stothard, J.R.; Kabatereine, N.B.; Tukahebwa, E.M.; Kazibwe, F.; Rollinson, D.; Mathieson, W.; Webster, J.P.; Fenwick, A. Use of circulating cathodic antigen (CCA) dipsticks for detection of intestinal and urinary schistosomiasis. *Acta Trop.* **2006**, *97*, 219–228. [CrossRef] [PubMed]
51. Colley, D.G.; Binder, S.; Campbell, C.; King, C.H.; Tchuem Tchuenté, LA.; N'Goran, E.K. A Five-Country Evaluation of a Point-of-Care Circulating Cathodic Antigen Urine Assay for the Prevalence of *Schistosoma mansoni*. *Am. J. Trop. Med. Hyg.* **2013**, *88*, 426–432. [CrossRef] [PubMed]
52. Tchuem Tchuenté, L.A.; Kueté Fouodo, C.J.; Kamwa Ngassam, R.I.; Sumo, L.; Dongmo Noumedem, C.; Mérimé Kenfack, C.; Gipwe, N.F.; Dankoni Nana, E.; Stothard, J.R.; Rollinson, D. Evaluation of Circulating Cathodic Antigen (CCA) Urine-Tests for Diagnosis of *Schistosoma mansoni* Infection in Cameroon. *PLoS Negl. Trop. Dis.* **2012**, *6*, e1758. [CrossRef] [PubMed]
53. Ratard, R.C.; Kouemeni, L.E.; Ekani Bessala, M.M.; Ndamkou, K.N.; Greer, G.J.; Spilsbury, J.; Cline, B.L. Human schistosomiasis in Cameroon. I. Distribution of schistosomiasis. *Am. J. Trop. Med. Hyg.* **1990**, *42*, 561–572. [CrossRef] [PubMed]
54. WHO. *Prevention and Control of Schistosomiasis and Soil-Transmitted Helminthiasis*; World Health Organisation: Geneva, Switzerland, 2002.
55. Garba, A.; Campagne, G.; Tassie, J.M.; Barkire, A.; Vera, C.; Sellin, B.; Chippaux, J.P. Evaluation à long terme d'un traitement de masse par praziquantel sur la morbidité due à *Schistosoma haematobium* dans deux villages hyper-endémiques du Nige. *Bull. Soc. Pathol. Exot.* **2004**, *97*, 7–11. [PubMed]
56. Nsowah-Nuamah, N.N.; Aryeetey, M.E.; Jolayemi, E.T.; Yagatsuma, Y.; Mensah, G.; Dontwi, I.K.; Nkrumah, F.K.; Kojima, S. Predicting the timing of second praziquantel treatment and its effect on reduction of egg counts in southern Ghana. *Acta Trop.* **2004**, *90*, 263–720. [CrossRef] [PubMed]
57. Frenzel, K.; Grigull, L.; Odongo-Aginya, E.; Ndugwa, C.M.; Loroni-Lakwo, T.; Schweigmann, U.; Vester, U.; Spannbrucker, N.; Doehring, E. Evidence for a long-term effect of a single dose of praziquantel on *Schistosoma mansoni*–induced hepatosplenic lesions in Northern Uganda. *Am. J. Trop. Med. Hyg.* **1999**, *60*, 927–931. [CrossRef] [PubMed]
58. Keizer, J.; Utzinger, J. Efficacity of current drugs against Soil Transmitted Helminthiasis infections: Systematic review and meta-analysis. *JAMA* **2008**, *299*, 1937–1948.
59. Albonico, M.; Bickle, Q.; Ramsan, M.; Montresor, A.; Savioli, L.; Taylor, M. Efficacy of mebendazole and levamisole alone or in combination against intestinal nematode infections after repeated targeted mebendazole treatment in Zanzibar. *Bull. World Health Organ.* **2003**, *81*, 343–352. [PubMed]

Tropical Medicine and Infectious Disease

MDPI

Article

Low Praziquantel Treatment Coverage for *Schistosoma mansoni* in Mayuge District, Uganda, Due to the Absence of Treatment Opportunities, Rather Than Systematic Non-Compliance

Moses Adriko [1,†], Christina L. Faust [2,*,†], Lauren V. Carruthers [2], Arinaitwe Moses [1], Edridah M. Tukahebwa [1] and Poppy H. L. Lamberton [2,*]

1 Vector Control Division, Ministry of Health, Plot 15 Bombo Road, P.O. Box 1661, Kampala, Uganda; adrikomoses@gmail.com (M.A.); moses0772359814@gmail.com (A.M.); edmuheki@gmail.com (E.M.T.)

2 Institute of Biodiversity, Animal Health and Comparative Medicine and Wellcome Centre for Molecular Parasitology, University of Glasgow, Glasgow G12 8QQ, UK; l.carruthers.1@research.gla.ac.uk

* Correspondence: christina.faust@glasgow.ac.uk (C.L.F.); poppy.lamberton@glasgow.ac.uk (P.H.L.L.); Tel.: +44-(0)14-1330-6993 (C.L.F.); +44-(0)14-1330-5571 (P.H.L.L.)

† Joint first authors, listed in alphabetical order.

Received: 5 September 2018; Accepted: 26 September 2018; Published: 8 October 2018

Abstract: The World Health Organization (WHO) recommends praziquantel mass drug administration (MDA) to control schistosomiasis in endemic regions. We aimed to quantify recent and lifetime praziquantel coverage, and reasons for non-treatment, at an individual level to guide policy recommendations to help Uganda reach WHO goals. Cross-sectional household surveys ($n = 681$) encompassing 3208 individuals (adults and children) were conducted in 2017 in Bugoto A and B, Mayuge District, Uganda. Participants were asked if they had received praziquantel during the recent MDA (October 2016) and whether they had ever received praziquantel in their lifetime. A multivariate logistic regression analysis with socio-economic and individual characteristics as covariates was used to determine factors associated with praziquantel uptake. In the MDA eligible population (≥5 years of age), the most recent MDA coverage was 48.8%. Across individuals' lifetimes, 31.8% of eligible and 49.5% of the entire population reported having never taken praziquantel. Factors that improved individuals' odds of taking praziquantel included school enrolment, residence in Bugoto B and increasing years of village-residency. Not being offered (49.2%) and being away during treatment (21.4%) were the most frequent reasons for not taking the 2016 praziquantel MDA. Contrary to expectations, chronically-untreated individuals were rarely systematic non-compliers, but more commonly not offered treatment.

Keywords: Mayuge; MDA coverage; praziquantel; *S. mansoni*; systematic non-compliance; treatment-opportunities; Uganda

---

1. Introduction

Schistosomiasis is a severe, debilitating, neglected tropical disease that is often associated with poverty [1]. *Schistosoma* parasites are transmitted in areas with limited infrastructure and minimal access to, or use of, improved water, sanitation and hygiene (WASH) facilities [2,3]. The disease is endemic in 78 countries, causing an estimated 1.864 million disability adjusted life years lost (DALYs) in the over 250 million people infected, of whom >90% live in sub-Saharan Africa [4–7]. Improvements in diagnostics show that prevalence may be even higher than previously thought [8].

Currently, schistosomiasis control in endemic regions focuses heavily on regular praziquantel mass drug administration (MDA), which aims to prevent morbidity in later life by reducing infection intensities and prevalence [9]. The World Health Organization (WHO) recommends community-wide MDA in areas where prevalence in school-aged children (SAC; enrolled and non-enrolled children between the ages of 5–14) is >50% [9]. To achieve WHO goals to reduce schistosomiasis morbidity by 2020, countries need to reach targets of at least 75% preventive chemotherapy (PC) coverage of SAC and at-risk adults annually in these highly-endemic communities [10]. At-risk adults range from entire communities living in endemic areas to special groups (i.e., occupations involving frequent contact with infested water such as fishermen or irrigation workers). Models show that high PC coverage in both SAC and at-risk adults may be required for up to 15 years for successful morbidity control [11]. Models highlight that the required duration of annual MDA depends heavily on baseline intensity and the proportion of systematic non-compliance versus untreated people being randomly distributed each year [11]. However, there are few data regarding treatment across an individual's lifetime and how non-treatment is distributed across communities [12]. Annual MDA has been successful at reducing the prevalence and intensity of infections in several areas [13–16], but hotspots remain in others [13,17]. Preventive chemotherapy is the mainstay component of schistosomiasis control, but other supportive strategies such as provision of safe water and adequate sanitation, hygiene education and snail control will be essential for the achievement of the WHO 2020 goal of elimination as a public health problem.

Coverage data at country and regional levels is often aggregated across implementation units (IUs) [12,18], whereas schistosomiasis transmission is highly focal [19]. Data on geographic coverage helps to improve tracking towards WHO goals, but there is a gap in our understanding of MDA coverage across time within individuals. Crucially, current policies are based on mathematical models that assume that coverage is homogeneous across the landscape and individuals are randomly treated each time [20]. Recent research highlights the importance of systematically untreated individuals in maintaining transmission: the effect of this group is exacerbated when overall treatment coverage is low and parasites are long-lived (i.e., *Schistosoma mansoni*) [21,22]. These models demonstrate that these untreated individuals can maintain transmission in low endemic communities even after 20 rounds of MDA [22], highlighting the importance of identifying if, and how many, individuals are untreated across their lifetime.

In 2002, Uganda was the first country in sub-Saharan Africa to begin schistosomiasis MDA. Out of 122 districts in Uganda, urogenital schistosomiasis (caused by *Schistosoma haematobium*) is found in four districts, and intestinal schistosomiasis (caused by *S. mansoni*) is found in 82 districts (synonymous with IUs in Uganda) [23,24]. In Uganda, 11.6 million people are infected, with 16.7 million at risk of infection [23,24], representing nearly 6.0% of the global population requiring schistosomiasis PC [25]. In 2018, 46 districts will receive praziquantel MDA through the national control programme [24].

Few previous studies have evaluated praziquantel coverage at an individual level or reasons for non-treatment [12,26–30]. In a study in 17 villages across Mayuge District, Uganda, an average coverage of 56.7% was reported, with a range of 10.9–86.6%, whilst compliance ranged from 67.8–99.1% [26]. Predictors for not being treated included Islamic religion, being a minority tribe and having lived in the village for longer [27]. Untreated individuals were also more likely to have lower socioeconomic markers such as having a low home quality, drinking unpurified water, having no home latrine and not being socially linked to people in village governments [27]. Social and physical proximity networks were also shown to be important predictors of praziquantel coverage and compliance within Uganda [26]. Similar low coverages were also observed in Côte d'Ivoire, with only 27.7% and 52.3% of people treated across two communities despite the study using door-to-door praziquantel administration [30]. Reasons reported for not taking praziquantel during that treatment round included being busy with agricultural activities, the bitter taste of the drug and/or previous adverse side effects [30]. Mixed methods studies on Koome Islands, Uganda, reported 44.7% coverage, with people more likely to have taken the last MDA if they had knowledge about schistosomiasis and general health education [28]. In this study, drug shortages and loss of health workers were identified as reasons for low coverage [28]. Higher coverages have been reported in Zanzibar, particularly in school-based treatments; however, reasons for not taking the last praziquantel still included being absent during

MDA, not being visited by a drug distributor, being busy, fear of adverse events or feeling healthy [29]. Studies on other neglected tropical diseases controlled by MDA have also reported multiple complex reasons for low coverage and non-compliance [12,31]. Despite these studies on the coverage of recent praziquantel and reasons for not taking it, data on lifetime coverage and systematic non-compliance remain limited for schistosomiasis treatment [12].

We undertook household surveys of praziquantel coverage in two villages of Mayuge District, Uganda, to test model assumptions and better inform control interventions. We collected comprehensive data on praziquantel coverage, socio-economic indicators and individual-level factors that could influence praziquantel uptake. Our specific objectives were to (1) quantify praziquantel coverage, (2) determine reasons for not taking praziquantel during the last MDA round of treatment and (3) identify socio-economic and individual factors that influence praziquantel uptake in (a) the past year and (b) over a person's lifetime. The goal was to identify and quantify drug coverage and reasons for non-treatment during recent MDA praziquantel drug coverage at an individual level. The findings may help to guide future research, interventions and targeted policy recommendations to help Uganda and other countries reach WHO 2020 goals.

2. Materials and Methods

2.1. Ethical Approval and Study Setting

The methods used in this study were reviewed and approved by the Vector Control Division Research Ethics Committee (VCDREC/062), the Uganda National Council of Science and Technology (UNCST-HS 2193) and the University of Glasgow Medical, Veterinary and Life Sciences Research Ethics Committee (200160068).

The study was conducted in two villages in Mayuge District, Uganda: Bugoto A and Bugoto B. These communities are on a peninsula on the shores of Lake Victoria approximately 25 km from the Mayuge District Headquarters, where MDA distribution is overseen. The area is a *S. mansoni* hotspot, with prevalence >90% in primary-school children [32,33]. Mayuge District was one of the first 38 IUs where MDA was carried out in 2003. From 2003 to date, there was an annual MDA administered at the district level. Interventions are implemented through the local government structure managed by the district health officer. The district health officer oversees the district health teams. These teams are responsible for the training of teachers and community medicine distributors to implement MDA; the teams also supervise them and provide a progress report [15,34]. Interventions for schistosomiasis control in Uganda using MDA began to be rolled out in 2003 in 38 of the 56 IUs with the support of the Schistosomiasis Control Initiative [35]. This has since expanded to the treatment of over 4.5 million SAC and at-risk adults annually [36], with significant reductions in *S. mansoni* prevalence, intensity and associated morbidity [37,38].

2.2. Survey Methodology

We conducted a census-style survey across both villages over a four-week period beginning in February 2017 (Figure S1). Before interviews began, an advocacy meeting was held with Mayuge District officials to discuss the study and obtain district approval and support. Meetings were held with the local council, chairpersons from both villages and the village health teams (VHTs). During mobilization meetings, community members were asked to provide information when the researchers arrived in their homes, but were informed that they had no obligation to do so. Households were visited door-to-door; if residents were absent, teams returned to the house at least twice for follow-up. Informed and written consent from the head of household and adults was obtained. The study respondents included any individual present in the home and above the age of 16. Both head of household and respondents were noted in the interview; however, they did not have an effect on the answers given. The main interviewers were the Ministry of Health Vector Control Officers or the District Health Drug Distributor. Each team had a member of the village health team from the respective village. There were three teams performing interviews; team members rotated between groups to ensure uniform questioning across the community.

2.3. Outcomes and Explanatory Variables

Our main outcomes of interest were individual praziquantel uptake in the most recent MDA (October 2016) and across an individual's lifetime. We focused on treatment coverage (proportion of MDA target population (≥5 years) treated), but epidemiological coverage (proportion of total population) is also reported and clearly specified. Eligible individuals in this context (i.e., target population in this high endemic region) are those that are aged 5 years or older. If an individual recalled praziquantel treatment, the location of treatment was recorded. Individuals were asked to provide a reason if they were untreated in the recent MDA. Households and individual data were collected as explanatory variables for treatment coverage. We collected household information on religion, bed ownership, mosquito net ownership, house structure (materials of floor, walls and roof), water sources (for drinking, bathing and washing) and latrine structure (materials of floor, walls and roof) and usage. We also asked individuals for details of their sex, age, occupation (or current school enrolment, encompassing all levels of education) and residence time in the village. Residence time was evaluated as a continuous variable (number of years), but also as a categorical variable split into: not present during MDA (0–0.75 years), short-term residence (0.76–4 years), intermediate term residence (5–9 years) and long-term residence (10 years or more).

2.4. Data Analysis

Household and individual survey data were cleaned and checked for consistency using custom scripts in R v. 3.2.1 [39] (Text S1). Ninety-five percent confidence intervals (95% CI) for proportions were calculated using the Agresti–Coull method [40]. Multivariate logistic mixed effects models were created with the function glmer from the lme4 package using the binomial family to evaluate two binomial outcome variables: receiving praziquantel in the last year and receiving praziquantel during lifetime. Models were created for the target population (≥5 years). Models were created with all possible explanatory variables initially; then, insignificant predictors were removed in a stepwise manner. Best-fit models were selected using the Akaike information criteria (AIC) [41]. Adjusted odds ratios (aORs) were calculated for the best-fit multivariate models, and the Wald method was used to calculate 95% CI.

3. Results

We conducted 681 household interviews encompassing 3208 individuals. This covered 90.8% (95% CI: 88.0–93.0%) of Bugoto A and 90.8% (86.2–94.0%) of Bugoto B households according to estimates from Uganda's 2014 census. According to 2014 census population projections for 2017, data were collected from 92.4% (91.3–93.5%) of individuals in Bugoto A and 92.1% (90.4–93.5%) of individuals in Bugoto B. The mean age of individuals was 17.3 years, and median age was 13 years. The main economic activities in the area were linked to fisheries, farming and small-scale business (Figure S2).

3.1. Self-Reported Praziquantel Uptake in Bugoto A and Bugoto B

Amongst surveyed individuals, 77.2% (75.7–78.6%) were eligible to receive praziquantel PC (five years or older). In the last MDA, treatment coverage was 46.5% (44.5–48.5%), whereas lifetime MDA treatment coverage was higher at 64.7% (62.8–66.7%). This means that 35.3% (33.4–37.2%) of the target population and 50.1% (48.4–51.9%) of the entire population reported never taking praziquantel. Treatment coverage among age groups in the last MDA ranged from 11.7% (eligible pre-SAC; 7.3–17.8%) to 70.7% (SAC; 67.6–73.6%) (Figure 1). If eligible pre-SAC are omitted (coverage is the same as in the last year), lifetime MDA praziquantel coverage within age groups ranged from 57.3% (20s; 52.7–61.9%) to 77.3% (SAC; 74.4–80.0%) (Figure 1).

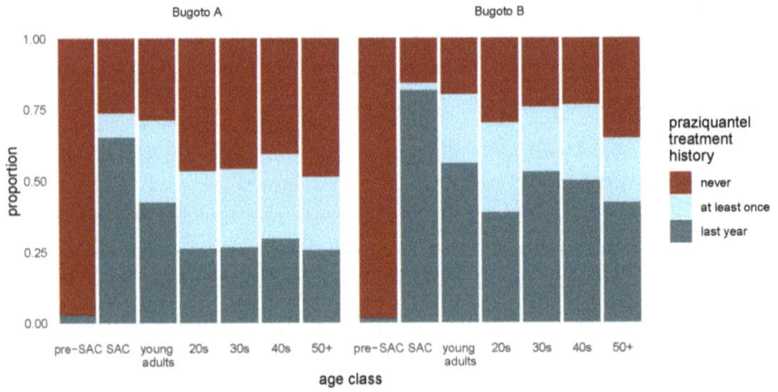

Figure 1. Praziquantel treatment across lifetime. The proportion of individuals in each age class that recalled receiving praziquantel treatment in 2016 (dark blue), not in 2016, but at least once in their lifetime (light blue), or never (red) are shown. For the ease of visualizing data, individuals were grouped into age groups: children were classified into pre-school-aged children (pre-SAC) (0–5 years) and SAC (6–14 years), whereas individuals who were 15 years and older were classified either as young adults (15–19 years) or by decade. Bugoto A is shown on the left, whereas Bugoto B is on the right.

3.2. *Self-Reported Reasons for Not Receiving Praziquantel during the Last MDA Round*

People offered nine reasons for not taking praziquantel in the last MDA (Figure 2, Table S1). The most common reason was that they were not offered treatment (44.1%; 41.3–46.9%); this included many individuals who had not known about the MDA. Absence during MDA was also common, with 19.2% (17.1–21.6%) of respondents giving this as a reason. Only 4.1% (3.1–5.4%) of respondents indicated fear of side effects/active treatment refusal as the reason for not taking praziquantel.

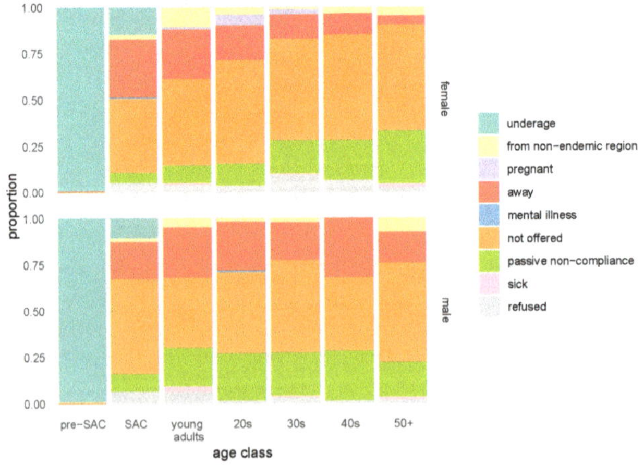

Figure 2. Reasons for not taking praziquantel in 2016. The proportion of individuals that reported a specific reason for not taking praziquantel is shown for both females (top) and males (bottom). For the ease of visualizing data, individuals were grouped into age groups: children were classified into pre-school-aged children (pre-SAC) (0–5 years) and SAC (6–14 years), whereas individuals who were 15 years and older were classified either as young adults (15–19 years) or by decade.

3.3. *Socio-Economic and Individual Risk Factors Influence Praziquantel Uptake*

Mixed effects models were used to investigate significant predictors of praziquantel treatment during MDA amongst the eligible population (five years and older). The best-fit model for taking praziquantel in 2016 included age group, residence time (as a categorical variable; see Materials and Methods), village residence, school enrolment and household ownership of a mosquito net (Figure 3). There were very similar predictors for lifetime praziquantel treatment (Figure S3). In all models, household identity was included as a random effect.

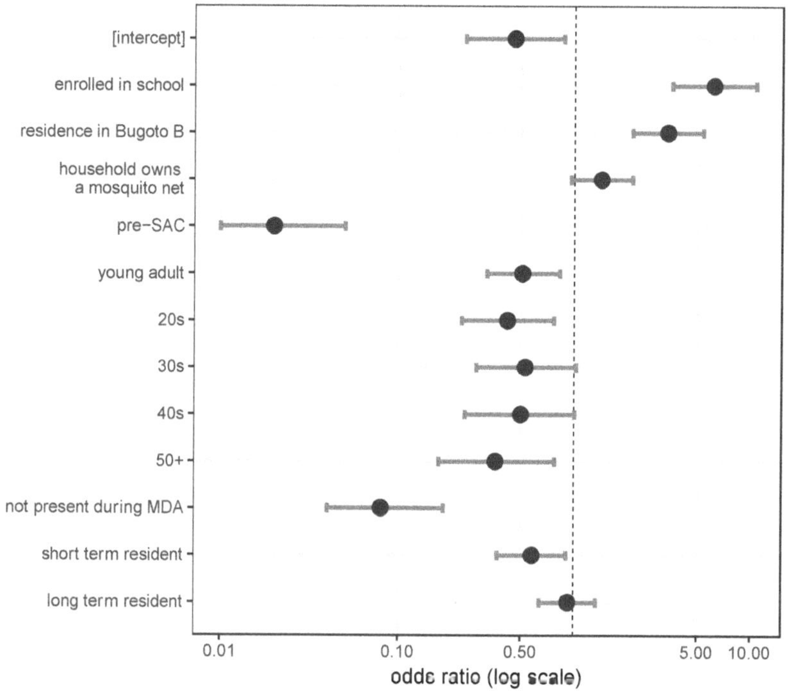

Figure 3. Multivariate analysis of socio-economic and individual factors that influence praziquantel uptake in the last year. Individuals were grouped into age groups: children were classified into pre-school-aged children (pre-SAC) (0–5 years) and SAC (6–14 years), whereas individuals who were 15 years and older were classified either as young adults (15–19 years) or by decade. The intercept represents an unenrolled SAC that resides in Bugoto A without a mosquito net and has lived in the village an intermediate time (5–9 years). Adjusted odds ratios are plotted on a log scale, with coloured dots indicating the estimate, and grey lines indicate 95% CI for each estimate.

Specifically, the odds of an individual receiving praziquantel in 2016 was highest in SAC, with the majority of age groups having significantly lower odds: pre-SAC (adjusted odds ratio (aOR): 0.02, 95% CI: 0.01–0.05), young adults (aOR: 0.51, 95% CI: 0.32–0.83), 20s (aOR: 0.42, 95% CI: 0.23–0.77), 30s (aOR: 0.53, 95% CI: 0.28–1.03), 40s (aOR: 0.50, 95% CI: 0.24–1.01) and 50s (aOR: 0.36, 95%CI: 0.17–0.78). Enrolment at a school, including primary, secondary or any graduate education, increased odds of taking praziquantel (aOR: 6.17, 95% CI: 3.58–10.64), as did residing in Bugoto B (aOR: 3.39, 95% CI: 2.15–5.35). Having a mosquito net at home could increase the odds of taking praziquantel in the last year (aOR: 1.44, 95% CI: 0.96–2.15). Although this predictor was not significant at $p = 0.05$, including this variable improved the fit of the model and was retained for the final model. Residence time was also an important factor in determining whether an individual received praziquantel in the last year. Intermediate residence time (5–9 years) was similar to long-term residence (aOR: 0.93, 95% CI: 0.64–1.35). However, if individuals were not living in Bugoto during the previous MDA campaign, their odds of receiving treatment elsewhere were low (aOR: 0.08, 95% CI: 0.04, 0.18), and short-term residence also decreased the odds of receiving praziquantel (aOR: 0.58, 95% CI: 0.37, 0.91). There were no significant interactions between the variables in this model.

Predictors of taking praziquantel treatment across lifetime were similar to the last year, but the direction and magnitude of the predictors often varied (Figure S3). However, mosquito net ownership was no longer included in the best fit model, but there was a significant interaction between age and residence time. The odds of receiving praziquantel across one's lifetime increased with school enrolment (aOR: 3.62, 2.13–6.15), residence in Bugoto B (aOR: 2.23, 1.53–3.24) and residence time in the village (for each year, aOR: 1.38, 1.29–1.47). Unlike praziquantel in the last year, most adults had higher odds of being treated with praziquantel than children (YA, aOR: 3.22, 1.40–7.39; 20s, aOR: 6.06, 2.83–12.97; 30s, aOR: 10.12, 4.37–23.40; 40s, aOR: 10.91, 4.37–23.40). Pre-SAC were less likely to receive praziquantel compared with SAC (aOR: 0.04, 0.00–0.61), whereas older (50s) individuals had similar odds as SAC (aOR: 2.29, 0.72–7.29). There was a significant interaction between age and residence; often times reducing the odds of taking praziquantel (i.e., residence years* 20s (interaction denoted by *), aOR: 0.77, 0.72–0.82).

4. Discussion

Our results highlight that annual praziquantel uptake rates are well below the WHO targets in Mayuge District, Uganda. Treatment coverage during the most recent MDA (2016) was only 46.5% of eligible residents, and 35.3% of eligible residents reported having never taken the drug. To achieve the WHO's goal of controlling schistosomiasis morbidity by 2020 and ultimately eliminating it as a public health problem, at least 75% treatment coverage is needed annually for over 10 years [18]. A key assumption of this goal is that the majority of individuals untreated each year are randomly distributed. Therefore, as annual MDA is repeated, untreated people are 'mopped up'. This would result in the number of people who have never received praziquantel diminishing over time. In our study communities, in a country where MDA has been going on for longer than all other sub-Saharan African countries, a third of eligible individuals reported that they have never taken praziquantel. These untreated individuals are not randomly distributed and are at risk of chronic schistosomiasis and associated morbidity. They also act as reservoirs for reinfection of treated individuals [21,22].

Low MDA treatment coverage, annually and over an individual's lifetime, has serious implications for national disease control and prevention programmes and the sustainable control of schistosomiasis morbidity and transmission. The self-reported uptake in our villages was on the lower end of coverage compared to other studies, especially amongst adults [26–29,42,43]. Adult coverage in 2016 was 34.8% (95% CI: 32.3%, 37.3%), whereas 70.7% (95% CI: 67.6–73.6%) of SAC were treated. Levels were similar on Koome Island, Uganda (44.7%, 95% CI: 40.8–48.7%), but islanders have been identified as national priorities for improved interventions [28]. To the authors' knowledge, only one published study in sub-Saharan Africa has observed lower treatment uptake at 28.2% (95% CI: 22.9, 33.6%), in the city of Jinja, Uganda [44], where advocacy was lacking.

Across Uganda, only 1/3 of the population requiring PC was treated in 2016, partly due to some completely untreated districts [36]. Mayuge District has previously reported low praziquantel coverage in 2009 (35%) [45], but attributed it to a lack of praziquantel stock. Our study focused on two geographically-close communities, but data reflect similar trends across the district and country since the control programme began.

The majority of studies have focused on recent treatment coverage [26,28,29,42,43,46], but have not addressed lifetime treatment data and the important issue of systematic non-treatment rates [11,12]. We show that a third of the at-risk population has never been treated despite 14 years of MDA. Using these data to parameterise models could have a significant effect on the predicted duration that repeated MDA is needed to control morbidity. Using just our coverage rates of 70.7% in SAC and 34.8% in adults, the sensitivity analyses by Turner and colleagues (2017) indicate that MDA is needed for 6–9 years with a 20% systematic non-compliance [11]. Our finding of 35.3% systematically non-treated eligible individuals, and 49.5% of the entire population never receiving treatment, likely explains the high infection prevalence and intensity still observed in these communities after 14 years of MDA [33,47]. If these low annual treatment rates and high lifetime MDA non-treatment continue, MDA programmes in districts such as this may potentially never control morbidity.

Despite low coverage, several individual and community factors were significantly correlated with praziquantel uptake. Current school enrolment status significantly increased the chance of receiving praziquantel, both within primary school children and adults enrolled in secondary and tertiary education. Residence in Bugoto B increased chances of praziquantel treatment in the last year and over lifetime. Bugoto B has a smaller total population and is more spread out than Bugoto A. This potentially makes it easier for distributors in Bugoto B to keep track of who has, and has not, received treatment and possibly makes it more likely to identify and include newcomers in the MDA. The higher praziquantel uptake may also be a product of established and stable social networks in Bugoto B; these social ties have been shown to be important in other settings [26]. Bugoto B has more long-term residents (residents have spent an average of 69% of their life in the village) compared to Bugoto A (average of 56% of their life in the village). In our study, the longer an individual had lived in the village, the more likely he/she was to receive treatment, especially across a person's lifetime (but this is slightly mitigated by residence time). Lastly, mosquito net ownership can increase the likelihood of taking praziquantel in the last year, which could be interpreted as a proxy for health-seeking behaviour. These factors are important to consider when modifying programmes to increase praziquantel uptake.

The term systematic non-compliers is often used instead of systematically non-treated. Praziquantel MDA coverage can be significantly lower than other MDA programmes locally and nationally and is commonly attributed to the fear of side effects [48]. Despite this common belief, residents in our study were significantly more likely to have not been offered praziquantel, to have been away during treatment or to have been passive non-compliers than to have actively refused it. Of the target population that had not taken the drug in the last MDA, only 4.6% refused treatment. This is similar to other praziquantel studies [29,49] indicating that the belief that fear of side effects reduces treatment uptake is unfounded and unhelpful.

The most common reason for not taking praziquantel in the last year was not being offered, with rates much higher than other studies [29]. Increasing the number of community drug distributors (CDD) could increase drug coverage. In these villages, each drug distributor covers 150 households, well above the recommended 25–30 households [50]. If each CDD is responsible for fewer households, MDA coverage increases significantly [45,51]. Encouraging house-to-house administration in these communities should also increase coverage [45,46]. In general, most adults taking praziquantel in the last year received treatment at central locations rather than their household. However, a higher proportion of Bugoto B residents compared to Bugoto A residents reported receiving praziquantel treatment at home in 2016, which may partly explain the higher coverage in Bugoto B. The second most common reason for not taking praziquantel was being away during MDA, compounded by the absence of praziquantel in almost all Ugandan frontline health facilities. Similar findings were reported for lymphatic filariasis, where MDAs were reported to be too short and not lasting long enough to reach the whole communities [31]. Leaving drugs at health centres or with key personnel after each MDA may enable a significant mop up of these mobile populations. Many reasons given for not taking praziquantel in the last MDA suggest that improved educational campaigns and effective mobilization could increase health-seeking behaviour and improve community-wide MDA. A recent study supports these conclusions with findings that anytime was suitable for treatments if people were informed in advance [30]. They also reported that knowledge of the disease was a positive predictor of treatment, highlighting that communication is key at all levels. In addition, the dry season was suggested as the best time of year to go with people less likely to be in the fields and absent during treatment than in the rainy season. They further found that in a large village, house-to-house treatment was preferred, but this was not important in a smaller village where people possibly all lived closer to a drug distribution point [30]; this could also further support our findings of higher praziquantel success in the smaller population of Bugoto B, although this is a geographically dispersed population.

Anecdotal evidence during our surveys suggested that individuals believed they were cured after one round of treatment and therefore did not take praziquantel in subsequent MDAs (i.e., passive non-complier). In Côte d'Ivoire, three-quarters of people treated during the study said they would not take the drug again, despite a significant proportion of people saying they felt better after treatment [30]. In Zanzibar, treatment fatigue was reported [29], which also may explain our interaction between age and duration in the village and the reduction of treatment uptake in the last MDA. Others believe praziquantel MDA is for SAC only or had simply never heard of the MDA. Studies in Nigeria show that obtaining community support and involvement before praziquantel MDA implementation contributes to an effective treatment strategy for schistosomiasis [52]. However, knowledge of schistosomiasis transmission and prevention that increases the likelihood of taking praziquantel MDA has not successfully reached the intended communities as suggested [42].

The key limitations of this study were that only two villages were surveyed and that the source of data on participants' past treatment with praziquantel was through interviews, which may be prone to recall bias. Participants might not be in a position to differentiate praziquantel from other medicines they have taken, and this might be exacerbated by the time between the most recent MDA and the survey date. This was minimised where possible by showing images of praziquantel and describing its bitter taste to the interviewees. Thus, if individuals were to confuse treatments with other MDA programmes, it would likely result in a higher recall of the wrong drug rather than no recall at all. If people had taken the drug many years before and forgotten, then this could lower the lifetime coverage, which could be better inferred as coverage within memory. In addition, MDA has only been occurring in Mayuge for 14 years, and so, lifetime refers more to the lifetime of the national control programme, rather than, for example, the full extent of an adult's life. Furthermore, if someone had taken praziquantel once a long time ago, at the start of the national programme, but is now systematically untreated, then the effect on transmission and morbidity may remain relatively unchanged if they are still being exposed in these highly endemic communities. However, similar low coverages in recent treatments have been reported across Mayuge [53], indicating that our data for recent treatment are in line with other studies and provide additional information regarding long-term treatment exposure, which other studies rarely address, despite it being highlighted by modellers as an important knowledge gap [11,12].

The communities involved in this study are incredibly diverse, and there are factors that were not measured that are also likely to influence praziquantel uptake. For example, additional household characteristics, ethnicity and social networks have also been shown to influence likelihood of praziquantel treatment [26,53]. We therefore recommend further studies into the social and cultural factors influencing long-term praziquantel uptake and schistosomiasis transmission in these communities. This will help highlight which targeted mobilization approaches are feasible and are most successful in increasing praziquantel coverage and reducing transmission.

5. Conclusions

Schistosomiasis is associated with low socio-economic status, poor sanitation, lack of access to healthcare systems and frequent contact with infected water bodies [54,55]. Annual MDA has been successful at reducing prevalence and intensity of infections in several areas [14,16,37,38], but hotspots remain in others [13,17]. While PC is an important component of schistosomiasis control, other supportive strategies such as provision of safe water and adequate sanitation, hygiene education and snail control will be essential for the control and elimination of schistosomiasis. However, improvements in MDA can impact disease morbidity and improve short-term outcomes for stakeholders. Based on community surveys, praziquantel uptake could be improved by leaving supplies of praziquantel at health facilities or with CDDs, improving awareness that people can get re-infected post-treatment and emphasizing that praziquantel is recommended for adults in these communities, not just children. This study supports the notion that bottlenecks for schistosomiasis control by MDA are occurring at the level of distribution and are not driven by non-compliance.

Supplementary Materials: The following are available online at http://www.mdpi.com/2414-6366/3/4/111/s1: Text S1: Supplementary methods; Figure S1: Community survey template, Figure S2: Occupations of individuals in each village above the age of fourteen by gender, Figure S3: Multivariate analysis of socio-economic and individual factors that influence praziquantel uptake across one's lifetime, Table S1: Self-reported reasons for not receiving praziquantel during the last MDA (2016).

Author Contributions: Conceptualization, E.M.T. and P.H.L.L. Data curation, M.A., C.L.F., L.V.C., A.M. and P.H.L.L. Formal analysis, C.L.F. Funding acquisition, P.H.L.L. Methodology, C.L.F. and P.H.L.L. Project administration, C.L.F., E.M.T. and P.H.L.L. Visualization, C.L.F. Writing, original draft, M.A., C.L.F. and P.H.L.L. Writing, review and editing, M.A., C.L.F., L.V.C., A.M., E.M.T. and P.H.L.L.

Funding: The research was funded by the European Research Council Starting Grant (SCHISTO_PERSIST_680088).

Acknowledgments: We are grateful to the District Vector Control Officer, Juma Nabonge, and the village chairpersons for their efforts in mobilizing the communities for this study. We also thank the Village Health Teams for their assistance in data collection.

Conflicts of Interest: The authors declare no conflict of interest. The funders had no role in the design of the study; in the collection, analyses or interpretation of data; in the writing of the manuscript; nor in the decision to publish the results.

References

1. WHO. *Schistosomiasis: Progress Report 2001–2011, Strategic Plan 2012–2020*; WHO: Geneva, Switzerland, 2013.
2. Savioli, L.; Albonico, M.; Colley, D.G.; Correa-Oliveira, R.; Fenwick, A.; Green, W.; Kabatereine, N.; Kabore, A.; Katz, N.; Klohe, K.; et al. Building a global schistosomiasis alliance: An opportunity to join forces to fight inequality and rural poverty. *Infect. Dis. Poverty* **2017**, *6*, 65. [CrossRef] [PubMed]
3. Hotez, P.J.; Molyneux, D.H.; Fenwick, A.; Kumaresan, J.; Sachs, S.E.; Sachs, J.D.; Savioli, L. Control of neglected tropical diseases. *N. Engl. J. Med.* **2007**, *357*, 1018–1027. [CrossRef] [PubMed]
4. Hotez, P.J.; Alvarado, M.; Basanez, M.G.; Bolliger, I.; Bourne, R.; Boussinesq, M.; Brooker, S.J.; Brown, A.S.; Buckle, G.; Budke, C.M.; et al. The Global Burden of Disease Study 2010: Interpretation and implications for the neglected tropical diseases. *PLoS Negl. Trop. Dis.* **2014**, *8*, e2865. [CrossRef] [PubMed]
5. GBD 2015 Maternal Mortality Collaborators. Global, regional, and national levels of maternal mortality, 1990–2015: A systematic analysis for the Global Burden of Disease Study 2015. *Lancet* **2016**, *388*, 1775–1812. [CrossRef]
6. GBD 2016 DALYs and HALE Collaborators. Global, regional, and national disability-adjusted life-years (DALYs) for 333 diseases and injuries and healthy life expectancy (HALE) for 195 countries and territories, 1990–2016: A systematic analysis for the Global Burden of Disease Study 2016. *Lancet* **2017**, *390*, 1260–1344. [CrossRef]
7. Lo, N.C.; Addiss, D.G.; Hotez, P.J.; King, C.H.; Stothard, J.R.; Evans, D.S.; Colley, D.G.; Lin, W.; Coulibaly, J.T.; Bustinduy, A.L.; et al. A call to strengthen the global strategy against schistosomiasis and soil-transmitted helminthiasis: The time is now. *Lancet Infect. Dis.* **2017**, *17*, e64–e69. [CrossRef]
8. Colley, D.G.; Andros, T.S.; Campbell, C.H., Jr. Schistosomiasis is more prevalent than previously thought: What does it mean for public health goals, policies, strategies, guidelines and intervention programs? *Infect. Dis. Poverty* **2017**, *6*, 63. [CrossRef] [PubMed]
9. WHO. *Preventive Chemotherapy in Human Helminthiasis: Coordinated Use of Anthelminthic Drugs in Control Interventions: A Manual for Health Professionals and Programme Managers*; WHO: Geneva, Switzerland, 2006.
10. WHO. *Accelerating Work to Overcome the Global Impact of Neglected Tropical Diseases—A Roadmap for Implementation*; WHO: Geneva, Switzerland, 2012.
11. Turner, H.C.; Truscott, J.E.; Bettis, A.A.; Farrell, S.H.; Deol, A.K.; Whitton, J.M.; Fleming, F.M.; Anderson, R.M. Evaluating the variation in the projected benefit of community-wide mass treatment for schistosomiasis: Implications for future economic evaluations. *Parasit. Vectors* **2017**, *10*, 213. [CrossRef] [PubMed]
12. Shuford, K.V.; Turner, H.C.; Anderson, R.M. Compliance with anthelmintic treatment in the neglected tropical diseases control programmes: A systematic review. *Parasit. Vectors* **2016**, *9*, 29. [CrossRef] [PubMed]

13. French, M.D.; Churcher, T.S.; Webster, J.P.; Fleming, F.M.; Fenwick, A.; Kabatereine, N.B.; Sacko, M.; Garba, A.; Toure, S.; Nyandindi, U.; et al. Estimation of changes in the force of infection for intestinal and urogenital schistosomiasis in countries with schistosomiasis control initiative-assisted programmes. *Parasit. Vectors* **2015**, *8*, 558. [CrossRef] [PubMed]
14. Rollinson, D.; Knopp, S.; Levitz, S.; Stothard, J.R.; Tchuem Tchuente, L.A.; Garba, A.; Mohammed, K.A.; Schur, N.; Person, B.; Colley, D.G.; et al. Time to set the agenda for schistosomiasis elimination. *Acta Trop.* **2013**, *128*, 423–440. [CrossRef] [PubMed]
15. Kabatereine, N.B.; Tukahebwa, E.; Kazibwe, F.; Namwangye, H.; Zaramba, S.; Brooker, S.; Stothard, J.R.; Kamenka, C.; Whawell, S.; Webster, J.P.; et al. Progress towards countrywide control of schistosomiasis and soil-transmitted helminthiasis in Uganda. *Trans. R. Soc. Trop. Med. Hyg.* **2006**, *100*, 208–215. [CrossRef] [PubMed]
16. Standley, C.J.; Adriko, M.; Arinaitwe, M.; Atuhaire, A.; Kazibwe, F.; Fenwick, A.; Kabatereine, N.B.; Stothard, J.R. Epidemiology and control of intestinal schistosomiasis on the Sesse Islands, Uganda: Integrating malacology and parasitology to tailor local treatment recommendations. *Parasit. Vectors* **2010**, *3*, 64. [CrossRef] [PubMed]
17. Standley, C.J.; Adriko, M.; Besigye, F.; Kabatereine, N.B.; Stothard, R.J. Confirmed local endemicity and putative high transmission of *Schistosoma mansoni* in the Sesse Islands, Lake Victoria, Uganda. *Parasit. Vectors* **2011**, *4*, 29. [CrossRef] [PubMed]
18. Bockarie, M.J.; Kelly-Hope, L.A.; Rebollo, M.; Molyneux, D.H. Preventive chemotherapy as a strategy for elimination of neglected tropical parasitic diseases: Endgame challenges. *Philos. Trans. R. Soc. Lond. B* **2013**, *368*, 20120144. [CrossRef] [PubMed]
19. WHO. *Helminth Control in School-Age Children. A Guide for Managers for Control Programmes*; WHO: Geneva, Switzerland, 2011.
20. Truscott, J.; Gurarie, D.; Alsallaq, R.; Toor, J.; Yoon, N.; Farrell, S.; Turner, H.; Phillips, A.; Aurelio, H.; Ferro, J. A Comparison of two mathematical models of the impact of mass drug administration on the transmission and control of schistosomiasis. *Epidemics* **2017**, *18*, 29–37. [CrossRef] [PubMed]
21. Dyson, L.; Stolk, W.A.; Farrell, S.H.; Hollingsworth, T.D. Measuring and modelling the effects of systematic non-adherence to mass drug administration. *Epidemics* **2017**, *18*, 56–66. [CrossRef] [PubMed]
22. Farrell, S.H.; Truscott, J.E.; Anderson, R.M. The importance of patient compliance in repeated rounds of mass drug administration (MDA) for the elimination of intestinal helminth transmission. *Parasit. Vectors* **2017**, *10*, 291. [CrossRef] [PubMed]
23. Ministry of Health Republic of Uganda. *Uganda Master Plan for National Neglected Tropical Diseases Programmes*; Government of Uganda: Kampala, Uganda, 2014.
24. Ministry of Health Republic of Uganda. *Uganda Master Plan for National Neglected Tropical Diseases Programmes: 2017–2022*; Government of Uganda: Kampala, Uganda, 2017.
25. WHO. *Schistosomiasis and Soil-Transmitted Helminthiases: Number of People Treated in 2016*; WHO: Geneva, Switzerland, 2017.
26. Chami, G.F.; Kontoleon, A.A.; Bulte, E.; Fenwick, A.; Kabatereine, N.B.; Tukahebwa, E.M.; Dunne, D.W. Community-directed mass drug administration is undermined by status seeking in friendship networks and inadequate trust in health advice networks. *Soc. Sci. Med.* **2017**, *183*, 37–47. [CrossRef] [PubMed]
27. Chami, G.F.; Kontoleon, A.A.; Bulte, E.; Fenwick, A.; Kabatereine, N.B.; Tukahebwa, E.M.; Dunne, D.W. Profiling nonrecipients of mass drug administration for schistosomiasis and hookworm infections: A comprehensive analysis of praziquantel and albendazole coverage in community-directed treatment in Uganda. *Clin. Infect. Dis.* **2015**, *62*, 200–207. [CrossRef] [PubMed]
28. Tuhebwe, D.; Bagonza, J.; Kiracho, E.E.; Yeka, A.; Elliott, A.M.; Nuwaha, F. Uptake of mass drug administration programme for schistosomiasis control in Koome Islands, Central Uganda. *PLoS ONE* **2015**, *10*, e0123673. [CrossRef] [PubMed]
29. Knopp, S.; Person, B.; Ame, S.M.; Ali, S.M.; Muhsin, J.; Juma, S.; Khamis, I.S.; Rabone, M.; Blair, L.; Fenwick, A.; et al. Praziquantel coverage in schools and communities targeted for the elimination of urogenital schistosomiasis in Zanzibar: A cross-sectional survey. *Parasit. Vectors* **2016**, *9*, 5. [CrossRef] [PubMed]

30. Coulibaly, J.; Ouattara, M.; Barda, B.; Utzinger, J.; N'Goran, E.; Keiser, J. A rapid appraisal of factors influencing praziquantel treatment compliance in two communities endemic for schistosomiasis in Côte d'Ivoire. *Trop. Med. Infect. Dis.* **2018**, *3*, 69. [CrossRef] [PubMed]
31. Krentel, A.; Fischer, P.U.; Weil, G.J. A review of factors that influence individual compliance with mass drug administration for elimination of lymphatic filariasis. *PLoS Negl. Trop. Dis.* **2013**, *7*, e2447. [CrossRef] [PubMed]
32. Lamberton, P.H.; Kabatereine, N.B.; Oguttu, D.W.; Fenwick, A.; Webster, J.P. Sensitivity and specificity of multiple Kato-Katz thick smears and a circulating cathodic antigen test for *Schistosoma mansoni* diagnosis pre- and post-repeated-praziquantel treatment. *PLoS Negl. Trop. Dis.* **2014**, *8*, e3139. [CrossRef] [PubMed]
33. Crellen, T.; Walker, M.; Lamberton, P.H.; Kabatereine, N.B.; Tukahebwa, E.M.; Cotton, J.A.; Webster, J.P. Reduced efficacy of praziquantel against *Schistosoma mansoni* is associated with multiple rounds of mass drug administration. *Clin. Infect. Dis.* **2016**, *63*, 1151–1159. [PubMed]
34. Fleming, F.M.; Fenwick, A.; Tukahebwa, E.M.; Lubanga, R.G.; Namwangye, H.; Zaramba, S.; Kabatereine, N.B. Process evaluation of schistosomiasis control in Uganda, 2003 to 2006: Perceptions, attitudes and constraints of a national programme. *Parasitology* **2009**, *136*, 1759–1769. [CrossRef] [PubMed]
35. Fenwick, A.; Webster, J.P.; Bosque-Oliva, E.; Blair, L.; Fleming, F.M.; Zhang, Y.; Garba, A.; Stothard, J.R.; Gabrielli, A.F.; Clements, A.C.; et al. The Schistosomiasis Control Initiative (SCI): Rationale, development and implementation from 2002–2008. *Parasitology* **2009**, *136*, 1719–1730. [CrossRef] [PubMed]
36. Global Health Observatory Data Repository. Available online: http://www.who.int/gho/en/ (accessed on 11 April 2018).
37. French, M.D.; Churcher, T.S.; Gambhir, M.; Fenwick, A.; Webster, J.P.; Kabatereine, N.B.; Basáñez, M.G. Observed Reductions in *Schistosoma mansoni* transmission from large-scale administration of praziquantel in Uganda: A Mathematical modelling study. *PLoS Negl. Trop. Dis.* **2010**, *4*, e897. [CrossRef] [PubMed]
38. Kabatereine, N.B.; Brooker, S.; Koukounari, A.; Kazibwe, F.; Tukahebwa, E.M.; Fleming, F.M.; Zhang, Y.; Webster, J.P.; Stothard, J.R.; Fenwick, A. Impact of a national helminth control programme on infection and morbidity in Ugandan schoolchildren. *Bull. World Health Organ.* **2007**, *85*, 91–99. [PubMed]
39. The R Development Core Team. *R: A Language and Environment for Statistical Computing*; V 3.2; R Foundation for Statistical Computing: Vienna, Austria, 2015.
40. Agresti, A.; Coull, B. Approximate is better than 'exact' for interval estimation of binomial proportions. *Am. Stat.* **1998**, *52*, 119–126.
41. Akaike, H. Factor analysis and AIC. *Psychometrika* **1987**, *52*, 371–386. [CrossRef]
42. Muhumuza, S.; Katahoire, A.; Nuwaha, F.; Olsen, A. Increasing teacher motivation and supervision is an important but not sufficient strategy for improving praziquantel uptake in *Schistosoma mansoni* control programs: Serial cross sectional surveys in Uganda. *BMC Infect. Dis.* **2013**, *13*, 590. [CrossRef] [PubMed]
43. Parker, M.; Allen, T. Does mass drug administration for the integrated treatment of neglected tropical diseases really work? Assessing evidence for the control of schistosomiasis and soil-transmitted helminths in Uganda. *Health Res. Policy. Syst.* **2011**, *9*, 3. [CrossRef] [PubMed]
44. Muhumuza, S.; Olsen, A.; Katahoire, A.; Nuwaha, F. Uptake of preventive treatment for intestinal schistosomiasis among school children in Jinja district, Uganda: A cross-sectional study. *PLoS ONE* **2013**, *8*, e63438. [CrossRef] [PubMed]
45. Fleming, F.M.; Matovu, F.; Hansen, K.S.; Webster, J.P. A mixed methods approach to evaluating community drug distributor performance in the control of neglected tropical diseases. *Parasit. Vectors* **2016**, *9*, 345. [CrossRef] [PubMed]
46. Sangho, H.; Dabo, A.; Sidibe, A.; Dembele, R.; Diawara, A.; Diallo, A.; Konate, S. Coverage rate and satisfaction of populations after mass treatment with praziquantel and albendazole in Mali. *Mali Med.* **2009**, *24*, 21–24. [PubMed]
47. Kabatereine, N.; Fleming, F.; Thuo, W.; Tinkitina, B.; Tukahebwa, E.M.; Fenwick, A. Community perceptions, attitude, practices and treatment seeking behaviour for schistosomiasis in L. Victoria Islands in Uganda. *BMC Res. Notes* **2014**, *7*, 900. [CrossRef] [PubMed]
48. Parker, M.; Allen, T.; Hastings, J. Resisting control of neglected tropical diseases: Dilemmas in the mass treatment of schistosomiasis and soil-transmitted helminths in north-west Uganda. *J. Biosoc. Sci.* **2008**, *40*, 161–181. [CrossRef] [PubMed]

49. Dabo, A.; Bary, B.; Kouriba, B.; Sankare, O.; Doumbo, O. Factors associated with coverage of praziquantel for schistosomiasis control in the community-direct intervention (CDI) approach in Mali (West Africa). *Infect. Dis. Poverty* **2013**, *2*, 11. [CrossRef] [PubMed]
50. Ministry of Health Republic of Uganda. *Village Health Teams: Guide for Training the Trainers of Village Health Teams*; Government of Uganda: Kampala, Uganda, 2010.
51. Katabarwa, M.; Habomugisha, P.; Eyamba, A.; Agunyo, S.; Mentou, C. Monitoring ivermectin distributors involved in integrated health care services through community-directed interventions—A comparison of Cameroon and Uganda experiences over a period of three years (2004–2006). *Trop. Med. Int. Health* **2010**, *15*, 216–223. [CrossRef] [PubMed]
52. Adeneye, A.K.; Akinwale, O.P.; Idowu, E.T.; Adewale, B.; Manafa, O.U.; Sulyman, M.A.; Omotola, B.D.; Akande, D.O.; Mafe, M.A.; Appelt, B. Sociocultural aspects of mass delivery of praziquantel in schistosomiasis control: The Abeokuta experience. *Res. Soc. Adm. Pharm.* **2006**, *3*, 183–198. [CrossRef] [PubMed]
53. Chami, G.F.; Kontoleon, A.A.; Bulte, E.; Fenwick, A.; Kabatereine, N.B.; Tukahebwa, E.M.; Dunne, D.W. Diffusion of treatment in social networks and mass drug administration. *Nat. Commun.* **2017**, *8*, 1929. [CrossRef] [PubMed]
54. Woolhouse, M.E.; Dye, C.; Etard, J.-F.; Smith, T.; Charlwood, J.; Garnett, G.; Hagan, P.; Hii, J.; Ndhlovu, P.; Quinnell, R. Heterogeneities in the transmission of infectious agents: Implications for the design of control programs. *Proc. Natl. Acad. Sci. USA* **1997**, *94*, 338–342. [CrossRef] [PubMed]
55. Lwambo, N.; Siza, J.; Brooker, S.; Bundy, D.; Guyatt, H. Patterns of concurrent hookworm infection and schistosomiasis in schoolchildren in Tanzania. *Trans. R. Soc. Trop. Med. Hyg.* **1999**, *93*, 497–502. [CrossRef]

Tropical Medicine and Infectious Disease

MDPI

Article

A Rapid Appraisal of Factors Influencing Praziquantel Treatment Compliance in Two Communities Endemic for Schistosomiasis in Côte d'Ivoire

Jean T. Coulibaly [1,2,3,4,*], Mamadou Ouattara [3,4], Beatrice Barda [1,2], Jürg Utzinger [1,2], Eliézer K. N'Goran [3,4] and Jennifer Keiser [1,2]

1 Swiss Tropical and Public Health Institute, P.O. Box, CH-4002 Basel, Switzerland; beatrice.barda@gmail.com (B.B.); juerg.utzinger@swisstph.ch (J.U.); jennifer.keiser@swisstph.ch (J.K.)

2 University of Basel, P.O. Box, CH-4001 Basel, Switzerland

3 Unité de Formation et de Recherche Biosciences, Université Félix Houphouët-Boigny, 01 BP 770, Abidjan 01, Côte d'Ivoire; mamadou_ouatt@yahoo.fr (M.O.); eliezerngoran@yahoo.fr (E.K.N.)

4 Centre Suisse de Recherches Scientifiques en Côte d'Ivoire, 01 BP 1303, Abidjan 01, Côte d'Ivoire

* Correspondence: couljeanvae@yahoo.fr; Tel.: +225-2347-2790

Received: 13 April 2018; Accepted: 14 June 2018; Published: 19 June 2018

Abstract: Over the past decade, a significant reduction in the prevalence of schistosomiasis has been achieved, partially explained by the large-scale administration of praziquantel. Yet, the burden of schistosomiasis remains considerable, and factors influencing intervention coverage are important. This study aimed to deepen the understanding of low treatment coverage rates observed in two schistosomiasis-endemic villages in Côte d'Ivoire. The research was conducted in August 2015, in Moronou and Bigouin, two villages of Côte d'Ivoire that are endemic for *Schistosoma haematobium* and *S. mansoni*, respectively. After completion of a clinical trial, standard praziquantel treatment (single 40 mg/kg oral dose) was offered to all village inhabitants by community health workers using a house-to-house approach. Factors influencing treatment coverage were determined by a questionnaire survey, randomly selecting 405 individuals. The overall treatment coverage rate was only 47.6% (2730/5733) with considerable intervillage heterogeneity (27.7% in Bigouin (302/1091) versus 52.3% in Moronou (2428/4642)). Among the 200 individuals interviewed in Moronou, 50.0% were administered praziquantel, while only 19.5% of the 205 individuals interviewed in Bigouin received praziquantel. The main reasons for low treatment coverage were work-related (agricultural activities), the bitter taste of praziquantel and previous experiences with adverse events. The most suitable period for treatment campaigns was reported to be the dry season. More than three-quarter of the interviewees who had taken praziquantel (overall, 116/140; Moronou, 84/100; Bigouin, 32/40) declared that they would not participate in future treatments ($p < 0.001$). In order to enhance praziquantel treatment coverage, careful consideration should be given to attitudes and practices, such as prior or perceived adverse events and taste of praziquantel, and appropriate timing, harmonized with agricultural activities. Without such understanding, breaking the transmission of schistosomiasis remains a distant goal.

Keywords: Côte d'Ivoire; coverage rate; praziquantel; preventive chemotherapy; *Schistosoma haematobium*; *Schistosoma mansoni*

---

1. Introduction

Schistosomiasis is a widespread neglected tropical disease with a considerable public health impact. Indeed, 779 million people are at risk of schistosomiasis, more than 250 million people are infected with blood flukes of the genus *Schistosoma*, and the global burden in 2016 was estimated at 1.864 million disability-adjusted life years [1–3]. More than 90% of schistosome infections are concentrated in Africa [1,4]. There is growing evidence of a positive relationship between schistosome infections and subtle morbidity, including educational, learning and memory deficits [5]. The global strategy is morbidity control, emphasizing periodic administration of praziquantel to at-risk populations without prior diagnosis. This strategy is phrased 'preventive chemotherapy' with the declared aim to achieve at least 75% of treatment coverage among school-aged children in schistosome-endemic areas [6]. Efforts are underway to eliminate schistosomiasis as a public health problem by 2025 [7–9]. In order to reach this ambitious goal, treatment with praziquantel needs to be administered repetitively with high coverage, in concert with ancillary measures, such as water, sanitation and hygiene (WASH), information, education and communication (IEC) and snail control [10–15].

In Côte d'Ivoire, schistosomiasis control efforts have been intensified since 2006, yet were challenged during periods of social unrest, armed conflict and war [16,17]. Starting in 2013, with financial support from the Schistosomiasis Control Initiative (SCI) and other donors, regular large-scale administration of praziquantel is under way, including sporadic assessment of treatment coverage. However, factors influencing coverage rates and reasons for noncompliance have yet to be systematically evaluated in Côte d'Ivoire.

In general, investigations that systematically evaluate treatment coverage and compliance of the community are scarce [18–20]. Recent studies carried out in Uganda [18] and Zanzibar [19] determined underlying factors responsible for low treatment compliance. The main reasons identified by Knopp and colleagues for communities in Zanzibar not receiving or taking praziquantel were: absence during drug distribution, no drug distributor reached the household, fear of adverse events, pregnancy, breastfeeding or feeling healthy [19]. Moreover, lack of motivation or professional expertise of drug distributors and limited information of the target population were associated with low compliance of local communities with preventive chemotherapy [21,22]. Chami and colleagues identified additional reasons for low compliance: They found that individuals of low socioeconomic status, religious minorities and small tribes showed particularly low compliance rates with preventive chemotherapy [18].

Within the frame of a randomized controlled trial conducted in two villages of central and western Côte d'Ivoire that assessed the efficacy and safety of potential new treatments (i.e., Synriam®, moxidectin and Synriam®–praziquantel) against schistosomiasis [12], there was an opportunity to determine praziquantel treatment coverage rates. Indeed, after completion of the clinical trial, a single 40 mg/kg oral dose of praziquantel was offered to the communities. Low compliance was observed, and hence, a questionnaire survey was conducted to identify reasons that might explain lack of compliance. Here we present findings on attitudes and practices towards treatment of schistosomiasis in the two study communities. Results and lessons might help to overcome current challenges in order to achieve effective control and elimination of schistosomiasisin Côte d'Ivoire and other countries.

2. Material and Methods

2.1. Ethical Approval and Study Setting

The study was conducted in August 2015 during the rainy season, following completion of a clinical trial assessing the efficacy and safety of Synriam® and moxidectin [12] against urogenital and intestinal schistosomiasis in 256 school-aged children and adolescents (age: 12–17 years) in the villages of Moronou (central Côte d'Ivoire) and Bigouin (western Côte d'Ivoire). As described elsewhere, Moronou and Bigouin are highly endemic for *Schistosoma haematobium* and *S. mansoni*, respectively [12]. The clinical trial was approved by the Ethics Committee of Northwestern and Central Switzerland (EKNZ; reference no. 15/01) and the Comité National d'Éthique et de la Recherche (CNER; reference no. 026, approval date: 16 June 2015) of the Ministry of Health in Côte d'Ivoire. According to the last national census carried out in 2014, there were 4642 and 1091 inhabitants in Moronou and Bigouin, respectively [23]. Informed oral consent was obtained from all participants for the questionnaire survey.

2.2. Sample Size Calculation

The sample size was assessed as recommended by Lemeshow et al. [24]. Briefly, we assumed that 90% (P) of the individuals approached would answer the questionnaire with a relative precision (d) of 5% and a level of confidence of 95% (Z = 1.96). The minimum sample size for each setting was 138 individuals, calculated as follows: $n = Z^2{}_{1-\alpha/2}P(1 - P)/d^2$.

Allowing for 30% of absence during the door-to-door visit, approximately 200 individuals (school-aged children, 6–15 years and adolescents/adults, ≥16 years) were randomly selected in each village with equal numbers of treated and nontreated individuals during the door-to-door treatment (as described below).

2.3. Praziquantel Treatment

Praziquantel tablets (Cesol® 600 mg) were offered free of charge to both communities following the completion of a clinical trial (Figure 1). Communities were informed about the treatment days, and the objectives, procedures and potential risks and benefits were explained. Village chiefs and community leaders conducted an information meeting and, subsequently, the information was passed on to the entire population. In both villages, a door-to-door approach was employed to administer praziquantel over two consecutive days. In each village, a community health worker (CHW) was recruited per neighborhood (six in Moronou and four in Bigouin). The CHWs were trained to treat community members using a dose pole [25,26]. Villagers were invited to swallow the drug in front of the CHWs. Related data, including name, sex, age and number of tablets administered, were recorded in a register used by the national schistosomiasis control programme.

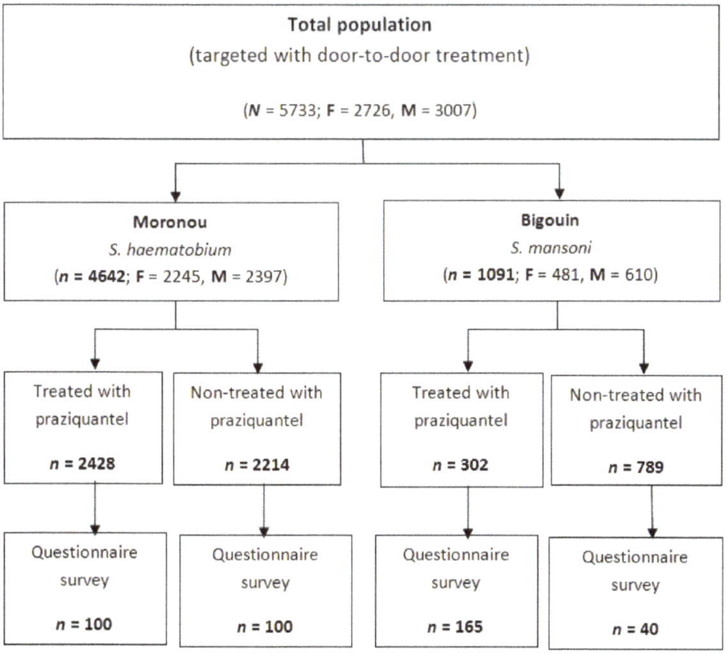

Figure 1. Study profile.

2.4. Questionnaire Assessing Factors Influencing Treatment Compliance

A structured questionnaire was created, including data on demographics, main activities of the participants, whether they had accepted the recent praziquantel treatment and factors that influenced treatment compliance (Supplementary file 1). We also gathered suggestions on how to improve the distribution and administration of treatment in order to increase compliance. The questionnaire was pretested in Abidjan, the economic capital of Côte d'Ivoire, among 15 randomly selected children aged 9–12 years. CHWs were trained to implement the questionnaire. They were fluent in the local language (i.e., Baoulé in Moronou and Yacouba in Bigouin). Translation of the questionnaire into local languages was done for each study location. The questionnaire was implemented over 7 days in each village, after the house-to-house treatment.

2.5. Statistical Analysis

Data were double entered into a database using EpiInfo version 3.5.1. (Centers for Disease Control and Prevention, Atlanta, GA, USA). Data analysis was done using STATA version 12.1 (StataCorp., College Station, TX, USA). Qualitative (e.g., reasons for noncompliance) and quantitative data (e.g., age and sex) were expressed as proportions and means, respectively. Proportions were compared using Pearson's chi-squared test (χ^2). A p-value less than or equal to 0.05 was considered as statistically significant.

3. Results

3.1. Treatment Compliance

Table 1 shows the praziquantel treatment coverage rate in Moronou and Bigouin. The overall coverage rate was 47.6% (2730/5733) with considerable difference between the two villages (27.7% in Bigouin (302/1091) versus 52.3% in Moronou (2428/4642)). While males reported significantly higher treatment compliance in Bigouin ($\chi^2 = 19.96$, $p < 0.001$), no sex difference was observed in Moronou ($\chi^2 = 0.16$, $p = 0.104$).

3.2. Factors Associated with Coverage of Praziquantel Treatment

Table 2 summarizes sex, age and occupation of the participants interviewed. The factors influencing treatment compliance and suggestions on how treatment programmes could be improved are presented in Table 3. In both settings we interviewed more males than females (248 versus 157) with a statistically-significant difference observed in Bigouin (145 males versus 60 females; $\chi^2 = 23.95$, $p < 0.001$). The main activity of the participants was farming with cash crops, particularly coffee, cacao and hevea (53.5% in Moronou and 48.8% in Bigouin), followed by vegetables and rice (20.5% and 19.5%, respectively).

Table 1. Praziquantel treatment coverage in Moronou and Bigouin, endemic respectively for *Schistosoma haematobium* and *S. mansoni*, in Côte d'Ivoire. The denominators for the treatment coverage rate were derived from the 2014 national census.

Characteristic	Total Population	χ^2	p	No. of People Treated	Treatment Coverage %	χ^2	p
Bigouin							
Male	610			212	34.8		
Female	481	10.19	0.001	90	18.7	19.96	<0.001
Total	1091			302	27.7		
Moronou							
Male	2397			1266	52.8		
Female	2245			1162	51.8	0.16	0.104
Total	4642	3.32	0.069	2428	52.3		
Total	5733			2730	47.6	85.39	<0.001

Table 2. Characteristics of study participants.

Participant Characteristics	Moronou (n = 200)			Bigouin (n = 205)			Total (N = 405)		
	n (%)	χ^2	p	n (%)	χ^2	p	n (%)	χ^2	p
Sex									
Female	97 (48.5)			60 (29.3)			157 (38.8)		
Male	103 (51.5)	0.12	0.729	145 (70.7)	23.95	<0.001	248 (61.2)	13.71	<0.001
Average Age (SD)									
6–15 years	11.9 (2.5)			11.3 (2.2)			11.6 (2.4)		
≥16 years	36.6 (14.0)			40.1 (14.3)			38.4 (14.3)		
Occupation									
Cash crops (cocoa, coffee, hevea) (1)	107 (53.5)			100 (48.8)			207 (51.1)		
Vegetable and rice crops (2)	41 (20.5)			40 (19.5)			81 (20.0)		
Combined activities (1 & 2)	18 (9.0)			50 (24.4)			68 (16.8)		
Other activity (trade, civil servant, etc.)	34 (17.0)	66.84	<0.001	15 (7.3)	57.15	<0.001	49 (12.1)	109.87	<0.001

Table 3. Factors associated with praziquantel treatment coverage rates in Moronou and Bigouin, Côte d'Ivoire.

Associated Factor	Moronou (n = 200)			Bigouin (n = 205)			Total (N = 405)		
	n (%)	χ^2	p	n (%)	χ^2	p	n (%)	χ^2	p
Accepted Praziquantel Treatment (MDA)									
Yes	100 (50.0)			40 (19.5)			140 (34.6)		
No	100 (50.0)	n.a.	n.a.	165 (80.5)	53.00	<0.001	265 (65.4)	26.00	<0.001
Reason for Denial of Treatment	n = 100			n = 165			n = 265		
Not sick	4 (4.0)			13 (7.9)			17 (6.4)		
Adverse events of previous treatment	25 (25.0)			3 (1.8)			28 (10.6)		
Busy with field activities	70 (70.0)			148 (89.7)			218 (82.3)		
Not informed about the treatment	1 (1.0)	87.42	<0.001	1 (0.6)	237.48	<0.001	2 (0.7)	306.93	<0.001
Reason of Treatment's Acceptance	n = 100			n = 40			n = 140		
Sick	7 (7.0)			2 (5.0)			9 (6.4)		
Knowledge on schistosomiasis/disease	68 (68.0)			11 (27.5)			79 (56.4)		
Emulation	25 (25.0)	42.57	<0.001	27 (67.5)	17.86	<0.001	52 (37.1)	43.33	<0.001
What you did not like with the drug?	n = 100			n = 40			n = 140		
The taste	26 (26.0)			15 (37.5)			41 (29.3)		
The size of the tablet	12 (12.0)			4 (10.0)			16 (11.4)		
Adverse events	62 (62.0)	28.69	<0.001	21 (52.5)	8.98	<0.008	63 (45.0)	22.06	<0.001
Impact of the drug on your wellbeing	n = 100			n = 40			n = 140		
No effect	15 (15.0)			4 (10.0)			19 (13.6)		
Improvement	85 (85.0)	34.55	<0.001	36 (90.0)	18.37	<0.001	121 (86.4)	52.65	<0.001
Could you accept a new treatment?	n = 100			n = 40			n = 140		
Yes	16 (16.0)			8 (20.0)			24 (9.2)		
No	84 (84.0)	32.50	<0.001	32 (80.0)	10.00	<0.002	116 (44.4)	48.61	<0.001
Appropriate period for the treatment	n = 200			n = 205			n = 405		
Rainy season	2 (1.0)			7 (3.4)			9 (2.2)		
Dry season	198 (99.0)	143.35	<0.001	198 (96.6)	131.30	<0.001	396 (97.8)	274.37	<0.001
Appropriate time for the treatment	n = 200			n = 205			n = 405		
Early in the morning	15 (7.5)			2 (1.0)			17 (4.2)		
In the evening	14 (7.0)			26 (12.7)			40 (9.9)		
At any time, if I am informed	171 (85.5)	164.12	<0.001	177 (86.3)	179.78	<0.001	348 (85.9)	340.58	<0.001
What is the best place to facilitate treatment?	n = 200			n = 205			n = 405		
Central part of the village	16 (8.0)			78 (38.0)			94 (23.2)		
House-to-house distribution	137 (68.5)			55 (26.8)			192 (47.4)		
Health centre	47 (23.5)	84.39	<0.001	72 (35.1)	3.19	0.200	119 (29.4)	27.90	<0.001

Half of the interviewees in Moronou (n = 100, 50%) and four out of five interviewees in Bigouin (n = 165, 80.5%) did not take praziquantel during the treatment campaign. Farming activities were stated as the main reason for not participating in the treatment (70%, 70/100 in Moronou; 89.7%, 148/165 in Bigouin). Other factors were adverse events experienced in previous treatment campaigns (25.0%, 25/100 in Moronou) and a lack of treatment need (7.9%, 13/165 in Bigouin). Additionally, 26.0% (26/100) of the participants in Moronou and 37.5% (15/40) in Bigouin complained about the bitter taste of praziquantel as a reason for refusing treatment. Among the participants who accepted the treatment, 62.0% (62/100) in Moronou and 52.5% (21/40) in Bigouin complained about adverse events.

We were also interested in learning whether interviewees would accept another round of praziquantel treatment and if so, whether they could give us some indications on the most appropriate approach and timing for treatment. In both villages, among the individuals who were willing to accept another treatment, three-quarters (overall 116/140; Moronou 84/100; Bigouin 32/40) declared that they would not participate in a future treatment round ($p < 0.001$). Study participants recorded that in both villages the most suitable period of the year for treatment campaigns would be the dry season. There was no preferable time during the course of the day for the treatment. When asked about the most suitable approach for the treatment delivery, in Moronou, two-third (68.5%, 137/200) suggested a house-to-house approach as used in the current study ($p < 0.001$). There was no specific preference in Bigouin ($p = 0.200$).

4. Discussion

Schistosomiasis is a neglected tropical disease that remains of considerable public health relevance [3,27]. The cornerstone of schistosomiasis control is preventive chemotherapy, emphasising periodic treatment of school-aged children with the declared aim to treat at least 75% of this age group in schistosomiasis-endemic areas [7,8]. In view of new aspirations to eliminate schistosomiasis as a public health problem and to break transmission, a range of activities, including broadening of preventive chemotherapy along with WASH, IEC and snail control, are required [15,28,29]. Expanding preventive chemotherapy programmes to the adult population calls for investigations of low treatment coverage and compliance issues observed in several endemic areas that might undermine the success of preventive chemotherapy [30].

Assessment of treatment compliance has been done mainly for mass drug administration against lymphatic filariasis [21,31]. Only a few studies focused on schistosomiasis and intestinal helminthiases [19,32,33]. Moreover, in Côte d'Ivoire, the factors influencing praziquantel coverage rates have yet to be investigated.

We pursued a cross-sectional questionnaire survey to study factors that might explain low treatment coverage in two selected villages in which a small clinical trial had been conducted before the current study [12]. We employed a door-to-door approach with previously trained CHWs. While the treatment compliance in Bigouin was very low (27.7%), it was considerably higher in Moronou (52.3%). The main reason for not having received or taken praziquantel was farming activities at the time of drug administration. Additional reasons were experience with adverse events from previous treatments and the bitter taste of praziquantel. Although the bitter taste of praziquantel and adverse events are well acknowledged in the literature [34–37], to our knowledge, studies evaluating the impact of these issues on treatment compliance are scarce [35].

Previous studies assessing praziquantel treatment coverage reported varying compliance rates and a host of factors influencing coverage. It might be worth highlighting that most of the data reported thus far are based on systematic reviews, but only few have considered coverage as a study objective and assessed it thoroughly using a questionnaire approach [19,38]. However, a standard questionnaire used by the research teams to evaluate the factors influencing the treatment coverage is lacking, rendering comparison from one location to another difficult [39–41].

Advice has been given by the interviewed population to preferably implement preventive chemotherapy in the dry season when farming activities are significantly reduced. Note that in Côte d'Ivoire, as in other African countries, the rainy season is a period of intense farming activities. In that period, a high proportion of the population is staying in small temporary hamlets, often inaccessible to CHWs. It is clear that, while schoolchildren can be easily reached through the education system [42], when extending the treatment to the entire community, socio–cultural issues, accessibility and main occupational activities should be considered through a participatory approach [21]. Another factor to be taken into account might be the duration of the intervention. Krentelet al. reported that in some settings, the scheduled time for drug distribution was not sufficient to cover the entire target population. Hence, one option would be to increase time dedicated to preventive chemotherapy and to increase the number of CHWs distributing praziquantel. Yet, this suggestion was not made by the people interviewed in the current investigation.

Our study has several limitations. First, the research was restricted to two rural settings of central and western Côte d'Ivoire. In previous studies, distinctively different treatment compliance rates were observed when comparing rural and urban settings; usually compliance in urban areas is lower [21,31]. This was attributed mostly to a high proportion of migrants and mobile population, private health institutions that discourage people from participating in preventive chemotherapy and lack of a specific urban health strategy. Second, the treatment approach used by CHWs might differ based on the size of the location. We found that in Moronou, which is approximately three times larger than Bigouin, the population prefers a house-to-house approach. On the other hand, in Bigouin, no preferable drug distribution emerged, as revealed by our questionnaire survey. As expected, treatment needs by different populations vary and further investigations are required to elucidate this issue. Third, we evaluated the current praziquantel treatment coverage rates shortly after the completion of a small clinical trial in adolescents, assessing the efficacy and safety of different novel treatments and treatment combinations against schistosomiasis, including praziquantel. Of note, during this trial only a few participants from each community experienced adverse events, most of which were mild and transient. Yet, it is conceivable that people experiencing adverse events or complaining of the bitter taste of praziquantel might have influenced the willingness of the community members to participate in the current mass treatment.

Only a few studies determined the impact of repeated preventive chemotherapy on treatment compliance with praziquantel. In settings that underwent several years of mass drug administration, such as in Zanzibar [19], Knopp et al. speculated on 'treatment fatigue' of the population being only marginally infected, but repeatedly given medications. Similarly, in our study, we found that most of the interviewees denied a subsequent treatment. This is an important issue, which needs careful attention by disease control programme managers, since predictive models taking into account prevalence and treatment coverage have shown that to reach elimination with mass drug administration, at least 10 years of regular treatment with high treatment coverage (>70%) is required [43]. In settings that aim at breaking transmission, integrated control approaches are warranted, complementing preventive chemotherapy with WASH, IEC and snail control [44–46]. Such integrated control programmes require long-term commitment [47].

In conclusion, with schistosomiasis morbidity control progressively moving towards elimination, and hence broadening preventive chemotherapy from school-aged children to include preschool-aged children and adults, efforts should be made to regularly assess treatment coverage rates. Since morbidity of schistosomiasis is often subtle and individuals might not feel sick, sensitization prior to treatment should be carried out to diminish the reluctance of the population towards the treatment caused by adverse events and the bitter taste of praziquantel. Particular attention should be given to idiosyncrasies of endemic areas by taking into account timing and the mix of the intervention.

Supplementary Materials: Available online http://www.mdpi.com/2414-6366/3/2/69/s1.

Author Contributions: J.T.C. and M.O. designed the study. J.T.C. and M.O. implemented the study. J.T.C., M.O., B.B., J.U., E.K.N. and J.K. analysed and interpreted the data. J.T.C. and J.K. wrote the first draft of the report. B.B., J.U. and E.K.N. revised the manuscript. All authors read and approved the final version of the report prior to submission.

Funding: This work was supported by a grant of the European Research Council (ERC) (grant number, ERC-2013-CoG 614739-A_HERO) held by Jennifer Keiser and a grant from the 'Programme d'Appui Stratégique à la Recherche Scientifique' (PASRES) (grant number, 113) held by Jean T. Coulibaly. The funders had no role in study design, data collection, analysis and decision to publish the work.

Acknowledgments: We thank all participating children, adolescents and adults from the study villages for their availability despite farming activities and the national schistosomiasis control programme for providing praziquantel free of charge.

Conflicts of Interest: The authors have declared that no conflicts interests exist.

References

1. Steinmann, P.; Keiser, J.; Bos, R.; Tanner, M.; Utzinger, J. Schistosomiasis and water resources development: Systematic review, meta-analysis, and estimates of people at risk. *Lancet Infect. Dis.* **2006**, *6*, 411–425. [CrossRef]
2. Hotez, P.J.; Alvarado, M.; Basáñez, M.G.; Bolliger, I.; Bourne, R.; Boussinesq, M.; Brooker, S.J.; Brown, A.S.; Buckle, G.; Budke, C.M.; et al. The Global Burden of Disease study 2010: Interpretation and implications for the neglected tropical diseases. *PLoS Negl. Trop. Dis.* **2014**, *8*, e2865. [CrossRef] [PubMed]
3. GBD 2016 DALYs and HALE Collaborators. Global, regional, and national disability-adjusted life-years (DALYs) for 333 diseases and injuries and healthy life expectancy (HALE) for 195 countries and territories, 1990–2016: A systematic analysis for the Global Burden of Disease study 2016. *Lancet* **2017**, *390*, 1260–1344.
4. Hotez, P.J. Mass drug administration and integrated control for the world's high-prevalence neglected tropical diseases. *Clin. Pharmacol. Ther.* **2009**, *85*, 659–664. [CrossRef] [PubMed]
5. Ezeamama, A.E.; Bustinduy, A.L.; Nkwata, A.K.; Martinez, L.; Pabalan, N.; Boivin, M.J.; King, C.H. Cognitive deficits and educational loss in children with schistosome infection-a systematic review and meta-analysis. *PLoS Negl. Trop. Dis.* **2018**, *12*, e0005524. [CrossRef] [PubMed]
6. World Health Organization (WHO). Prevention and control of schistosomiasis and soil-transmitted helminthiasis: Report of a WHO expert committee. *WHO Tech. Rep. Ser.* **2002**, *912*, 1–57.
7. Savioli, L.; Gabrielli, A.F.; Montresor, A.; Chitsulo, L.; Engels, D. Schistosomiasis control in Africa: 8 years after World Health Assembly resolution 54.19. *Parasitology* **2009**, *136*, 1677–1681. [CrossRef] [PubMed]
8. World Health Organization (WHO). *Schistosomiasis: Progress Report 2001–2011 and Strategic Plan 2012–2020*; WHO: Geneva, Switzerland, 2013.
9. World Health Organization (WHO). Schistosomiasis and soil-transmitted helminthiases: Number of people treated in 2016. *Wkly. Epidemiol. Rec.* **2017**, *92*, 749–760.
10. Parker, M.; Allen, T.; Hastings, J. Resisting control of neglected tropical diseases: Dilemmas in the mass treatment of schistosomiasis and soil-transmitted helminths in north-west Uganda. *J. Biosoc. Sci.* **2008**, *40*, 161–181. [CrossRef] [PubMed]
11. Stothard, J.R.; Chitsulo, L.; Kristensen, T.K.; Utzinger, J. Control of schistosomiasis in sub-Saharan Africa: Progress made, new opportunities and remaining challenges. *Parasitology* **2009**, *136*, 1665–1675. [CrossRef] [PubMed]
12. Barda, B.; Coulibaly, J.T.; Puchkov, M.; Huwyler, J.; Hattendorf, J.; Keiser, J. Efficacy and safety of moxidectin, synriam, synriam-praziquantel versus praziquantel against *Schistosoma haematobium* and *S. mansoni* infections: A randomized, exploratory phase 2 trial. *PLoS Negl. Trop. Dis.* **2016**, *10*, e0005008. [CrossRef] [PubMed]
13. Utzinger, J.; Keiser, J. Research and development for neglected diseases: More is still needed, and faster. *Lancet Glob. Health* **2013**, *1*, e317–e318. [CrossRef]
14. Ross, A.G.P.; Chau, T.N.; Inobaya, M.T.; Olveda, R.M.; Li, Y.; Harn, D.A. A new global strategy for the elimination of schistosomiasis. *Int. J. Infect. Dis.* **2017**, *54*, 130–137. [CrossRef] [PubMed]
15. Sokolow, S.H.; Wood, C.L.; Jones, I.J.; Lafferty, K.D.; Kuris, A.M.; Hsieh, M.H.; De Leo, G.A. To reduce the global burden of human schistosomiasis, use 'old fashioned' snail control. *Trends Parasitol.* **2018**, *34*, 23–40. [CrossRef] [PubMed]

16. Bonfoh, B.; Raso, G.; Koné, I.; Dao, D.; Girardin, O.; Cissé, G.; Zinsstag, J.; Utzinger, J.; Tanner, M. Research in a war zone. *Nature* **2011**, *474*, 569–571. [CrossRef] [PubMed]
17. Tchuem Tchuenté, L.A.; N'Goran, E.K. Schistosomiasis and soil-transmitted helminthiasis control in Cameroon and Côte d'Ivoire: Implementing control on a limited budget. *Parasitology* **2009**, *136*, 1739–1745. [CrossRef] [PubMed]
18. Chami, G.F.; Kontoleon, A.A.; Bulte, E.; Fenwick, A.; Kabatereine, N.B.; Tukahebwa, E.M.; Dunne, D.W. Profiling nonrecipients of mass drug administration for schistosomiasis and hookworm infections: A comprehensive analysis of praziquantel and albendazole coverage in community-directed treatment in Uganda. *Clin. Infect. Dis.* **2016**, *62*, 200–207. [CrossRef] [PubMed]
19. Knopp, S.; Person, B.; Ame, S.M.; Ali, S.M.; Muhsin, J.; Juma, S.; Khamis, I.S.; Rabone, M.; Blair, L.; Fenwick, A.; et al. Praziquantel coverage in schools and communities targeted for the elimination of urogenital schistosomiasis in Zanzibar: A cross-sectional survey. *Parasit Vectors* **2016**, *9*, 5. [CrossRef] [PubMed]
20. Ross, A.G.P.; Olveda, R.M.; Chy, D.; Olveda, D.U.; Li, Y.; Harn, D.A.; Gray, D.J.; McManus, D.P.; Tallo, V.; Chau, T.N.P.; et al. Can mass drug administration lead to the sustainable control of schistosomiasis? *J. Infect. Dis.* **2015**, *211*, 283–289. [CrossRef] [PubMed]
21. Krentel, A.; Fischer, P.U.; Weil, G.J. A review of factors that influence individual compliance with mass drug administration for elimination of lymphatic filariasis. *PLoS Negl. Trop. Dis.* **2013**, *7*, e2447. [CrossRef] [PubMed]
22. Shuford, K.V.; Turner, H.C.; Anderson, R.M. Compliance with anthelmintic treatment in the neglected tropical diseases control programmes: A systematic review. *Parasit Vectors* **2016**, *9*, 29. [CrossRef] [PubMed]
23. Recensement général de la population et de l'habitat 2014 (RGPH). 2014, p. 26. Available online: http://www.ins.ci/n/documents/RGPH2014_expo_dg.pdf (accessed on 6 June 2018).
24. Lemeshow, S.; Hosmer, D.W.J.; Klar, J.; Lwanga, S.K. *Adequacy of Sample Size in Health Studies*; Wiley: Chichester, UK, 1990; p. 233.
25. World Health Organization (WHO). *Helminth Control in School-Age Children. A Guide for Managers of Control Programmes*; WHO: Geneva, Switzerland, 2011.
26. Montresor, A.; Engels, D.; Chitsulo, L.; Bundy, D.A.P.; Brooker, S.; Savioli, L. Development and validation of a 'tablet pole' for the administration of praziquantel in sub-Saharan Africa. *Trans. R. Soc. Trop. Med. Hyg.* **2001**, *95*, 542–544. [CrossRef]
27. Colley, D.G.; Bustinduy, A.L.; Secor, W.E.; King, C.H. Human schistosomiasis. *Lancet* **2014**, *383*, 2253–2264. [CrossRef]
28. Lo, N.C.; Addiss, D.G.; Hotez, P.J.; King, C.H.; Stothard, J.R.; Evans, D.S.; Colley, D.G.; Lin, W.; Coulibaly, J.T.; Bustinduy, A.L.; et al. A call to strengthen the global strategy against schistosomiasis and soil-transmitted helminthiasis: The time is now. *Lancet Infect. Dis.* **2017**, *17*, e64–e69. [CrossRef]
29. Rollinson, D.; Knopp, S.; Levitz, S.; Stothard, J.R.; Tchuem Tchuenté, L.A.; Garba, A.; Mohammed, K.A.; Schur, N.; Person, B.; Colley, D.G.; et al. Time to set the agenda for schistosomiasis elimination. *Acta Trop.* **2013**, *128*, 423–440. [CrossRef] [PubMed]
30. Parker, M.; Allen, T. Does mass drug administration for the integrated treatment of neglected tropical diseases really work? Assessing evidence for the control of schistosomiasis and soil-transmitted helminths in Uganda. *Health Res. Policy Syst.* **2011**, *9*, 3. [CrossRef] [PubMed]
31. Babu, B.V.; Babu, G.R. Coverage of, and compliance with, mass drug administration under the programme to eliminate lymphatic filariasis in India: A systematic review. *Trans. R. Soc. Trop. Med. Hyg.* **2014**, *108*, 538–549. [CrossRef] [PubMed]
32. Colley, D.G.; Andros, T.S.; Campbell, C.H., Jr. Schistosomiasis is more prevalent than previously thought: What does it mean for public health goals, policies, strategies, guidelines and intervention programs? *Infect. Dis. Poverty* **2017**, *6*, 63. [CrossRef] [PubMed]
33. Burnim, M.; Ivy, J.A.; King, C.H. Systematic review of community-based, school-based, and combined delivery modes for reaching school-aged children in mass drug administration programs for schistosomiasis. *PLoS Negl. Trop. Dis.* **2017**, *11*, e0006043. [CrossRef] [PubMed]
34. Coulibaly, J.T.; N'Gbesso, Y.K.; Knopp, S.; Keiser, J.; N'Goran, E.K.; Utzinger, J. Efficacy and safety of praziquantel in preschool-aged children in an area co-endemic for *Schistosoma mansoni* and *S. haematobium*. *PLoS Negl. Trop. Dis.* **2012**, *6*, e1917. [CrossRef] [PubMed]

35. Meyer, T.; Sekljic, H.; Fuchs, S.; Bothe, H.; Schollmeyer, D.; Miculka, C. Taste, a new incentive to switch to (*R*)-praziquantel in schistosomiasis treatment. *PLoS Negl. Trop. Dis.* **2009**, *3*, e357. [CrossRef] [PubMed]
36. Danso-Appiah, A.; Olliaro, P.L.; Donegan, S.; Sinclair, D.; Utzinger, J. Drugs for treating *Schistosoma mansoni* infection. *Cochrane Database Syst. Rev.* **2013**, CD000528. [CrossRef] [PubMed]
37. Kramer, C.V.; Zhang, F.; Sinclair, D.; Olliaro, P.L. Drugs for treating urinary schistosomiasis. *Cochrane Database Syst. Rev.* **2014**, CD000053. [CrossRef] [PubMed]
38. Tuhebwe, D.; Bagonza, J.; Kiracho, E.E.; Yeka, A.; Elliott, A.M.; Nuwaha, F. Uptake of mass drug administration programme for schistosomiasis control in Koome islands, central Uganda. *PLoS ONE* **2015**, *10*, e0123673. [CrossRef] [PubMed]
39. Dabo, A.; Bary, B.; Kouriba, B.; Sankare, O.; Doumbo, O. Factors associated with coverage of praziquantel for schistosomiasis control in the community-direct intervention (CDI) approach in Mali (West Africa). *Infect. Dis. Poverty* **2013**, *2*, 11. [CrossRef] [PubMed]
40. Sangho, H.; Dabo, A.; Sidibe, A.; Dembele, R.; Diawara, A.; Diallo, A.; Konate, S. Coverage rate and satisfaction of populations after mass treatment with praziquantel and albendazole in Mali. *Mali Med.* **2009**, *24*, 21–24. [PubMed]
41. Tallo, V.L.; Carabin, H.; Alday, P.P.; Balolong, E., Jr.; Olveda, R.M.; McGarvey, S.T. Is mass treatment the appropriate schistosomiasis elimination strategy? *Bull. World Health Organ.* **2008**, *86*, 765–771. [CrossRef] [PubMed]
42. Coulibaly, J.T.; N'Gbesso, Y.K.; N'Guessan, N.A.; Winkler, M.S.; Utzinger, J.; N'Goran, E.K. Epidemiology of schistosomiasis in two high-risk communities of south Côte d'Ivoire with particular emphasis on pre-school-aged children. *Am. J. Trop. Med. Hyg.* **2013**, *89*, 32–41. [CrossRef] [PubMed]
43. Gurarie, D.; Yoon, N.; Li, E.; Ndeffo-Mbah, M.; Durham, D.; Phillips, A.E.; Aurelio, H.O.; Ferro, J.; Galvani, A.P.; King, C.H. Modelling control of *Schistosoma haematobium* infection: Predictions of the long-term impact of mass drug administration in Africa. *Parasit Vectors* **2015**, *8*, 529. [CrossRef] [PubMed]
44. Asaolu, S.O.; Ofoezie, I.E. The role of health education and sanitation in the control of helminth infections. *Acta Trop.* **2003**, *86*, 283–294. [CrossRef]
45. Utzinger, J.; Bergquist, R.; Xiao, S.H.; Singer, B.H.; Tanner, M. Sustainable schistosomiasis control—The way forward. *Lancet* **2003**, *362*, 1932–1934. [CrossRef]
46. Ziegelbauer, K.; Speich, B.; Mäusezahl, D.; Bos, R.; Keiser, J.; Utzinger, J. Effect of sanitation on soil-transmitted helminth infection: Systematic review and meta-analysis. *PLoS Med.* **2012**, *9*, e1001162. [CrossRef] [PubMed]
47. Yuan, H.; Jiang, Q.; Zhao, G.; He, N. Achievements of schistosomiasis control in China. *Mem. Inst. Oswaldo Cruz* **2002**, *97* (Suppl. 1), 187–189. [CrossRef] [PubMed]

Tropical Medicine and Infectious Disease

MDPI

Article

Young Adults in Endemic Areas: An Untreated Group in Need of School-Based Preventive Chemotherapy for Schistosomiasis Control and Elimination

Harrison K. Korir [1,2], Diana K. Riner [3], Emmy Kavere [1], Amos Omondi [1,4], Jasmine Landry [5], Nupur Kittur [3], Eric M. Ndombi [1,6], Bartholomew N. Ondigo [1,7], W. Evan Secor [8], Diana M. S. Karanja [1] and Daniel G. Colley [2,9,*]

1 Centre for Global Health Research, Kenya Medical Research Institute, Kisumu 40100, Kenya; cheriyotharrison9@gmail.com (H.K.K.); awinoemmy01@gmail.com (E.K.); amosomondi2@gmail.com (A.O.); emakuto@gmail.com (E.M.N.); ondigo2002@gmail.com (B.N.O.); diana@cohesu.org (D.M.S.K.)

2 School of Public Health, Department of Biomedical Sciences, Maseno University, Kisumu 40100 Kenya

3 Center for Tropical and Emerging Global Diseases, University of Georgia, Athens, GA 30602, USA; dianariner@yahoo.com (D.K.R); nupur.kittur@gmail.com (N.K.)

4 Institute of Tropical Medicine and Infectious Diseases, Jomo Kenyatta University of Agriculture and Technology, Nairobi 56100, Kenya

5 Albany Medical College, Albany, NY 12208, USA; landryj1@amc.edu

6 Department of Pathology, Kenyatta University, Nairobi 00609, Kenya

7 Department of Biochemistry and Molecular Biology, Egerton University, Nakuru 20115, Kenya

8 Division of Parasitic Diseases and Malaria, Centers for Disease Control and Prevention, Atlanta, GA 30333, USA; was4@cdc.gov

9 Department of Microbiology, University of Georgia, Athens, GA 30602, USA

* Correspondence: dcolley@uga.edu; Tel.: +1-706-542-4112

Received: 24 July 2018; Accepted: 31 August 2018; Published: 5 September 2018

Abstract: Parasitologic surveys of young adults in college and university settings are not commonly done, even in areas known to be endemic for schistosomiasis and soil-transmitted helminths. We have done a survey of 291 students and staff at the Kisumu National Polytechnic in Kisumu, Kenya, using the stool microscopy Kato-Katz (KK) method and the urine point-of-care circulating cathodic antigen (POC-CCA) test. Based on three stools/two KK slides each, in the 208 participants for whom three consecutive stools were obtained, *Schistosoma mansoni* prevalence was 17.8%. When all 291 individuals were analyzed based on the first stool, as done by the national neglected tropical disease (NTD) program, and one urine POC-CCA assay (n = 276), the prevalence was 13.7% by KK and 23.2% by POC-CCA. Based on three stools, 2.5% of 208 participants had heavy *S. mansoni* infections ($\geq$400 eggs/gram feces), with heavy *S. mansoni* infections making up 13.5% of the *S. mansoni* cases. The prevalence of the soil-transmitted helminths (STH: *Ascaris lumbricoides*, *Trichuris trichiura* and hookworm) by three stools was 1.4%, 3.1%, and 4.1%, respectively, and by the first stool was 1.4%, 2.4% and 1.4%, respectively. This prevalence and intensity of infection with *S. mansoni* in a college setting warrants mass drug administration with praziquantel. This population of young adults is 'in school' and is both approachable and worthy of inclusion in national schistosomiasis control and elimination programs.

Keywords: schistosomiasis; Kato-Katz; POC-CCA; young adults; soil-transmitted helminths

1. Introduction

The effort to control and eventually eliminate schistosomiasis has gained considerable momentum since the adoption of the World Health Assembly (WHA) Resolution 54.19 in 2001 [1] and WHA

Resolution 65.21 in 2012 [2]. These efforts have largely been by primary school-based implementation of preventive chemotherapy through annual or biennial mass drug administration (MDA) of praziquantel (PZQ) along with albendazole or mebendazole for treatment of soil-transmitted helminths (STH; *Ascaris lumbricoides*, *Trichuris trichiura*, and hookworm). While effective in bringing down the prevalence and intensity of these helminth infections [3,4], this approach alone fails to eliminate transmission of schistosomiasis and almost universally fails to treat young adults in secondary school, college or university. The need and advantage of extending MDA to students in secondary schools have been demonstrated recently [3], and we sought to determine if the same might be true in regard to young adults attending a technical college, Kisumu National Polytechnic (KNP) located in a schistosomiasis endemic area of western Kenya. Such students comprise a population that is associated with given institutions and could be incorporated into national 'school-based' preventive chemotherapy programs. If ignored they may represent a danger to themselves in terms of morbidity and a danger to the control and elimination programs being rolled out across sub-Saharan Africa. Our results indicate that young adults in college or university settings in endemic areas need treatment for their schistosomiasis and their STHs.

2. Materials and Methods

This cross-sectional study was conducted among students and staff of Kisumu National Polytechnic (KNP), which is situated within the lakeside city of Kisumu about three km east of the city center, latitude 0°6′13.7″ (0.1038°) south and longitude 34°46′23″ (34.7731°) east, in western Kenya. At the time of this study KNP had 3106 students and 134 teaching and non-teaching staff. This parasitologic survey was a part of a larger immunologic study [5]. Recruitment inclusion criteria were that they must be student or staff at the college, be willing to provide stool and urine specimens, undergo validated testing and counseling for HIV at the local HIV Volunteer Counseling and Testing center and sign a detailed consent form. The consideration of HIV status was critical for the immunologic portions of the study but did not impact the parasitologic data presented herein. At least one stool and one urine specimen were collected from each participant, and when feasible, three consecutive stools were collected. Specimens in plastic containers labeled with unique identification numbers were delivered to the Centre for Global Health Research of the Kenya Medical Research Institute laboratory in cooler boxes within 3–5 h of collection for parasitologic processing.

Stools were examined for *S. mansoni* and STH eggs by microscopically evaluating two slides by the Kato-Katz (KK) thick smear method [6]. The number of *S. mansoni* eggs were counted, recorded and multiplied by 24 to determine the number of eggs per gram of feces (epg). Infection intensity was classified as light (1–99 epg), medium (100–399 epg), or heavy (≥400 epg) according to World Health Organization (WHO) guidelines [7]. Urine specimens were assayed for circulating cathodic antigen (CCA) by the point-of-care circulating cathodic antigen (POC-CCA) test, as described by the manufacturer (Rapid Diagnostics, Inc., Pretoria, South Africa). STH eggs were recorded as positive or negative.

Study procedures were approved by the institutional review boards of the University of Georgia (Protocol 2012-1-10145), the Scientific Steering Committee of the Kenya Medical Research Institute (KEMRI) and the KEMRI National Ethics Review Committee of Kenya (Protocol 2303) and reviewed by the institutional review board of the Centers for Disease Control and Prevention (CDC), which deemed CDC personnel to be non-engaged. All study participants found positive for *S. mansoni* were provided PZQ treatment (40 mg/kg body weight) and all those positive for STH were provided with albendazole (400 mg).

3. Results

The study population consisted of 291 students or staff at KNP who volunteered and were enrolled, consented and provided at least one stool specimen. Of these, 208 provided all three requested stool specimens. All stool specimens were examined by the Kato-Katz (KK) method [6] for the presence or absence of STH eggs, and the eggs of *S. mansoni* were counted to determine infection intensity. In addition, 276 of these participants also provided single urine specimens, and these were tested for CCA by the POC-CCA test (Rapid Diagnostics Inc., Pretoria, South Africa). The demographic and parasitologic data of the participants are given in Table 1. There were no significant demographic differences by Chi square analyses between those who provided three stools and those who provided fewer. The median age of the 291 participants was 22 years, and males constituted 45.5% of this study population. Ninety-two percent were students, 4% (n = 12) were staff, and the status data on the other 4% were missing.

Table 1. Characteristics of study participants.

Characteristic	Number of Participants (%)		
Age, median (range) years	22 (17–41)		
Male sex	132 (45.4%)		
Prevalence of helminth infections	**1 urine sample (CCA) (n = 276)**	**1 stool sample (n = 291)**	**3 stool samples (n = 208)**
Schistosoma mansoni prevalence (%)	64 (23.2%)	40 (13.7%)	37 (17.8%)
Ascaris lumbricoides prevalence (%)	N/A	4 (1.4%)	4 (1.4%)
Trichuris trichiura prevalence (%)	N/A	7 (2.4%)	9 (3.1%)
Hookworm prevalence (%)	N/A	4 (1.4%)	12 (4.1%)

Stool examinations by the Kato-Katz method; CCA assays by the point of care circulating cathodic antigen urine test.

Based on examination of the first stool by the KK method (n = 291), the prevalence of *S. mansoni* was 13.7% (Table 1). The prevalence based on a single urine assay by the POC-CCA test (n = 276) was 23.2%. The prevalence of *A. lumbricoides*, *T. trichiura*, and hookworm based on a single stool was 1.4%, 2.4%, and 1.4%, respectively. For the 208 participants who provided all three stools, the prevalence of *S. mansoni* rose to 17.8% and the prevalence of *A. lumbricoides*, *T. trichiura* and hookworm was 1.4%, 3.1%, and 4.1%, respectively. There were no significant differences in terms of prevalence or prevalence of heavy infection based on gender.

When the intensity of *S. mansoni* infection, based on the number of eggs per gram of feces (epg) was calculated based on all three stools (n = 208), 2.5% of this population were categorized as heavy infections (≥400 epg of stool) [as categorized by the WHO] [7] (Figure 1), 5.3% had moderate infections (100–399 epg), and 10.1% had light infections (1–99 epg). Within the *S. mansoni*-infected population 13.5% had heavy infections, another 29.7% had moderate intensity infections, and the remaining infected individuals (56.8%) had light infections. Chi square analyses showed no significant difference in *S. mansoni* prevalence or prevalence of heavy infection between students and staff (p = 0.765).

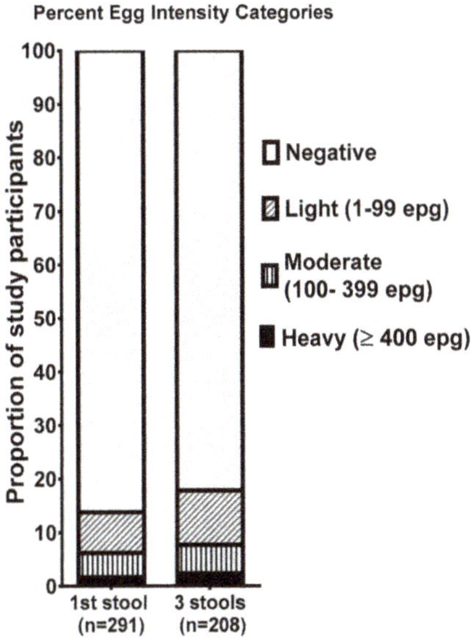

Figure 1. Proportion of the study participants with schistosomiasis, stratified by World Health Organization (WHO) intensity categories based on either the first stool examined (**left bar**) or three stools when available (**right bar**).

4. Discussion

We have previously shown that extending school-based MDA beyond primary schools to include secondary schools, is highly effective in rapidly dropping the prevalence and intensity of *S. mansoni* and STHs in secondary school students [3]. We have now demonstrated that there is also a need to extend national neglected tropical disease (NTD) program MDA for schistosomiasis to include college- and university-attending young adults in school-based programs in endemic areas. Such colleges and universities often have nurses staffing on-site health clinics and health science-related students who participate in health education groups, both of whom proved to be a great assistance in our study, and who could likewise be capitalized upon by national programs that wish to extend into these venues. We acknowledge that this study was conducted only at one such site and the study population was not randomly selected, but rather comprises only those who volunteered and consented to participate by providing stools and urine, as well as blood samples for the larger immunologic study [5]. Nevertheless, a substantial number of college-age students participated and a notable number of them had *S. mansoni* infections, and some of those had heavy infections.

The discrepancy between the prevalence of *S. mansoni* based on a single stool exam compared to a single urine POC-CCA assay is within the expected relative ranges of sensitivity, with the more sensitive POC-CCA always providing a higher prevalence in areas of low to moderate *S. mansoni* prevalence [8–10]. The increase in prevalence seen when three stools are evaluated compared to a single stool, is also to be expected, as the sensitivity increases when multiple stools from different days are tested [11–13].

It is clear, based on WHO guidelines, that an overall prevalence of >10% and even a prevalence of >1% heavy infection by *S. mansoni* meets the requirement for MDA in school-aged children [14]. Both of these criteria are satisfied in the population studied here although they are a different age group. While it is impossible to extrapolate and state that the same is true in other colleges and universities in endemic regions, these findings strongly suggest that this might be true and begs the question for further surveys of such populations. This is important both for the health of the infected students and in regard to control and elimination of schistosomiasis. Such heavy infections with *S. mansoni* are associated with the chronic development of severe morbidity [15], and the presence of low-to-moderate intensity infections is associated with both physical and cognitive subtle or functional morbidities [16,17]. It may be true that this population is less likely to further transmit schistosomiasis because they have more routine access to sanitation facilities; however, we previously reported that students in the KNP population who were *S. mansoni*-positive were more likely to report contact with water from Lake Victoria while in their home villages [5]. Upon returning home for holidays or other visits, they may revert to the conditions available and periodically reintroduce eggs into the environment, serving as a source of contamination that can infect vector snails and continue the life-cycle of *S. mansoni*.

5. Conclusions

This study demonstrates that a substantial number of young adults attending KNP harbor *S. mansoni* and STH infections. That the prevalence of *S. mansoni* and the prevalence of heavy infections with *S. mansoni* were as high as was found in this upwardly mobile, young adult population, was somewhat surprising. It is true that KNP is in western Kenya, along the shores of Lake Victoria, an area that is known to be highly endemic for *S. mansoni*, and while its students are drawn from across the country, a majority of the student body and this study group is from western Kenya. However, the highest burden of *S. mansoni* is usually in children, and the focus of national NTD schistosomiasis programs is most often on primary school children. In an earlier study, we demonstrated that high prevalence and high prevalence of heavy infections was also to be found in secondary schools in this area and noted that, likewise, this population is usually ignored in national schistosomiasis programs [3]. While these are relatively small studies, we propose that both the secondary school and college or university populations in endemic areas need to be more extensively surveyed and included in national schistosomiasis control and elimination programs. To do otherwise is to leave a population from 14–25 years of age at risk for morbidity and as a potential risk to their communities in terms of continued transmission. In addition, in areas endemic for *S. mansoni*, surveys should consider assaying urine by POC-CCA to detect low intensity *S. mansoni* infections that may be missed by a single Kato-Katz assay. Collection of stool to test for the presence of STH as well as *S. mansoni* eggs would also be useful.

Author Contributions: Conceptualization, D.G.C., W.E.S., D.M.S.K.; Methodology, D.G.C., W.E.S., D.M.S.K., D.K.R.; Validation, D.G.C., D.K.R.; Formal Analyses, N.K.; Investigation, H.K.K., D.K.R., E.K., A.O., J.L., E.M.N.; Resources, D.G.C.; E.K., D.K.R.; Data Curation, N.K.; Writing-Original Draft, D.G.C.; Preparation, H.K.K., B.N.O., E.M.N., N.K.; Writing–Review and editing, D.G.C., H.K.K., N.K., B.N.O., E.M.N., D.K.R., W.E.S., D.M.S.K., E.M.N.; Visualization, N.K., D.G.C.; Supervision, D.G.C., W.E.S., D.M.S.K.; Project administration, D.G.C., D.M.S.K.; Funding acquisition, D.G.C., W.E.S., D.M.S.K.

Funding: This research received funding from the National Institutes of Health, USA, grant number R01 AI53695.

Acknowledgments: We thank the administration, faculty, staff and students of Kisumu Polytechnic College for their willingness to participate in this study. We also acknowledge the many contributions of the CGHR/KEMRI NTD field, laboratory and data staff. The findings and conclusions in this report are those of the authors and do not necessarily represent the views of the Centers for Disease Control and Prevention. This work is published with the permission of the Office of the Director of the Kenya Medical Research Institute.

Conflicts of Interest: The authors declare no conflicts of interest.

References

1. World Health Organization. World Health Assembly Resolution WHA 54.19 Elimination of Schistosomiasis. 2001. Available online: http://www.who.int/entity/neglected_diseases/mediacentre/WHA_54.19_Eng.pdf?ua=1 (accessed on 10 February 2017).
2. World Health Organization. World Health Assembly Resolution WHA 65.21 Elimination of Schistosomiasis. 2012. Available online: http://www.who.int/neglected_diseases/mediacentre/WHA_65.21_Eng.pdf (accessed on 15 February 2017).

3. Abudho, B.O.; Ndombi, E.M.; Guya, B.; Carter, J.M.; Riner, D.K.; Kittur, N.; Karanja, D.M.S.; Secor, W.E.; Colley, D.G. Impact of four years of annual mass drug administration on prevalence and intensity of schistosomiasis among primary and high school children in Western Kenya: A repeated cross-sectional study. *Am. J. Trop. Med. Hyg.* **2018**, *98*, 1397–1402. [CrossRef] [PubMed]
4. Masaku, M.F.; Gichuki, P.M.; Okoyo, C.; Njenga, S.M. High prevalence of helminths infection and associated risk factors among adults living in a rural setting, central Kenya: A cross-sectional study. *Trop. Med. Health* **2017**, *45*, 15. [CrossRef] [PubMed]
5. Riner, D.K.; Ndombi, E M.; Carter, J.M.; Omondi, A.; Kittur, N.; Kavere, E.; Korir, H.K.; Flaherty, B.; Karanja, D.; Colley, D.G. Schistosoma mansoni infection can jeopardize the duration of protective levels of antibody responses to immunizations against hepatitis B and tetanus toxoid. *PLoS Negl. Trop. Dis.* **2016**, *10*, e0005180.
6. Katz, N.; Chaves, A.; Pellegrino, J. A simple device for quantitative stool thick-smear technique in *Schistosomiasis mansoni*. *Rev. Inst. Med. Trop. Sao Paulo* **1972**, *14*, 397–400. [PubMed]
7. World Health Organization. Helminth Control in School Age Children. A Guide for Control Managers. 2011. Available online: http://apps.who.int/iris/bitstream/handle/10665/44671/9789241548267_eng.pdf;jsessionid=1906846F5DDE37F11A805DE0E5BD5F44?sequence=1 (accessed on 23 May 2013).
8. Clements, M.N.; Donnelly, C.A.; Fenwick, A.; Kabatereine, N.B.; Knowles, S.C L.; Meité, A.; N'Goran, E.K.; Nalule, Y.; Nogaro, S.; Phillips, A.E.; et al. Interpreting ambiguous 'trace' results in *Schistosoma mansoni* CCA Tests: Estimating sensitivity and specificity of ambiguous results with no gold standard. *PLoS Negl. Trop. Dis.* **2017**, *11*, e0006102. [CrossRef] [PubMed]
9. Colley, D.G.; Andros, T.S.; Campbell, C.H. Schistosomiasis is more prevalent than previously thought: What does it mean for public health goals, policies, strategies, guidelines and intervention programs? *Infect. Dis. Poverty* **2017**, *6*, 63. [CrossRef] [PubMed]
10. Ogongo, P.; Kariuki, T.M.; Wilson, R.A. Diagnosis of schistosomiasis mansoni: An evaluation of existing methods and research towards single worm pair detection. *Parasitology* **2018**. [CrossRef] [PubMed]
11. Danso-Appiah, A.; Minton, J.; Boamah, D.; Otchere, J.; Asmah, R.H.; Rodgers, M.; Bosompem, K.M.; Eusebi, P.; De Vlas, S.J. Accuracy of point-of-care testing for circulatory cathodic antigen in the detection of schistosome infection: Systematic review and meta-analysis. *Bull. World Health Organ.* **2016**, *94*, 522–533. [CrossRef] [PubMed]
12. Kittur, N.; Castleman, J.D.; Campbell, C.H.; King, C.H.; Colley, D.G. Comparison of *Schistosoma mansoni* prevalence and intensity of infection, as determined by the circulating cathodic antigen urine assay or by the Kato-Katz fecal assay: A systematic review. *Am. J. Trop. Med. Hyg.* **2016**, *94*, 605–610. [CrossRef] [PubMed]
13. Utzinger, J.; Raso, G.; Brooker, S.; De Savigny, D.; Tanner, M.; Ornbjerg, N.; Singer, B.H.; N'goran, E.K. Schistosomiasis and neglected tropical diseases: Towards integrated and sustainable control and a word of caution. *Parasitology* **2009**, *136*, 1859–1874. [CrossRef] [PubMed]
14. World Health Organization. Prevention and Control of Schistosomiasis and Soil-Transmitted Helminthiasis. 2002. Available online: http://apps.who.int/iris/bitstream/handle/10665/42588/WHO_TRS_912.pdf?sequence=1&isAllowed=y (accessed on 31 July 2018).
15. Vennervald, B.J.; Dunne, D.W. Morbidity in schistosomiasis: an update. *Curr. Opin. Infect. Dis.* **2004**, *17*, 439–447. [CrossRef] [PubMed]
16. Ezeamama, A.E.; He, C.L.; Shen, Y.; Yin, X.P.; Binder, S.C.; Campbell, C.H.; Rathbun, S.; Whalen, C.C.; N'Goran, E.K.; Utzinger, J.; et al. Gaining and sustaining schistosomiasis control: Study protocol and baseline data prior to different treatment strategies in five African countries. *BMC Infect. Dis.* **2016**, *16*, 229. [CrossRef] [PubMed]
17. King, C.H.; Sturrock, R.F.; Kariuki, H.C.; Hamburger, J. Transmission control for schistosomiasis—Why it matters now. *Trends Parasitol.* **2006**, *22*, 575–582. [CrossRef] [PubMed]

Tropical Medicine and Infectious Disease

MDPI

Review

DNA Diagnostics for Schistosomiasis Control

Kosala G. Weerakoon [1,2,3,*], Catherine A. Gordon [1] and Donald P. McManus [1,*]

1 Molecular Parasitology Laboratory, Infectious Diseases Division, QIMR Berghofer Medical Research Institute, Brisbane 4006, Australia; Catherine.Gordon@qimrberghofer.edu.au
2 School of Public Health, University of Queensland, Brisbane 4006, Australia
3 Department of Parasitology, Faculty of Medicine and Allied Sciences, Rajarata University of Sri Lanka, Saliyapura 50008, Sri Lanka
* Correspondence: kosala.weerakoon@qimrberghofer.edu.au (K.G.W.); Don.McManus@qimrberghofer.edu.au (D.P.M.); Tel.: +61-7-3362-0405 (K.G.W.); +61-7-3362-0401 (D.P.M.)

Received: 24 June 2018; Accepted: 30 July 2018; Published: 1 August 2018

Abstract: Despite extensive efforts over the last few decades, the global disease burden of schistosomiasis still remains unacceptably high. This could partly be attributed to the lack of accurate diagnostic tools for detecting human and animal schistosome infections in endemic areas. In low transmission and low prevalence areas where schistosomiasis elimination is targeted, case detection requires a test that is highly sensitive. Diagnostic tests with low sensitivity will miss individuals with low infection intensity and these will continue to contribute to transmission, thereby interfering with the efficacy of the control measures operating. Of the many diagnostic approaches undertaken to date, the detection of schistosome DNA using DNA amplification techniques including polymerase chain reaction (PCR) provide valuable adjuncts to more conventional microscopic and serological methods, due their accuracy, high sensitivity, and the capacity to detect early pre-patent infections. Furthermore, DNA-based methods represent important screening tools, particularly in those endemic areas with ongoing control where infection prevalence and intensity have been reduced to very low levels. Here we review the role of DNA diagnostics in the path towards the control and elimination of schistosomiasis.

Keywords: schistosomiasis; diagnosis; control and elimination; DNA; polymerase chain reaction

1. Introduction

The public health and socioeconomic impact of schistosomiasis is such that, to date, over 230 million people have acquired the disease, including many children, mainly in the tropics and subtropics. Further, this chronic debilitating disease leads to around 11,500 deaths a year and it is responsible for the loss of over 3.5 million DALYs, the majority (more than 80%) from sub-Saharan Africa [1,2]. The major schistosome species that cause infection in humans include *S. haematobium*, the agent of urinary schistosomiasis, and *S. mansoni*, *S. japonicum*, *S. mekongi*, *S. intercalatum* and *S. guineensis*, which cause intestinal schistosomiasis. These blood-feeding flukes are responsible for substantial long-term clinical complications with multiple organ involvement including the liver, intestine, and urinary bladder. Infective cercariae in fresh water sources penetrate the host skin and enter the blood circulation as schistosomules and inhabit mesenteric or vesical (intestinal and urinary schistosomiasis respectively) venous plexuses after pulmonary and hepatic migrations. Mature female worms lay eggs in these sites, and eggs then penetrate the intestinal walls (in intestinal schistosomiasis) to be excreted in stool or penetrate the bladder wall (in urinary schistosomiasis) to be excreted in urine while some of the eggs migrate towards ectopic sites such as the liver and other organs, leading to chronic inflammation and fibrosis. The eggs released to the environment hatch in fresh water sources releasing miracidia that penetrate specific snail hosts within which they undergo asexual reproduction and become cercariae to continue the life cycle.

Successful disease prevention and elimination programs for schistosomiasis involve the implementation of intensive intervention and efficient monitoring measures, with different countries having their own modified approaches tailored to the sociocultural and economic situations prevailing [3–5]. For example, in China the number of human schistosomiasis cases was reduced by 90% over the decade from 2004 through human case detection and treatment, health education and snail control [6]. Additionally, China has had a strong political will for many decades to eliminate schistosomiasis, since control options were first instigated by Chairman Mao in 1956, who made its elimination a national health priority [7]. In general, accurate community diagnosis of the infection and continued surveillance is helpful in the control of transmission of schistosomiasis, while prompt treatment following early detection can minimize the associated morbidity and mortality [8,9]. With continuing multiple prevention and control efforts, the prevalence and intensity of schistosomiasis in many endemic regions have gone down, so that in many infected individuals, the disease may go undetected with commonly-used conventional diagnostic tools such as the Kato-Katz fecal smear (KK) test or urine egg filtration methods, due to their low sensitivity [10–13]. As a result, a schistosomiasis-endemic area may appear to be free of the disease infection whereas in reality transmission continues and may even spread to other communities, thereby increasing the time for control and eventual elimination. A recent World Health Organization (WHO) expert committee report [12] highlighted the significance of a One Health approach focusing on preventive chemotherapy, improvement of water, sanitation and hygiene (WASH), health promotion, snail control, and detection and treatment of animal reservoirs for the sustained control and elimination of Asian schistosomiasis [12]. This further emphasizes the importance and essential need for accurate diagnostics, if the target goals of transmission interruption by 2025 and elimination of transmission by 2030 are to be achieved.

2. A General Overview of Diagnostics for Schistosomiasis

Procedures that have been commonly applied in schistosomiasis diagnosis include conventional microscopy-based tests, different antibody-based serological assays, parasite antigen detection assays and DNA detection methods including polymerase chain reaction (PCR)-based procedures (Figure 1). As considered earlier, the KK and microscopy-based egg detection in urine have the major drawbacks of low sensitivity and can be labor intensive [14–17]. Antibody detection assays also have low diagnostic accuracy, particularly in terms of test specificity, as well as being unable to distinguish between past and current infections [16]. Recent improvements in circulating parasite antigen detection assays have resulted in relatively higher accuracy in comparison with microscopic and antibody detection methods but frequent fluctuations in assay replicates have suggested the need for multiple testing to improve diagnostic accuracy [18,19].

Furthermore, the circulating antigen (circulating anodic antigen (CAA) and circulating cathodic antigen (CCA))-based assays are not currently applicable for all schistosome species. The CCA-based assay is used as a point of care test to diagnose *S. mansoni* but does not work for *S. haematobium* [20]. CAA-based lateral flow assays combined with up-converting phosphor reporter technology, work for both *S. mansoni* and *S. haematobium*. However, they have not as yet proven as effective with other schistosome species [20–22]. As a result, DNA, especially PCR-based parasite DNA detection assays, have stimulated much interest as alternative options due to their proven diagnostic accuracy, higher sensitivity, and wider range of applicability, including the ability to detect early pre-patent infections. Here we review the different DNA detection methods that have been employed in the diagnosis of human and animal schistosomiasis, discuss their application in control programs and consider their value in surveillance leading to elimination goals.

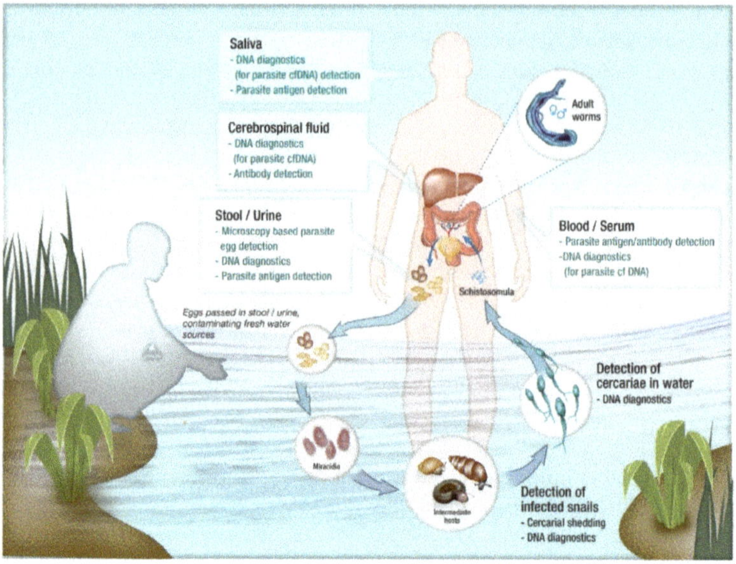

Figure 1. Applicability of diagnostic tools for the detection of different lifecycle stages of schistosomes.

3. DNA-Based Diagnostics for Schistosomiasis

Technological advances and the substantial genomic data now available for schistosomes [23–25] have opened up new avenues for the development of novel diagnostics as well as identifying new therapeutic and vaccine targets. Recent advances in DNA amplification assays include the application of real-time quantitative PCR (qPCR) and droplet digital PCR (ddPCR) for the detection of circulating cell-free parasite DNA using different clinical samples and the development of isothermal amplification assays such as loop-mediated isothermal amplification (LAMP) and recombinase polymerase amplification (RPA) techniques [26–29]. Measures of accuracy including diagnostic sensitivity and specificity of DNA detection assays vary depending on the type of the assay, target gene sequence used, as well as the type of sample tested [30]. Some of the key advantages and limitations of these different DNA detection assays along with the relative costs involved are summarized in Table 1. One of the key factors in the development of a highly sensitive DNA amplification assay is the selection of a specific amplification target sequence with numerous copies that is available in abundance within a single parasite cell; such sequences include both nuclear and mitochondrial genes [27,30–33]. In addition to being highly abundant, a target gene sequence for diagnostic DNA amplification needs to be highly specific for the targeted species so that the resulting assay is highly sensitive and specific. The *SjR2* retrotransposon [34–36] and the *nad1* mitochondrial gene [37,38] are two target sequences that have been commonly used in the diagnosis of *S. japonicum* infection. Similarly, the *SM1-7* tandem repeat sequence [39] and 18S rDNA are two targets used in the diagnosis of *S. mansoni* while mitochondrial *cox1* [40] and the *Dra1* repeat sequence [41] have been utilized for *S. haematobium* detection.

Table 1. Advantages and limitations of different DNA diagnostics.

Assay Type	Advantages	Limitations	Relative Cost *	References
cPCR	- Low cost compared to qPCR and ddPCR - Can be multiplexed when target amplicon sizes are different	- Requires post PCR processing—running PCR products in a gel—which allows high chance of contamination - More time consuming and labor intensive compared to most other PCR methods - Prone to potential laboratory contamination with the need of manual handling of PCR products	$$	[42–44]
nPCR	- Use of two sets of primers improves the specificity while the need of two rounds of cPCR provide a higher sensitivity	- Relatively time consuming and complicated initial optimization process - Need to complete two rounds of cPCR amplifications, hence more time consuming and labor intensive - Prone to contamination with amplified PCR products	$$	[45,46]
qPCR	- Higher sensitivity compared to cPCR - Higher specificity, specifically when probes are used - No post PCR processing (such as running a gel in cPCR) required for final results - No manual handling of PCR products which limits the potential laboratory contamination - Can quantify the amount of amplicons (relative quantification) - Can be multiplexed for the detection of multiple species within a single reaction - Less time consuming and less labor intensive compared to cPCR	- Relatively time consuming and complicated initial optimization process in multiplexed assays - Requires triplicate reactions to improve the accuracy of final calculations - More expensive than cPCR, LAMP, direct PCR	$$$	[13,29,38]
LAMP	- Cost effective - Less equipment required - Can visualize the end products directly without running in a gel - Faster procedures compared to other types of PCR	- Relatively time consuming and complicated initial optimization process - Prone to carryover contamination	$	[47,48]

Table 1. *Cont.*

Assay Type	Advantages	Limitations	Relative Cost *	References
RPA	- Cost effective - Less equipment required - End products can be visualized on a chip/lateral flow device - Has a great potential to be developed as a point of care diagnostic tool	- Relatively time consuming and complicated initial optimization process - Prone to contamination with the need of transferring amplified products to a detection device	$	[49–51]
ddPCR	- Higher sensitivity compared to most other types of PCR - Higher specificity, specifically when probes are used - Can quantify the amount of amplicons (absolute quantification) - No manual handling of PCR products which limits the potential laboratory contamination - Can be multiplexed for the detection of multiple species within a single reaction	- Requires specific and expensive machinery for the initial establishment - Relatively time consuming and complicated initial optimization process in multiplexed assays	$$$	[35,52,53]
Direct PCR	- Raw sample is used as the template for PCR amplification, eliminating the need of a DNA extraction step - Less time consuming and convenient	- Initial development and optimization is relatively complicated and time consuming, as it is required to overcome PCR inhibitors in raw samples.	$	[54]

* The cost of diagnostics is given as a relative scale to each other: $—low, $$—moderate, $$$—high. The individual cost of DNA diagnostics can be variable depending on factors such as the type and brand of commercial reagents used and the regional source where these reagents are purchased. Abbreviations: cPCR: conventional PCR, ddPCR: droplet digital PCR, LAMP: Loop mediated isothermal amplification, nPCR: nested PCR, RPA: Recombinase polymerase amplification.

3.1. Sample Preservation and DNA Isolation for DNA Amplification Assays

DNA extraction is a key procedure but it can be a methodological bottleneck in PCR-based diagnostic assays since the yield and quality of DNA directly affects the outcome of the amplification procedure; it is also often the most expensive part of DNA-based diagnosis, particularly when using commercially-available extraction kits [55,56]. Furthermore, sample collection and preservation techniques have a significant influence on DNA extraction and amplification outcomes. DNA extraction from fresh clinical samples is not feasible in the field and generally needs to be performed in a central laboratory. Hence appropriate measures are required to preserve samples until DNA extraction can be undertaken. These methods can vary depending on the type of clinical sample involved [56,57]. For example, common methods used in plasma sample preservation and storage include addition of K3EDTA at the time of blood sampling, and freezing [57]. K3EDTA is preferred over heparin as it stabilizes DNA and, unlike heparin, does not inhibit downstream amplification reactions [57]. Similarly, fecal samples for parasite DNA extraction can be readily preserved by immediate freezing, storage with alcohol, addition of commercial solutions such as RNA later and PAXgene, and preservation on Whatman FTA cards [58]. However, these preservation/storage reagents need to be carefully removed prior to DNA extraction since they can interfere with DNA yield as well as downstream assay procedures [58].

Major aims of DNA isolation for PCR include the removal of PCR inhibitors and nucleases, and maximizing DNA recovery and quality of DNA. In the diagnosis of schistosomiasis, stool and urine are the most commonly used clinical samples for DNA isolation; other bio-fluids (serum, saliva, and cerebrospinal fluid) are also used, particularly for cell-free DNA (cfDNA) detections assays. Conventional DNA extraction methods include precipitation techniques with phenol-chloroform and ethanol or isopropanol. However, the feasibility of applying these methods has in the past been affected by the potential for direct exposure of hazardous chemicals to operators and the significant time involved. However, the availability of commercial DNA extraction kits has markedly reduced these limitations and improved the quality and yield of isolated DNA [59,60]. The protocols involve techniques such as spin column-based purification and magnetic bead DNA separation. Furthermore, these kits have been developed for use on different clinical sample types to overcome the unique challenges related to each. Moreover, recent advances in DNA purification technology have resulted in high-throughput automated platforms minimizing the time spent, the labor involved and manual handling, making the process convenient, efficient and accurate [61–63]. However, as is common to most high-tech applications these automated techniques involve costly equipment, and are currently not suitable for field application in disease-endemic, resource-poor settings.

Most DNA amplification methods generally need to be performed in well-equipped centralized facilities that are generally located distant from the clinical specimen collection site. Therefore, under these circumstances it is important that feasible and rapid sample preservation methods are available prior to DNA extraction and amplification. Potential solutions to these issues include the preservation of clinical specimens such as fingerprick blood, urine, or stool on filter papers as dried spots for convenient transportation to a central laboratory for DNA extraction and amplification, or for direct PCR [45,64–66].

3.2. Conventional and Quantitative Real Time PCR

Of nucleic acid amplification tests, conventional PCR (cPCR) was developed first. A key advantage of the technique is the ability to observe the amplification products corresponding to appropriate base pair size that can be conveniently used in specific genomic detection through sequencing. cPCR has been applied in different surveys including the evaluation of therapeutic responses in schistosomiasis [16,67]. Another important aspect of cPCR is the feasibility to develop a multiplex assay to detect multiple infections within a single clinical sample [68]. Multiplexing in cPCR requires differing target amplicon sizes to be distinctively identified in gel electrophoresis. Specific target gene segment detection in stool or urine samples using cPCR has been widely applied in the diagnosis of schistosomiasis [42–44]. The method is highly sensitive compared with conventional microscopy methods, particularly with low intensity infections [33,43,69,70]. The accuracy of cPCR assays has been improved with the combination of other techniques, such as PCR-ELISA analysis [71] and restriction fragment length polymorphism analysis of PCR amplified fragments (PCR-RFLP) for the diagnosis of schistosome infections. The PCR-RFLP technique involves restriction endonucleases digestion of the PCR amplicon, giving rise to different electrophoretic patterns thereby providing a method for simultaneous analysis of multiple species/strains [72]. This technique has been used in characterization of snails as well as in the detection of schistosomiasis and other helminth infections [72–75].

Nested PCR (nPCR) is a more sensitive and a specific approach than cPCR, and has been successfully applied in different instances in the diagnosis of schistosomiasis [46,76]. However, the procedure includes duplication of cPCR for the initial amplification of a larger gene fragment and then another sequence within the initial fragment, which involves more labor and a higher cost.

qPCR has been widely applied in the detection of human schistosome infections of different species including large-scale epidemiological surveys and monitoring of the therapeutic response. The qPCR technique is generally more sensitive than cPCR and, importantly, can provide a measurement of infection intensity. Additionally, the procedures involved with qPCR are streamlined compared with cPCR which needs an additional electrophoresis step to detect PCR end-products [27,77,78]. Another important characteristic of qPCR is that, like cPCR, it has the ability to utilise multiplex assays to detect multiple infections within a single clinical sample using specific DNA probes. Generally, however, qPCR assays are preferred over cPCR in the development of multiplex assays, having the additional advantage of improved specificity with the use of probes and convenience in high-throughput applications. Moreover, recent studies have demonstrated the ability to detect a very high spectrum of parasites in a single sample (multi-parallel PCR) further improving multiplex qPCR assays [79–82]. Multiplexing capability has clear practical significance largely in terms of cost-effective application in epidemiological studies and for monitoring of schistosomiasis control programs, particularly in co-endemic settings, an example being the detection of *S. mansoni* and *S. haematobium* in human fecal or urine samples in areas where both species are present [27,83].

3.3. Loop-Mediated Isothermal Amplification (LAMP)

The LAMP technique is a relatively simple, cost-effective and rapid DNA detection approach compared with the commonly-used PCR-based assays and is more field-friendly. Application of the assay does not require specific equipment such as a thermocycler, electrophoresis apparatus or gel documentation units [84]; hence it is simple, and applicable in resource-poor settings once optimized. Moreover, the use of specific inner and outer primer sets makes the assay highly specific to the intended target sequence, combined with high sensitivity [85,86]. However, the initial optimization process is complicated and time consuming with the use of multiple primers. Furthermore, it is known that the LAMP technique, being highly sensitive, is highly vulnerable to carryover contamination of LAMP products from previous reactions, which can be re-amplified leading to false-positive results [87,88].

LAMP assays have demonstrated high sensitivity in the detection of *S. mansoni* and *S. haematobium* infections in co-endemic areas using urine samples, indicating the possible use of the technique as a point of care (POC) diagnostic [65]. Furthermore, a LAMP assay has been used in the sensitive detection of early pre-patent schistosome infection in an animal model [89]. In a recent field survey to detect *S. mansoni* infection in a low-transmission area, a LAMP assay was successfully applied in both snail and human stool samples and the study emphasized the potential application of this molecular approach for the identification of transmission foci and for building risk maps in support of control programs [48]. Furthermore, the LAMP method was successfully used recently in China for surveillance, including in snail surveys, indicating its usefulness, and applicability as a rapid screening and environmental risk assessment tool to identify areas suitable for targeted intervention [12].

Recent research has raised the possibility of developing multiplex LAMP assays, a concept that could be adapted for the diagnosis of multiple parasitic species, including different schistosomes, in infected individuals. Multiplex LAMP procedures incorporate an additional endpoint readout option to discriminate between amplified products, such as melting curve analysis to test for different melting temperatures or detection of distinctive gel-electrophoretic banding patterns reflecting different species characters [90,91]. The LAMP technique could provide an effective method, applicable in resource-poor endemic communities, to diagnose co-infections of *S. mansoni* and *S. haematobium*, multiple co-infections of soil-transmitted helminths (STH), or co-infections of intestinal protozoa and schistosomes, as achieved using qPCR [27,92–94].

3.4. Recombinase Polymerase Amplification (RPA)

The RPA technique is another isothermal amplification technique usually conducted under lower temperatures (around 40 °C). In RPA, DNA sequences are amplified with the use of DNA polymerase, DNA binding proteins and recombinase; primer binding to the template DNA is facilitated by nucleoprotein complexes made of recombinase proteins and oligonucleotide primers [49,95]. Similar to LAMP, the application of the RPA technique is straight forward and applicable in resource-poor settings since it does not require specific equipment such as a thermocycler, electrophoresis apparatus or gel documentations units. This novel technique has now been integrated with a chip and lateral flow devices making it a convenient portable application as a point of care diagnostic tool [95,96]. RPA has been applied in the diagnosis of both intestinal and urinary schistosomiasis, including its use in field evaluation, and has been shown to be superior to microscopy and serology in terms of convenience, detection time and diagnostic sensitivity [49–51]. However, the technique does have some practical limitations such as the need for transferring amplified products to the detection device, which can lead to potential nucleic acid contamination resulting in false positives [50,96].

3.5. Droplet Digital PCR (ddPCR)

Due to a recent advance in PCR technology, ddPCR is proving to be more sensitive and precise compared with qPCR [97–99]. ddPCR has been successfully used in the detection of cfDNA and in the diagnosis of infections and other clinical conditions, including cancer [53,97,100–104]. Moreover, it was recently applied in the diagnosis of *S. japonicum* in both an animal model and in diverse human clinical samples, and was able to quantify intensity of infection in terms of direct target gene copy number [35,53]. The technique can also be used for multiple target testing, thereby providing an effective diagnostic approach for detecting multiple parasites in an infected individual [105,106].

3.6. Direct PCR

The need for a prior DNA isolation step is a major limitation in routine PCR analysis, resulting in the requirement for additional resources and costs, delays in obtaining a result, and added complexity. Attempts have been made to overcome this constraint by optimizing PCR protocols so that clinical specimens can be added directly into the PCR reaction. However, the initial development and optimization of a 'direct PCR' assay has multiple challenges, particularly the potential negative effect of PCR inhibitors present in clinical samples. Application of modified, inhibitor-resistant polymerases and inclusion of additional reagents such as chelating agents and protease inhibitors are some strategies used to overcome these effects [107,108]. Direct application of the PCR technique has been undertaken in clinical diagnosis, including the identification of parasitic infections, with the use of conveniently preserved clinical samples such as dry blood spots [109,110]. This technique has been tested for applicability in schistosomiasis diagnosis using animal models [54], and its further improvement and evaluation would be a helpful advance for undertaking molecular diagnostics directly under field conditions rather than in a central laboratory, far from the disease-endemic community.

3.7. Parasite cfDNA Detection in Clinical Samples

Application of the PCR technique was mostly restricted to schistosome egg DNA detection until the recent development of parasite cfDNA detection methods in different clinical samples. Compared with the DNA originating from schistosome eggs in stool or urine samples, cfDNA is generally homogenously distributed in plasma and other bodily fluids, which potentially eliminates one of the major sampling problems associated with copro PCR or urine PCR, where eggs are the primary source of DNA [16,33,35,53,111,112]. Parasite cfDNA is released from schistosome stages (schistosomula, adult worms and eggs) within the mammalian host, and could possibly be the result of dead or decaying parasites within the circulation and tissues, active shedding from the parasite or from disintegrating inactive eggs [29,113,114]. Infections with all the three major human schistosomes have been diagnosed using DNA amplification-based cfDNA detection assays, and parasite cfDNA can be detected in host serum in early prepatent schistosomiasis [115–117]. In addition to serum/plasma, parasite cfDNA can be excreted in bodily fluids such as urine, saliva, and cerebrospinal fluid, and can be effectively quantified using qPCR and ddPCR assays [33,53,112,118,119].

As it is likely that the amount of parasite cfDNA in a given clinical sample will be low compared with one containing parasite eggs, a higher level of detection sensitivityis imperative. Of the different PCR-based DNA detection methods available, ddPCR and qPCR are optimal for this purpose [35,52,53]. Recent studies have demonstrated the successful amplification of the *SjR2* retrotransposon gene and *nad1* mitochondrial gene for the detection of both early pre-patent and late *S. japonicum* infection [35,53]. Furthermore, detection of cfDNA using ddPCR and qPCR has proven to be effective in individual case detection, in large scale field application and for monitoring therapeutic responses [111,118,120].

4. Applications of DNA Diagnostics for Schistosomiasis

4.1. Individual Case Detection

Early confirmation of the diagnosis of acute schistosome infection is imperative for early intervention and to achieve a good prognosis for the patient with minimum complications. Acute schistosomiasis cases include returned travelers, immigrants, and refugees [121,122], where patients present to health care facilities with early clinical manifestations such as cercarial dermatitis. These patients need to be carefully clinically evaluated and investigated but most of the commonly applied diagnostics are unable to detect these pre-patent schistosome infections. Schistosome cfDNA detection is an ideal option to diagnose these cases either using serum or non-invasive clinical samples like urine [114]. Furthermore, cfDNA detection is helpful in situations such as neuroschistosomiasis, where parasite DNA can be detected in host cerebrospinal fluid [46,120].

4.2. Diagnosis of Zoonotic Schistosomiasis in Animal Reservoirs

Accurate diagnosis of *S. japonicum*-infected mammalian reservoirs is key to achievingthe elimination of zoonotic schistosomiasis in China and the Philippines [42,123,124]. Similar to the diagnosis of human cases, insensitive conventional microscopy-based diagnostic procedures often do not detect infected animals that continue to contribute to schistosomiasis transmission. DNA amplification-based methods have now been shown to be highly effective in the diagnosis of animal reservoirs of Asian schistosomiasis. Recent surveys undertaken on carabao in the Philippines disclosed a substantially higher prevalence of schistosomiasis using qPCR on fecal samples, compared with copro-microscopic diagnosis [42,125]. Moreover, a recently-developed nPCR assay has also shown potential for field application in the sensitive diagnosis of early cases of schistosomiasis in domestic animals, using serum samples [45].

4.3. Detection of Infected Snail Hosts

Bulinus spp., *Biomphalaria* spp., and *Oncomelania* spp. act as the intermediate hosts of *S. haematobium*, *S. mansoni* and *S. japonicum* respectively. Detection of infected snail hosts—xeno-monitoring—is a pivotal indicator of an existence of schistosomiasis in a particular area, and the potential for transmission. Furthermore, xeno-monitoring is important in identifying infection risk areas to guide surveillance and necessary interventions, and represents a critical measure for achieving schistosomiasis elimination goals [126–128]. The example of Japan is one of the best to show the importance of snail control in schistosomiasis elimination, where the main control strategy was to target susceptible snail colonies using chemical molluscicides and environmental modifications [129].

Commonly used techniques in xeno-monitoring include cercarial shedding with light exposure, microscopic detection of sporocysts and cercariae in crushed snails. These traditional methods have detection limitations particularly in situations where there is a low parasite burden, or where there is aborted development of sporocysts [130]. Moreover, the labor-intensive nature of these procedures, including the collection and handling of snails and the associated costs, are both major disadvantages [131].

Molecular tools are now being widely applied in the detection of schistosome-infected snail hosts, providing promising results in support of control and elimination efforts particularly with large scale screening programs [132]. One early study described the detection of *S. haematobium* in *Bulinus truncatus* snails using cPCR targeting the *DraI* repeat sequence [128]. As well as demonstrating high sensitivity, the study highlighted the cost-effective application of the assay through the grouping and pooling of snails in the analysis. Moreover, PCR and LAMP assays were used in recent studies to detect *S. mansoni* DNA in *Biomphalaria* snails [133,134]. One of the studies showed that the LAMP assay could detect one infected snail within a pool of a thousand uninfected snails [133]. Hence this approach can provide an important low cost, rapid and highly sensitive tool for the monitoring of infected snails to provide important information required before appropriate control measures are undertaken [133]. Similar efforts have also been successful in the detection of *S. japonicum*-infected *Oncomelania* snails using LAMP-based DNA detection [135]. The application of multiplex qPCR assays have the additional advantage of identifying both snail and infecting schistosome species, another helpful consideration for successful schistosome and snail control programs [136]. Furthermore, molecular methods are of considerable help in developing transmission risk maps prior to the instigation of control efforts [48,135].

4.4. Surveillance of Environmental Sources

In addition to xeno-monitoring, the other important surveillance measure to determine the existence of environmental contamination with schistosomes is the detection of miracidia and cercariae in water sources. Evaluating the presence of cercariae is an important factor in detecting infection transmission sites. Commonly used conventional microscopic methods lack sensitivity and are highly labor-intensive [137,138]. Testing for the presence of cercariae is helpful in determining their diurnal variation, seasonal patterns, and spatial distribution. PCR-based molecular tools are now being increasingly applied to this area of surveillance [131,139,140]. qPCR has been successfully used in quantitative detection of *S. japonicum* cercariae in water samples, showing potential for the rapid and high throughput analysis of environmental samples and its application in the field [140,141].

4.5. Assessment of Progress of Control Measures

One of the key elements of sustained efforts on control and elimination measures is the frequent monitoring and surveillance of the effects/progress of the strategies already implemented. While effective control measures need to be continued with high priority, identification of less effective interventions are important in early application of appropriate modifications to improve the effect on control and elimination efforts. Application of highly sensitive and accurate diagnostics is imperative for this purpose since the ongoing control measures lead to lowered prevalence of infection and lowered infection intensity in the community [6,131,142,143]. Further, these assays also need to have the capability to perform in a short time period, with a minimum requirement of equipment and expertise and they have to be cost-effective [144]. The equipment, reagents, and setup required for conventional diagnostics, particularly parasitological methods, are relatively inexpensive, but they can be laborious especially as they need to be repeated multiple times to reach a certain diagnostic accuracy, which can also affect the costs involved. Both molecular and serological diagnostics performed in specific laboratories are more expensive, particularly with the requirements of costly equipment and reagents, specific maintenance requirements, and the need of trained personnel to carry out the tests. Field/community applicable POC immunodiagnostics are simple to use and require only a minimum amount of labor and equipment, but may involve a higher production cost [145,146]. As a result, despite being highly sensitive and accurate, DNA diagnostics cannot currently completely replace the conventional diagnostic methods for community, field, and environmental surveillance. However, the combined application of different techniques is a reasonable approach whereby, for example, an initial diagnosis is undertaken with traditional methods followed by further screening of any test-negatives with molecular tools to capture any missed infections.

5. Challenges and the Way Forward

While there has been substantial focus on mass drug administration (MDA) as a measure to control and eliminate schistosomiasis, efforts to establish accurate, field-deployable novel diagnostics, particularly in resource-poor endemic settings, have been comparatively limited. Microscopy-basedprocedures are recognized as being imprecise, making it important that more sensitive diagnostic tools are developed and deployed. Parasite DNA amplification-based molecular tools are showing encouraging promise towards reaching the level of sensitivity and specificity required to monitor the effectiveness of control programs that will lead to the elimination of schistosomiasis. These molecular assays have a wide range of applications including human case detection, detection of infection in animal reservoir hosts and snails, and in environmental surveillance, which are essential requirements to achieve elimination targets.

Despite the fact that highly sensitive and accurate, ddPCR technology is not yet at the level where it can be used routinely in the field. This is likely in the near future as it can be readily applied for the diagnosis of many other pathogens such as HIV and *Mycobacterium tuberculosis*, which are also endemic in many areas endemic for schistosomiasis. Hence the development of central laboratories that are able to undertake molecular diagnostics targeting multiple infections in these regions would be a cost-effective approach for infection control, and rather than relying on less sensitive, less accurate diagnostics which miss infected individuals, thereby hindering control efforts. Other promising advances include the diagnostic application of the LAMP and RPA techniques, which are applicable to resource-poor settings. Simplifying available DNA extraction procedures, so that they are more convenientand less expensive, and the increased use of fingerprick blood spots and urine filtrates on filter papers [65], should be advocated for field-friendly DNA detection-based molecular diagnosis. Furthermore, improvement and adaption of direct PCR approaches, without the need for DNA extraction, modifications to nucleic acid amplification procedures making them simpler, reducing equipment requirements and expertise while maintaining accuracy, would invariably favor the field use of molecular assays. Altogether these advances have the potential to provide a mechanism for the wider application of more accurate and convenient DNA detection methods that will be invaluable in future schistosomiasis control and elimination efforts.

Funding: Our studies on schistosomiasis receive financial support from The National Health and Medical Research Council (NHMRC) of Australia.

Acknowledgments: We thank Madeleine Flynn, QIMR Berghofer Medical Research Institute, for preparing the figure.

Conflicts of Interest: The authors declare no conflict of interest.

Abbreviations

cfDNA	Cell-free DNA
CAA	Circulating anodic antigen
CCA	Circulating cathodic antigen
PCR	Polymerase chain reaction
cPCR	Conventional PCR

ddPCR	Droplet digital PCR
KK	Kato-Katz fecal smear
LAMP	Loop-mediated isothermal amplification
MDA	Mass drug administration
nPCR	Nested PCR
PCR-RFLP	Restriction fragment length polymorphism analysis of PCR products
POC	Point of care
qPCR	Real time quantitative PCR
RPA	Recombinase polymerase amplification
STH	Soil transmitted helminths
WASH	Water, sanitation and hygiene

References

1. Hotez, P.J.; Alvarado, M.; Basáñez, M.G.; Bolliger, I.; Bourne, R.; Boussinesq, M.; Brooker, S.J.; Brown, A.S.; Buckle, G.; Budke, C.M.; et al. The global burden of disease study 2010: Interpretation and implications for the neglected tropical diseases. *PLoS Negl. Trop. Dis.* **2014**, *8*, e2865. [CrossRef] [PubMed]
2. WHO. *Prevention and Control of Schistosomiasis and Soil-Transmitted Helminthiasis: WHO Technical Report Series (912)*; WHO: Geneva, Switzerland, 2002.
3. WHO. *Schistosomiasis: Progress Report 2001–2011 and Strategic Plan 2012–2020*; WHO: Geneva, Switzerland, 2013.
4. Ross, A.G.P.; Olveda, R.M.; Acosta, L.; Harn, D.A.; Chy, D.; Li, Y.; Gray, D.J.; Gordon, C.A.; McManus, D.P.; Williams, G.M. Road to the elimination of schistosomiasis from Asia: The journey is far from over. *Microbes Infect.* **2013**, *15*, 858–865. [CrossRef] [PubMed]
5. Boatin, B.A.; Basáñez, M.G.; Prichard, R.K.; Awadzi, K.; Barakat, R.M.; García, H.H.; Gazzinelli, A.; Grant, W.N.; McCarthy, J.S.; N'Goran, E.K.; et al. A research agenda for helminth diseases of humans: Towards control and elimination. *PLoS Negl. Trop. Dis.* **2012**, *6*, e1547. [CrossRef] [PubMed]
6. Sun, L.P.; Wang, W.; Hong, Q.B.; Li, S.Z.; Liang, Y.S.; Yang, H.T.; Zhou, X.N. Approaches being used in the national schistosomiasis elimination programme in China: A review. *Infect. Dis. Poverty* **2017**, *6*, 55. [CrossRef] [PubMed]
7. Fan, K.; Lai, H. Mao Zedong's fight against schistosomiasis. *Perspect. Biol. Med.* **2008**, *51*, 176–187. [PubMed]
8. WHO. *Accelerating Work to Overcome the Global Impact of Neglected Tropical Diseases: A Roadmap for Implementation*; WHO: Geneva, Switzerland, 2012.
9. WHO. *Integrating Neglected Tropical Diseases into Global Health and Development: Fourth WHO Report on Neglected Tropical Diseases*; WHO: Geneva, Switzerland, 2017.
10. Bergquist, R.; Zhou, X.N.; Rollinson, D.; Reinhard-Rupp, J.; Klohe, K. Elimination of schistosomiasis: The tools required. *Infect. Dis. Poverty* **2017**, *6*, 158. [CrossRef] [PubMed]
11. Shiff, C. Accurate diagnostics for schistosomiasis: A new role for PCR? *Rep. Parasitol.* **2015**, *4*, 23–29. [CrossRef]
12. WHO. *Expert Consultation to Accelerate Elimination of Asian Schistosomiasis*; WHO: Shanghai, China, 2017.
13. He, P.; Gordon, C.A.; Williams, G.M.; Li, Y.; Wang, Y.; Hu, J.; Gray, D.J.; Ross, A.G.; Harn, D.; McManus, D.P. Real-time PCR diagnosis of *Schistosoma japonicum* in low transmission areas of China. *Infect. Dis. Poverty* **2018**, *7*, 8. [CrossRef] [PubMed]
14. Spear, R.C.; Seto, E.Y.W.; Carlton, E.J.; Liang, S.; Remais, J.V.; Zhong, B.; Qiu, D. The challenge of effective surveillance in moving from low transmission to elimination of schistosomiasis in China. *Int. J. Parasitol.* **2011**, *41*, 1243–1247. [CrossRef] [PubMed]
15. Kongs, A.; Marks, G.; Verlé, P.; Van der Stuyft, P. The unreliability of the Kato-Katz technique limits its usefulness for evaluating *S. mansoni* infections. *Trop. Med. Int. Health* **2001**, *6*, 163–169. [CrossRef] [PubMed]
16. Weerakoon, K.G.A.D.; Gobert, G.N.; Cai, P.; McManus, D.P. Advances in the diagnosis of human schistosomiasis. *Clin. Microbiol. Rev.* **2015**, *28*, 939–967. [CrossRef] [PubMed]
17. Xu, B.; Gordon, C.A.; Hu, W.; McManus, D.P.; Chen, H.G.; Gray, D.J.; Ju, C.; Zeng, X.J.; Gobert, G.N.; Ge, J.; et al. A novel procedure for precise quantification of *Schistosoma japonicum* eggs in bovine feces. *PLoS Negl. Trop. Dis.* **2012**, *6*, e1885. [CrossRef]

18. Legesse, M.; Erko, B. Field-based evaluation of a reagent strip test for diagnosis of *Schistosoma mansoni* by detecting circulating cathodic antigen in urine before and after chemotherapy. *Trans. R. Soc. Trop. Med. Hyg.* **2007**, *101*, 668–673. [CrossRef] [PubMed]
19. Stothard, J.R.; Kabatereine, N.B.; Tukahebwa, E.M.; Kazibwe, F.; Rollinson, D.; Mathieson, W.; Webster, J.P.; Fenwick, A. Use of circulating cathodic antigen (CCA) dipsticks for detection of intestinal and urinary schistosomiasis. *Acta Trop.* **2006**, *97*, 219–228. [CrossRef] [PubMed]
20. Ochodo, E.A.; Gopalakrishna, G.; Spek, B.; Reitsma, J.B.; van Lieshout, L.; Polman, K.; Lamberton, P.; Bossuyt, P.M.M.; Leeflang, M.M.G. Circulating antigen tests and urine reagent strips for diagnosis of active schistosomiasis in endemic areas. *Cochrane Database Syst. Rev.* **2015**, *11*, CD009579. [CrossRef] [PubMed]
21. Van Grootveld, R.; van Dam, G.J.; de Dood, C.; de Vries, J.J.C.; Visser, L.G.; Corstjens, P.L.A.M.; van Lieshout, L. Improved diagnosis of active *Schistosoma* infection in travellers and migrants using the ultra-sensitive in-house lateral flow test for detection of circulating anodic antigen (CAA) in serum. *Eur. J. Clin. Microbiol. Infect. Dis.* **2018**, in press. [CrossRef] [PubMed]
22. Knopp, S.; Corstjens, P.L.A.M.; Koukounari, A.; Cercamondi, C.I.; Ame, S.M.; Ali, S.M.; de Dood, C.J.; Mohammed, K.A.; Utzinger, J.; Rollinson, D.; et al. Sensitivity and specificity of a urine circulating anodic antigen test for the diagnosis of *Schistosoma haematobium* in low endemic settings. *PLoS Negl. Trop. Dis.* **2015**, *9*, e0003752. [CrossRef] [PubMed]
23. Liu, F.; Zhou, Y.; Wang, Z.Q.; Lu, G.; Zheng, H.; Brindley, P.J.; McManus, D.P.; Blair, D.; Zhang, Q.H.; Zhong, Y.; et al. *Schistosoma japonicum* genome sequencing and functional analysis consortium the *Schistosoma japonicum* genome reveals features of host-parasite interplay. *Nature* **2009**, *460*, 345–351.
24. Young, N.D.; Jex, A.R.; Li, B.; Liu, S.; Yang, L.; Xiong, Z.; Li, Y.; Cantacessi, C.; Hall, R.S.; Xu, X.; et al. Whole-genome sequence of *Schistosoma haematobium*. *Nat. Genet.* **2012**, *44*, 221–225. [CrossRef] [PubMed]
25. Le, T.H.; Blair, D.; Agatsuma, T.; Humair, P.F.; Campbell, N.J.; Iwagami, M.; Littlewood, D.T.; Peacock, B.; Johnston, D.A.; Bartley, J.; et al. Phylogenies inferred from mitochondrial gene orders—A cautionary tale from the parasitic flatworms. *Mol. Biol. Evol.* **2000**, *17*, 1123–1125. [CrossRef] [PubMed]
26. Lier, T.; Simonsen, G.S.; Wang, T.; Lu, D.; Haukland, H.H.; Vennervald, B.J.; Hegstad, J.; Johansen, M.V. Real-time polymerase chain reaction for detection of low-intensity *Schistosoma japonicum* infections in China. *Am. J. Trop. Med. Hyg.* **2009**, *81*, 428–432. [PubMed]
27. Ten Hove, R.J.; Verweij, J.J.; Vereecken, K.; Polman, K.; Dieye, L.; van Lieshout, L. Multiplex real-time PCR for the detection and quantification of *Schistosoma mansoni* and *S. haematobium* infection in stool samples collected in northern Senegal. *Trans. R. Soc. Trop. Med. Hyg.* **2008**, *102*, 179–185. [CrossRef] [PubMed]
28. Obeng, B.B.; Aryeetey, Y.A.; Amoah, A.S.; Larbi, I.A.; Deelder, A.M.; Yazdanbakhsh, M.; Hartgers, F.C.; Boakye, D.A.; Verweij, J.J.; van Dam, G.J.; et al. Application of a circulating-cathodic-antigen (CCA) strip test and real-time PCR, in comparison with microscopy, for the detection of *Schistosoma haematobium* in urine samples from Ghana. *Ann. Trop. Med. Parasitol.* **2008**, *102*, 625–633. [CrossRef] [PubMed]
29. Cnops, L.; Soentjens, P.; Clerinx, J.; Van Esbroeck, M. A *Schistosoma haematobium*-specific real-time PCR for diagnosis of urogenital schistosomiasis in serum samples of international travelers and migrants. *PLoS Negl. Trop. Dis.* **2013**, *7*, e2413. [CrossRef] [PubMed]
30. He, P.; Song, L.G.; Xie, H.; Liang, J.Y.; Yuan, D.Y.; Wu, Z.D.; Lv, Z.Y. Nucleic acid detection in the diagnosis and prevention of schistosomiasis. *Infect. Dis. Poverty* **2016**, *5*, 25. [CrossRef] [PubMed]
31. Lier, T.; Johansen, M.V.; Hjelmevoll, S.O.; Vennervald, B.J.; Simonsen, G.S. Real-time PCR for detection of low intensity *Schistosoma japonicum* infections in a pig model. *Acta Trop.* **2008**, *105*, 74–80. [CrossRef] [PubMed]
32. Gobert, G.N.; Chai, M.; Duke, M.; McManus, D.P. Copro-PCR based detection of *Schistosoma* eggs using mitochondrial DNA markers. *Mol. Cell. Probes* **2005**, *19*, 250–254. [CrossRef] [PubMed]
33. Pontes, L.A.; Dias-Neto, E.; Rabello, A. Detection by polymerase chain reaction of *Schistosoma mansoni* DNA in human serum and feces. *Am. J. Trop. Med. Hyg.* **2002**, *66*, 157–162. [CrossRef] [PubMed]
34. Laha, T.; Brindley, P.J.; Smout, M.J.; Verity, C.K.; McManus, D.P.; Loukas, A. Reverse transcriptase activity and untranslated region sharing of a new RTE-like, non-long terminal repeat retrotransposon from the human blood fluke, *Schistosoma japonicum*. *Int. J. Parasitol.* **2002**, *32*, 1163–1174. [CrossRef]
35. Weerakoon, K.G.; Gordon, C.A.; Cai, P.; Gobert, G.N.; Duke, M.; Williams, G.M.; McManus, D.P. A novel duplex ddPCR assay for the diagnosis of schistosomiasis japonica: Proof of concept in an experimental mouse model. *Parasitology* **2017**, *144*, 1005–1015. [CrossRef] [PubMed]

36. Xu, X.; Zhang, Y.; Lin, D.; Zhang, J.; Xu, J.; Liu, Y.M.; Hu, F.; Qing, X.; Xia, C.; Pan, W. Serodiagnosis of *Schistosoma japonicum* infection: Genome-wide identification of a protein marker, and assessment of its diagnostic validity in a field study in China. *Lancet Infect. Dis.* **2014**, *14*, 489–497. [CrossRef]
37. Lier, T.; Simonsen, G.S.; Haaheim, H.; Hjelmevoll, S.O.; Vennervald, B.J.; Johansen, M.V. Novel real-time PCR for detection of *Schistosoma japonicum* in stool. *Southeast Asian J. Trop. Med. Public Health* **2006**, *37*, 257–264. [PubMed]
38. Gordon, C.; Acosta, L.P.; Gobert, G.N.; Olveda, R.M.; Ross, A.G.; Williams, G.M.; Gray, D.J.; Harn, D.; Li, Y.; McManus, D.P. Real-time PCR demonstrates high prevalence of *Schistosoma japonicum* in the Philippines: Implications for surveillance and control. *PLoS Negl. Trop. Dis.* **2015**, *9*, e0003483. [CrossRef] [PubMed]
39. Espírito-Santo, M.; Alvarado-Mora, M.; Dias-Neto, E.; Botelho-Lima, L.; Moreira, J.; Amorim, M.; Pinto, P.; Heath, A.R.; Castilho, V.; Gonçalves, E.; et al. Evaluation of real-time PCR assay to detect *Schistosoma mansoni* infections in a low endemic setting. *BMC Infect. Dis.* **2014**, *14*, 558. [CrossRef] [PubMed]
40. Umar, S.; Shinkafi, S.H.; Hudu, S.A.; Neela, V.; Suresh, K.; Nordin, S.A.; Malina, O. Prevalence and molecular characterisation of *Schistosoma haematobium* among primary school children in Kebbi State, Nigeria. *Ann. Parasitol.* **2017**, *63*, 133–139. [PubMed]
41. Lodh, N.; Naples, J.M.; Bosompem, K.M.; Quartey, J.; Shiff, C.J. Detection of parasite-specific DNA in urine sediment obtained by filtration differentiates between single and mixed infections of *Schistosoma mansoni* and *S. haematobium* from endemic areas in Ghana. *PLoS ONE* **2014**, *9*, e91144. [CrossRef] [PubMed]
42. Gordon, C.A.; Acosta, L.P.; Gray, D.J.; Olveda, R.M.; Jarilla, B.; Gobert, G.N.; Ross, A.G.; McManus, D.P. High prevalence of *Schistosoma japonicum* infection in Carabao from Samar Province, the Philippines: Implications for transmission and control. *PLoS Negl. Trop. Dis.* **2012**, *6*, e1778. [CrossRef] [PubMed]
43. Pontes, L.A.; Oliveira, M.C.; Katz, N.; Dias-Neto, E.; Rabello, A. Comparison of a polymerase chain reaction and the Kato-Katz technique for diagnosing infection with *Schistosoma mansoni*. *Am. J. Trop. Med. Hyg.* **2003**, *68*, 652–656. [PubMed]
44. Ibironke, O.A.; Phillips, A.E.; Garba, A.; Lamine, S.M.; Shiff, C. Diagnosis of *Schistosoma haematobium* by detection of specific DNA fragments from filtered urine samples. *Am. J. Trop. Med. Hyg.* **2011**, *84*, 998–1001. [CrossRef] [PubMed]
45. Zhang, X.; He, C.C.; Liu, J.M.; Li, H.; Lu, K.; Fu, Z.Q.; Zhu, C.G.; Liu, Y.P.; Tong, L.B.; Zhou, D.-B.; et al. Nested-PCR assay for detection of *Schistosoma japonicum* infection in domestic animals. *Infect. Dis. Poverty* **2017**, *6*, 86. [CrossRef] [PubMed]
46. Bruscky, I.S.; de Melo, F.L.; de Medeiros, Z.M.; Albuquerque, F.F.; Wanderley, L.B.; da Cunha-Correia, C. Nested polymerase chain reaction in cerebrospinal fluid for diagnosing spinal cord schistosomiasis: A promising method. *J. Neurol. Sci.* **2016**, *366*, 87–90. [CrossRef] [PubMed]
47. Mwangi, I.N.; Agola, E.L.; Mugambi, R.M.; Shiraho, E.A.; Mkoji, G.M. Development and evaluation of a loop-mediated isothermal amplification assay for diagnosis of *Schistosoma mansoni* infection in faecal samples. *J. Parasitol. Res.* **2018**, *2018*, 1267826. [CrossRef] [PubMed]
48. Gandasegui, J.; Fernández-Soto, P.; Muro, A.; Simões Barbosa, C.; Lopes de Melo, F.; Loyo, R.; de Souza Gomes, E.C. A field survey using LAMP assay for detection of *Schistosoma mansoni* in a low-transmission area of schistosomiasis in Umbuzeiro, Brazil: Assessment in human and snail samples. *PLoS Negl. Trop. Dis.* **2018**, *12*, e0006314. [CrossRef] [PubMed]
49. Poulton, K.; Webster, B. Development of a lateral flow recombinase polymerase assay for the diagnosis of *Schistosoma mansoni* infections. *Anal. Biochem.* **2018**, *546*, 65–71. [CrossRef] [PubMed]
50. Xing, W.; Yu, X.; Feng, J.; Sun, K.; Fu, W.; Wang, Y.; Zou, M.; Xia, W.; Luo, Z.; He, H.; et al. Field evaluation of a recombinase polymerase amplification assay for the diagnosis of *Schistosoma japonicum* infection in Hunan province of China. *BMC Infect. Dis.* **2017**, *17*, 164. [CrossRef] [PubMed]
51. Rosser, A.; Rollinson, D.; Forrest, M.; Webster, B.L. Isothermal recombinase polymerase amplification (RPA) of *Schistosoma haematobium* DNA and oligochromatographic lateral flow detection. *Parasit. Vectors* **2015**, *8*, 446. [CrossRef] [PubMed]
52. Weerakoon, K.G.; Gordon, C.A.; Gobert, G.N.; Cai, P.; McManus, D.P. Optimisation of a droplet digital PCR assay for the diagnosis of *Schistosoma japonicum* infection: A duplex approach with DNA binding dye chemistry. *J. Microbiol. Methods* **2016**, *125*, 19–27. [CrossRef] [PubMed]

53. Weerakoon, K.G.; Gordon, C.A.; Williams, G.M.; Cai, P.; Gobert, G.N.; Olveda, R.M.; Ross, A.G.; Olveda, D.U.; McManus, D.P. Droplet digital PCR diagnosis of human schistosomiasis: Parasite cell-free DNA detection in diverse clinical samples. *J. Infect. Dis.* **2017**, *216*, 1611–1622. [CrossRef] [PubMed]
54. Eraky, M.; Aly, N.M. Assessment of diagnostic performance of a commercial direct blood PCR kit for the detection of *Schistosoma mansoni* infection in mice compared with the pre-extracted PCR assay. *Parasitol. United J.* **2016**, *9*, 13. [CrossRef]
55. Silva, M.A.L.D.; Medeiros, Z.; Soares, C.R.P.; Silva, E.D.D.; Miranda-Filho, D.B.; Melo, F.L. De. A comparison of four DNA extraction protocols for the analysis of urine from patients with visceral leishmaniasis. *Rev. Soc. Bras. Med. Trop.* **2014**, *47*, 193–197. [CrossRef] [PubMed]
56. Van den Broeck, F.; Geldof, S.; Polman, K.; Volckaert, F.A.M.; Huyse, T. Optimal sample storage and extraction procotols for reliable multilocus genotyping of the human parasite *Schistosoma mansoni*. *Infect. Genet. Evol.* **2011**, *11*, 1413–1418. [CrossRef] [PubMed]
57. El Messaoudi, S.; Rolet, F.; Mouliere, F.; Thierry, A.R. Circulating cell free DNA: Preanalytical considerations. *Clin. Chim. Acta* **2013**, *424*, 222–230. [CrossRef] [PubMed]
58. Papaiakovou, M.; Pilotte, N.; Baumer, B.; Grant, J.; Asbjornsdottir, K.; Schaer, F.; Hu, Y.; Aroian, R.; Walson, J.; Williams, S.A. A comparative analysis of preservation techniques for the optimal molecular detection of hookworm DNA in a human fecal specimen. *PLoS Negl. Trop. Dis.* **2018**, *12*, e0006130. [CrossRef] [PubMed]
59. Gutiérrez-López, R.; Martínez-de la Puente, J.; Gangoso, L.; Soriguer, R.C.; Figuerola, J. Comparison of manual and semi-automatic DNA extraction protocols for the barcoding characterization of hematophagous louse flies (Diptera: Hippoboscidae). *J. Vector Ecol.* **2015**, *40*, 11–15. [CrossRef] [PubMed]
60. Warton, K.; Graham, L.J.; Yuwono, N.; Samimi, G. Comparison of 4 commercial kits for the extraction of circulating DNA from plasma. *Cancer Genet.* **2018**, in press. [CrossRef] [PubMed]
61. Mathay, C.; Hamot, G.; Henry, E.; Mommaerts, K.; Thorlaksdottir, A.; Trouet, J.; Betsou, F. Method validation for extraction of nucleic acids from peripheral whole blood. *Biopreserv. Biobank.* **2016**, *14*, 520–529. [CrossRef] [PubMed]
62. Kang, S.H.; Lee, E.H.; Park, G.; Jang, S.J.; Moon, D.S. Comparison of MagNA Pure 96, Chemagic MSM1, and QIAamp MinElute for hepatitis B virus nucleic acid extraction. *Ann. Clin. Lab. Sci.* **2012**, *42*, 370–374. [PubMed]
63. Lee, J.H.; Park, Y.; Choi, J.R.; Lee, E.K.; Kim, H.S. Comparisons of three automated systems for genomic DNA extraction in a clinical diagnostic laboratory. *Yonsei Med. J.* **2010**, *51*, 104–110. [CrossRef] [PubMed]
64. Schunk, M.; Kebede Mekonnen, S.; Wondafrash, B.; Mengele, C.; Fleischmann, E.; Herbinger, K.H.; Verweij, J.J.; Geldmacher, C.; Bretzel, G.; Löscher, T.; et al. Use of occult blood detection cards for real-time PCR-based diagnosis of *Schistosoma mansoni* infection. *PLoS ONE* **2015**, *10*, e0137730. [CrossRef] [PubMed]
65. Lodh, N.; Mikita, K.; Bosompem, K.M.; Anyan, W.K.; Quartey, J.K.; Otchere, J.; Shiff, C.J. Point of care diagnosis of multiple schistosome parasites: Species-specific DNA detection in urine by loop-mediated isothermal amplification (LAMP). *Acta Trop.* **2017**, *173*, 125–129. [CrossRef] [PubMed]
66. Zainabadi, K.; Adams, M.; Han, Z.Y.; Lwin, H.W.; Han, K.T.; Ouattara, A.; Thura, S.; Plowe, C.V.; Nyunt, M.M. A novel method for extracting nucleic acids from dried blood spots for ultrasensitive detection of low-density *Plasmodium falciparum* and *Plasmodium vivax* infections. *Malar. J.* **2017**, *16*, 377. [CrossRef] [PubMed]
67. Fung, M.S.; Xiao, N.; Wang, S.; Carlton, E.J. Field evaluation of a PCR test for *Schistosoma japonicum* egg detection in low-prevalence regions of China. *Am. J. Trop. Med. Hyg.* **2012**, *87*, 1053–1058. [CrossRef] [PubMed]
68. Moreira, O.C.; Verly, T.; Finamore-Araujo, P.; Gomes, S.A.O.; Lopes, C.M.; de Sousa, D.M.; Azevedo, L.R.; da Mota, F.F.; D'Avila-Levy, C.M.; Santos-Mallet, J.R.; et al. Development of conventional and real-time multiplex PCR-based assays for estimation of natural infection rates and *Trypanosoma cruzi* load in triatomine vectors. *Parasit. Vectors* **2017**, *10*, 404. [CrossRef] [PubMed]
69. Sandoval, N.; Siles-Lucas, M.; Pérez-Arellano, J.L.; Carranza, C.; Puente, S.; López-Abán, J.; Muro, A. A new PCR-based approach for the specific amplification of DNA from different *Schistosoma* species applicable to human urine samples. *Parasitology* **2006**, *133*, 581–587. [CrossRef] [PubMed]
70. Oliveira, L.M.A.; Santos, H.L.C.; Gonçalves, M.M.L.; Barreto, M.G.M.; Peralta, J.M. Evaluation of polymerase chain reaction as an additional tool for the diagnosis of low-intensity *Schistosoma mansoni* infection. *Diagn. Microbiol. Infect. Dis.* **2010**, *68*, 416–421. [CrossRef] [PubMed]

71. Gomes, L.I.; Dos Santos Marques, L.H.; Enk, M.J.; de Oliveira, M.C.; Coelho, P.M.Z.; Rabello, A. Development and evaluation of a sensitive PCR-ELISA system for detection of *Schistosoma* infection in feces. *PLoS Negl. Trop. Dis.* **2010**, *4*, e664. [CrossRef] [PubMed]
72. Sørensen, E.; Bøgh, H.O.; Johansen, M.V.; McManus, D.P. PCR-based identification of individuals of *Schistosoma japonicum* representing different subpopulations using a genetic marker in mitochondrial DNA. *Int. J. Parasitol.* **1999**, *29*, 1121–1128. [CrossRef]
73. Mikaeili, F.; Mathis, A.; Deplazes, P.; Mirhendi, H.; Barazesh, A.; Ebrahimi, S.; Kia, E.B. Differentiation of *Toxocara canis* and *Toxocara cati* based on PCR-RFLP analyses of rDNA-ITS and mitochondrial *cox1* and *nad1* regions. *Acta Parasitol.* **2017**, *62*, 549–556. [CrossRef] [PubMed]
74. González, L.M.; Montero, E.; Morakote, N.; Puente, S.; Díaz De Tuesta, J.L.; Serra, T.; López-Velez, R.; McManus, D.P.; Harrison, L.J.S.; Parkhouse, R.M.E.; et al. Differential diagnosis of *Taenia saginata* and *Taenia saginata asiatica* taeniasis through PCR. *Diagn. Microbiol. Infect. Dis.* **2004**, *49*, 183–188. [CrossRef] [PubMed]
75. Caldeira, R.L.; Teodoro, T.M.; Jannotti-Passos, L.K.; Lira-Moreira, P.M.; Goveia, C.D.O.; Carvalho, O.D.S. Characterization of South American snails of the genus *Biomphalaria* (Basommatophora: Planorbidae) and *Schistosoma mansoni* (Platyhelminthes: Trematoda) in molluscs by PCR-RFLP. *BioMed Res. Int.* **2016**, *2016*, 1045391. [CrossRef] [PubMed]
76. Gray, D.J.; Ross, A.G.; Li, Y.S.; McManus, D.P. Diagnosis and management of schistosomiasis. *BMJ* **2011**, *342*, d2651. [CrossRef] [PubMed]
77. Gomes, A.L.D.V.; Melo, F.L.; Werkhauser, R.P.; Abath, F.G.C. Development of a real time polymerase chain reaction for quantitation of *Schistosoma mansoni* DNA. *Mem. Inst. Oswaldo Cruz* **2006**, *101* (Suppl. 1), 133–136. [CrossRef] [PubMed]
78. Pillay, P.; Taylor, M.; Zulu, S.G.; Gundersen, S.G.; Verweij, J.J.; Hoekstra, P.; Brienen, E.A.T.; Kleppa, E.; Kjetland, E.F.; van Lieshout, L. Real-time polymerase chain reaction for detection of *Schistosoma* DNA in small-volume urine samples reflects focal distribution of urogenital schistosomiasis in primary school girls in KwaZulu-Natal, South Africa. *Am. J. Trop. Med. Hyg.* **2014**, *90*, 546–552. [CrossRef] [PubMed]
79. Easton, A.V.; Oliveira, R.G.; O'Connell, E.M.; Kepha, S.; Mwandawiro, C.S.; Njenga, S.M.; Kihara, J.H.; Mwatele, C.; Odiere, M.R.; Brooker, S.J.; et al. Multi-parallel qPCR provides increased sensitivity and diagnostic breadth for gastrointestinal parasites of humans: Field-based inferences on the impact of mass deworming. *Parasit. Vectors* **2016**, *9*, 38. [CrossRef] [PubMed]
80. Mejia, R.; Vicuña, Y.; Broncano, N.; Sandoval, C.; Vaca, M.; Chico, M.; Cooper, P.J.; Nutman, T.B. A novel, multi-parallel, real-time polymerase chain reaction approach for eight gastrointestinal parasites provides improved diagnostic capabilities to resource-limited at-risk populations. *Am. J. Trop. Med. Hyg.* **2013**, *88*, 1041–1047. [CrossRef] [PubMed]
81. Cimino, R.O.; Jeun, R.; Juarez, M.; Cajal, P.S.; Vargas, P.; Echazú, A.; Bryan, P.E.; Nasser, J.; Krolewiecki, A.; Mejia, R. Identification of human intestinal parasites affecting an asymptomatic peri-urban Argentinian population using multi-parallel quantitative real-time polymerase chain reaction. *Parasit. Vectors* **2015**, *8*, 380. [CrossRef] [PubMed]
82. Pilotte, N.; Papaiakovou, M.; Grant, J.R.; Bierwert, L.A.; Llewellyn, S.; McCarthy, J.S.; Williams, S.A. Improved PCR-based detection of soil transmitted helminth infections using a next-generation sequencing approach to assay design. *PLoS Negl. Trop. Dis.* **2016**, *10*, e0004578. [CrossRef] [PubMed]
83. Sady, H.; Al-Mekhlafi, H.M.; Ngui, R.; Atroosh, W.M.; Al-Delaimy, A.K.; Nasr, N.A.; Dawaki, S.; Abdulsalam, A.M.; Ithoi, I.; Lim, Y.A.L.; et al. Detection of *Schistosoma mansoni* and *Schistosoma haematobium* by real-time PCR with high resolution melting analysis. *Int. J. Mol. Sci.* **2015**, *16*, 16085–16103. [CrossRef] [PubMed]
84. Tomita, N.; Mori, Y.; Kanda, H.; Notomi, T. Loop-mediated isothermal amplification (LAMP) of gene sequences and simple visual detection of products. *Nat. Protoc.* **2012**, *3*, 877–882. [CrossRef] [PubMed]
85. Notomi, T.; Okayama, H.; Masubuchi, H.; Yonekawa, T.; Watanabe, K.; Amino, N.; Hase, T. Loop-mediated isothermal amplification of DNA. *Nucleic Acids Res.* **2000**, *28*, E63. [CrossRef] [PubMed]
86. Xu, J.; Rong, R.; Zhang, H.Q.; Shi, C.J.; Zhu, X.Q.; Xia, C.M. Sensitive and rapid detection of *Schistosoma japonicum* DNA by loop-mediated isothermal amplification (LAMP). *Int. J. Parasitol.* **2010**, *40*, 327–331. [CrossRef] [PubMed]

87. Hsieh, K.; Mage, P.L.; Csordas, A.T.; Eisenstein, M.; Soh, H.T. Simultaneous elimination of carryover contamination and detection of DNA with uracil-DNA-glycosylase-supplemented loop-mediated isothermal amplification (UDG-LAMP). *Chem. Commun. (Camb.)* **2014**, *50*, 3747–3749. [CrossRef] [PubMed]
88. Ma, C.; Wang, F.; Wang, X.; Han, L.; Jing, H.; Zhang, H.; Shi, C. A novel method to control carryover contamination in isothermal nucleic acid amplification. *Chem. Commun. (Camb.)* **2017**, *53*, 10696–10699. [CrossRef] [PubMed]
89. Fernández-Soto, P.; Gandasegui Arahuetes, J.; Sánchez Hernández, A.; López Abán, J.; Vicente Santiago, B.; Muro, A. A loop-mediated isothermal amplification (LAMP) assay for early detection of *Schistosoma mansoni* in stool samples: A diagnostic approach in a murine model. *PLoS Negl. Trop. Dis.* **2014**, *8*, e3126. [CrossRef] [PubMed]
90. Nyan, D.C.; Swinson, K.L. A novel multiplex isothermal amplification method for rapid detection and identification of viruses. *Sci. Rep.* **2015**, *5*, 17925. [CrossRef] [PubMed]
91. Liu, N.; Zou, D.; Dong, D.; Yang, Z.; Ao, D.; Liu, W.; Huang, L. Development of a multiplex loop-mediated isothermal amplification method for the simultaneous detection of *Salmonella* spp. and *Vibrio parahaemolyticus*. *Sci. Rep.* **2017**, *7*, 45601. [CrossRef] [PubMed]
92. Llewellyn, S.; Inpankaew, T.; Nery, S.V.; Gray, D.J.; Verweij, J.J.; Clements, A.C.A.; Gomes, S.J.; Traub, R.; McCarthy, J.S. Application of a multiplex quantitative PCR to assess prevalence and intensity of intestinal parasite infections in a controlled clinical trial. *PLoS Negl. Trop. Dis.* **2016**, *10*, e0004380. [CrossRef] [PubMed]
93. Gordon, C.A.; McManus, D.P.; Acosta, L.P.; Olveda, R.M.; Williams, G.M.; Ross, A.G.; Gray, D.J.; Gobert, G.N. Multiplex real-time PCR monitoring of intestinal helminths in humans reveals widespread polyparasitism in Northern Samar, the Philippines. *Int. J. Parasitol.* **2015**, *45*, 477–483. [CrossRef] [PubMed]
94. Haque, R.; Roy, S.; Siddique, A.; Mondal, U.; Rahman, S.M.M.; Mondal, D.; Houpt, E.; Petri, W.A. Multiplex real-time PCR assay for detection of *Entamoeba histolytica*, *Giardia intestinalis*, and *Cryptosporidium* spp. *Am. J. Trop. Med. Hyg.* **2007**, *76*, 713–717. [PubMed]
95. Piepenburg, O.; Williams, C.H.; Stemple, D.L.; Armes, N.A. DNA detection using recombination proteins. *PLoS Biol.* **2006**, *4*, e204. [CrossRef] [PubMed]
96. Zanoli, L.M.; Spoto, G. Isothermal amplification methods for the detection of nucleic acids in microfluidic devices. *Biosensors* **2013**, *3*, 18–43. [CrossRef] [PubMed]
97. Yang, R.; Paparini, A.; Monis, P.; Ryan, U. Comparison of next-generation droplet digital PCR (ddPCR) with quantitative PCR (qPCR) for enumeration of *Cryptosporidium* oocysts in faecal samples. *Int. J. Parasitol.* **2014**, *44*, 1105–1111. [CrossRef] [PubMed]
98. Sze, M.A.; Abbasi, M.; Hogg, J.C.; Sin, D.D. A Comparison between droplet digital and quantitative PCR in the analysis of bacterial 16S load in lung tissue samples from control and COPD GOLD 2. *PLoS ONE* **2014**, *9*, e110351. [CrossRef] [PubMed]
99. Hindson, C.M.; Chevillet, J.R.; Briggs, H.A.; Gallichotte, E.N.; Ruf, I.K.; Hindson, B.J.; Vessella, R.L.; Tewari, M. Absolute quantification by droplet digital PCR versus analog real-time PCR. *Nat. Methods* **2013**, *10*, 1003–1005. [CrossRef] [PubMed]
100. Manokhina, I.; Singh, T.K.; Peñaherrera, M.S.; Robinson, W.P. Quantification of cell-free DNA in normal and complicated pregnancies: Overcoming biological and technical issues. *PLoS ONE* **2014**, *9*, e101500. [CrossRef] [PubMed]
101. Sedlak, R.H.; Cook, L.; Cheng, A.; Magaret, A.; Jerome, K.R. Clinical utility of droplet digital PCR for human cytomegalovirus. *J. Clin. Microbiol.* **2014**, *52*, 2844–2848. [CrossRef] [PubMed]
102. Olmedillas-López, S.; García-Arranz, M.; García-Olmo, D. Current and emerging applications of droplet digital PCR in Oncology. *Mol. Diagn. Ther.* **2017**, *21*, 493–510. [CrossRef] [PubMed]
103. Hudecova, I. Digital PCR analysis of circulating nucleic acids. *Clin. Biochem.* **2015**, *48*, 948–956. [CrossRef] [PubMed]
104. Hall Sedlak, R.; Jerome, K.R. The potential advantages of digital PCR for clinical virology diagnostics. *Expert Rev. Mol. Diagn.* **2014**, *14*, 501–507. [CrossRef] [PubMed]
105. Jongthawin, J.; Intapan, P.M.; Lulitanond, V.; Sanpool, O.; Thanchomnang, T.; Sadaow, L.; Maleewong, W. Detection and quantification of *Wuchereria bancrofti* and *Brugia malayi* DNA in blood samples and mosquitoes using duplex droplet digital polymerase chain reaction. *Parasitol. Res.* **2016**, *115*, 2967–2972. [CrossRef] [PubMed]

106. Srisutham, S.; Saralamba, N.; Malleret, B.; Rénia, L.; Dondorp, A.M.; Imwong, M. Four human *Plasmodium* species quantification using droplet digital PCR. *PLoS ONE* **2017**, *12*, e0175771. [CrossRef] [PubMed]
107. Hall, D.E.; Roy, R. An evaluation of direct PCR amplification. *Croat. Med. J.* **2014**, *55*, 655–661. [CrossRef] [PubMed]
108. Chin, W.H.; Sun, Y.; Høgberg, J.; Quyen, T.L.; Engelsmann, P.; Wolff, A.; Bang, D.D. Direct PCR—A rapid method for multiplexed detection of different serotypes of *Salmonella* in enriched pork meat samples. *Mol. Cell. Probes* **2017**, *32*, 24–32. [CrossRef] [PubMed]
109. Silbermayr, K.; Eigner, B.; Duscher, G.G.; Joachim, A.; Fuehrer, H.-P. The detection of different *Dirofilaria* species using direct PCR technique. *Parasitol. Res.* **2014**, *113*, 513–516. [CrossRef] [PubMed]
110. Echeverry, D.F.; Deason, N.A.; Davidson, J.; Makuru, V.; Xiao, H.; Niedbalski, J.; Kern, M.; Russell, T.L.; Burkot, T.R.; Collins, F.H.; et al. Human malaria diagnosis using a single-step direct-PCR based on the *Plasmodium* cytochrome oxidase III gene. *Malar. J.* **2016**, *15*, 128. [CrossRef] [PubMed]
111. Wichmann, D.; Poppert, S.; Von Thien, H.; Clerinx, J.; Dieckmann, S.; Jensenius, M.; Parola, P.; Richter, J.; Schunk, M.; Stich, A.; et al. Prospective European-wide multicentre study on a blood based real-time PCR for the diagnosis of acute schistosomiasis. *BMC Infect. Dis.* **2013**, *13*, 55. [CrossRef] [PubMed]
112. Wichmann, D.; Panning, M.; Quack, T.; Kramme, S.; Burchard, G.-D.; Grevelding, C.; Drosten, C. Diagnosing schistosomiasis by detection of cell-free parasite DNA in human plasma. *PLoS Negl. Trop. Dis.* **2009**, *3*, e422. [CrossRef] [PubMed]
113. Xu, J.; Liu, A.; Guo, J.; Wang, B.; Qiu, S.J.; Sun, H.; Guan, W.; Zhu, X.Q.; Xia, C.M.; Wu, Z.D. The sources and metabolic dynamics of *Schistosoma japonicum* DNA in serum of the host. *Parasitol. Res.* **2013**, *112*, 129–133. [CrossRef] [PubMed]
114. Weerakoon, K.G.; McManus, D.P. Cell-Free DNA as a diagnostic tool for human parasitic infections. *Trends Parasitol.* **2016**, *32*, 378–391. [CrossRef] [PubMed]
115. Suzuki, T.; Osada, Y.; Kumagai, T.; Hamada, A.; Okuzawa, E.; Kanazawa, T. Early detection of *Schistosoma mansoni* infection by touchdown PCR in a mouse model. *Parasitol. Int.* **2006**, *55*, 213–218. [CrossRef] [PubMed]
116. Xia, C.-M.; Rong, R.; Lu, Z.-X.; Shi, C.-J.; Xu, J.; Zhang, H.-Q.; Gong, W.; Luo, W. *Schistosoma japonicum*: A PCR assay for the early detection and evaluation of treatment in a rabbit model. *Exp. Parasitol.* **2009**, *121*, 175–179. [CrossRef] [PubMed]
117. Kato-Hayashi, N.; Kirinoki, M.; Iwamura, Y.; Kanazawa, T.; Kitikoon, V.; Matsuda, H.; Chigusa, Y. Identification and differentiation of human schistosomes by polymerase chain reaction. *Exp. Parasitol.* **2010**, *124*, 325–329. [CrossRef] [PubMed]
118. Kato-Hayashi, N.; Yasuda, M.; Yuasa, J.; Isaka, S.; Haruki, K.; Ohmae, H.; Osada, Y.; Kanazawa, T.; Chigusa, Y. Use of cell-free circulating schistosome DNA in serum, urine, semen, and saliva to monitor a case of refractory imported schistosomiasis hematobia. *J. Clin. Microbiol.* **2013**, *51*, 3435–3438. [CrossRef] [PubMed]
119. Kato-Hayashi, N.; Leonardo, L.R.; Arevalo, N.L.; Tagum, M.N.B.; Apin, J.; Agsolid, L.M.; Chua, J.C.; Villacorte, E.A.; Kirinoki, M.; Kikuchi, M.; et al. Detection of active schistosome infection by cell-free circulating DNA of *Schistosoma japonicum* in highly endemic areas in Sorsogon Province, the Philippines. *Acta Trop.* **2015**, *141*, 178–183. [CrossRef] [PubMed]
120. Härter, G.; Frickmann, H.; Zenk, S.; Wichmann, D.; Ammann, B.; Kern, P.; Fleischer, B.; Tannich, E.; Poppert, S. Diagnosis of neuroschistosomiasis by antibody specificity index and semi-quantitative real-time PCR from cerebrospinal fluid and serum. *J. Med. Microbiol.* **2014**, *63*, 309–312. [CrossRef] [PubMed]
121. Kincaid-Smith, J.; Rey, O.; Toulza, E.; Berry, A.; Boissier, J. Emerging schistosomiasis in Europe: A need to quantify the risks. *Trends Parasitol.* **2017**, *33*, 600–609. [CrossRef] [PubMed]
122. Leblanc, C.; Pham, L.L.; Mariani, P.; Titomanlio, L.; El Ghoneimi, A.; Paris, L.; Escoda, S.; Lottmann, H.; Toubiana, J.; Paugam, A.; et al. Imported schistosomiasis in children: Clinical, diagnostic aspects and outcome in 5 tertiary hospitals in France. *Pediatr. Infect. Dis. J.* **2017**, *36*, e349–e351. [CrossRef] [PubMed]
123. Olveda, D.U.; Li, Y.; Olveda, R.M.; Lam, A.K.; McManus, D.P.; Chau, T.N.P.; Harn, D.A.; Williams, G.M.; Gray, D.J.; Ross, A.G.P. Bilharzia in the Philippines: Past, present, and future. *Int. J. Infect. Dis.* **2014**, *18*, 52–56. [CrossRef] [PubMed]
124. Cao, Z.G.; Zhao, Y.E.; Lee Willingham, A.; Wang, T.P. Towards the elimination of schistosomiasis japonica through control of the disease in domestic animals in the People's Republic of China: A tale of over 60 years. *Adv. Parasitol.* **2016**, *92*, 269–306. [PubMed]

125. Wu, H.W.; Qin, Y.F.; Chu, K.; Meng, R.; Liu, Y.; McGarvey, S.T.; Olveda, R.; Acosta, L.; Ji, M.-J.; Fernandez, T.; et al. High prevalence of *Schistosoma japonicum* infection in water buffaloes in the Philippines assessed by real-time polymerase chain reaction. *Am. J. Trop. Med. Hyg.* **2010**, *82*, 646–652. [CrossRef] [PubMed]
126. Hamburger, J.; Hoffman, O.; Kariuki, H.C.; Muchiri, E.M.; Ouma, J.H.; Koech, D.K.; Sturrock, R.F.; King, C.H. Large-scale, polymerase chain reaction-based surveillance of *Schistosoma haematobium* DNA in snails from transmission sites in coastal Kenya: A new tool for studying the dynamics of snail infection. *Am. J. Trop. Med. Hyg.* **2004**, *71*, 765–773. [PubMed]
127. King, C.H.; Sturrock, R.F.; Kariuki, H.C.; Hamburger, J. Transmission control for schistosomiasis—Why it matters now. *Trends Parasitol.* **2006**, *22*, 575–582. [CrossRef] [PubMed]
128. Amarir, F.; Sebti, F.; Abbasi, I.; Sadak, A.; Fellah, H.; Nhammi, H.; Ameur, B.; El Idrissi, A.L.; Rhajaoui, M. *Schistosoma haematobium* detection in snails by *DraI* PCR and *Sh110/Sm-Sl* PCR: Further evidence of the interruption of schistosomiasis transmission in Morocco. *Parasit. Vectors* **2014**, *7*, 288. [CrossRef] [PubMed]
129. Tanaka, H.; Tsuji, M. From discovery to eradication of schistosomiasis in Japan: 1847–1996. *Int. J. Parasitol.* **1997**, *27*, 1465–1480. [CrossRef]
130. Abbasi, I.; King, C.H.; Muchiri, E.M.; Hamburger, J. Detection of *Schistosoma mansoni* and *Schistosoma haematobium* DNA by loop-mediated isothermal amplification: Identification of infected snails from early prepatency. *Am. J. Trop. Med. Hyg.* **2010**, *83*, 427–432. [CrossRef] [PubMed]
131. Abath, F.G.C.; Gomes, A.L.D.V.; Melo, F.L.; Barbosa, C.S.; Werkhauser, R.P. Molecular approaches for the detection of *Schistosoma mansoni*: Possible applications in the detection of snail infection, monitoring of transmission sites, and diagnosis of human infection. *Mem. Inst. Oswaldo Cruz* **2006**, *101* (Suppl. 1), 145–148. [CrossRef] [PubMed]
132. Melo, F.L.; Gomes, A.L.D.V.; Barbosa, C.S.; Werkhauser, R.P.; Abath, F.G.C. Development of molecular approaches for the identification of transmission sites of schistosomiasis. *Trans. R. Soc. Trop. Med. Hyg.* **2006**, *100*, 1049–1055. [CrossRef] [PubMed]
133. Caldeira, R.L.; Jannotti-Passos, L.K.; Dos Santos Carvalho, O. Use of molecular methods for the rapid mass detection of *Schistosoma mansoni* (Platyhelminthes: Trematoda) in *Biomphalaria* spp. (Gastropoda: Planorbidae). *J. Trop. Med.* **2017**, *2017*, 8628971. [CrossRef] [PubMed]
134. Gandasegui, J.; Fernández-Soto, P.; Hernández-Goenaga, J.; López-Abán, J.; Vicente, B.; Muro, A. Biompha-LAMP: A new rapid loop-mediated isothermal amplification assay for detecting *Schistosoma mansoni* in *Biomphalaria glabrata* snail host. *PLoS Negl. Trop. Dis.* **2016**, *10*, e0005225. [CrossRef] [PubMed]
135. Tong, Q.; Chen, R.; Zhang, Y.; Yang, G.-J.; Kumagai, T.; Furushima-Shimogawara, R.; Lou, D.; Yang, K.; Wen, L.; Lu, S.; et al. A new surveillance and response tool: Risk map of infected *Oncomelania hupensis* detected by loop-mediated isothermal amplification (LAMP) from pooled samples. *Acta Trop.* **2015**, *141*, 170–177. [CrossRef] [PubMed]
136. Jannotti-Passos, L.K.; Magalhães, K.G.; Carvalho, O.S.; Vidigal, T.H.D.A. Multiplex PCR for both identification of Brazilian *Biomphalaria* species (Gastropoda: Planorbidae) and diagnosis of infection by *Schistosoma mansoni* (Trematoda: Schistosomatidae). *J. Parasitol.* **2006**, *92*, 401–403. [CrossRef] [PubMed]
137. Muhoho, N.D.; Katsumata, T.; Kimura, E.; Migwi, D.K.; Mutua, W.R.; Kiliku, F.M.; Habe, S.; Aoki, Y. Cercarial density in the river of an endemic area of schistosomiasis haematobia in Kenya. *Am. J. Trop. Med. Hyg.* **1997**, *57*, 162–167. [CrossRef] [PubMed]
138. Aoki, Y.; Sato, K.; Muhoho, N.D.; Noda, S.; Kimura, E. Cercariometry for detection of transmission sites for schistosomiasis. *Parasitol. Int.* **2003**, *52*, 403–408. [CrossRef]
139. Hertel, J.; Kedves, K.; Hassan, A.H.M.; Haberl, B.; Haas, W. Detection of *Schistosoma mansoni* cercariae in plankton samples by PCR. *Acta Trop.* **2004**, *91*, 43–46. [CrossRef] [PubMed]
140. Worrell, C.; Xiao, N.; Vidal, J.E.; Chen, L.; Zhong, B.; Remais, J. Field detection of *Schistosoma japonicum* cercariae in environmental water samples by quantitative PCR. *Appl. Environ. Microbiol.* **2011**, *77*, 2192–2195. [CrossRef] [PubMed]
141. Hung, Y.W.; Remais, J. Quantitative detection of *Schistosoma japonicum* cercariae in water by real-time PCR. *PLoS Negl. Trop. Dis.* **2008**, *2*, e337. [CrossRef] [PubMed]
142. Utzinger, J.; Becker, S.L.; van Lieshout, L.; van Dam, G.J.; Knopp, S. New diagnostic tools in schistosomiasis. *Clin. Microbiol. Infect.* **2015**, *21*, 529–542. [CrossRef] [PubMed]

143. Hawkins, K.R.; Cantera, J.L.; Storey, H.L.; Leader, B.T.; de Los Santos, T. Diagnostic tests to support late-stage control programs for schistosomiasis and soil-transmitted helminthiases. *PLoS Negl. Trop. Dis.* **2016**, *10*, e0004985. [CrossRef] [PubMed]
144. Feldmeier, H.; Poggensee, G. Diagnostic techniques in schistosomiasis control. A review. *Acta Trop.* **1993**, *52*, 205–220. [CrossRef]
145. TchuemTchuenté, L.A. Control of soil-transmitted helminths in sub-Saharan Africa: Diagnosis, drug efficacy concerns and challenges. *Acta Trop.* **2011**, *120* (Suppl 1), S4–S11. [CrossRef] [PubMed]
146. Stothard, J.R.; Stanton, M.C.; Bustinduy, A.L.; Sousa-Figueiredo, J.C.; Van Dam, G.J.; Betson, M.; Waterhouse, D.; Ward, S.; Allan, F.; Hassan, A.A.; et al. Diagnostics for schistosomiasis in Africa and Arabia: A review of present options in control and future needs for elimination. *Parasitology* **2014**, *141*, 1947–1961. [CrossRef] [PubMed]

Tropical Medicine and Infectious Disease

MDPI

Article

Field Evaluation of a Loop-Mediated Isothermal Amplification (LAMP) Platform for the Detection of *Schistosoma japonicum* Infection in *Oncomelania hupensis* Snails

Zhi-Qiang Qin [1], Jing Xu [1], Ting Feng [1], Shan Lv [1], Ying-Jun Qian [1], Li-Juan Zhang [1], Yin-Long Li [1], Chao Lv [1], Robert Bergquist [2], Shi-Zhu Li [1] and Xiao-Nong Zhou [1,*]

1. Key Laboratory of Parasite and Vector Biology, Ministry of Health; National Institute of Parasitic Diseases, Chinese Center for Disease Control and Prevention, Shanghai 200025, China; qinzq1008@hotmail.com (Z.-Q.Q.); xujing@nipd.chinacdc.cn (J.X.); fengting@nipd.chinacdc.cn (T.F.); lvshan@nipd.chinacdc.cn (S.L.); yjqiancn@163.com (Y.-J.Q.); zhanglj@nipd.chinacdc.cn (L.-J.Z.); liyl@nipd.chinacdc.cn (Y.-L.L.); lvchao@nipd.chinacdc.cn (C.L.); lisz@chinacdc.cn (S.-Z.L.)
2. Ingerod, SE-454 94 Brastad, Sweden; robert.bergquist@outlook.com

* Correspondence: zhouxn1@chinacdc.cn; Tel.: +86-21-6437-8058; Fax: +86-021-6433-2670

Received: 20 October 2018; Accepted: 11 December 2018; Published: 15 December 2018

Abstract: *Schistosoma* infection in snails can be monitored by microscopy or indirectly by sentinel mice. As both these approaches can miss infections, more sensitive tests are needed, particularly in low-level transmission settings. In this study, loop-mediated isothermal amplification (LAMP) technique, designed to detect a specific 28S ribosomal *Schistosoma japonicum* (Sj28S) gene with high sensitivity, was compared to microscopy using snail samples from 51 areas endemic for schistosomiasis in five Chinese provinces. In addition, the results were compared with those from polymerase chain reaction (PCR) by adding DNA sequencing as a reference. The testing of pooled snail samples with the LAMP assay showed that a dilution factor of 1/50, i.e., one infected snail plus 49 non-infected ones, would still result in a positive reaction after the recommended number of amplification cycles. Testing a total of 232 pooled samples, emanating from 4006 snail specimens, showed a rate of infection of 6.5%, while traditional microscopy found only 0.4% positive samples in the same materials. Parallel PCR analysis confirmed the diagnostic accuracy of the LAMP assay, with DNA sequencing even giving LAMP a slight lead. Microscopy and the LAMP test were carried out at local schistosomiasis-control stations, demonstrating that the potential of the latter assay to serve as a point-of-care (POC) test with results available within 60–90 min, while the more complicated PCR test had to be carried out at the National Institute of Parasitic Diseases (NIPD) in Shanghai, China. In conclusion, LAMP was found to be clearly superior to microscopy and as good as, or better than, PCR. As it can be used under field conditions and requires less time than other techniques, LAMP testing would improve and accelerate schistosomiasis control.

Keywords: *Schistosoma japonicum*; *Oncomelania hupensis*; snail; 28S ribosomal DNA; PCR; loop-mediated isothermal amplification (LAMP); pooled samples; China

1. Introduction

Schistosomiasis, one of the neglected tropical diseases (NTDs), is a public health problem caused by one of six species of the *Schistosoma* parasite that affects >200 million people in Africa, South America and Southeast Asia. However, the prevalence of schistosomiasis, based on stool examination and urine filtration, strongly understates the presumed real figure, as indicated by more sensitive techniques [1,2]. In China, the Philippines and three small pockets of the Indonesian island Sulawesi, the disease is a zoonosis caused by *Schistosoma japonicum* [1–3]. In China, the required intermediate snail host, *Oncomelania hupensis*, is widely distributed in the country's endemic areas, ranging from the Yangtze River Valley and the southern plains, to the mountainous regions of Sichuan and Yunnan in the west [4]. In 2004, a new integrated control strategy was introduced [5,6] involving reduction of infection sources by fencing off transmission sites, the replacement of water buffaloes (an important reservoir) with tractors for agricultural work and improved sanitation via access to clean water and latrines. These approaches have markedly reduced the infection rate in humans, domestic animals and the intermediate snail host [7]. The changes accomplished are so profound that it has become difficult to monitor the remaining transmission sites by only testing humans and domestic animals [8]. Conversely, snail diagnosis by microscopy or the use of the sentinel mice approach [9] are not only labor-intensive and time-consuming, but are also not sufficiently sensitive. To sustain the success achieved with regard to schistosomiasis elimination in China, highly sensitive snail-monitoring systems capable of assessing residual transmission in real time are now needed.

Due to its high sensitivity, molecular diagnosis has emerged as a promising approach for the detection of a suspected, low-level presence of pathogens [10–13]. However, a lack of the resources essential for this kind of diagnostics—such as bio-safety cabinets, a stable supply of electricity and well-experienced technicians, which are rare in peripheral laboratories in developing countries—limits the implementation of sophisticated technology.

The loop-mediated isothermal amplification (LAMP) technology employs a polymerase that amplifies the target DNA gene sequence with high specificity and rapidity under isothermal conditions [14]. Hamburger and colleagues investigated the use of this technique for the detection of infections due to *S. mansoni* and *S. haematobium*, showing excellent results, not only confirming that the LAMP technique works in the laboratory, but also in the field in Africa [15]. The usefulness and high sensitivity of LAMP-assisted snail diagnosis was later confirmed in Brazil by Gandasegui et al. [16] and in China by Kumagai et al. [17]. The latter research group developed a diagnostic platform based on a target 28S ribosomal DNA (rDNA) specific for *S. japonicum* (not reacting with *S. mansoni*) and showed that snails experimentally infected with only one miracidium could be detected less than 24 h after infection. As part of this study, we explored the application of LAMP using pooled snail samples, i.e., instead of testing each snail separately, we combined snails, however never in numbers exceeding 50 snails per pooled sample, based on preliminary dilution tests (see Results). The protocol used was derived from a visual LAMP-detection method developed by Tomita et al. [18], where the amplification of the pyrophosphate ion by-product combines with a divalent metal ion to form an insoluble salt. Adding calcein, a bivalent fluorescein/manganese complex, to the reaction solution results in a strong fluorescent signal from positive reactions, enabling visual discrimination by the naked eye without specialized equipment. We compared the results of the LAMP assay with the outcome using a polymerase chain reaction (PCR), applying DNA sequencing to determine the identity of the amplified product.

The purpose of the present study was not only to confirm the sensitivity of the LAMP method when used for the detection of *S. japonicum* DNA in infected snails in known endemic settings, but also to investigate and validate its application under field conditions soon after snail collection. An added aim was to determine if the LAMP procedure could be speeded up by testing pooled DNA samples in place of testing the snails individually.

2. Materials and Methods

This study constitutes an evaluation of LAMP-based snail diagnosis with the eventual aim of being part of a platform integrating different kinds of data and, thereby, enabling improved surveillance of schistosomiasis transmission. *O. hupensis* snails were collected during the spring over a period of three years (2013–2015) from all endemic regions in China, covering five provinces. The LAMP approach used is shown schematically in the form of a flow chart (Figure 1). As we were interested to see if the field work could be accelerated by testing samples consisting of pooled snails, DNA from various numbers of snails was investigated before the main study was undertaken.

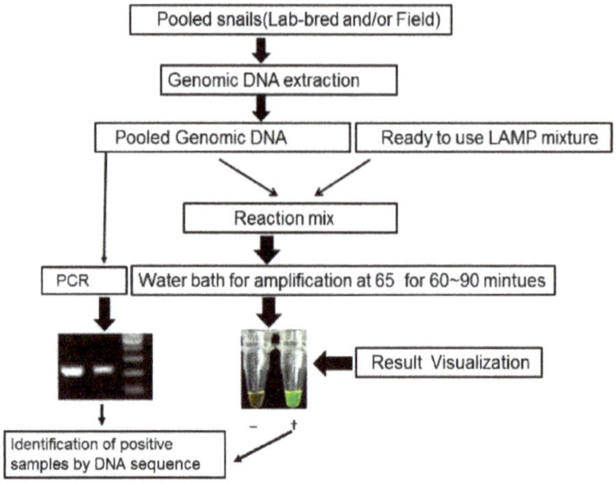

Figure 1. Flow chart of loop-mediated isothermal amplification (LAMP) and PCR for detecting *S. japonicum*-infected snails.

2.1. Ethical Statement

Although this study did not include human sera or experimental animal data, an ethical statement is required to initiate any research project. Thus, we hereby state that all procedures performed within this study were conducted following animal husbandry guidelines of the Chinese Academy of Medical Sciences and with permission from the Experimental Animal Committee (National Institute of Parasitic Diseases (NIPD), Chinese Center for Diseases Control and Prevention, (China CDC) with ethical clearance number IPD-2012-5.

2.2. Snail Sampling Procedure

O. hupensis snails were collected from areas with known human schistosomiasis infection rates varying between 0.9% and 2.8% [19]. We used snails collected in April/May each year from 51 villages in 15 counties in Hunan, Hubei, Jiangxi, Anhui and Yunnan provinces. Most collection spots were in marshlands, except in Yunnan Province, where the snails were found in irrigation and drainage ditches. Systematic sampling was applied for snail investigation using survey frames of 250 m^2 in the marshlands and smaller areas spaced 50 m apart along the ditches [20,21]. All live snails found, together numbering 4006 specimens, were kept and transferred to the laboratory for testing.

2.3. Microscopy Testing and DNA Extraction

After having been crushed by pressure between clean glass plates and the pieces of shell removed, the snails were examined individually under the microscope at low magnification (generally 10×) to certify whether cercariae and/or sporocysts were present. After microscopy testing, 232 pooled snail samples from the 4006 single snails, were collected for further genomic DNA extraction. The snail soft tissues were pooled in clean 2.0 or 10.0 mL tubes (not exceeding 50 snail bodies in each) with 400–1000 μL of DNA lysis buffer (Qiagen, Valencia, CA, USA) added into each tube and the tissue collections homogenized. Subsequently, 20–50 μL of ProteinK (Qiagen, Valencia, CA, USA) was added to the snail homogenates with the tubes kept in a water bath at 56 °C, for 2–3 h, after which the supernatant of snail homogenates was saved and passed through a DNA binding column (Qiagen, Valencia, CA, USA). Finally, the dedicated DNA binding column was washed by the washing buffer

(Qiagen, Valencia, CA, USA) and the genomic DNA recovered by eluting the DNA-binding column with nuclease-free water. The recovered DNA samples were used for further testing by the LAMP assay and conventional PCR.

2.4. PCR Assay

A conventional PCR assay (PCR kit purchased from Takara Biotech, Dalian, China) was carried out in parallel with the LAMP assay (see below). Paired primer strands, i.e., 5′-GGTTTGACTATTAT TGTTGAGC-3′ and 5′-CTCACCTTAGTTCGGACTGA-3′ targeting the *S. japonicum* 28S (Sj28S) rDNA (Accession:EU835689.1) were used [17]. The ingredients were 1 μL of each primer (10 pmol/L each), 3 μL DNA template, 0.2 mM deoxynucleotide (dNTP) solution, 1.25 units of highly thermostable DNA polymerase from the thermophilic bacterium *Thermus aquaticus* (Taq DNA) and 2.5 μL 10× buffer (pH 8.8 Tris-HCl, KCl and $MgCl_2$). The initial activation (cycle 1) was set for 3 min at 94 °C followed by 33 cycles of 30 s at 94 °C, 56 °C for 50 s and 72 °C for 1 min. The final extension step was carried out for 7 min at 72 °C. The amplified product was visualized by agarose gel electrophoresis (1.5%) with ethidium bromide staining.

2.5. DNA Sequencing

In order to make sure that the PCR product of all 14 positive samples exactly matched the target sequence, the 330 bp band of each PCR product was separated by gel electrophoresis, cloned into the Pmd19-T vector (Takara Biotech, Dalian, China), transferred into *E. coli* cells, strain DH5α, and then cultured in Luria-Bertani (LB) medium with ampicillin (100 μg/mL) at 37 °C in a 5.0 mL tube. After 12–16 h of culture, plasmid DNA was extracted from the bacterial colonies using a DNA extraction kit. The purified plasmid DNA was sent to a commercial company (Sangon Biotech, Co., Ltd., Shanghai, China) for sequence analysis, confirming the sample to be a complete match to Sj28S rDNA when compared with the National Center for Biotechnology Information (NCBI) database. One sample found to be positive by LAMP but negative by PCR, was subjected to an additional agarose gel analysis, thus we isolated the target band and sent the purified product for DNA sequence analysis to Sangon Biotech.

2.6. LAMP Assay

(A) Reagent stock solution set-up and primer sequence

a. The 2× reaction mixture: pH 8.8 Tris buffer (40 mM), KCl (20 M), $MgSO_4$ (16 mM), $(NH_4)_2SO_4$ (20 mM), Tween 20 (0.2%), betaine (1.6 M), dNTPs (2.8 mM each).
b. Calcein working solution (2 × composition): Calcein (50 μM), $MnCl_2$ (1 mM).
c. Sj28S gene primers [17], (5′-3′, Sangon; HPLC purification): F3 (GCTTTGTCCTTCGGG CATTA), B3 (GGTTTCGTAACGCCCAATGA), FIP (ACGCAACTGCCAACGTGACATACT GGTCGGCTTGTTACTAGC), BIP (TGGTAGACGATCCACCTGACCCCTCGCGCACATGT TAAACTC)

(B) Amplification (60–90 min)

We produced a reaction mixture of 7.5 μL nuclease-free water, 12.5 μL of 2× reaction buffer, 1.0 μL of 25× primer mixture, 1.0 μL (8 μ/μL) of Bst, a *Bacillus stearothermophilus* DNA polymerase homologue used for DNA strand displacement and 1.0 μL calcein. We used 0.2 mL reaction tubes dispensing 23 μL of the reaction mixture together with 2.0 μL of the sample to be tested into each tube. In addition, 23 μL of the reaction mixture was added to the Sj28S rDNA target in a second tube (the positive control) and also to the nuclease-free water in second tube (the negative control). All reaction tubes were incubated at 65 °C for 60~90 min, followed by the inactivation of the enzyme by the incubation of the tubes at 85 °C for 5 min. The tubes were then observed by the unaided eye to observe the color of the reaction changing from orange to yellow-green in the presence of LAMP (see Results).

2.6.1. Testing Samples with Life Cycle Stages of *S. japonicum*

Laboratory-bred *O. hupensis* snails were challenged with *S. japonicum* miracidia and the next life cycle stages of *S. japonicum* were thus transferred to the *O. hupensis* snails. To confirm whether DNA from different developing stage of *S. japonicum* could be detected by the LAMP assay, we performed the test with DNA collected from a mother sporocyst, a daughter sporocyst and a mature cercaria from these laboratory-based snails (infected and non-infected). Furthermore, to study whether DNA from other *Schistosoma* species would cross-react in the LAMP assay *Trichobilharzia* cercariae, emanating from a common bird-specific *Schistosoma* species, was also subjected to testing using the same procedure as described above under 2.5 and 2.6.

2.6.2. Pooled Snail Samples

To evaluate the detection limit of the LAMP method before the main study, we performed a preliminary test in which one schistosome-positive snail was mixed with different numbers of schistosome-negative snails at the following ratios: 1/4, 1/9, 1/19, 1/49, 1/99 and 1/199. For practical reasons, each snail pool in the main study came from the same area (though the different pools investigated contained different sets of snails). Depending on availability, the number of snails in the pools could not be standardized but it was always kept at $\leq$50. The result of this exercise was 232 snail pools made out of the total number of snails collected (4006). Depending on how many snails were pooled, the pools were kept in 2.0 mL or 10 mL centrifuge tubes together with 400 µL or 1.0 mL, of a lysis buffer from a DNeasy blood and tissue kit, (Qiagen, Valencia, CA, USA).

2.7. *Validation*

To assess the quality of the LAMP assay, a panel of nucleic acid extracts and test kits were dispatched to 28 separate testing health agency laboratories in the endemic areas at the provincial and county levels, where laboratory personnel were well-trained to operate the LAMP assay. Each nucleic acid sample was thawed, divided into 100 µL aliquots, coded and refrozen. The next day, all samples were packaged and sent by overnight shipment to the 28 separate laboratories. Each laboratory tested each sample 5 times using a standard LAMP protocol provided by National Institute of Parasitic Diseases (NIPD) at China CDC, based in Shanghai. The samples were validated against the true results, kept at the NIPD, which were unknown to the staff carrying out the testing in the health agency laboratories. The outcomes were scored according to a 0–100 scale, where 5 equal results were given a score of 100, 4 equal results were given a score of 80, and so on. To make sure that the LAMP test had the required specificity, it was applied (in parallel with the PCR assay) to 20 pools produced from a total of 1000 individual snails that had previously also been investigated by microscopy.

3. Results

As seen in Figure 2, the preliminary test of the snail pools in different ratios showed that large-scale testing could be carried out based on 50 snails without the risk of missing a positive result.

The ready-to-use LAMP test kit evaluated here detected 7.5 times more infected snails than microscopy, while the PCR results were consistent with those of the LAMP assay, except with respect to a single snail pool that was found to be positive by LAMP and negative by PCR. Out of the 232 pooled snail samples tested, 217 were found to be negative and 14 positive by both assays (Table 1), while the remaining single sample, found positive by LAMP but negative by PCR, was found to be positive by DNA sequence analysis, underlining LAMP's superiority. As can be seen in Table 2, none of the diagnostic approaches produced false positive results when applied to snail samples from non-endemic areas. The results further demonstrated that the schistosome DNA included in a single miracidium is sufficient to be amplified by the LAMP assay, making it possible to detect the schistosome infection already at the sporocyst stages in the snail, as well as when mature cercariae are ready for release.

The *Trichobilharzia* cercariae used to test the specificity were negative, confirming the specificity of the test (Figure 3).

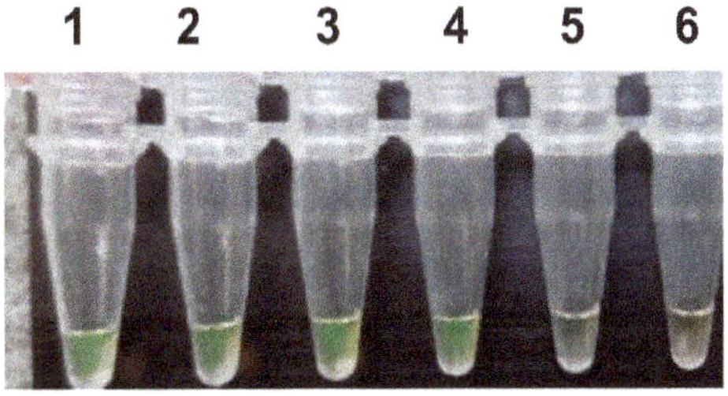

Figure 2. Investigation of the LAMP diagnostic capability by testing serial dilutions of the Sj28S gene component. The following dilutions of infected and uninfected snails are shown: 1/4 (tube no. 1); 1/9 (tube no. 2); 1/19 (tube no. 3); 1/49 (tube no. 4); 1/99 (tube no. 5) and 1/199 (tube no. 6).

Table 1. Comparison between microscopy, LAMP and PCR in screening snail samples.

Province	No. of Counties Included	No. of Villages Included	No. of Snails Tested	No. of Pooled Samples	Microscopy		LAMP		PCR	
					Pos. *	%	Pos. *	%	Pos. *	%
Hubei	2	5	599	38	1	0.5	3	7. 9	3	7.9
Hunan	2	6	716	80	0	0	2	2.5	2	2.5
Jiangxi	6	25	1183	34	0	0	5	14.7	4	11.8
Anhui	2	6	698	43	0	0	1	2.3	1	2.3
Yunnan	3	9	810	37	0	0	4	10.8	4	10.8
Total	**15**	**51**	**4006**	**232**	**1**	**0.4**	**15**	**6.5**	**14**	**6.0**

* Positive.

Table 2. Screening snail samples in three non-endemic areas: comparison between microscopy, LAMP and PCR.

Province	No. of Counties Included	No. of Villages Included	No. of Snails Tested	No. of Pooled Samples	Microscopy		LAMP		PCR	
					Pos. *	%	Pos. *	%	Pos. *	%
Shanghai	2	2	200	4	0	0	0	0	0	0
Zhejiang	2	2	500	10	0	0	0	0	0	0
Guangxi	2	2	300	6	0	0	0	0	0	0
Total	**6**	**6**	**1000**	**20**	**0**	**0**	**0**	**0**	**0**	**0**

* Positive.

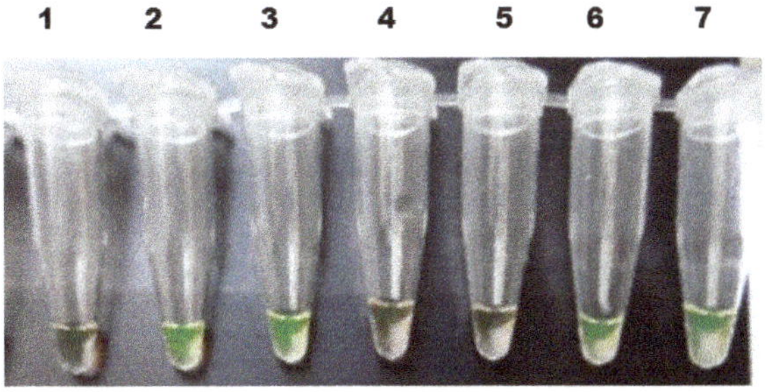

Figure 3. Detection of the Sj28S gene component in the different parasite developmental stages of *S. japonicum* in *O. hupensis* by the LAMP method. 1. Negative control (nuclease-free water); 2. Positive control (Sj28 plasmid DNA); 3. Cercariae; 4. Specificity control (*Trichobilharzia* cercariae); 5. Negative control (pooled snail DNA from a non-endemic area); 6. Mother sporocyst; 7. Daughter sporocyst.

The 28 different laboratories at the provincial and county health agency levels, belonging to the inter-laboratory panel, demonstrated an almost total agreement with respect to the results over the three reported years. Only four laboratories showed slightly lower scores, one with a score of 80 in

2013, two with a score of 60 in 2014, and one with a score of 80 in 2014 and a score of 90 in 2015 (Table 3). Importantly, with the exception of one laboratory, those with scores lower than 100 in one year did not have the same score in other years.

Table 3. Inter-laboratory comparison using LAMP for the detection of intermediate snail hosts infected by *S. japonicum*.

Province	Laboratory	Score 2013	Score 2014	Score 2015
Hunan	IPD	100	100	100
	Hanshou	-	100	100
	Yuanjiang	-	100	100
	Yueyang	-	100	100
Hubei	CDC	100	100	100
	Gongan	-	100	100
	Hanchuan	-	100	100
	Jiangling	-	100	100
Anhui	IPD	100	100	100
	Wuhu	-	100	100
	Anqin	-	100	100
	Guichi	-	100	100
Jiangxi	IPD	100	100	100
	Poyang	-	60	100
	Duchang	-	60	100
Jiangsu	IPD	100	100	100
	Qixia	-	100	100
Sichuan	CDC	100	100	100
	Renshou	-	100	100
	Guanghan	-	100	100
Yunnan	CDC	100	100	100
	Dali	-	80	90
	Eryuan	-	100	100
Shanghai	CDC	100	100	100
Guangdong	CDC	100	100	100
Fujian	CDC	100	100	100
Zhejiang	IPD	100	100	100
Guangxi	CDC	80	100	100

CDC = Center for Disease Control and Prevention; IPD= Provincial Institute of Parasitic Diseases; Scores are the levels of agreement between five tests. The number of samples from 2013 was not sufficient to be tested in all laboratories (signified with a dash in the table).

4. Discussion

Estimates of the prevalence of *S. japonicum* infection in its obligatory vector snail can be used as a proxy for areas at risk of schistosomiasis. As already pointed out by Hamburger et al. [12] and reiterated by Abbasi et al. [13], the snail infection rate provides a measure of the transmission from humans (and other definitive reservoir hosts) to the snail and can, therefore, serve as a marker of residual infection in an area. However, traditional snail diagnosis depends on the labor-intensive, time-consuming individual dissection of thousands of collected snails from the field and the results are not sufficiently sensitive to support this statement, but with the advent of molecular diagnostics this has changed. The successful use of the LAMP technique shown here promises to revolutionize snail surveillance, not only in the laboratory but also in field [13–17]. The reported results are timely, as the use of snail control as a complementary approach along with chemotherapy is again being proposed as a potentially necessary means to achieve the elimination of schistosomiasis [22].

PCR-based assays have been around since the mid-1970s [10], but were not used for schistosomiasis diagnosis until the end of the 1990s and the early 2000s, first for snails [12] and later also for human infections [23,24]. However, the instability and variability inherent in enzymatic processes, as well as the need for advanced equipment, limit PCR applications in the field. In this regard, the LAMP approach is superior, as it can be adapted for application in field laboratories [25] by using ready-mixed reagents suitable for shipment at ambient temperature, together with sample storage under minimal refrigeration [13–16]. The development of a surveillance platform based on molecular diagnostic techniques and characterized by simplicity and reliability, yet with high throughput, requires an approach that is adaptable to county-level laboratories with limited resources. The manganese/calcein method of Tomita et al. [18] is an important contribution in this regard as it enables the recognition of small quantities of DNA by means of a fluorescent signal emitted from the sample solution after amplification, and has been successfully used in China by Kumagai et al. [17]. Other attempts to increase readability and sensitivity include the use of various dyes, e.g., SYBR green (Singh et al., 2017) or hydroxyl napthol blue (Ali et al., 2017) which have also produced good results [26,27]. Dyes have the advantage of being independent of refrigeration.

Any increase of the dilution factor would considerably accelerate the area needed to be tested. We found a dilution ratio of 1/50 to be useful (Figure 2), but if the number of infected snails decreases, as it is supposed to do with the elimination program in force, the risk of mistakenly declaring an area free of transmission increases if the snail pool contains too few snails. This could be counteracted by using a higher number of snails in the pool and increasing the time of amplification for the test, however, the risk for false positives would then rise.

The strength of the present study is not only that it further improves the potential of the LAMP test that has already proved successful for snail diagnosis [16,17], but also that it targets a gene specific for *S. japonicum* and provides validation leading to the reliable use of the pooled-snail approach piloted by Hamburger et al. for *S. mansoni* [15] and Tong et al. for *S. japonicum* [20]. A further advantage of the LAMP technique is that although it is highly technical, it is easy to perform in basic laboratory settings common in rural areas. It is also easy to learn, as shown by the excellent agreement over three years in the many places included in this study. In addition, while sporocysts and parasite germ balls are easily missed by traditional microscopic methods, the snails containing mother or daughter sporocysts were both positive the day after infection. Therefore, the LAMP assay is an appropriate method for the detection of pre-patent infections. As seen in Table 1, the outcome of testing with PCR and the LAMP approach largely agreed, indicating that the sensitivity of the two techniques is the same in practice. However, theoretically the latter has an advantage since the one sample reacting negatively by PCR was positive when tested with the LAMP test. Comparison with microscopy, on the other hand, clearly showed that molecular testing is superior and should be used in the future. The excellent agreement between all 28 field laboratories (Table 3) shows that we are now ready to change from microscopy to molecular testing, preferably using LAMP, as it lends itself to use in the field. It is suggested that this kind of snail testing be included together with the diagnostic testing of humans and domestic animals in a joint surveillance and response platform based on only high-resolution techniques.

The risk of schistosomiasis still exists in China and snail control remains a significant challenge in the field [28]. In the present study, the LAMP results indicate that Hunan, Hubei, Jiangxi, Anhui, and Yunnan Provinces contain infected snails, underlining the risk of schistosomiasis transmission. The results can be used to guide further local investigations and snail control activities.

5. Conclusions

The LAMP platform is an effective method for monitoring snails in endemic field sites. Despite expensive reagents and the risk of contamination that requires specific training of the staff in charge, we recommend that the LAMP-based test replace microscopy for snail diagnosis due to its greater accuracy and reduced delay in delivering results.

Author Contributions: S.-Z.L. and X-N.Z. conceived and designed the project, and supervised the study. Z.-Q.Q. performed most of the experiments and analyzed the data and wrote the original draft. J.X. helped analyze the data, R.B. helped organize and write the article. T.F., C.L., Y.-L.L. and Y.-J.Q. helped with DNA extraction, PCR and LAMP experiments. S.L. and L.-J.Z. helped with snail samples collection in field. All authors reviewed and approved the manuscript.

Funding: This work was Sponsored by National Major Special Science and Technology Project of China (No. 2016ZX10004222), and a Research Project of Shanghai Municipal Health Bureau (No. 201440498).

Conflicts of Interest: The authors declare no competing financial interests.

References

1. McManus, D.P.; Dunne, D.W.; Sacko, M.; Utzinger, J.; Vennervald, B.J.; Zhou, X.N. Schistosomiasis. *Nat. Rev. Dis. Primers* **2018**, *4*, 13. [CrossRef]
2. Assaré, R.K.; Tra, M.B.I.; Ouattara, M.; Hürlimann, E.; Coulibaly, J.T.; N'Goran, E.K.; Utzinger, J. Sensitivity of the point-of-care circulating cathodic antigen urine cassette test for diagnosis of *Schistosoma mansoni* in low-endemicity settings in Côte d'Ivoire. *Am. J. Trop. Med. Hyg.* **2018**. [CrossRef]
3. Hadidjaja, P. Clinical study of Indonesian schistosomiasis at Lindu lake area, Central Sulawesi. *Southeast Asian J. Trop. Med. Public Health* **1984**, *15*, 507–514. [PubMed]
4. Zhu, G.; Fan, J.; Peterson, A.T. *Schistosoma japonicum* transmission risk maps at present and under climate change in mainland China. *PLoS Negl. Trop. Dis.* **2017**, *11*, e0006021. [CrossRef] [PubMed]
5. Wang, L.D.; Chen, H.G.; Guo, J.G.; Zeng, X.J.; Hong, X.L.; Xiong, J.J.; Wu, X.H.; Wang, X.H.; Wang, L.Y.; Xia, G.; et al. A strategy to control transmission of *Schistosoma japonicum* in China. *N. Engl. J. Med.* **2009**, *360*, 121–128. [CrossRef] [PubMed]
6. Wang, L.D.; Guo, J.G.; Wu, X.H.; Chen, H.G.; Wang, T.P.; Zhu, S.P.; Zhang, Z.H.; Steinmann, P.; Yang, G.J.; Wang, S.P.; et al. China's new strategy to block *Schistosoma japonicum* transmission: Experiences and impact beyond schistosomiasis. *Trop. Med. Int. Health* **2009**, *14*, 1475–1483. [CrossRef] [PubMed]
7. Sun, L.P.; Wang, W.; Hong, Q.B.; Li, S.Z.; Liang, Y.S.; Yang, H.T.; Zhou, X.N. Approaches being used in the national schistosomiasis elimination programme in China: A review. *Infect. Dis. Poverty* **2017**, *6*, 55. [CrossRef]
8. Spear, R.C.; Seto, E.Y.; Carlton, E.J.; Liang, S.; Remais, J.V.; Zhong, B.; Qiu, D. The challenge of effective surveillance in moving from low transmission to elimination of schistosomiasis in China. *Int. J. Parasitol.* **2011**, *41*, 1243–1247. [CrossRef]
9. Yang, K.; Sun, L.P.; Liang, Y.S.; Wu, F.; Li, W.; Zhang, J.F.; Huang, Y.X.; Hang, D.R.; Liang, S.; Bergquist, R.; et al. *Schistosoma japonicum* risk in Jiangsu province, People's Republic of China: Identification of a spatio-temporal risk pattern along the Yangtze River. *Geospat. Health* **2013**, *8*, 133–142. [CrossRef]
10. Erlich, H.A. Polymerase chain reaction. *J. Clin. Immunol.* **1989**, *9*, 437–447. [CrossRef]
11. Notomi, T.; Okayama, H.; Masubuchi, H.; Yonekawa, T.; Watanabe, K.; Amino, N.; Hase, T. Loop-mediated isothermal amplification of DNA. *Nucleic Acids Res.* **2000**, *28*, E63. [CrossRef] [PubMed]
12. Hamburger, J.; He-Na; Xin, X.Y.; Ramzy, R.M.; Jourdane, J.; Ruppel, A. A polymerase chain reaction assay for detecting snails infected with bilharzia parasites (*Schistosoma mansoni*) from very early prepatency. *Am. J. Trop. Med. Hyg.* **1998**, *59*, 872–876. [CrossRef] [PubMed]
13. Abbasi, I.; King, C.H.; Muchiri, E.M.; Hamburger, J. Detection of *Schistosoma mansoni* and *Schistosoma haematobium* DNA by loop-mediated isothermal amplification: Identification of infected snails from early prepatency. *Am. J. Trop. Med. Hyg.* **2010**, *83*, 427–432. [CrossRef] [PubMed]
14. Notomi, T.; Mori, Y.; Tomita, N.; Kanda, H. Loop-mediated isothermal amplification (LAMP): Principle, features, and future prospects. *J. Microbiol.* **2015**, *53*, 1–5. [CrossRef] [PubMed]
15. Hamburger, J.; Abbasi, I.; Kariuki, C.; Wanjala, A.; Mzungu, E.; Mungai, P.; Muchiri, E.; King, C.H. Evaluation of loop-mediated isothermal amplification suitable for molecular monitoring of schistosome-infected snails in field laboratories. *Am. J. Trop. Med. Hyg.* **2013**, *88*, 344–351. [CrossRef]
16. Gandasegui, J.; Fernández-Soto, P.; Muro, A.; Simões Barbosa, C.; Lopes de Melo, F.; Loyo, R.; de Souza Gomes, E.C. A field survey using LAMP assay for detection of *Schistosoma mansoni* in a low-transmission area of schistosomiasis in Umbuzeiro, Brazil: Assessment in human and snail samples. *PLoS Negl. Trop. Dis.* **2018**, *12*, e0006314. [CrossRef] [PubMed]

17. Kumagai, T.; Furushima-Shimogawara, R.; Ohmae, H.; Wang, T.P.; Lu, S.; Chen, R.; Wen, L.; Ohta, N. Detection of early and single infections of *Schistosoma japonicum* in the intermediate host snail, *Oncomelania hupensis*, by PCR and loop-mediated isothermal amplification (LAMP) assay. *Am. J. Trop. Med. Hyg.* **2010**, *83*, 542–548. [CrossRef]
18. Tomita, N.; Mori, Y.; Kanda, H.; Notomi, T. Loop-mediated isothermal amplification (LAMP) of gene sequences and simple visual detection of products. *Nat. Protoc.* **2008**, *3*, 877–882. [CrossRef]
19. Lei, Z.L.; Zhang, L.J.; Xu, Z.M.; Dang, H.; Xu, J.; Lv, S.; Cao, C.L.; Li, S.Z.; Zhou, X.N. Endemic status of schistosomiasis in People's Republic of China in 2014. *Zhongguo Xue Xi Chong Bing Fang Zhi Za Zhi* **2015**, *27*, 563–569. (In Chinese)
20. Tong, Q.B.; Chen, R.; Zhang, Y.; Yang, G.J.; Kumagai, T.; Furushima-Shimogawara, R.; Lou, D.; Yang, K.; Wen, L.Y.; Lu, S.H.; et al. A new surveillance and response tool: Risk map of infected *Oncomelania hupensis* detected by loop-mediated isothermal amplification (LAMP) from pooled samples. *Acta Trop.* **2015**, *141 Pt B*, 170–177. [CrossRef]
21. Xun-Ping, W.; An, Z. Study of spatial stratified sampling strategy of *Oncomelania hupensis* snail survey based on plant abundance. *Zhongguo Xue Xi Chong Bing Fang Zhi Za Zhi* **2017**, *29*, 420–425. (In Chinese) [PubMed]
22. Lo, N.C.; Gurarie, D.; Yoon, N.; Coulibaly, J.T.; Bendavid, E.; Andrews, J.R.; King, C.H. Impact and cost-effectiveness of snail control to achieve disease control targets for schistosomiasis. *Proc. Natl. Acad. Sci. USA* **2018**, *115*, E584–E591. [CrossRef] [PubMed]
23. Pontes, L.A.; Dias-Neto, E.; Rabello, A. Detection by polymerase chain reaction of *Schistosoma mansoni* DNA in human serum and feces. *Am. J. Trop. Med. Hyg.* **2002**, *66*, 157–162. [CrossRef] [PubMed]
24. He, P.; Gordon, C.A.; Williams, G.M.; Li, Y.; Wang, Y.; Hu, J.; Gray, D.J.; Ross, A.G.; Harn, D.; McManus, D.P. Real-time PCR diagnosis of *Schistosoma japonicum* in low transmission areas of China. *Infect. Dis. Poverty* **2018**, *7*, 8. [CrossRef] [PubMed]
25. Wilisiani, F.; Tomiyama, A.; Katoh, H.; Hartono, S.; Neriya, Y.; Nishigawa, H.; Natsuaki, T. Development of a LAMP assay with a portable device for real-time detection of begomoviruses under field conditions. *J. Virol. Methods* **2018**. [CrossRef] [PubMed]
26. Singh, R.; Singh, D.P.; Savargaonkar, D.; Singh, O.P.; Bhatt, R.M.; Valecha, N. Evaluation of SYBR green I based visual loop-mediated isothermal amplification (LAMP) assay for genus and species-specific diagnosis of malaria in *P. vivax* and *P. falciparum* endemic regions. *J. Vector Borne Dis.* **2017**, *54*, 54–60. [PubMed]
27. Ali, S.A.; Kaur, G.; Boby, N.; Sabarinath, T.; Solanki, K.; Pal, D.; Chaudhuri, P. Rapid and visual detection of leptospira in urine by LigB-LAMP assay with pre-addition of dye. *Mol. Cell. Probes* **2017**, *36*, 29–35. [CrossRef]
28. Yang, Y.; Zheng, S.B.; Yang, Y.; Cheng, W.T.; Pan, X.; Dai, Q.Q.; Chen, Y.; Zhu, L.; Jiang, Q.W.; Zhou, Y.B. The Three Gorges Dam: Does the flooding time determine the distribution of schistosome-transmitting snails in the middle and lower reaches of the Yangtze River, China? *Int. J. Environ. Res. Public Health* **2018**, *15*, 1304. [CrossRef]

Tropical Medicine and Infectious Disease

MDPI

Article

Phylogeography of *Bulinus truncatus* (Audouin, 1827) (Gastropoda: Planorbidae) in Selected African Countries

Eniola M. Abe [1,*], Yun-Hai Guo [1], Haimo Shen [1], Masceline J. Mutsaka-Makuvaza [2], Mohamed R. Habib [3], Jing-Bo Xue [1], Nicholas Midzi [2], Jing Xu [1], Shi-Zhu Li [1] and Xiao-Nong Zhou [1,*]

1 National Institute of Parasitic Diseases (NIPD), Chinese Centre for Disease Control and Prevention, Shanghai 200025, China; guoyunhaigy@163.com (Y.G.); shenhm@nipd.chinacdc.cn (H.S.); xuejb@nipd.chinacdc.cn (J.-B.X.); xujing@nipd.chinacdc.cn (J.X.); lisz@chinacdc.cn (S.-Z.L.)

2 Department of Medical Microbiology, College of Health Sciences, University of Zimbabwe, Harare 00263, Zimbabwe; mascelinejeni@gmail.com (M.M.-M.); midzinicholas@gmail.com (N.M.)

3 Medical Malacology Laboratory, Theodor Bilharz Research Institute, Giza 12411, Egypt; m_ramadanhabib@yahoo.com

* Correspondence: abeeniola11@126.com (E.M.A.); zhouxn1@chinacdc.cn (X.-N.Z.); Tel.: +86-21-6437-8058 (X.-N.Z.); Fax: +86-021-6433-2670 (X.-N.Z.)

Received: 27 September 2018; Accepted: 13 December 2018; Published: 19 December 2018

Abstract: The transmission of some schistosome parasites is dependent on the planorbid snail hosts. *Bulinus truncatus* is important in urinary schistosomiasis epidemiology in Africa. Hence, there is a need to define the snails' phylogeography. This study assessed the population genetic structure of *B. truncatus* from Giza and Sharkia (Egypt), Barakat (Sudan) and Madziwa, Shamva District (Zimbabwe) using mitochondrial cytochrome oxidase subunit 1 gene (COI) and internal transcribed spacer 1 (ITS 1) markers. COI was sequenced from 94 *B. truncatus* samples including 38 (Egypt), 36 (Sudan) and 20 (Zimbabwe). However, only 51 ITS 1 sequences were identified from Egypt (28) and Sudan (23) (because of failure in either amplification or sequencing). The unique COI haplotypes of *B. truncatus* sequences observed were 6, 11, and 6 for Egypt, Sudan, and Zimbabwe, respectively. Also, 3 and 2 unique ITS 1 haplotypes were observed in sequences from Egypt and Sudan respectively. Mitochondrial DNA sequences from Sudan and Zimbabwe indicated high haplotype diversity with 0.768 and 0.784, respectively, while relatively low haplotype diversity was also observed for sequences from Egypt (0.334). The location of populations from Egypt and Sudan on the *B. truncatus* clade agrees with the location of both countries geographically. The clustering of the Zimbabwe sequences on different locations on the clade can be attributed to individuals with different genotypes within the population. No significant variation was observed within *B. truncatus* populations from Egypt and Sudan as indicated by the ITS 1 tree. This study investigated the genetic diversity of *B. truncatus* from Giza and Sharkia (Egypt), Barakat area (Sudan), and Madziwa (Zimbabwe), which is necessary for snail host surveillance in the study areas and also provided genomic data of this important snail species from the sampled countries.

Keywords: phylogeography; *Bulinus truncatus*; planorbidae; Africa

---

1. Background

The snail intermediate hosts of the genus *Bulinus* play active roles in the epidemiology of urinary schistosomiasis. The schistosome parasites depend on these snails for the development of the asexual phase of their life cycle before the cercariae are released into the water bodies to look for unsuspecting human hosts for penetration, where they continue the sexual phase of their development [1–4].

Members of the genus *Bulinus* are hermaphroditic planorbid snails, and this genus includes 37 recognized species distributed in the tropic and sub-tropic regions of the world including Africa, Mediterranean countries, and parts of the Middle East [5]. They differ in their interaction with schistosome parasites and some are involved in the transmission of human and animal schistosomiasis [6].

These important snail species inhabit various types of freshwater bodies such as streams, ponds, rivers, and irrigation canals [7]. The genetic structure of snail hosts is mostly determined by their habitat distribution, which is largely influenced by the spatial and temporal fluctuations in water availability [8,9] leading to population bottlenecks [5].

Snails belonging to the *Bulinus* group have a great capacity to rapidly increase their population size through cross- or self-fertilization, but *B. truncatus* has a preference for self-fertilization [10]. Selfing and population bottlenecks increase genetic differentiation among snail population but reduce the amount of genetic diversity within a population [11].

Whilst morphological identification of snails helps with identifying snails at group or genus level, it cannot give further insights about their interaction with the parasites [12].

Assessment of snail hosts population structure using molecular markers and other genetic tools creates a robust system for species identification and differentiation [8,12–17]. This provides useful information about their genetic diversity and detailed elucidation of the host–parasite relationship [4], which can be applied to target effective integrated schistosomiasis control strategies in most endemic areas [18].

The use of different markers such as COI, microsatellites and ITS 1, has helped to achieve identification of *B. truncatus* sampled from few African countries including Senegal, Niger, Tanzania, Burkina Faso, and Cameroon [11,12]. Studies have also observed strong population subdivision and low diversity for hermaphroditic freshwater snails including *B. truncatus* [11,19–23].

It is, therefore, imperative to provide information on the diversity of important snail hosts including *B. truncatus* through assessing their phylogenic status in most countries endemic for schistosomiasis across Africa, to further improve our understanding about their phylogenetic relationships as well as the disease epidemiology.

This study provided information on the phylogeography of *B. truncatus* populations from Giza and Sharkia (Egypt), Barakat area (Sudan), and Madziwa, Shamva District (Zimbabwe), using partial mitochondrial DNA cytochrome oxidase subunit I (COI) and internal transcribed spacer 1 (ITS 1) to determine their phylogenetic relationship, which is important for epidemiological investigation and snail hosts surveillance.

2. Materials and Methods

2.1. Sample Collection

Bulinus snails were collected from different locations in freshwater bodies at Giza and Sharkia governorates (Egypt), Barakat area (Sudan) and Madziwa area, Shamva District (Zimbabwe). Snail sampling was done at selected sites along water bodies; these included water contact sites where people swim, carry out fishing activities, collect water for domestic purposes, bathing, and washing clothes and utensils. Sites with no apparent human water contact activities were also visited for snail collection. A total of 134 *Bulinus* snails was assessed from different locations across the three countries.

The snails were identified phenotypically using shell morphology [24]. Snails were then preserved in absolute ethanol. Information that includes snail collection and geographic coordinates of the study areas are shown in Table 1. A map of study areas is shown in Figure 1.

Table 1. Geographic coordinates of the study areas.

Country	Location	No. of Samples Collected	Time of Collection	Type of Water Body	Latitude	Longitude
Egypt	Giza (El-Nile river, Gezerite El-Warrak)	25	October, 2016	River	30.102	31.243
	Sharkia (El-Salam canal, El-Hesenia district)	30	November, 2016	Canal	31.258	32.270
Sudan	Barakat area, Wad Madani	14	July, 2016	Canal	14.33673	33.52736
	Barakat area, Wad Madani	22	August, 2016	Canal	14.31780	33.53167
	Barakat area, Wad Madani	5	August, 2016	Canal	14.29210	33.55261
	Barakat area, Wad Madani	8	August, 2016	Canal	14.25122	33.59070
Zimbabwe	Madziwa, Shamva District	11	March, 2016	River	16.93642	31.44603
	Madziwa	6	March, 2016	River	16.91498	31.42868
	Madziwa	10	June, 2016	River	16.85695	31.49413
	Madziwa	3	June, 2016	River	16.88070	31.49083

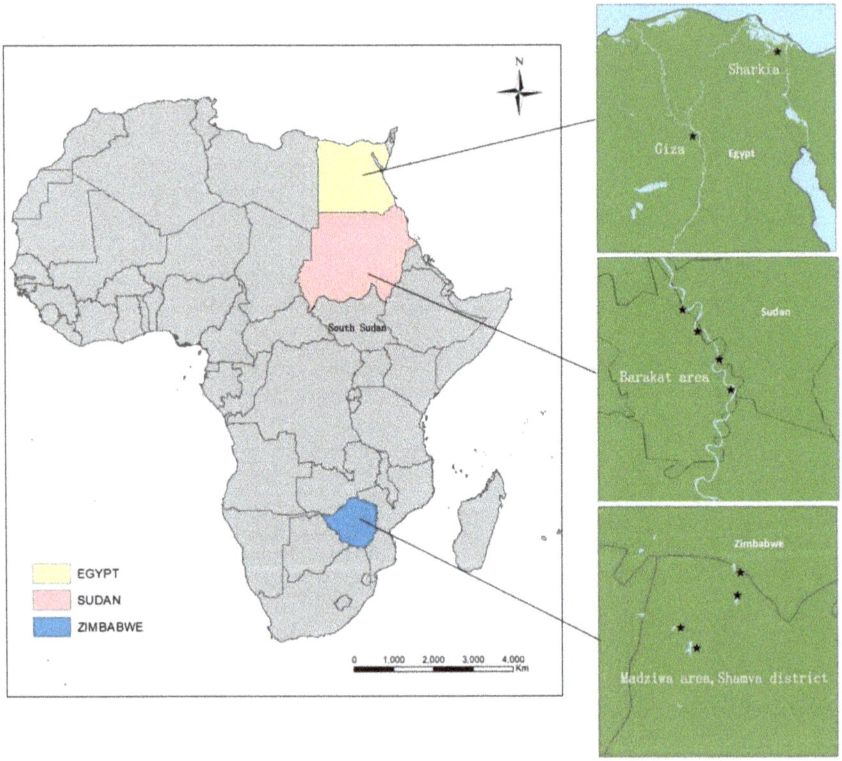

Figure 1. Map of Africa showing countries where snail samples were collected.

2.2. Sample Preparation and DNA Extraction

The specimens were recounted, identified by morphological characters, and re-spirited (absolute ethanol) upon arrival at the National Institute of Parasitic Diseases, Shanghai, schistosomiasis laboratory [25]. Specimens were placed in TE buffer (10 mM Tris, 0.1 mM EDTA) pH 7.4 for 1 h to remove the remaining alcohol from within the tissue, which might interfere with subsequent extraction techniques. Total genomic DNA was isolated from head-foot snail tissue using the DNeasy Blood and Tissue kit (Qiagen, Crawley, UK) according to the manufacturer's instructions. DNA was eluted into 200 μL AE buffer. The snails' genomic DNA concentration was quantified using the Nanodrop

ND-1000 Spectrophotometer (Nanodrop Technologies Inc., Thermo Fisher Scientific, Wilmington, DE, USA).

2.3. Polymerase Chain Reaction (PCR) Amplification of COI and ITS 1 Fragments

IllustraPuRe Taq Ready-To-Go PCR beads (GE Healthcare) were used for the amplification of the COI and ITS 1 fragments using the methods outlined in Kane et al. [12] with 0.4 μM each of Bulcox 5 (5′CCT TTA AGA GGN CCT ATT GC 3′) (forward primer) and Bulcox 14 (5′GGA AAT CAG TAM AYA AAA CCA GC 3′) (reverse primer) while ETTS10 (5′ GCA TAC TGC TTT GAA CAT CG 3′) (forward primer) and ETTS1(5′GC TTA AGT TCA GCG GGT 3′) (reverse primer) were used for *B. truncatus* amplification. A DNA template of 1 μL was added to each tube that contained 22 μL double distilled water, 1 μL each of forward and reverse primers. The total reaction volume was 25 μL. Double distilled water was used as the negative control. PCR amplification of snail genomic DNA was done using Applied Biosystems GeneAmp Thermal Cycler 2700 version 2.08. Cycling conditions for COI and ITS 1 reactions are as follows: one cycle of 95 °C for 5 min, 45 cycles of 95 °C for 30 s, 54.3 °C for 30 s, 72 °C for 45 s and 72 °C for 10 min and one cycle of 95 °C for 5 min, 45 cycles of 95 °C for 30 s, 42 °C for 30 s, 72 °C for 45 s and 72 °C for 10 min respectively. PCR fragments were separated on 1% agarose gel and visualization was performed using a gel documentation and analysis system (UVP, EpiChem II darkroom). Sequencing was performed on an Applied Biosystems 3730XL analyser (Life Technologies, Northumberland, UK).

2.4. Phylogenetic Analysis of Sequence Data

Nucleotide sequences were visually edited using Bioedit software v 7.0. [26]. BLAST searches via the National Centre for Biotechnology Information (http://www.ncbi.nlm.nih.gov/) were performed for the obtained sequences against Genbank database to ensure that contaminant sequences had not been obtained by error [27] and aligned with the reference materials [12] using the Clustal W algorithm [28]. We performed the maximum-likelihood analyses for the COI and ITS 1 sequences using the program RAxML [29]. The maximum-likelihood estimates were bootstrapped for 1000 replicates based on the GTRGAMMA substitution model. Downloaded *B. truncatus* sequences deposited in Genbank from Niger (AM286316.2), Senegal (AM921807.1 and AM921806.1) Portugal (AM286314), Italy (AM286312.3), Burkina Faso (AM286315.2), and Tanzania (AM286313.2) [12] were used as reference isolates for COI sequences, while *B. truncatus* isolates from Tanzania (AM921983), Niger (AM921965) [16], and Cameroon (KJ157504.1, KJ157503.1, KJ157500.1, KJ157501.1, KJ157502.1) [13] were used as reference isolates for ITS 1 sequences. Sequence data from other *Bulinus* species on Genbank (detailed information on accession number and origin provided as Supplementary Data) were also included in constructing the maximum likelihood phylogenetic trees. Additionally, *Bulinus forskalii* (AM286306.2) was used as an outgroup for *Bulinus truncatus* group assessed with COI marker. *Bulinus forskalii* (AM921961.1) was used as the outgroup for the *Bulinus truncatus* group assessed with ITS 1 marker.

We also estimated the phylogenetic relationships of the COI and ITS 1 *B. truncatus* dataset using Bayesian inference in MrBayes version 3.2.0 programs [30] (Figures S1 and S2). Prior to Bayesian inference, the best fit nucleotide substitution models (HKY for COI and TrN for ITS 1) were determined using a hierarchical likelihood ratio test in jMODELTEST version 0.1.1 [31]. The posterior probabilities were calculated via 1,000,000 generations using Markov chain Monte Carlo (MCMC) simulations, and the chains were sampled every 1000 generations. At the end of this run, the average standard deviation of split frequencies was below 0.01, and the potential scale reduction factor was reasonably close to 1.0 for all parameters. A consensus tree was summarized and visualized in FigTree version 1.4.3 [32].

B. truncatus sequences from the three populations, reference isolates, and other *Bulinus* species sequences used for constructing ML trees were repeated for the construction of the Bayes ML trees Clade comprising *B. forskalii* (AM286308, AM286293.2, and AM286306.2) was used as the outgroup for COI *B. truncatus* sequences while *B. forskalii* (AM921961.1) was used the outgroup for ITS 1 *B. truncatus* sequences.

The minimum spanning tree was built using NETWORK 5.0.0.0 [33] (Figure S3). We built the network to support the COI ML tree and it showed the torso of the genetic structure.

DNA sequences have been submitted to the National Centre for Biotechnology Information Archive with accession numbers MG759386–MG759479 (*B. truncatus* group assessed with COI marker) and MG757840-757890 (*B. truncatus* group assessed with ITS 1 marker).

2.5. Determination of Haplotype and Nucleotide Diversity

The level of sequence diversity, which includes number of haplotype (h), haplotype diversity (hd), nucleotide diversity (π), Tajima's D (D), and theta per site statistics, were calculated for *B. truncatus* populations assessed with both COI and ITS 1 markers in Arlequin software version 3.5 [34]. In addition, we compared Fst of *B. truncatus* studied populations using Arlequin software version 3.5 [34].

3. Results

3.1. Phylogeny

Altogether, 94 individual snail samples including 38 (Giza and Sharkia; Egypt), 36 (Barakat area; Sudan), and 20 (Madziwa, Shamva District; Zimbabwe) were successfully sequenced at the COI region (Table 2), and 51 including 28 (Egypt) and 23 (Sudan) were sequenced at the ITS 1 locus (Table 2), because of failure in either amplification or sequencing. Following the sequencing alignment and trimming of all the sequences, the final fragments of 737 bp (COI) and 580 bp (ITS 1) were obtained. Among these, 6, 11, and 6 unique COI haplotypes of *B. truncatus* sequences were observed from Giza and Sharkia (Egypt), Barakat area (Sudan) and Madziwa, Shamva district (Zimbabwe), respectively (Table 2). In Egypt and Sudan, respectively, 3 and 2 unique ITS 1 haplotypes of *B. truncatus* sequences were observed (Table 2). No information on *B. truncatus* ITS 1 sequences from Zimbabwe was recorded in this study due to failure in either amplification or sequencing.

Table 2. Estimation of nucleotide diversity and summary statistics of *Bulinus truncatus* identified using COI I and ITS 1 markers.

		N	H	Hd	π	S.D.π	Θ_S	s.d.S	Tajima's D	*p*-Value
COI	Egypt	38	6	0.334	0.00205	0.001445	0.002916	0.001299	−0.85621	0.24
	Sudan	36	11	0.768	0.009359	0.005067	0.009602	0.003341	−0.08761	0.538
	Zimbabwe	20	6	0.784	0.014701	0.007859	0.011655	0.004442	1.01745	0.898
ITS 1	Egypt	28	3	0.14	0.005589	0.003362	0.020107	0.006909	−2.69592	0
	Sudan	23	2	0.443	0.00169	0.001367	0.001034	0.000769	1.41416	0.923

Number of sequences (N), number of haplotypes (h), haplotype diversity (Hd), nucleotide diversity (pi), theta per site (Θ_S), standard deviation (s.d.).

Phylogenetic analyses indicated some measures of variation in the genetic population structure of *B. truncatus* population from Giza and Sharkia (Egypt), Barakat area (Sudan), and Madziwa (Zimbabwe). A large quantity of COI sequence data from Giza and Sharkia (Egypt) and Barakat area (Sudan) cluster together on the *B. truncatus* clade but the COI sequence data of Madziwa (Zimbabwe) *B. truncatus* population cluster at different locations on the tree (Figure 2 and Figure S1). No significant variation was observed between *B. truncatus* populations from Giza and Sharkia (Egypt) and Barakat area (Sudan) (Figure 3 and Figure S2). The minimum spanning tree indicated the torso of *B. truncatus* populations genetic structure (Figure S3). The tree showed five haplotypes for *B. truncatus* obtained from Zimbabwe, while five and two haplotypes were indicated for Sudan and Egypt *B. truncatus* populations respectively. Cryptic lineages or other known species of *B. truncatus* were not detected.

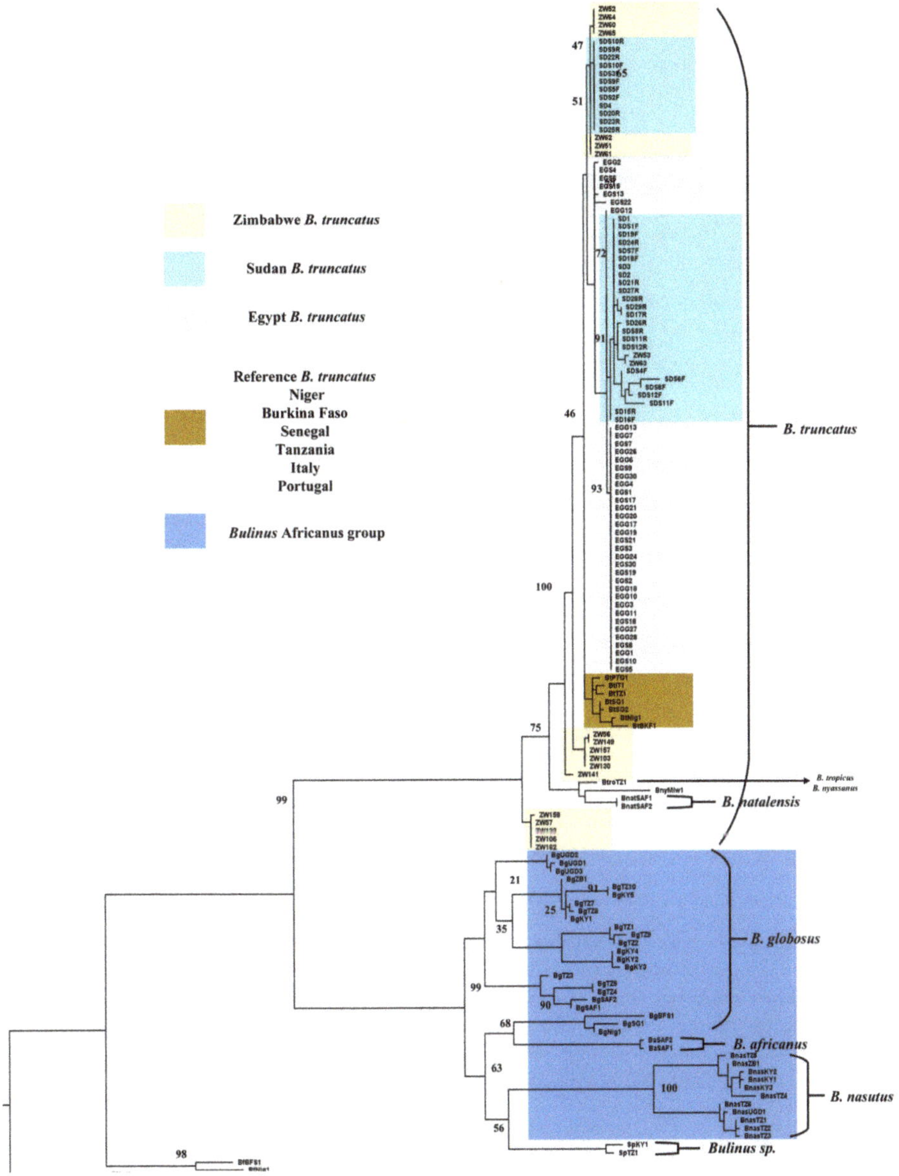

Figure 2. A rooted maximum likelihood tree of *Bulinus truncatus* for CO1 sequences. Maximum likelihood tree of a 737 bp fragment of the cytochrome oxidase subunit 1 (CO1) gene for *B. truncatus* in this study with an additional 51 published Genbank sequences including *B. truncatus* reference isolates. Values on the branches are bootstrap support based on 1000 replications. *B. forskalii* (AM286306.2) was defined as outgroup. * UGD-Uganda, TZ-Tanzania, SAF-South Africa, KY-Kenya, ZB-Zanzibar, SG-Senegal, BFS, Burkina Faso, Nig-Niger, Agl-Angola, Mlw-Malawi.

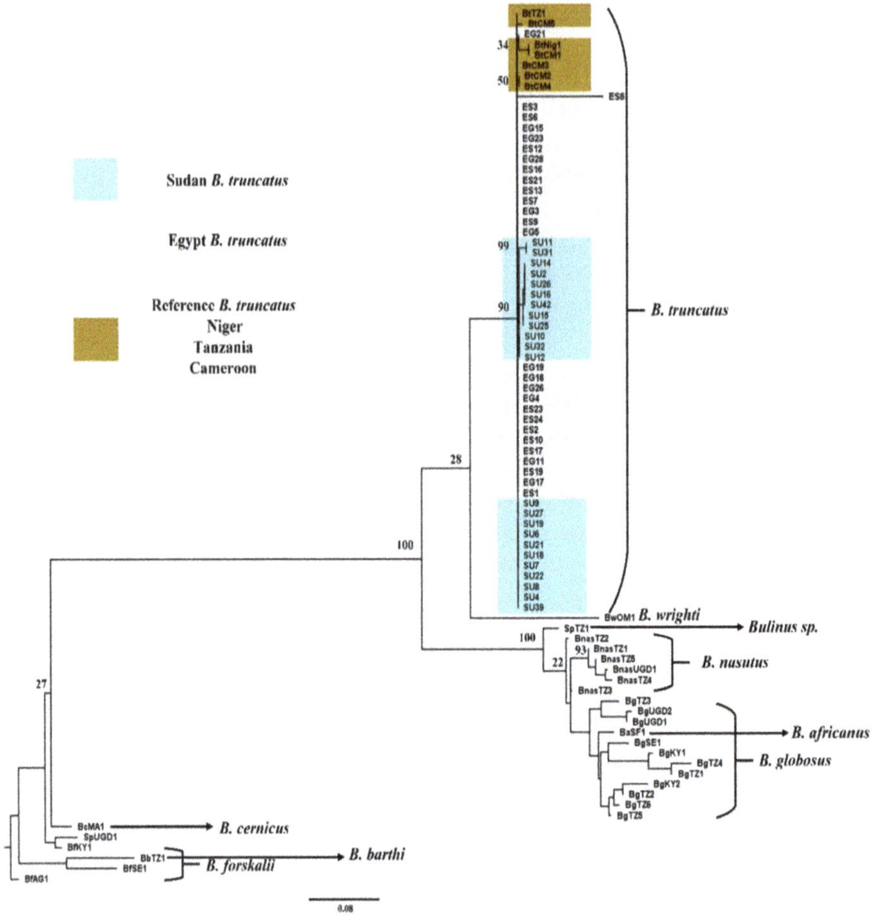

Figure 3. A rooted maximum likelihood tree of *Bulinus truncatus* for ITS 1 sequences. Maximum likelihood tree of a 580 bp fragment of the internal transcribed spacer 1 (ITS 1) for *B. truncatus* in this study with an additional 33 published Genbank sequences including *B. truncatus* reference isolates. Values on the branches are bootstrap support based on 1000 replications. *B. forslkalii* (AM921961.1) was defined as outgroup. * UGD-Uganda, TZ-Tanzania, SF-South Africa, KY-Kenya, SE-Senegal, BFS, Burkina Faso, Nig-Niger, AG-Angola, MA-Mauritius, OM-Oman.

3.2. Haplotype and Nucleotide Diversity

Nucleotide polymorphism obtained for all *B. truncatus* sequences assessed in this study is shown in Table 2. Haplotype diversity observed of sequences from the three populations assessed with COI includes 0.334 (Giza and Sharkia, Egypt), 0.768 (Barakat area, Sudan), and 0.784 (Madziwa, Zimbabwe) while their nucleotide diversity includes 0.00205 (s.d. = 0.001445), 0.009359 (s.d. = 0.005067), and 0.014701 (s.d. = 0.007859) for Egypt, Sudan, and Zimbabwe, respectively (Table 2). Haplotype diversity for the two populations assessed with ITS 1 is 0.14 and 0.443 while nucleotide diversity includes 0.005589 (s.d. π 0.003362) and 0.00169 (s.d. π 0.001367) for (Giza and Sharkia, Egypt) and (Barakat area, Sudan), respectively. F_{ST} values in the pairwise population comparisons are shown in Table 3.

Table 3. Population pairwise Φst.

	Egypt	Sudan
Sudan	0.34860 *	
Zimbabwe	0.59653 *	0.36160 *

* Significant p value < 0.05.

4. Discussion

Urinary schistosomiasis burden is widely reported in Africa and this is a consequence of the unabated distribution of the important snail intermediate hosts of the genus *Bulinus* that serves as host to the schistosome parasite [4]. The *Bulinus* group is made up of about 37 recognized species and has been divided into four different groups for convenience [5].

This study assessed the genetic diversity of *B. truncatus* populations, the snail host implicated in the transmission of *S. haematobium* in Africa using mitochondrial cytochrome oxidase 1 (COI) gene and internal transcribed spacer (ITS 1).

Snail host identification using morphological characters is unreliable and sometimes ambiguous but the development and application of molecular techniques have been helpful, providing good species discrimination [4,5].

We observed that mitochondrial DNA sequences from Barakat area (Sudan) and Madziwa, Shamva (Zimbabwe) indicated high haplotype diversity including 0.768 and 0.784, respectively, a similar observation was earlier reported by Zein-Eddine et al. [14]. The level of haplotype diversity observed from the two populations in our study is less than the values reported by Zein-Eddine et al. [14]. However, relatively low haplotype diversity was also observed for sequences from Giza and Sharkia (Egypt), with 0.334. Nevertheless, the low levels of haplotype diversity observed for *B. truncatus* in this study were similar to findings by Zein-Eddine et al. [11] and those observed by Goodall-Copestake et al. [19,35], with low diversity species.

Our findings indicated some degree of variation in the *Bulinus* species population structure across Africa. *Bulinus* species populations on both COI and ITS 1 trees (Figures 2 and 3, Figures S1 and S2) separated into populations that correspond to *Bulinus* species groups [12,36]. However, we observed that *B. globosus* from West Africa clusters separately from the East African species as indicated by the COI sequence data.

Kane et al. [12] reported the division between *B. globosus* from the two regions in Africa and that *Bulinus africanus* has a close affinity with West African *B. globosus* species. This is also evident from the information provided by our COI sequence data (Figure 2).

Some levels of segregation were observed within the COI *B. truncatus* populations. The location of populations from Giza and Sharkia (Egypt) and Barakat area (Sudan) on the *B. truncatus* clade agrees with the location of both countries geographically (Figure 2). The clustering of the Madziwa, Shamva (Zimbabwe) sequences in different locations on the *B. truncatus* clade can be attributed to individuals with different genotypes within the population (Figure 2).

Findings from this study using COI identified two reciprocally monophyletic *B. truncatus* sister subclades and this corresponds to *B. truncatus* and *B. tropicus* respectively [12,36]. Nalugwa et al. [36] also obtained similar results from findings on the *B. truncatus/tropicus* complex collected from Albertine Rift freshwater bodies in Uganda. Brown and Shaw [37] have shown that *B. truncatus* is a tetraploid and *B. tropicus* is diploid; however, it is difficult to distinguish *B. truncatus* and *B. tropicus* morphologically.

The minimum spanning network was constructed to support the ML tree and this informed our decision to include some outgroup sequences. The network did not indicate a substantial difference from the information on the tree (Figure S3).

Although *Bulinus* species populations separated distinctly into groups as earlier indicated [12], no significant variation was observed within *B. truncatus* populations from Giza and Sharkia (Egypt) and Barakat area (Sudan) as indicated by the ITS 1 tree (Figure 3). Kane et al. [12] stated that

Bulinus wrighti has a characteristic COI sequence that positions the species and other members of the *Bulinus reticulatus* group close to the *Bulinus truncatus* complex. This was also observed from our ITS 1 result (Figure 3).

This study is not unique; however, it has investigated the genetic diversity of *B. truncatus* from Giza and Sharkia (Egypt), Barakat area (Sudan), and Madziwa (Zimbabwe), which is necessary for snail host surveillance in the study areas and it has also provided genomic data of this important snail species from the sampled countries.

Although no infection was detected from the snails when screened for patent and prepatent infection, the presence and distribution of *B. truncatus* in the studied areas poses a threat to the inhabitants of these areas should an infected person visit the water bodies and urinate inside or near enough for the schistosome eggs released with the urine to have contact with the water bodies, especially water contact sites such as the Nile River and El-Salam Canal (Egypt), where inhabitants engage in a lot of fishing activities, and the river at Madziwa (Zimbabwe) that people visit frequently to carry out their domestic chores as well as engage in activities such as swimming.

Previous studies implicated *B. truncatus* as the only *Bulinus* species that transmits *S. haematobium* in Egypt and other parts of northern Africa, while *Bulinus globosus* is implicated for schistosomiasis transmission in Zimbabwe [4]. The presence of *B. truncatus* in the southern African country can be attributed to the favorable environmental factors and migration of snail population; however, human activities have also increased the number of snail hosts of *S. haematobium*. This is a cause for concern and there is a need to improve measures for effective snail control strategies.

Differentiating snail host populations to assess their diversity should be prioritized in Africa, where host snails' genome data is scarce for most schistosomiasis endemic countries [18]. Efforts should be made to initiate a continent-wide snail host genome project to help develop a more comprehensive and robust snail host genome database for the African continent.

5. Conclusions

This study identified *B. truncatus*, the snail host of *S. haematobium* obtained from Giza and Sharkia (Egypt), Barakat area (Sudan), and Madziwa, Shamva District (Zimbabwe) using COI and ITS 1 markers, as well as provided information on their genetic diversity.

With the increasing global call that effective schistosomiasis control programmes should target snail control, there is a need to prioritize snail studies for effective mapping of schistosomiasis transmission [38], as well as to strengthen surveillance strategies.

Supplementary Materials: The following are available online at http://www.mdpi.com/2414-6366/3/4/127/s1. S1A–S1J, data were used to prepare Table 2, S1A: Egypt B. truncatus COI.out, S1B: Egypt B. truncatus COI Tajima D.out, S1C: Egypt B. truncatus Fu_Li Test.out, S1D: Egypt_SUD_ZWE B. truncatus COI final.out, S1E: Fu_Li Egypt_SUD_ZWE B. truncatus COI.out, S1F: Sudan B. truncatus COI.out, S1G: Sudan B. truncatus COI Tajima D.out, S1H: Sudan B. truncatus Fu_Li test.out, S1I: Zimbabwe B. truncatus.out, S1J: Zimbabwe B. truncatus COI Tajima D.out, S2A–S2F data were used to prepare Table 3, S2A: Egypt B. truncatus ITS Fu_Li test.out, S2B: Egypt B. truncatus ITS Tajima D.out, S2C: Egypt B. truncatus ITS.out, S2D: Sudan B. truncatus ITS.out, S2E: Sudan B. truncatus ITS Fu_Li test.out, S2F: Sudan B. truncatus ITS Tajima D.out, S3A–S3M were used to prepare Figure 2A,B, S3A: Egypt Bulinus truncatus GENBANK PROTEIN SEQ NEW.fas, S3B: Egypt Bulinus truncatus GENBANK SEQ NEW.d.txt, S3C: Egypt B. truncatus GENBANK SEQ NEW.fas, S3D: SUDAN B. truncatus COI Protein SEQ1.fas, S3E: SUDAN B. truncatus COI genbankSEQ.fas, S3F: SUDAN B. truncatus Genbank SEQ COI.txt, S3G: Zimbabwe B.truncatus COI protein SEQ for genbank submission.fas, S3H: Zimbabwe B. truncatus COI SEQ for genbank submission.fas, S3I: Zimbabwe B. truncatus COI SEQ for genbank submission.txt, S3J: ZWE_SUDAN_EGYPT_BT_REF_COI_OUTGROUP.txt, S3K.ZWE_SUDAN_EGYPT_BT_REF_COI_OUTGROUP2-v2NEW.fas, S3L: Summary of the STRUCTURE analysis for B. truncatus COI.docx, S3M: Table 1. Information on B. truncatus sequences submitted to genbank, S4A–S4H were used to prepare Figure 3A,B, S4A: Information B. truncatus ITS 1 sequences submitted to genbank.xls, S4B: Egypt B. truncatus ITS.fas, S4C: Egypt B. truncatus ITS.txt, S4D: Egypt_Sudan_REF B. truncatus ITS.fas, S4E: Egypt_Sudan_REF_Outgroup B. truncatus ITS.txt, S4F: SUDAN B. truncatus ITS.fas, S4G: SUDAN B. truncatus ITS.txt, S4H: Summary of STRUCTURE analysis for B truncatus.docx.

Author Contributions: E.M.A. and X.N.Z. conceived the study; E.M.A., M.J.M. and Y.H.G. carried out laboratory analysis; H.S., X.J.B. and E.M.A. carried out data analysis; M.M., M.H. and N.M. conducted fieldwork; J.X. and S.Z.L. contributed reagents, materials, and analysis tools; E.M.A., S.Z.L. and X.N.Z. wrote the paper.

Funding: This research received no external funding.

Acknowledgments: E.M.A. acknowledges the funding and support received from the National Institute of Parasitic Diseases, WHO Collaborating Centre for Tropical Diseases, and the China CDC for the postdoctoral fellowship.

Conflicts of Interest: Authors declare there is no conflict of interest.

References

1. WHO. *Country Profile: Preventive Chemotherapy and Transmission Control*; World Health Organization: Geneva, Switzerland, 2010; Available online: http://www.who.int/neglected_diseases/preventive_chemotherapy/databank/CP (accessed on 10 February 2018).
2. Hanington, P.C.; Forys, M.A.; Loker, E.S. A somatically diversified defense factor, FREP3, is a determinant of snail resistance to schistosome infection. *PLoS Negl. Trop. Dis.* **2012**. [CrossRef] [PubMed]
3. Gordy, M.A.; Kish, L.; Tarrabain, M.; Hanington, P.C. A comprehensive survey of larval digenean trematodes and their snail hosts in central Alberta, Canada. *Parasitol. Res.* **2016**. [CrossRef] [PubMed]
4. Rollinson, D.; Stothard, J.R.; Southgate, V.R. Interactions between intermediate snail hosts of the genus *Bulinus* and schistosomes of the *Schistosoma haematobium* group. *Parasitology* **2001**, *123*, S245–S260. [CrossRef] [PubMed]
5. Brown, D.S. *Fresh Water Snails of Africa and Their Medical Importance*, 2nd ed.; Taylor and Francis: London, UK, 1994; p. 609.
6. Akinwale, O.P.; Kane, R.A.; Rollinson, D.; Stothard, J.R.; Ajayi, M.B.; Akande, D.O.; Ogungbemi, M.O.; Duker, C.; Gyang, P.V.; Adeleke, M.A. Molecular approaches to the identification of *Bulinus* species in south-west Nigeria and observations on natural snail infections with schistosomes. *J. Helminthol.* **2010**, *85*, 283–293. [CrossRef] [PubMed]
7. Jarne, P. Mating system, bottlenecks and genetic-polymorphism in hermaphroditic animals. *Genet. Res.* **1995**, *65*, 193–207. [CrossRef]
8. Djuikwo-Teukenga, F.F.; Da Silva, A.; Njiokou, F.; Kamgang, B.; Same Ekobo, A.; Dreyfuss, G. Significant population genetic structure of the Cameroonian freshwater snail, *Bulinus globosus*, (Gastropoda: Planorbidae) revealed by nuclear microsatellite loci analysis. *Acta Trop.* **2014**, *137*, 111–117. [CrossRef] [PubMed]
9. Brown, D.S. *Freshwater Snails of Africa and Their Medical Importance*; Taylor and Francis: London, UK, 1980; p. 487.
10. Jarne, P.; Charlesworth, D. The evolution of the selfing rate in functionally hermaphrodite plants and animals. *Annu. Rev. Ecol. Syst.* **1993**, *24*, 441–466. [CrossRef]
11. Zein-Eddine, R.; Djuikwo-Teukeng, F.F.; Dar, Y.; Dreyfuss, G.; Van den Broeck, F. Population genetics of the *Schistosoma* snail host *Bulinus truncatus* in Egypt. *Acta Trop.* **2017**, *172*, 36–43. [CrossRef]
12. Kane, R.A.; Stothard, J.R.; Emery, A.M.; Rollinson, D. Molecular characterization of freshwater snails in the genus *Bulinus*: A role for bar codes? *Parasites Vectors* **2008**, *1*, 15. [CrossRef]
13. Standley, C.J.; Goodacre, S.L.; Wade, C.M.; Stothard, J.R. The population genetic structure of *Biomphalaria choanomphala* in Lake Victoria, East Africa: Implications for schistosomiasis transmission. *Parasites Vectors* **2014**, *7*, 524. [CrossRef]
14. Zein-Eddine, R.; Djuikwo-Teukeng, F.F.; Al-Jawhari, M.; Senghor, B.; Huyse, T.; Dreyfuss, G. Phylogeny of seven *Bulinus* species originating from endemic areas in three African countries, in relation to the human blood fluke *Schistosoma haematobium*. *BMC Evol. Biol.* **2014**, *14*, 271. [CrossRef] [PubMed]
15. Mohamed, A.H.; Sharaf El-Din, A.T.; Mohamed, A.M.; Habib, M.R. The relationship between genetic variability and the susceptibility of *Biomphalaria alexandrina* snails to *Schistosoma mansoni* infection. *Mem. Inst. Oswaldo Cruz* **2012**, *107*, 326–337. [CrossRef] [PubMed]
16. Abdel-Hamid, Z.A.; Rawi, S.M.; Arafa, A.F. Identification of a genetic marker associated with the resistance to *Schistosoma mansoni* infection using random amplified polymorphic DNA analysis. *Mem. Inst. Oswaldo Cruz* **2006**, *101*, 863–868. [CrossRef] [PubMed]
17. Emery, A.M.; Loxton, N.J.; Stothard, J.R.; Jones, C.S.; Spinks, J.; Llewellyn-Hughes, J.; Noble, L.R.; Rollinson, D. Microsatellites in the freshwater snail *Bulinus globosus* (Gastropoda: Planorbidae) from Zanzibar. *Mol. Ecol. Notes* **2003**, *3*, 108–110. [CrossRef]

18. Abe, E.M.; Guan, W.; Guo, Y.H.; Kassegne, K.; Qin, Z.Q.; Xu, J.; Chen, J.H.; Ekpo, U.F.; Li, S.Z.; Zhou, X.N. Differentiating snail intermediate hosts of *Schistosoma* spp. using molecular approaches: Fundamental to successful integrated control mechanism in Africa. *Infect. Dis. Poverty* **2018**. [CrossRef] [PubMed]
19. Djuikwo-Teukeng, F.F.; Njiokou, F.; Nkengazong, L.; De Meeus, T.; SameEkobo, A.; Dreyfuss, G. Strong genetic structure in Cameroonian populations of *Bulinus truncatus* (Gastropoda: Planorbidae), intermediate host of *Schistosoma haematobium*. *Infect. Genet. Evol.* **2001**, *11*, 17–22. [CrossRef] [PubMed]
20. Viard, F.; Bremond, P.; Labbo, R.; Justy, F.; Delay, B.; Jarne, P. Microsatellites and the genetics of highly selfing populations in the freshwater snail *Bulinus truncatus*. *Genetics* **1996**, *142*, 1237–1247.
21. Viard, F.; Justy, F.; Jarne, P. Population dynamics inferred from temporal variation at microsatellite loci in the selfing snail *Bulinus truncatus*. *Genetics* **1997**, *146*, 973–982.
22. Chlyeh, G.; Henry, P.Y.; Jarne, P. Spatial and temporal variation of life-history traits documented using capture-mark-recapture methods in the vector snail *Bulinus truncatus*. *Parasitology* **2003**, *127*, 243–251. [CrossRef]
23. Jarne, P.; Viard, F.; Delay, B.; Cuny, G. Variable microsatellites in the highly selfing snail *Bulinus truncatus* (Basommatophora: Planorbidae). *Mol. Ecol.* **1994**, *3*, 527–528. [CrossRef]
24. Brown, D.S.; Kristensen, T.K. *A Fish Guide to Fresh Water Snails*; Danish Bilharziasis Laboratory: DK-2920 Charlottenlund, Denmark, 1993.
25. Emery, A.M.; Allan, F.E.; Rabone, M.E.; Rollinson, D. Schistosomiasis collection at NHM (SCAN). *Parasit Vectors* **2012**, *5*, 185. [CrossRef] [PubMed]
26. Hall, T.A. BioEdit: A user-friendly biological sequence alignment editor and analysis program for Windows 95/98/NT. In *Nucleic Acids Symposium Series*; Information Retrieval Ltd.: London, UK, 1999; pp. 95–98.
27. Altschul, S.F.; Gish, W.; Miller, W.; Myers, E.W.; Lipman, D.J. Basic local alignment search tool. *J. Mol. Biol.* **1990**, *215*, 403–410. [CrossRef]
28. Thompson, J.D.; Higgins, D.G.; Gibson, T.J. CLUSTALW: Improving the sensitivity of progressive multiple sequence alignment through sequence weighting, position-specific gap penalties and weight matrix choice. *Nucleic Acids Res.* **1994**, *22*, 4673–4680. [CrossRef] [PubMed]
29. Stamatakis, A. RAxML version 8: A tool for phylogenetic analysis and post-analysis of large phylogenies. *Bioinformatics* **2014**, *30*, 1312–1313. [CrossRef] [PubMed]
30. Ronquist, F.; Teslenko, M.; van der Mark, P.; Avres, D.L.; Darling, A.; Hohna, S.; Larget, B.; Liu, L.; Suchard, M.A.; Huelsenbeck, J.P. MrBayes 3.2: Efficient Bayesian phylogenetic inference and model choice across a large model space. *Syst. Biol.* **2012**, *61*, 539–542. [CrossRef] [PubMed]
31. Posada, D. jModelTest: Phylogenetic model averaging. *Mol. Biol. Evol.* **2008**, *25*, 1253–1256. [CrossRef] [PubMed]
32. Rambaut, A. Evolution and phylogenetics software. FigTree version 1.4.3. Available online: http://tree.bio.ed.ac.uk/software/figtree/ (accessed on 8 December 2018).
33. Polzin, T.; Daneshmand, S.V. On Steiner trees and minimum spanning trees in hypergraphs. *Oper. Res. Lett.* **2003**, *31*, 12–20. [CrossRef]
34. Excoffier, L.; Laval, G.; Schneider, S. Arlequin ver.3.1: An integrated software package for population genetics data analysis. *Evol. Bioinform.* **2005**, *1*, 47–50. [CrossRef]
35. Goodall-Copestake, W.P.; Tarling, G.A.; Murphy, E.J. On the comparison of population-level estimates of haplotype and nucleotide diversity: A case study using the gene *cox1* in animals. *Heredity* **2012**, *109*, 50–56. [CrossRef]
36. Nalugwa, A.; Jørgensen, A.; Nyakaana, S.; Kristensen, TK. Molecular phylogeny of *Bulinus* (Gastropoda: Planorbidae) reveals the presence of three species complexes in the Albertine Rift freshwater bodies. *Int. J. Genet. Mol. Biol.* **2010**, *2*, 130–139.
37. Brown, D.S.; Shaw, K.M. Freshwater snails of thee *Bulinus truncatus/tropicus* complex in Kenya: Tetraploid species. *J. Mollus. Stud.* **1989**, *55*, 509–532. [CrossRef]
38. Allan, F.; Sousa-Figueiredo, J.C.; Emery, A.M.; Paulo, R.; Mirante, C.; Sebastião, A.; Brito, M.; Rollinson, D. Mapping freshwater snails in north-western Angola: Distribution, identity and molecular diversity of medically important taxa. *Parasites Vectors* **2017**, *10*, 460. [CrossRef] [PubMed]

Tropical Medicine and Infectious Disease

MDPI

Review

Treading the Path towards Genetic Control of Snail Resistance to Schistosome Infection

Damilare O. Famakinde

Department of Medical Microbiology and Parasitology, College of Medicine, University of Lagos, Idi-Araba, Surulere, Lagos 100254, Nigeria; damfam.joe@gmail.com; Tel.: +234-703-330-2069

Received: 18 July 2018; Accepted: 13 August 2018; Published: 15 August 2018

Abstract: Schistosomiasis remains the most important tropical snail-borne trematodiasis that threatens many millions of human lives. In achieving schistosomiasis elimination targets, sustainable control of the snail vectors represents a logical approach. Nonetheless, the ineffectiveness of the present snail control interventions emphasizes the need to develop new complementary strategies to ensure more effective control outcomes. Accordingly, the use of genetic techniques aimed at driving resistance traits into natural vector populations has been put forward as a promising tool for integrated snail control. Leveraging the *Biomphalaria-Schistosoma* model system, studies unraveling the complexities of the vector biology and those exploring the molecular basis of snail resistance to schistosome infection have been expanding in various breadths, generating many significant discoveries, and raising the hope for future breakthroughs. This review provides a compendium of relevant findings, and without neglecting the current existing gaps and potential future challenges, discusses how a transgenic snail approach may be adapted and harnessed to control human schistosomiasis.

Keywords: schistosomiasis; vector control; snail resistance; gene drive; transgenic snail

1. Introduction

It is presently more than a century since malacological discoveries established that various genera of freshwater snails (Mollusca: Gastropoda) serve as biological vectors of human diseases caused by parasitic trematodes. These findings have made the study of snail biology an important aspect of infectious disease research, particularly in tropical helminthology. Among these human snail-borne trematodiases, schistosomiasis (bilharziasis) ranks as the most important disease, afflicting more than 206 million humans [1], and being responsible for over 3.51 million disability-adjusted life years (DALYs) [2], most prominently in the tropics. Most cases of human schistosomiasis are caused by three parasitic schistosomes (blood flukes): *Schistosoma haematobium*, *S. mansoni,* and *S. japonicum* [3]. Both *S. haematobium* and *S. mansoni* are found in Africa and the Middle East; only *S. mansoni* occurs in the Americas, and *S. japonicum* is a major disease-causing species in China, Indonesia, and the Philippines [3]. However, the geographical distribution of these flukes is synchronous to, and importantly determined by, the local distribution of their snail vectors. *S. haematobium* is transmitted by *Bulinus* snails, *S. mansoni* by *Biomphalaria* snails, and *S. japonicum* by *Oncomelania* snails [4].

The human-to-snail-to-human transmission of *Schistsosoma* occurs when adult male and female living in copula within the human host mate and produce fertilized eggs. Some of the eggs are voided with urine (in *S. haematobium*) or feces (in *S. mansoni* and *S. japonicum*) into the environment. The eggs that reach the vectors' freshwater habitats hatch and release the enclosed miracidia larvae, which swim actively to locate and infect their snail vectors. A miracidium that successfully infects a susceptible vector undergoes intramolluscan polyembryonic development to produce thousands of actively-swimming tailed cercariae larvae that emerge continuously from the snail host for the rest of the its lifetime (spanning months) [3–6]. Human infection with schistosomes is acquired through skin contact with, and subsequent penetration by, the cercariae during recreational, domestic, or occupational activities with contaminated water [5]. Following penetration, the worms transform into immature schistosomes (schistosomulae) and are carried in body circulation, from where they enter the portal veins and mature in about 5–7 weeks [3,5]. Mature worm pairs migrate to their preferred host sites—*S. mansoni* and *S. japonicum* to the mesenteric venules of the bowel or rectum, and *S. haematobium* to the venous plexus of the bladder, where they mate and the females lay eggs to repeat the cycle [4,5]. Adult schistosomes have an average lifespan of 3–10 years, but they may also live as long as 30–40 years in their human hosts [3–5]. The eggs are highly immunogenic and are majorly responsible for disease outcomes by triggering localized pathologic reactions within the human host [4,7,8]. Although human infection with *Schistosoma* species may cause non-specific but incapacitating systemic morbidities such as malnutrition, anemia, and impaired physical and cognitive development in children, poor birth outcomes in infected pregnant women, and neurological aberrations, *S. haematobium* is specifically responsible for urogenital pathologies, while other *Schistosoma* species majorly cause gastrointestinal complications, but also hepatosplenic enlargement, ascites, and portal hypertension in advanced cases [3,7,9,10]. Again, there is growing evidence that female urogenital schistosomiasis poses an increased risk of HIV transmission and/or progression [11–13].

Taking a leap towards the beginning of the end human schistosomiasis requires an integrated control approach that cuts across both the vector and the human cycles. Current strategy in the fight against the disease co-implements ongoing preventive chemotherapy through mass drug administration (MDA), with complementary public-health interventions. This approach, as defined by WHO/AFRO, is known as PHASE—preventive chemotherapy, health education, access to clean water, sanitation improvement, and environmental snail control and focal mollusciciding [14]. Recent efforts made to evaluate the degree of importance of snail control in schistosomiasis elimination [15–18] clearly showed that sustainable snail control is pivotal in achieving targeted disease elimination. This is especially true in the present era of highly challenging anti-schistosome vaccine development, as well as the monochemotherapeutic availability of praziquantel and its feared resistance by schistosomes [19–21]. Strategies currently in use for controlling schistosomiasis snail vectors are: biocontrol using competitors or predators, modification of snail habitats, and application of molluscicides. These approaches, used either singly or in combination, have evidently contributed to many successful schistosomiasis control efforts in different localities and countries [15,22–27]; however, each approach is not without limitations [24]. The application of chemical molluscicides has been mostly exploited. Among other chemical molluscicidal agents, niclosamide has a long track record of being successful against snail hosts, and is often regarded as the molluscicide of choice. Nevertheless, apart from its expensiveness, toxicity of niclosamide to a variety of non-target aquatic life forms (plants, invertebrates and vertebrates including amphibians) has led to its decreased acceptability. Again, the inability of niclosamide to prevent snail recolonization, especially in large permanent water bodies, necessitates repeated applications that result in high cost [24,28–30].

In view of the present challenges facing schistosomiasis control efforts, coupled with the endorsement by the World Health Assembly Resolution 65.21 to take full advantage of non-drug-based interventions to prevent schistosomiasis transmission [31], it will be timely to adapt new strategies in order to interrupt snail-mediated schistosome transmission, and thus, forestall human infection. The use of genetic techniques to manipulate snail vectors of schistosomiasis has long been stressed as a novel biocontrol strategy with the potential to constitute an important complementary tool for transmission reduction or breaking. Embracing all the means to actualize this potential, studies unraveling the complexities of the vector biology and those exploring the molecular underpinnings of snail resistance/susceptibility to schistosome infection have been expanding in various breadths, generating many significant discoveries and raising the hope for future breakthroughs. The aim of this review is to provide a compendium of relevant findings, and discuss how transgenic snail approach may be adapted and harnessed to control human schistosomiasis.

2. Biology of Snail Resistance/Susceptibility to *Schistosoma* Infections–Major Exploits so Far

The first groundbreaking discovery on the identification of intermediate snail hosts of schistosomes was made by Miyairi and Suzuki, who observed stages of *S. japonicum* in *Oncomelania* snails in Japan in 1913 [32,33]. This was followed by the achievements of Robert Leiper, who also demonstrated the complete life cycles of *S. haematobium* and *S. mansoni* in their respective snail hosts in Egypt [34,35]. Subsequent to these watershed moments in the long history of schistosomiasis, investigations on the interactions between schistosomes and their snail vectors became kinetic. The genetic study of snail-schistosome compatibility was pioneered by Newton [36,37], who demonstrated that susceptibility of snail vectors to *Schistosoma* infections is fundamentally genetic and a heritable character. This was later underscored by other investigators who revealed that resistance character, which is acquired at the maturity phase in the adults of resistant snail stocks, is monogenic, dominant, and heritable by a simple Mendelian pattern of inheritance [38–41]. This genetic dominance of the resistance trait has been confirmed by various crossbreeding experiments in *Biomphalaria* species [42–46]. Be that as it may, Rosa et al. [45] showed that resistance in *B. tenagophila* is determined by two dominant genes. In contrast, in juvenile *B. glabrata*, resistance is a complex trait governed by a minimum of four genes, each having multiple alleles (alternative forms of the same gene) [40,47]. From these various lines of evidence, it could be understood that genetic determinism of resistance is governed by a single major locus (position of a particular gene or allele on a chromosome) to a potentially high number of loci, and snails with significantly increased resistance could be artificially selected in the laboratory; meanwhile, molecular markers mapped to resistance could be identified in genetic crosses.

Thus far, work has been done most extensively using the *Biomphalaria-Schistosoma* model, and has led to the nomenclature of some stocks known for resistance (e.g., pigmented BS-90 [48], black-eye 10-R2 [49], and 13-16-IR [50]) or susceptibility (e.g., the albino M-line and NMRI [51], and BB02 [52]) to *S. mansoni* infection, which are now maintained in the laboratory for research purposes. In contrast to the 10-R2 and 13-16-IR strains, however, BS-90 demonstrates unflinching resistance stability, irrespective of age (juvenile or adult), under laboratory conditions [40,53].

A major physiological determinant of snail resistance/susceptibility to infections, which is also under genetic influence, is the snail internal defense system (IDS). The IDS comprises the cellular elements (hemocytes) and the humoral (plasma) factors of the hemolymph that work independently or in concert to recognize, encapsulate, kill, and clear intruding trematodes [6,54–56]. Establishment of the *B. glabrata* embryonic (*Bge*) cell line in 1976 [57] provided an enabling avenue for investigators to delve into the molecular and cellular aspects of the complex snail immune functions against schistosomes by using an *in vitro* culture model, rather than using the whole intact animal, which could have resulted in a rudimentary understanding of the complex biological events. Moreover, major advances in *Biomphalaria* omic studies, such as the recent availability of the whole genome sequence of *B. glabrata* [58], provide a useful resource in deciphering complex functions of the snail biology that were previously obscure. Using various strain and species combinations of the *Biomphalaria-Schistosoma* model system, robust molecular studies have been carried out, leveraging various techniques to identify and characterize endogenous effector protein/gene candidates that are functional in the snail internal defense machinery against schistosomes. Table 1 below presents a synopsis of various endogenous factors that have been implicated in *Biomphalaria* resistance to schistosomes.

Table 1. Putative genes and proteins conferring *Biomphalaria* resistance to *Schistosoma* infection.

Resistance Factor	Snail spp.	*Schistosoma* spp.	Function	Reference(s)
40S ribosomal protein S9	*B. glabrata*	*S. mansoni*	Protein translation in hemocytes.	[59]
*Bg*AIF	*B. glabrata*	*S. mansoni*	Modulates hemocyte activation.	[60]
*Bg*GRN	*B. glabrata*	*S. mansoni*	Production of adherent hemocytes.	[61]
*Bg*MIF	*B. glabrata*	*S. mansoni*	Induces hemocyte proliferation.	[62]
*Bg*TLR	*B. glabrata*	*S. mansoni*	Parasite recognition and activation of effector functions.	[63]
Biomphalysin	*B. glabrata*	*S. mansoni*	Binds to the sporocyst surface and lyses it.	[54,64]
Cathepsin B	*B. glabrata*	*S. mansoni*	Lysis of encapsulated sporocyst.	[65]
Cathepsin L	*B. glabrata*	*S. mansoni*	Lysis of encapsulated sporocyst.	[66]
Copine 1	*B. glabrata*	*S. mansoni*	Involves in signaling processes.	[66]
CREPs	*B. glabrata*	*S. mansoni*	Pattern recognition receptors/adhesion proteins.	[67]
Cu/Zn SOD (SOD1)	*B. glabrata*	*S. mansoni*	Catalyzes the production of H_2O_2 which is cytotoxic to sporocyst.	[50,68,69]
Cystatin 2	*B. glabrata*	*S. mansoni*	Protease inhibitor.	[70,71]
Cytidine deaminase	*B. glabrata*	*S. mansoni*	Nucleobase, nucleoside, nucleotide, and nucleic acid metabolism.	[47]
Cytochrome b	*B. glabrata*	*S. mansoni*	Mitochondrial respiration.	[70]
Cytochrome C oxidase subunits	*B. glabrata*	*S. mansoni*	Mitochondrial respiration.	[70,71]
Dermatopontin2	*B. glabrata*	*S. mansoni*	Participates in hemocyte adhesion and encapsulation responses.	[59,67,70]
Elastase2	*B. glabrata*	*S. mansoni*	Lysis of encapsulated sporocyst.	[66,70]
Elongation factors 1α & 2	*B. glabrata*	*S. mansoni*	Transcription enzymes (bind t-RNA to ribosomes).	[59,67]
Endo-1,4-β-glucanase	*B. glabrata*	*S. mansoni*	Carbohydrate metabolism.	[70]
Ferritin	*B. glabrata*	*S. mansoni*	Stores and transport iron in non-toxic form.	[70,71]
FREP1, 2, 3 & 12	*B. glabrata*	*S. mansoni*	Pattern recognition receptors/adhesion proteins.	[67,70,72,73]
Fribillin	*B. glabrata*	*S. mansoni*	Participates in hemocyte adhesion and encapsulation responses.	[70]
GlcNAc ↓	*B. tenagophila*	*S. mansoni*	Increases hemocyte binding to sporocyst.	[74]
GPCR kinase 2	*B. glabrata*	*S. mansoni*	Signal transduction.	[70]
Grctm6	*B. glabrata*	*S. mansoni*	Modulates cercarial shedding.	[75]
GREPs	*B. glabrata*	*S. mansoni*	Pattern recognition receptors/adhesion proteins.	[67]
GSTs	*B. glabrata*	*S. mansoni*	Prevent cellular damage to the hemocytes.	[70]
Hsp40, 60 & 70 #	*B. glabrata*	*S. mansoni*	Housekeeping cell repair activities.	[66,67,70,76–78]
Importin 7	*B. glabrata*	*S. mansoni*	Involves in signaling processes.	[66]
Inferred phagocyte oxidase	*B. glabrata*	*S. mansoni*	Production of superoxide anions.	[60]
Interleukin 1	*B. glabrata*	*S. mansoni*	Stimulates hemocyte defense response.	[79]
LPS-binding protein	*B. glabrata*	*S. mansoni*	Adhesion protein.	[67]
Matrilin	*B. glabrata*	*S. mansoni*	Participates in hemocyte adhesion and encapsulation responses.	[59,70]

Table 1. *Cont.*

Resistance Factor	Snail spp.	*Schistosoma* spp.	Function	Reference(s)
Metalloproteases	*B. glabrata*	*S. mansoni*	Tissue morphogenesis/remodeling.	[67]
MPEG 1	*B. glabrata*	*S. mansoni*	Participates in hemocyte defense responses.	[47]
Neo-calmodulin	*B. glabrata*	*S. mansoni*	Cacium signaling and homeostasis.	[67]
NF-kB	*B. glabrata*	*S. mansoni*	Downstream transcription in the TLR pathway.	[59,63,70,80]
NADH dehydrogenase subunis	*B. glabrata*	*S. mansoni*	Mitochondrial respiration.	[70]
Peroxiredoxines 1 & 4	*B. glabrata*	*S. mansoni*	Neutralize ROS and RNS that can damage cellular functions.	[60,81]
PGRP 1	*B. glabrata*	*S. mansoni*	Pattern recognition receptor.	[70]
PKC receptor	*B. glabrata*	*S. mansoni*	Signal transduction.	[47]
TEPs	*B. glabrata*	*S. mansoni*	Pattern recognition receptors/adhesion proteins.	[67]
TNF-α	*B. glabrata*	*S. mansoni*	Stimulates hemocyte defense response.	[82]

Symbols: $^{\downarrow}$ in lower concentrations; $^{\#}$ contrasting reports (see [67,78] for some details). Abbreviations: *Bg*AIF, *B. glabrata* allograft inflammatory factor; *Bg*GRN, *B. glabrata* granulin; *Bg*MIF, *B. glabrata* macrophage migration-inhibitory factor; *Bg*TLR, *B. glabrata* Toll-like receptor; CREP, C-type lectin-related protein; Cu/Zn SOD, copper/zinc superoxide dismutase; FREP, fibrinogen-related protein; GlcNac, N-acetyl-D-glucosamine; GPCR, G-protein coupled receptor; Grctm, Guadeloupe resistance complex transmembrane; GREP, galectin-related proteins; GSTs, glutathione-S-transferases; H_2O_2, hydrogen peroxide; Hsp, heat shock protein; LPS, lipopolysaccharide; MPEG, macrophage expressed gene; NADH, reduced nicotinamide adenine dinucleotide; NF-kB, nuclear factor kappa B; PKC, protein kinase C; PGRP, peptidoglycan recognition protein; RNS, reactive nitrogen species; ROS, reactive oxygen species; t-RNA, transfer ribonucleic acid; TEP, thioester-containing protein; TNF-α, tumor necrosis factor-alpha.

3. Transgenic Snail Methods for Schistosomiasis Control

The use of genetically engineered vectors to either suppress (reduce) or modify (replace) the natural populations of the biological vectors of some globally important infectious diseases has been a convincing concept that is now on the verge of deployment to control disease transmission. This rapidly emerging genetic control approach is distinguished from other biocontrol strategies (such as the use of natural parasitoids, predators, competitors, and infectious microbial agents), as it is mating-based, highly species-specific, and capable of being transmitted or inherited vertically [83]. In this context, suppression or elimination of natural local vector populations could be achieved by releasing transgenic vectors carrying sterile or detrimental characters into the local populations, while the population modification approach requires the release of transgenic pathogen-resistant vector strains or species. Depending on their characteristics or specific configurations, genetic methods for transgenic vector control may be self-limiting with transient persistence among subsequent vector generations unless replenished by repeated release of engineered vectors, or self-sustaining with indefinite persistence from the initial target population to the subsequent ones [83]. With revolutions in biotechnology, the use of gene drive systems (self-sustaining, selfish genetic elements that are inherited by progenies at frequencies largely exceeding those expected in Mendelian inheritance) has become an attractive method for vector control applications, as gene drivers are invasive wherever present, and so may overcome some evolutionary constraints [83,84].

As first proposed in 1958 [85], much emphasis has been placed on the use of genetic biocontrol for schistosomiasis vector control. To select a suitable transgenic vector method for schistosomiasis control however, the basics of the biology of the snail vectors must be taken into account. Although a wealth of genetic studies has been centered on the production of transgenic mosquito vectors of human diseases, biological differences between these dipterans and schistosomiasis molluscan vectors create the need for selective transgenic vector strategies for schistosomiasis control application. For example, unlike in mosquitoes where only females are capable of transmitting pathogens, *Biomphalaria* and *Bulinus* are hermaphrodites capable of self- or cross-fertilization [86], and all mating types serve as hosts for schistosomes. *Oncomelania* has separate sexes [86] but nevertheless, both sexes can also carry *S. japonicum*, only perhaps at varying degree of susceptibility [87,88]. These biological peculiarities render population reduction strategies unsuitable for genetic control of the snail hosts. This is because the newly released transgenic snails carrying harmful characters would remain susceptible to *Schistosoma* infections, therefore intensifying parasite transmission. Consequently, present focus in the genetic control of schistosomiasis vectors is set on strategies to modify the natural snail populations. According to Hubendick [85], population of the resistant strains can displace that of the susceptible ones in the field by natural selection. Although this scenario is plausible, it can be realized only through the application of self-sustaining transgenic vector systems (Figure 1).

Promoted by its advantages over other gene drive systems—such as transcription activator-like effector nucleases (TALENs) and zinc finger nucleases (ZFNs)—used in genome editing technology, and over other genetic techniques such as RNA interference (RNAi) [84,89,90], the recently-discovered CRISPR/Cas9 (clustered regularly-interspaced short palindromic repeats/CRISPR-associated protein 9) system has flowered, and is being widely used in current research trials and applications to modify genome sequences in diverse species spanning microbes, plants, animals, to even humans [89–93]. In parallel, the use of CRISPR/Cas9 to drive anti-*Schistosoma* effector genes into the genome of naturally susceptible snail strains is being envisioned, and has become an important subject in current discussions [17,75,94,95]. Fascinatingly, a proof-of-concept study [96] has demonstrated the possibility of CRISPR/Cas9-mediated gene editing in molluscs; indeed, more insights into the possible ways by which this may be achieved for schistosomiasis vector control, as well as the current and potential future challenges, will constitute a key guide for the scientific community in the appropriate fostering of this tantalizing approach in snail molecular research.

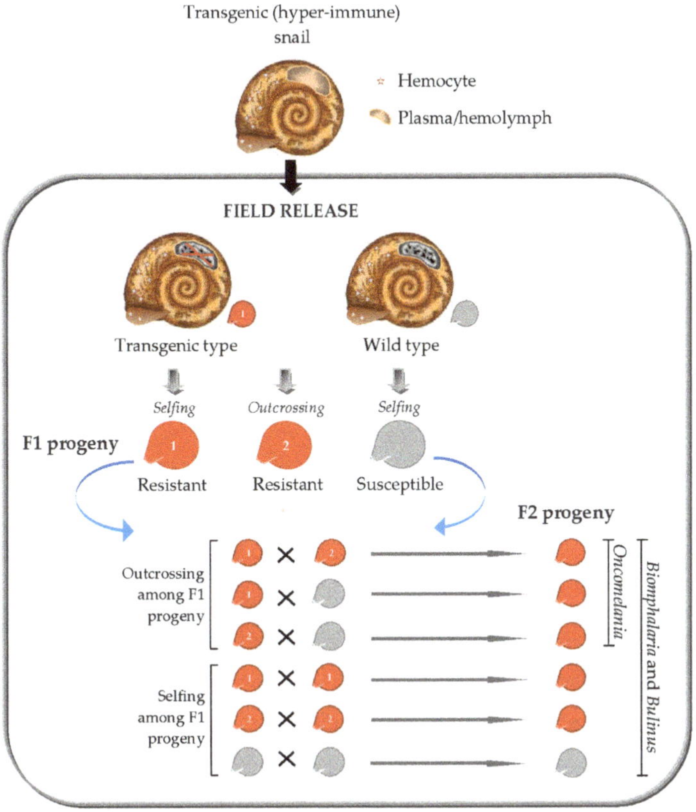

Figure 1. Transgenic snail system for field control of schistosomiasis transmission.

The three basic requirements for a CRISPR-based precise gene knock-in editing are Cas9 endonuclease, single-guide RNA (sgRNA), and repair template DNA (donor). The Cas9 enzyme combs through the genome of the host organism, acting as the 'molecular scissors' that cuts a specific DNA sequence at a genomic locus. The sgRNA (~20 nucleotides) is designed to match and target the desired DNA sequence to be deleted, while the donor DNA provides a template for genomic repair of the cleaved locus [92,97]. In the case of schistosomiasis snail vectors, Cas9-mediated introgression of refractoriness into susceptible strains will require an engineered donor DNA encoding a locus known to confer resistance. The anti-*Schistosoma* donor DNA can be tightly anchored to the Cas9/sgRNA complex, and the entire cassette is co-injected with a viral vector, such as lentivirus [98], into the early single-cell stage embryos of the snail vectors (Figure 2). In essence, the viral vector ensures safe and effective delivery of these components into the nuclei of the target cells. Suitable sites for the driver–cargo system injection may include the ovotestis of *Biomphalaria*/*Bulinus* snails and the ovary of female *Oncomelania* snails. In *Biomphalaria*, the ovotestis is located at the tip of the shell spire [99] and the driver–cargo system insertion into the ovotestis will be more appealing in the albino strain, as the transparency of the snail shell allows easy visibility of internal organs. Further analyses to assess targeting efficiency or screen for transgenic mutants among progenies may be done by T7 endonuclease I (T7E1) assay, restriction enzyme assay, next generation sequencing or direct PCR assay as applicable (Figure 2).

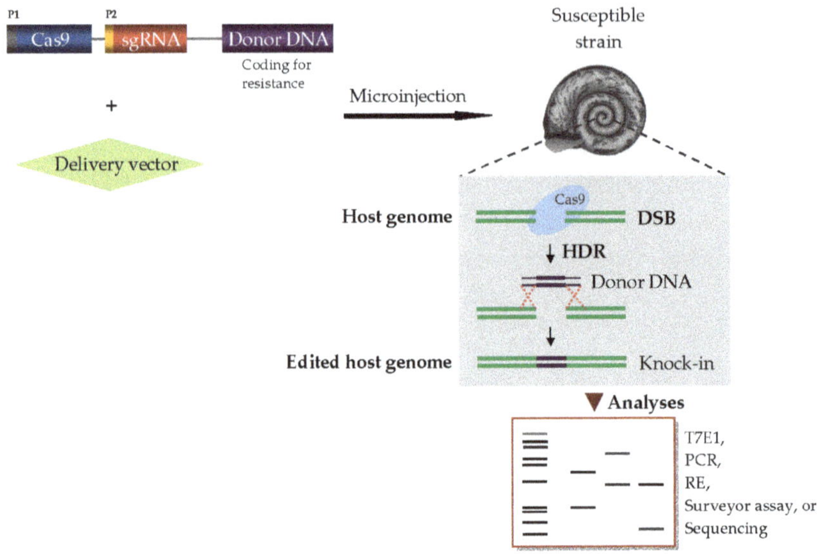

Figure 2. A schematic representation of CRISPR/Cas9 genome editing system in a snail vector of schistosome. Abbreviations: DSB, double-strand break; HDR, homology-directed repair; P1 & P2, promoters; PCR, polymerase chain reaction; RE, restriction enzyme; T7E1, T7 endonuclease I.

To date, the main genetic loci that have been identified in association with *B. glabrata* resistance to schistosome are *Sod1* and *RADres* (a restricted-site associated DNA-determined resistance locus) [50,68,69], and a *GRC* (Guadeloupe Resistance Complex) genomic region (<1 Mb) [69]. In combination with other known and yet unknown resistance genes, *Sod1* and *RADres* occupy haplotype blocks of >2 Mb genomic region [69,100]. Although putative functional gene candidates have been identified in the *GRC* region [75,95], the *Sod1* and *RADres* regions appear to demonstrate a wider spectrum of snail resistance [69]. Nevertheless, there is still a need to further narrow down these regions to the embedding causative genes, and to understand their immune stability and functions under different genetic backgrounds and environmental conditions.

4. Further Considerations

An early investigator [101] stated that the genetic factors controlling snail insusceptibility to schistosomes must first be clarified, and snail strains ferrying only refractory traits must be developed before we can gainfully engage genetic control methods. The first criterion has largely been met through relentless research unveiling resistance-determining proteins and genes. Despite these advances, current stumbling blocks involve developing snail strains that are reliably recalcitrant to schistosome infection. One major bottleneck is the highly variable strain-by-strain interaction—compatibility polymorphism—that is well-documented to occur in snail-schistosome systems [102,103]. As a consequence, developing a transgenic target for individual strain-to-strain combinations becomes cumbersome, but can be circumvented only if genetic loci with wide-spectrum resistance activities conserved across various strain-to-strain combinations could be identified and characterized. The BS-90 strain of *B. glabrata* (isolated in Salvadore, Brazil) has been bred in the laboratory for many years and has been shown to be steadily resistant; however, its relative performance in the field remains unpredictable. A tenable reason for this is that generations of the laboratory-bred strains are poor representatives of the genetic variations that actually occur in the original wild populations [103]. Another caveat in the future use of either the resistant BS-90 or transgenic snail strains is global warming, characterized by an increasing earth's average surface temperature. In sharp contrast to what was earlier known, Knight et al. [78] showed that snail resistance to schistosomes is also temperature-dependent, and even the naturally resistant BS-90 strain could be rendered susceptible at 32 °C. Other local environmental factors such as altitude, water level, soil, and vegetation may also cause differential gene expression and regulation among snails of the same species as a result of local adaptation mechanisms [104].

Organism biodiversity and signatures of interactions between other organisms and the snail vectors living in the same habitat may also impact the outcome of transgenic snail application. In an ecological milieu where natural predators [e.g., *Macrobrachium vollenhovenii* (a freshwater prawn), *Procambarus clarkia* (a freshwater crayfish), *Marisa cornuarietis* (an ampullarid snail), and cichlid fishes such as *Trematocranus placodon* and *Geophagus brasiliensis*] or competitors [e.g., thiarid snails such as *Melanoides tuberculata* and *Tarebia granifera*] of the snail vectors of schistosomiasis [4,24] exist in meaningful abundance, there is a possibility that the population of the released transgenic snails becomes reduced below levels required to displace that of the naturally susceptible vectors as a result of a more biased killing/eating of the transgenic snails (and eating of their egg masses) or deprivation of resources. When such a scenario operates, the resistance effect tapers off. Given this contingency, the release of transgenic snails may be chosen only in lieu of introducing predators or competitors of snail vectors; co-implementation of both methods in the same freshwater focus may not always complement the transgenic snail approach. In foci where populations of predators or competitors already occur in significant abundance, one-off niclosamide application prior to the release of transgenic snails may offer a more palatable approach in reducing the probability of diluted effect of the transgenic snail release. These phenomena highlight the importance of sampling water habitats for species diversity prior to, and periodically after, releasing transgenic snails.

The merits of using schistosome-resistant transgenic snails beat the limitations of other biological and environmental interventions. For instance, populations of molluscivorous fishes and prawns large enough to eat the snail vectors may rapidly diminish due to indiscriminate fishing by residents of communities where schistosomiasis is endemic, since these molluscivores are also a major source of food for humans. Moreover, introduction of competitor species of snails could greatly endanger agriculture and the ecosystem. On the other hand, environmental modifications (such as removal of vegetation on which the snail vectors feed, lining canals with cement, or draining water habitats) are very expensive and impractical for resource-constrained areas. Meanwhile, vegetation removal poses an increased risk of infection to workers who may not have protective tools [24]. Generally, however, certain issues concerning the use of gene drive systems have come into view. The most important of all include potential off-target mutations that may result in unpredictable effects, development of drive resistance in populations, fitness and competitiveness of released strains compared to wild populations, and possible difficulty in the containment, reversal, or adjustment of gene drive spread [83,84,105]. Nevertheless, it is somewhat relieving that a good number of these limitations can feasibly be overcome through the meticulous design of more specific sgRNAs, and development of reversal drive systems [84,89,91,92,97,105]. Moreover, the majority of the current issues regarding the application of gene drives for the control of disease vectors arose from studies focusing on mosquitoes, implying that some of the risk issues, such as vector dispersal beyond intended political boundaries [84], may be of lesser concern in other non-insect vector control systems. Conversely however, the significant body of research on mosquitoes may have also overcome some series of technical challenges that may remain unresolved for other disease vectors.

Should a breakthrough on the use of CRISPR-based vector control occur, the fine line between mating/reproductive biology of *Oncomelania* and that of *Bulinus* or *Biomphalaria*, as well as the varying degree of selfing among species of the hermaphroditic (*Bulinus* and *Biomphalaria*) snail vectors, will also have important implications in schistosomiasis snail control application. As shown in Figure 1, CRISPR/Cas9-driven resistance traits may spread more rapidly among successive progeny of *Oncomelania* (being a dioecious outcrossing vector) than in *Bulinus* and *Biomphalaria* snail vectors. More precisely, in the two latter snail vectors, gene drive approach may not be effective in predominantly selfing species, such as *Bulinus truncatus*, *Bulinus forskalii*, and *Biomphalaria pfeifferi*.

5. Conclusions

The prospective use of genetically manipulated vectors to stop the spread of vector-borne diseases maintains its impressiveness and is awaited by the scientific community. In fast-tracking sustainable schistosomiasis elimination, the use of CRISPR-based vector modification strategy appears fascinating and potentially effective. However, this approach is currently still underdeveloped in snail molecular research. Finding the pertinent missing pieces in our jigsaw of knowledge of schistosome/snail biology, and identifying ways to bypass potential future challenges, are requisites for achieving this promising snail control strategy. Finally, the use of schistosome-resistant transgenic snails may have the propensity to singly interrupt schistosomiasis transmission when only outcrossing vector species are present, but in foci where both predominantly selfing species and outcrossing species of *Bulinus* or *Biomphalaria* snails coexist, the integration of additional suitable snail control methods will provide a way of complementing this genetic control method for more effective outcomes.

Funding: This research received no external funding.

Acknowledgments: The author would like to thank Officer Adewale Adeniyi of the Nigerian Customs Service (NCS) for his financial assistance.

Conflicts of Interest: The author declares no conflict of interest.

References

1. World Health Organization. Schistosomiasis and soil-transmitted helminthiasis: Number of people treated in 2016. *Wkly. Epidemiol. Rec.* **2017**, *92*, 49–60.
2. World Health Organization. *Global Health Estimates Summary Tables. DALYs by Cause, Age and Sex, by WHO Region, 2000–2015*; World Health Organization: Geneva, Switzerland, 2016.
3. Colley, D.G.; Bustinduy, A.L.; Secor, W.E.; King, C.H. Human schistosomiasis. *Lancet* **2014**, *383*, 2253–2264. [CrossRef]
4. Muller, R.; Wakelin, D. *Worms and Human Disease*, 2nd ed.; CABI Publishing: Oxon, UK; New York, NY, USA, 2002; pp. 1–300.
5. Adenowo, A.B.; Oyinloye, B.E.; Ogunyinka, B.I.; Kappo, A.B. Impact of human schistosomiasis in sub-Saharan Africa. *Braz. J. Infect. Dis.* **2015**, *19*, 196–205. [CrossRef] [PubMed]
6. Famakinde, D.O. Molecular context of *Schistosoma mansoni* transmission in the molluscan environments: A mini-review. *Acta Trop.* **2017**, *176*, 98–104. [CrossRef] [PubMed]
7. Olveda, D.U.; Li, Y.; Olveda, R.M.; Lam, A.K.; Chau, T.N.P.; Harn, D.A.; Williams, G.M.; Gray, D.J.; Ross, A.G.P. Bilharzia: Pathology, diagnosis, management and control. *Trop. Med. Surg.* **2013**, *1*, 135. [CrossRef] [PubMed]
8. Colley, D.G.; Secor, W.E. Immunology of human schistosomiasis. *Parasite Immunol.* **2014**, *36*, 347–357. [CrossRef] [PubMed]
9. Friedman, J.F.; Mital, P.; Kanzaria, H.K.; Olds, G.R.; Kurtis, J.D. Schistosomiasis and pregnancy. *Trends Parasitol.* **2007**, *23*, 159–164. [CrossRef] [PubMed]
10. Salawu, O.T.; Odaibo, A.B. Maternal schistosomiasis: A growing concern in sub-Saharan Africa. *Pathog. Glob. Health* **2014**, *108*, 263–270. [CrossRef] [PubMed]
11. Kjetland, E.F.; Ndhlovu, P.D.; Gomo, E.; Mduluza, T.; Midzi, N.; Gwanzura, L.; Mason, P.R.; Sandvik, L.; Friis, H.; Gunderseen, S.G. Association between genital schistosomiasis and HIV in rural Zimbabwean women. *AIDS* **2006**, *20*, 593–600. [CrossRef] [PubMed]
12. Mbabazi, P.S.; Andan, O.; Fitzgerald, D.W.; Chitsulo, L.; Engels, D.; Downs, J.A. Examining the relationship between urogenital schistosomiasis and HIV infection. *PLoS Negl. Trop. Dis.* **2011**, *5*, e1396. [CrossRef] [PubMed]
13. Bustinduy, A.; King, C.; Scott, J.; Appleton, S.; Sousa-Figueiredo, J.C.; Betson, M.; Stothard, J.R. HIV and schistosomiasis co-infection in African children. *Lancet Infect. Dis.* **2014**, *14*, 640–649. [CrossRef]

14. Tchuenté, L.-A.T.; Rollinson, D.; Stothard, J.R.; Molyneux, D. Moving from control to elimination of schistosomiasis in sub-Saharan Africa: Time to change and adapt strategies. *Infect. Dis. Poverty* **2017**, *6*, 42. [CrossRef] [PubMed]
15. King, C.H.; Sutherland, L.J.; Bertsch, D. Systematic review and meta-analysis of the impact of chemical-based mollusciciding for control of *Schistosoma mansoni* and *S. haematobium* transmission. *PLoS Negl. Trop. Dis.* **2015**, *9*, e0004290. [CrossRef] [PubMed]
16. Lo, N.C.; Gurarie, D.; Toon, N.; Coulibaly, J.T.; Bendavid, E.; Andrews, J.R.; King, C.H. Impact and cost-effectiveness of snail control to achieve disease control targets for schistosomiasis. *Proc. Natl. Acad. Sci. USA* **2018**, *115*, E584–E591. [CrossRef] [PubMed]
17. Sokolow, S.H.; Wood, C.L.; Jones, I.J.; Lafferty, K.D.; Kuris, A.M.; Hseih, M.H.; De Loe, G.A. To reduce the global burden of human schistosomiasis, use 'old fashioned' snail control. *Trends Parasitol.* **2018**, *34*, 23–40. [CrossRef] [PubMed]
18. Sokolow, S.H.; Wood, C.L.; Jones, I.J.; Swartz, S.J.; Lopez, M.; Hseih, M.H.; Lafferty, K.D.; Kuris, A.M.; Rickards, C.; De Leo, G.A. Global assessment of schistosomiasis control over the past century shows targeting the snail intermediate host works best. *PLoS. Negl. Trop. Dis.* **2016**, *10*, e0004794. [CrossRef] [PubMed]
19. Alsaqabi, S.M.; Lofty, W.M. Praziquantel: A review. *J. Vet. Sci. Technol.* **2014**, *5*, 1000200. [CrossRef]
20. Cioli, D.; Pica-Mattoccia, L.; Basso, A.; Guidi, A. Schistosomiasis control: Praziquantel forever? *Mol. Biochem. Parasitol.* **2014**, *195*, 23–29. [CrossRef] [PubMed]
21. Tebeje, B.M.; Harvie, M.; You, H.; Loukas, A.; McManus, D.P. Schistosomiasis vaccines: Where do we stand? *Parasit. Vectors* **2016**, *9*, 528. [CrossRef] [PubMed]
22. Ebisawa, I. Epidemiology and eradication of schistosomiasis japonica in Japan. *J. Travel Med.* **1998**, *5*, 33–35. [CrossRef] [PubMed]
23. Barakat, R.M.R. Epidemiology of schistosomiasis in Egypt: Travel through time: Review. *J. Adv. Res.* **2013**, *4*, 425–432. [CrossRef] [PubMed]
24. Secor, W.E. Water-based interventions for schistosomiasis control. *Pathog. Glob. Health* **2014**, *108*, 246–254. [CrossRef] [PubMed]
25. Tlamçani, Z.; Er-Rami, M. Schistosomiasis control: Moroccan experience compared to other endemic countries. *Asian Pac. J. Trop. Dis.* **2014**, *4*, 329–332. [CrossRef]
26. King, C.H.; Bertsch, D. Historical perspective: Snail control to prevent schistosomiasis. *PLoS Negl. Trop. Dis.* **2015**, *9*, e0003657. [CrossRef] [PubMed]
27. Sun, L.P.; Wang, W.; Hong, Q.B.; Li, S.Z.; Liang, Y.S.; Yang, H.T.; Zhou, X.N. Approaches being used in the national schistosomiasis elimination programme in China: A review. *Infect. Dis. Poverty* **2017**, *6*, 55. [CrossRef] [PubMed]
28. Lardans, V.; Dissous, C. Snail control strategies for reduction of schistosomiasis transmission. *Parasitol. Today* **1998**, *14*, 413–417. [CrossRef]
29. Huang, D.; Zhen, J.; Quan, S.; Liu, M.; Liu, L. Risk assessment for niclosamide residues in water and sediments from Nan Ji Shan Island within Poyang Lake region, China. *Adv. Mat. Res.* **2013**, *721*, 608–612. [CrossRef]
30. World Health Organization. *Field Use of Molluscicides in Schistosomiasis Control Programmes: An Operational Manual for Programme Managers*; World Health Organization: Geneva, Switzerland, 2017.
31. World Health Assembly. Elimination of Schistosomiasis. In *Sixty-fifth World Health Assembly: Resolutions and Decisions*; World Health Organization: Geneva, Switzerland, 2012; pp. 36–37.
32. Miyairi, K.; Suzuki, M. On the development of *Schistosoma japonicum*. *Tokyo Med. J.* **1913**, *1836*, 1961–1965.
33. Tanaka, H.; Tsuji, M. From discovery to eradication of schistosomiasis in Japan: 1847–1996. *Int. J. Parasitol.* **1997**, *27*, 1465–1480. [CrossRef]
34. Leiper, R.T. On the relation between the terminal-spined and lateral-spined eggs of bilharzia. *Br. Med. J.* **1916**, *1*, 411. [CrossRef] [PubMed]
35. Leiper, R.T. Report on the results of the bilharzias mission in Egypt, 1915. *J. R. Army Med. Corps* **1918**, *30*, 235–260.
36. Newton, W.L. The comparative tissue reaction of two strains of *Australorbis glabratus* to infection with *Schistosoma mansoni*. *J. Parasitol.* **1952**, *38*, 362–366. [CrossRef] [PubMed]

37. Newton, W.L. The inheritance of susceptibility to infection with *Schistosoma mansoni* in *Australorbis glabratus*. *Exp. Parasitol.* **1953**, *2*, 242–257. [CrossRef]
38. Richards, C.S. Genetic studies of a molluscan vector of schistosomiasis. *Nature* **1970**, *227*, 231–241. [CrossRef]
39. Richards, C.S. Genetic factors in susceptibility of *Biomphalaria glabrata* for different strains of *Schistosoma mansoni*. *Parasitology* **1975**, *70*, 231–241. [CrossRef] [PubMed]
40. Richards, C.S. *Schistosoma mansoni*: susceptibility reversal with age in the snail host. *Exp. Parasitol.* **1977**, *42*, 165–168. [CrossRef]
41. Richards, C.S.; Knight, M.; Lewis, F.A. Genetics of *Biomphalaria glabrata* and its effects on the outcome of *Schistosoma mansoni* infection. *Parasitol. Today* **1992**, *8*, 171–174. [CrossRef]
42. Abou-El-Naga, I.F.; Eissa, M.M.; Mossallam, S.F.; El-Halim, S.I.A. Inheritance of *Schistosoma mansoni* infection incompatibility in *Biomphalaria alexandrina* snails. *Mem. do Inst. Oswaldo Cruz* **2010**, *105*, 149–154. [CrossRef]
43. Dos Santos, M.B.L.; Freitas, J.R.; Correia, M.C.R.; Coelho, P.M.Z. Susceptibility of *Biomphalaria tenagophila* hybrids to *Schistosoma mansoni*: Crossing between strains from Taim (RS), Cabo Frio (RJ), and Belo Horizonte (MG), Brasil. *Rev. Inst. de Med. Trop. São Paulo* **1979**, *21*, 281–286.
44. Knight, M.; Miller, A.N.; Patterson, C.N.; Rowe, C.G.; Michaels, G.; Carr, D.; Richards, C.S.; Lewis, F.A. The identification of markers segregating with resistance to *Schistosoma mansoni* infection in the snail *Biomphalaria glabrata*. *Proc. Natl. Acad. Sci. USA* **1999**, *96*, 1510–1515. [CrossRef] [PubMed]
45. Rosa, F.M.; Godard, A.L.B.; Azevedo, V.; Coelho, P.M.Z. *Biomphalaria tenagophila*: dominant character of the resistance to *Schistosoma mansoni* in descendants of crossbreedings between resistant (Taim, RS) and susceptible (Joinville, SC) strains. *Mem. do Inst. Oswaldo Cruz* **2005**, *100*, 19–23. [CrossRef]
46. Haggag, S.H.; El-Sherbiny, M. Molecular markers associated with resistance to *Schistosoma mansoni* infection in the *Biomphalaria glabrata* snails. *Biotechnology* **2006**, *5*, 404–412.
47. Ittiprasert, W.; Miller, A.; Myers, J.; Nene, V.; El-Sayed, N.M.; Knight, M. Identification of immediate response genes dominantly expressed in juvenile resistant and susceptible *Biomphalaria glabrata* snails upon exposure to *Schistosoma mansoni*. *Mol. Biochem. Parasitol.* **2010**, *169*, 27–39. [CrossRef] [PubMed]
48. Paraense, W.L.; Correa, L.R. Variation in susceptibility of populations of *Australorbis glabratus* to a strain of *Schistosoma mansoni*. *Rev. Inst. Med. Trop. São Paulo* **1963**, *5*, 15–22. [PubMed]
49. Richards, C.S. Susceptibility of adult *Biomphalaria glabrata* to *Schistosoma mansoni* infection. *Am. J. Trop. Med. Hyg.* **1973**, *22*, 748–756. [CrossRef] [PubMed]
50. Goodall, C.P.; Bender, R.C.; Brooks, J.K.; Bayne, C.J. *Biomphalaria glabrata* cytosolic copper/zinc superoxide dismutase (SOD1) gene: Association of SOD1 alleles with resistance/susceptibility to *Schistosoma mansoni*. *Mol. Biochem. Parasitol.* **2006**, *147*, 207–210. [CrossRef] [PubMed]
51. Newton, W.L. The establishment of a strain of *Australorbis glabratus* which combines albinism and high susceptibility to infection with *Schistosoma mansoni*. *J. Parasitol.* **1955**, *41*, 526–528. [CrossRef] [PubMed]
52. Adema, C.M.; Luo, M.Z.; Hanelt, B.; Hertel, L.A.; Marshall, J.J.; Zhang, S.M.; DeJong, R.J.; Kim, H.R.; Kudrna, D.; Wing, R.A.; et al. A bacterial artificial chromosome library for *Biomphalaria glabrata*, intermediate snail host of *Schistosoma mansoni*. *Mem. Inst. Oswaldo Cruz* **2006**, *101*, S167–S177. [CrossRef]
53. Ittiprasert, W.; Myers, J.; Odoemelam, E.C.; Raghavan, N.; Lewis, F.; Bridger, J.M.; Knight, M. Advances in the genomics and proteomics of the freshwater intermediate snail host of *Schistosoma mansoni*, *Biomphalaria glabrata*. In *Biomphalaria Snails and Larval Trematodes*; Toledo, R., Fried, B., Eds.; Springer: New York, NY, USA, 2011; pp. 191–213.
54. Pinaud, S.; Portela, J.; Duval, D.; Nowacki, F.C.; Olive, M.A.; Allienne, J.F.; Galinier, R.; Dheilly, N.M.; Kieffer-Jaquinod, S.; Mitta, G.; et al. A shift from cellular to humoral responses contributes to innate immune memory in the vector snail *Biomphalaria glabrata*. *PLoS Pathog.* **2016**, *12*, e1005361. [CrossRef] [PubMed]
55. Yoshino, T.P.; Coustau, C. Immunobiology of *Biomphalaria*–trematode interactions. In *Biomphalaria Snails and Larval Trematodes*; Toledo, R., Fried, B., Eds.; Springer: New York, NY, USA, 2011; pp. 159–189.
56. Pila, E.A.; Li, H.; Hambrook, J.R.; Wu, X.; Hanington, P. Schistosomiasis from a snail's perspective: Advances in snail immunity. *Trends Parasitol.* **2017**, *33*, 845–857. [CrossRef] [PubMed]
57. Hansen, E.L. A cell line from embryos of *Biomphalaria glabrata* (Pulmonata): Establishment and characteristics. In *Invertebrate Tissue Culture: Research Applications*; Maramorosch, K., Ed.; Academic Press: New York, NY, USA, 1976; pp. 75–97.

58. Adema, C.M.; Hillier, L.D.W.; Jones, C.S.; Loker, E.S.; Knight, M.; Minx, P.; Oliveira, G.; Raghavan, N.; Shedlock, A.; do Amaral, L.R.; et al. Whole genome analysis of a schistosomiasis-transmitting freshwater snail. *Nat. Comm.* **2017**, *8*, 15451. [CrossRef] [PubMed]
59. Zahoor, Z.; Lockyer, A.E.; Davies, A.J.; Kirk, R.S.; Emery, A.M.; Rollinson, D.; Jones, C.S.; Noble, L.R.; Walker, A.J. Differences in the gene expression profiles of haemocytes from schistosome-susceptible and -resistant *Biomphalaria glabrata* exposed to *Schistosoma mansoni* excretory secretory products. *PLoS ONE* **2014**, *9*, e93215. [CrossRef] [PubMed]
60. Larson, M.K.; Bender, R.C.; Bayne, C.J. Resistance of *Biomphalaria glabrata* 13–16-R1 snails to *Schistosoma mansoni* PR1 is a function of haemocyte abundance and constitutive levels of specific transcripts in haemocytes. *Int. J. Parasitol.* **2014**, *44*, 343–353. [CrossRef] [PubMed]
61. Pila, E.A.; Gordy, M.A.; Phillips, V.K.; Kabore, A.L.; Rudkom, S.P.; Hanington, P.C. Endogenous growth factor stimulation of hemocyte proliferation induces resistance to *Schistosoma mansoni* challenge in the snail host. *Proc. Natl. Acad. Sci. USA* **2016**, *113*, 5305–5310. [CrossRef] [PubMed]
62. Garcia, A.B.; Pierce, R.J.; Gourbal, B.; Werkmeister, E.; Colinet, D.; Reichhart, J.; Dissous, C.; Coustau, C. Involvement of the cytokine MIF in the snail host immune response to the parasite *Schistosoma mansoni*. *PLoS Pathog.* **2010**, *6*, e1001115.
63. Pila, E.A.; Tarrabain, M.; Kabore, A.L.; Hanington, P.C. A novel toll-like receptor (TLR) influences compatibility between the gastropod *Biomphalaria glabrata*, and the digenean trematode *Schistosoma mansoni*. *PLoS Pathog.* **2016**, *12*, e1005513. [CrossRef] [PubMed]
64. Galinier, R.; Portela, J.; Mone, Y.; Allienne, J.F.; Henri, H.; Delbecq, S.; Mitta, G.; Gourbal, B.; Duval, D. Biomphalysin, a new β pore-forming toxin involved in *Biomphalaria glabrata* immune defense against *Schistosoma mansoni*. *PLoS Pathog.* **2013**, *9*, e1003216. [CrossRef] [PubMed]
65. Myers, J.; Ittiprasert, N.; Raghavan, N.; Miller, A.; Knight, M. Differences in cysteine protease activity in *Schistosoma mansoni*-resistant and -susceptible *Biomphalaria glabrata* and characterization of the hepatopancreas cathepsin B fulllength cDNA. *J. Parasitol.* **2008**, *94*, 659–668. [CrossRef] [PubMed]
66. Lockyer, A.E.; Spinks, J.; Kane, R.A.; Hoffmann, K.F.; Fitzpatrick, J.M.; Rollinson, D.; Noble, L.R.; Jones, C.S. *Biomphalaria glabrata* transcriptome: cDNA microarray profiling identifies resistant- and susceptible-specific gene expression in haemocytes from snail strains exposed to *Schistosoma mansoni*. *BMC Genomics* **2008**, *9*, 634. [CrossRef] [PubMed]
67. Wu, X.; Dinguirard, N.; Sabat, G.; Lui, H.; Gonzalez, L.; Gehring, M.; Bickham-Wright, U.; Yoshino, T.P. Proteomic analysis of *Biomphalaria glabrata* plasma proteins with binding affinity to those expressed by early developing larval *Schistosoma mansoni*. *PLoS Pathog.* **2017**, *13*, e1006081. [CrossRef] [PubMed]
68. Bonner, K.M.; Bayne, C.J.; Larson, M.K.; Blouin, M.S. Effects of Cu/Zn superoxide dismutase (*sod1*) genotype and genetic background on growth, reproduction and defense in *Biomphalaria glabrata*. *PLoS Negl. Trop. Dis.* **2012**, *6*, e1701. [CrossRef] [PubMed]
69. Tennessen, J.A.; Bonner, K.M.; Bollmann, S.R.; Johnstun, J.A.; Yeh, J.Y.; Marine, M.; Tavalire, H.F.; Bayne, C.J.; Blouin, M.S. Genome-wide scan and test of candidate genes in the snail *Biomphalaria glabrata* reveal new locus influencing resistance to *Schistosoma mansoni*. *PLoSNegl. Trop. Dis.* **2015**, *9*, e0004077. [CrossRef] [PubMed]
70. Lockyer, A.E.; Emery, A.M.; Kane, R.A.; Walker, A.J.; Mayer, C.D.; Mitta, G.; Coustau, C.; Adema, C.M.; Hanelt, B.; Rollinson, D.; et al. Early differential gene expression in haemocytes from resistant and susceptible *Biomphalaria glabrata* strains in response to *Schistosoma mansoni*. *PLoS ONE* **2012**, *7*, e51102. [CrossRef] [PubMed]
71. Nowak, T.S.; Woodards, A.C.; Jung, Y.; Adema, C.M.; Loker, E.S. Identification of transcripts generated during the response of resistant *Biomphalaria glabrata* to *Schistosoma mansoni* infection using suppression subtractive hybridization. *J. Parasitol.* **2004**, *90*, 1034–1040. [CrossRef] [PubMed]
72. Hanington, P.C.; Forys, M.A.; Dragoo, J.W.; Zhang, S.; Adema, C.M.; Loker, E.S. Role for a somatically diversified lectin in resistance of an invertebrate to parasite infection. *Proc. Natl. Acad. Sci. USA* **2010**, *107*, 21087–21092. [CrossRef] [PubMed]
73. Hanington, P.C.; Forys, M.A.; Loker, E.S. A somatically diversified defense factor, FREP3, is a determinant of snail resistance to schistosome infection. *PLoS Negl. Trop. Dis.* **2012**, *6*, e1591. [CrossRef] [PubMed]

74. Martins-Souza, R.L.; Pereira, C.A.J.; Rodrigues, L.; Araújo, E.S.; Coelho, P.M.Z.; Corrêa, A., Jr.; Negrão-Corrêa, D. Participation of N-acetyl-D-glucosamine carbohydrate moieties in the recognition of *Schistosoma mansoni* sporocysts by haemocytes of *Biomphalaria tenagophila*. *Mem. Inst. Oswaldo Cruz* **2011**, *106*, 884–891. [CrossRef] [PubMed]
75. Allan, E.R.O.; Tennessen, J.A.; Bollmann, S.R.; Hanington, P.C.; Bayne, C.J.; Blouin, M.S. Schistosome infectivity in the snail, *Biomphalaria glabrata*, is partially dependent on the expression of Grctm6, a Guadeloupe Resistance Complex protein. *PLoS Negl. Trop. Dis.* **2017**, *11*, e0005362. [CrossRef] [PubMed]
76. Ittiprasert, W.; Knight, M. Reversing the resistance phenotype of the *Biomphalaria glabrata* snail host *Schistosoma mansoni* infection by temperature modulation. *PLoS Pathog.* **2012**, *8*, e1002677. [CrossRef] [PubMed]
77. Ittiprasert, W.; Nene, R.; Miller, A.; Raghavan, N.; Lewis, F.; Hodgson, J.; Knight, M. *Schistosoma mansoni* infection of juvenile *Biomphalaria glabrata* induces a differential stress response between resistant and susceptible snails. *Exp. Parasitol.* **2009**, *123*, 203–211. [CrossRef] [PubMed]
78. Knight, M.; Elhelu, O.; Smith, M.; Haugen, B.; Miller, A.; Raghavan, N.; Wellman, C.; Cousin, C.; Dixon, F.; Mann, V.; et al. Susceptibility of snails to infection with schistosomes is influenced by temperature and expression of heat shock proteins. *Epidemiology* **2015**, *5*, 1–18.
79. Granath, W.O., Jr.; Connors, V.A.; Tarleton, R.L. Interleukin 1 activity haemolymph from strains of the snail *Biomphalaria glabrata* varying in susceptibility to the human blood fluke, *Schistosoma mansoni*: Presence, differential expression, and biological function. *Cytokine* **1994**, *6*, 21–27. [CrossRef]
80. Zhang, S.M.; Coultas, K.A. Identification and characterization of five transcription factors that are associated with evolutionarily conserved immune signaling pathways in the schistosome-transmitting snail *Biomphalaria glabrata*. *Mol. Immunol.* **2011**, *48*, 1868–1881. [CrossRef] [PubMed]
81. Knight, M.; Raghavan, N.; Goodal, C.; Cousin, C.; Ittiprasert, W.; Sayed, A.; Miller, A.; Williams, D.L.; Bayne, C. *Biomphalaria glabrata* peroxiredoxin: effect of *Schistosoma mansoni* infection on differential gene regulation. *Mol. Biochem. Parasitol.* **2009**, *167*, 20–31. [CrossRef] [PubMed]
82. Ouwe-Missi-Oukem-Boyer, O.; Porchet, E.; Capron, A.; Dissous, C. Characterization of immunoreactive TNF-α molecules in the gastropod *Biomphalaria glabrata*. *Dev. Comp. Immunol.* **1994**, *18*, 211–218. [CrossRef]
83. Alphey, L. Genetic control of mosquitoes. *Annu. Rev. Emtomol.* **2014**, *59*, 205–224. [CrossRef] [PubMed]
84. Macias, V.M.; Ohm, J.R.; Rasgon, J.L. Gene drive for mosquito control: Where did it come from and where are we headed? *Int. J. Environ. Res. Public Health* **2017**, *14*, 1006. [CrossRef] [PubMed]
85. Hubendick, B. A possible method of schistosome-vector control by competition between resistant and susceptible strains. *Bull. World Health Organ.* **1958**, *18*, 1113–1116. [PubMed]
86. Rozendaal, J.A.; World Health Organization. Freshwater snails. In *Vector Control: Methods for Use by Individuals and Communities*; World Health Organization: Geneva, Switzerland, 1997; pp. 337–356.
87. Claveria, F.G.; Etges, F.J. Differential susceptibility of male and female *Oncomelania hupensis quadrasi* infected with *Schistosoma japonicum*. *Int. J. Parasitol.* **1987**, *17*, 1273–1277. [CrossRef]
88. Moose, J.W.; Williams, J.E. Infection rates of *Schistosoma japonicum* in experimentally exposed female and male oncomelanid snails. *Jan. J. Med. Sci. Biol.* **1964**, *17*, 333–334. [CrossRef]
89. Sun, D.; Gou, Z.; Liu, Y.; Zhang, Y. Progress and prospects of CRISPR/Cas systems in insects and other arthropods. *Front. Physiol.* **2017**, *8*, 608. [CrossRef] [PubMed]
90. Zhang, Z.; Zhang, Y.; Gao, F.; Han, S.; Cheah, K.S.; Tse, H.F.; Lian, Q. CRISPR/Cas9 genome-editing system in human stem cells: Current status and future prospects. *Mol. Ther. Nucleic Acids* **2017**, *9*, 230–241. [CrossRef] [PubMed]
91. Singh, V.; Braddick, D.; Dhar, P.K. Exploring the potential of genome editing CRISPR-Cas9 technology. *Gene* **2017**, *599*, 1–18. [CrossRef] [PubMed]
92. Liu, X.; Wu, S.; Xu, J.; Suin, C.; Wei, J. Application of CRISPR/Cas9 in plant biology. *Acta Pharm. Sin. B* **2017**, *7*, 292–302. [CrossRef] [PubMed]
93. Cai, L.; Fisher, A.L.; Huang, H.; Xie, Z. CRISR-mediated genome editing and human diseases. *Genes Dis.* **2016**, *3*, 244–251. [CrossRef]
94. Mouahid, G.; Rognon, A.; de Carvalho-Augusto, R.; Driguez, P.; Geyer, K.; Karinshak, S.; Luviano, N.; Mann, V.; Quack, T.; Rawlinson, K.; et al. Transplantation of schistosome sporocysts between host snails: A video guide. *Wellcome Open Res.* **2018**, *3*, 3. [CrossRef] [PubMed]

95. Tennessen, J.A.; Théron, A.; Marine, M.; Yeh, J.Y.; Rognon, A.; Blouin, M.S. Hyperdiverse gene cluster in snail host conveys resistance to human schistosome parasites. *PLoS Genet.* **2015**, *11*, e1005067. [CrossRef] [PubMed]
96. Perry, K.J.; Henry, J.Q. CRISPR/Cas9-mediated genome modification in the mollusc, *Crepidula fornicata*. *Genesis* **2015**, *53*, 237–244. [CrossRef] [PubMed]
97. Bortesi, L.; Zhu, C.; Zischewski, J.; Perez, L.; Bassié, L.; Nadi, R.; Forni, G.; Lade, S.B.; Soto, E.; Jin, X.; et al. Patterns of CRISPR/Cas9 activity in plants, animals and microbes. *Plant Biotechnol. J.* **2016**, *14*, 2203–2216. [CrossRef] [PubMed]
98. Wang, L.; Li, F.; Dang, L.; Liang, D.; Wang, C.; He, B.; Liu, J.; Li, D.; Wu, X.; Xu, X.; et al. *In vivo* delivery systems for therapeutic genome editing. *Int. J. Mol. Sci.* **2016**, *17*, 626. [CrossRef] [PubMed]
99. Jarne, P.; Pointier, J.-P.; David, P. Biosystematics of *Biomphalaria* spp. with an emphasis on *Biomphalaria glabrata*. In *Biomphalaria Snails and Larval Trematodes*; Toledo, R., Fried, B., Eds.; Springer: New York, NY, USA, 2011; pp. 1–32.
100. Blouin, M.S.; Bonner, K.M.; Cooper, B.; Amarasinghe, V.; O'Donnell, R.P.; Bayne, C.J. Three genes involved in the oxidative burst are closely linked in the genome of the snail, *Biomphalaria glabrata*. *Int. J. Parasitol.* **2013**, *43*, 51–55. [CrossRef] [PubMed]
101. Berg, C.O. Biological control of snail-borne diseases: A review. *Exp. Parasitol.* **1973**, *33*, 318–330. [CrossRef]
102. Galinier, R.; Roger, E.; Moné, Y.; Duval, D.; Portet, A.; Pinaud, S.; Chaparro, C.; Grunau, C.; Genthon, C.; Dubois, E.; et al. A multistrain approach to studying the mechanisms underlying compatibility in the interaction between *Biomphalaria glabrata* and *Schistosoma mansoni*. *PLoS Negl. Trop. Dis.* **2017**, *11*, e0005398. [CrossRef] [PubMed]
103. Mitta, G.; Adema, C.M.; Gourbal, B.; Loker, E.S.; Theron, A. Compatibility polymorphism in snail/schistosome interactions: From field to theory to molecular mechanisms. *Dev. Comp. Immunol.* **2012**, *37*, 1–8. [CrossRef] [PubMed]
104. Zhao, J.S.; Wang, A.Y.; Zhao, H.B.; Chen, Y.H. Transcriptome sequencing and differential gene expression analysis of the schistosome-transmitting snail *Oncomelania hupensis* inhabiting hilly and marshland regions. *Sci. Rep.* **2017**, *7*, 15809. [CrossRef] [PubMed]
105. Esvelt, K.M.; Smidler, A.L.; Catteruccia, F.; Church, G.M. Concerning RNA-guided gene drives for the alteration of wild population. *eLife* **2014**, *3*, e03401. [CrossRef] [PubMed]

Tropical Medicine and Infectious Disease

MDPI

Article

Potential Impact of Climate Change on Schistosomiasis: A Global Assessment Attempt

Guo-Jing Yang [1,2,*] and Robert Bergquist [3]

1 Department of Epidemiology and Public Health, Swiss Tropical and Public Health Institute, Socinstrasse 57, CH-4002 Basel, Switzerland
2 University of Basel, CH-4002 Basel, Switzerland
3 Ingerod, SE-454 94 Brastad, Sweden; robert.bergquist@outlook.com
* Correspondence: guojingyang@hotmail.com

Received: 18 October 2018; Accepted: 27 October 2018; Published: 3 November 2018

Abstract: Based on an ensemble of global circulation models (GCMs), four representative concentration pathways (RCPs) and several ongoing and planned Coupled Model Intercomparison Projects (CMIPs), the Intergovernmental Panel on Climate Change (IPCC) predicts that global, average temperatures will increase by at least 1.5 °C in the near future and more by the end of the century if greenhouse gases (GHGs) emissions are not genuinely tempered. While the RCPs are indicative of various amounts of GHGs in the atmosphere the CMIPs are designed to improve the workings of the GCMs. We chose RCP4.5 which represented a medium GHG emission increase and CMIP5, the most recently completed CMIP phase. Combining this meteorological model with a biological counterpart model accounted for replication and survival of the snail intermediate host as well as maturation of the parasite stage inside the snail at different ambient temperatures. The potential geographical distribution of the three main schistosome species: *Schistosoma japonicum*, *S. mansoni* and *S. haematobium* was investigated with reference to their different transmission capabilities at the monthly mean temperature, the maximum temperature of the warmest month(s) and the minimum temperature of the coldest month(s). The set of six maps representing the predicted situations in 2021–2050 and 2071–2100 for each species mainly showed increased transmission areas for all three species but they also left room for potential shrinkages in certain areas.

Keywords: climate change; schistosomiasis; distribution; intermediate snail host; transmission; modelling

1. Introduction

Schistosomiasis, caused by trematode parasites with a predilection for intestinal and urogenital venous circulation in the human definitive host, is one of the neglected tropical diseases (NTDs) selected for increased attention by the World Health Organization (WHO) [1]. Six different species of *Schistosoma* are capable of infecting humans, each depending on a certain snail species as an intermediate host. Humans infect snails by depositing parasite eggs (excreted in feces or urine) in waterlogged areas and humans are infected or reinfected when in contact with water containing schistosome cercariae released from infected snails. The disease is generally chronic, although schistosomiasis is often a contributing factor to premature death, direct mortality is comparatively low. Transmission of schistosomiasis has been reported in 78 countries and more than 800 million people in Africa, Latin America, the Middle East and Southeast Asia live in areas endemic to schistosomiasis [2], with up to 250 million actually infected [3]. Chemotherapy in amounts sufficient for more than 100 million school age children per year has been pledged by the private sector and development partners, but there is still a large discrepancy between the number of people requiring preventive treatment and those actually receiving it [4]. In addition, the number of people suffering from this infection continues to rise as a reflection of ongoing population growth, which is particularly high in endemic areas.

Schistosomiasis is not as neglected as many other tropical diseases since it has a large research focus and still remains one of the most prevalent infections in the world, estimated to correspond to 4.5 million disability-adjusted life years (DALYs) by the WHO Expert Committee in 2002 [5]. However, this estimate was based on a wider range of pathologies than that used in the global burden of disease (GBD) study of 1990 [6]. It was also higher than the updated GBD in 2010 [7] that put the burden of schistosomiasis at 3.3 million DALYs. Importantly, however, the GBD figure of 2010 was high enough to put this disease as no. 3 after malaria and tuberculosis on the NTD list [3]. This increase was due to the inclusion of diarrhea, dysuria and anemia in the DALY score which was not counted before. While later updates [8] show a sharply lower DALY score for schistosomiasis, other authors [9–11] hold that the true impact of this disease is several-fold higher because of the low weight given by the GBD estimates to subtle symptoms and pathology in individuals with infections too light to be revealed by diagnostics based on parasite egg-detection. Indeed, high-definition circulating antigen tests, such as the point-of-care circulating cathodic antigen (POC-CCA) assay indicates that the current number of infections may be at least 10 times higher than that shown by egg-detection [12].

The epidemiology of schistosomiasis (and that of all other organisms) must be seen in the light of the perceived ongoing climate change. The latest half century has seen signs of global warming, mainly thought to be due to the burning of coal and oil at an increasingly large scale. From 1990, reports relevant for our understanding of climate change, including options for its mitigation, are regularly produced by the Intergovernmental Panel on Climate Change (IPCC) [13] for the United Nations Framework Convention on Climate Change (UNFCCC). IPCC bases its assessments on the published, scientific literature and opinions of invited independent researchers. An important part of its work is to do with global circulation models (GCMs), which are currently used to predict the climate for the next 80 years based on complex mathematical representations of the Earth's energy balance between atmosphere, total land mass, sea and ice cover. These components interact as a coupled system, whose status emerges from equations based on the dynamic values of various climate variables, e.g., temperature, winds, etc., at each point on the globe. Climate modelling uses current and historic data to attempt the prediction of future climate scenarios from the present time to the end of the 21st century.

The projections of the GCMs disagree due to various forms of natural variability included in the models. Fortuitously, this variability can be reduced by averaging an ensemble of simulations, resulting in universal agreement. Generally, such averaged model ensembles produce simulations of current and past large-scale climates that agree with observation. Further confidence comes from the fact that converging GCMs also produce an accurate 'hindcast' of previous climate change that took place in the 1900s. Evidence is already available in the form of a rising average global temperature and amplified warming of air and oceans, particularly in the Arctic, leading to rising sea levels, dry places becoming dryer and wet places wetter.

The fact, temperature changes impact snail distributions in general as well as the maturation of the intermediate stages of the parasite inside this intermediate host, makes a discussion of future changes in the distribution of schistosomiasis complex. However, it is useful to know that water temperature below freezing puts an absolute limit to snail survival. Indeed, the climate-dependent, long-term (as opposed to seasonal) movements of the 'frost line' at northern latitudes indicates a diffuse zone north of which schistosomiasis transmission cannot occur. Immediately south of this zone, transmission is governed by the prevailing temperature and the time it stays above a certain limit, a fact rooted in the relationship between the development of plants and the ambient temperature first mentioned in the 1700s by Réaumur who coined the 'degree-day unit' and used it as a measure of crop maturation [14]. This unit, now called the growing degree-day (GDD), is defined as the amount of heat an organism needs to accumulate to achieve full development. Although its main application remains in agriculture, the GDD concept has also been used for predicting the development of parasites [15], monitoring snail replication as well as the maturation of the schistosome sporocyst stages inside the snail [16,17].

The effect of temperature alterations with regard to the potential distribution of schistosomiasis has been addressed in China [17–19] and Africa [20,21], but a global picture of potential long-term transmission alterations ascribed to climate change is still missing. To address this question, we felt that it was warranted to theorize about the intermediate- and long-term global distribution possibilities of this disease considering possible future dispersion of the intermediate snail host into non-endemic areas. The IPCC focuses a lot on temperature predictions and this variable has a strong influence on snail survival. Importantly, even minor temperature increases play a role if they cover a sufficiently long period of the annual cycle. For these reasons, we used GDD as the key parameter to evaluate the potential, future transmission risk of schistosomiasis.

2. Materials and Methods

When preparing the risk maps, we only considered the predicted temperature increase in relation to two required needs. These were the needs of the snail (three species) and that of the parasite stages inside the snail (mother sporocyst, daughter sporocyst and cercaria). Naturally, this approach was highly theoretical as many parameters other than temperature govern the potential distribution of schistosomiasis. However, it represents a first step in an investigation that can be developed further.

2.1. Study Area

Aiming to give a global overview of potential risk areas, a digital map of the world with country boundaries was downloaded from ArcGIS (ESRI, Redlands, CA, USA). Areas of particular risk for the change in schistosomiasis transmission were the current northern limits of the infection and slopes bordering high-altitude mountains. The southern limit was the southernmost tip of Africa and Chile and Brazil in South America as the sea rather than temperature limiting transmission at all other longitudes.

2.2. Meteorological Model

Modelling future temperatures builds on four representative concentration pathways (RCPs) representing four greenhouse gas concentration (not emission) trajectories, which were adopted by the IPCC for its 5th assessment report (AR5) in 2014 [22]. These RCPs superseded the Special Report on Emissions Scenarios (SRES) projections published in 2000 and were previously used for this purpose. Unlike simpler models which make mixing assumptions regarding processes internal to a presumed cell, while other functions govern the interface between such cells, the GCMs describe four possible climate futures, which are all considered possible depending on how much greenhouse gases (GHGs) are emitted in the years to come (see Figure 1). The four RCPs, i.e., RCP2.6, RCP4.5, RCP6 and RCP8.5 are named after a possible range of 'radiative' forcing relative to pre-industrial values (+2.6, +4.5, +6.0, and +8.5 W/m^2, respectively) [23].

The IPCC relies also on Coupled Model Intercomparison Project (CMIP) experiments, a collaborative series of experiments designed to improve our knowledge of the GCMs and their interactions. The most recently completed phase of the project is CMIP5, which includes more metadata describing model simulations than previous phases. The findings are summarized in AR5 (https://cmip.llnl.gov/cmip5/index.html). In this study, all models were based on CMIP5 with RCP4.5, which represented a medium GHG emission increase. The temperature prediction data used were derived from GCMs created in a grid format of 0.5×0.5 degrees latitude and longitude by five well-known research centers representing the most generally accepted view of the world's major climate systems (Table 1). The datasets we used consisted of a baseline temperature based on the 1961–1990 period and predicted periods 2021–2050 and 2071–2100. These were based on an ensemble of the five predicted climate scenarios between 2006 and 2100 with special reference to the monthly mean temperature (T_{mean}), the maximum temperature of the warmest months (T_{max}) and the minimum temperature of the coldest months (T_{min}), which are reminiscent of the BIO_1, BIO_5 and BIO_6 variables of the 'WorldClim' dataset [24]. Thirty years of averaged monthly temperatures (T_{mean}, T_{max} and T_{min}) spanning the periods 2021–2050 and 2071–2100 were extracted.

Table 1. The five global circulation models used in this study.

GCM [a]	Characteristics	Developing Centre
ACCE-SS1-0	Based on the UK MetOffice UM atmosphere model, the GFDL MOM4p1 ocean model, the LANL CICE4.1 sea-ice model and the MOSES2 land surface model.	The Australian Community Climate and Earth-System Simulator (ACCESS) weather models
IPSL-CM5A_LR	An atmosphere-land-ocean-sea ice model with representations of the carbon cycle; the stratospheric chemistry and the tropospheric aerosol chemistry	Institut Pierre Simon Laplace Climate Modelling Centre (IPSL-CMC) of Centre National de la Recherche Scientifique (CNRS); Paris; France
HadGEM2-AO	A configuration of the HadGEM2 model which is an atmosphere-only simulation with other component interfaces replaced with ancillary file input.	UK Met Office Hadley Centre
CanESM2	The second generation Canadian Earth System Model (CanESM2) consists of the physical coupled atmosphere-ocean model CanCM4 coupled to a terrestrial carbon model (CTEM) and an ocean carbon model (CMOC).	Canadian Centre for Climate Modelling and Analysis
GISS-E2-H-CC	Based on Earth system models that include interactive atmospheric chemistry, aerosols, carbon cycle and other tracers, as well as the standard atmosphere, ocean, sea ice and land surface components.	National Aeronautics and Space Administration (NASA) Goddard Institute for Space Studies

[a] Global Circulation Model.

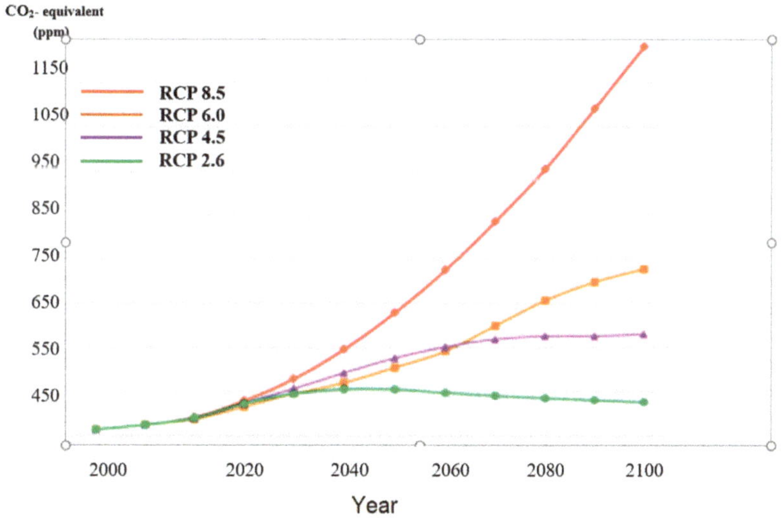

Figure 1. Estimated future equivalent atmospheric CO_2 concentrations including all 'forcing' agents according to the four representative concentration pathways (RCPs).

2.3. Biological Model

The GDD, being the temperature above a critical threshold multiplied by the duration needed, can be articulated as $T_{ave}-T_{base}$, where the former is the average daily temperature and the latter the base temperature or the lowest temperature at which development of an organism can occur. The annual sum of GDD, termed AGDD, determines fairly well the potential for the spatial distribution of living organisms. As the level of the GDD required to complete the development of an organism is fairly constant, organisms with high heat unit requirements are more likely to develop into mature stages in areas where AGDD is high. We found this unit useful for use as a means to define the geographical limits of schistosomiasis transmission, mainly based on the climate impact on the snail intermediate host but also on its effect on the development of the sporocyst inside the snail.

With the aim of assessing the effect of temperature on schistosomiasis development, we created biological models with reference to the parasites by calculating potential transmission indices (PTIs) derived from GDD and AGDD. The GDDs for *S. japonicum*, *S. mansoni* and *S. haematobium* were 853, 268 and 298 degree-days, respectively [17,25,26] and the efficient temperature ranges (T_{low} and T_{high}) for the development of *S. japonicum*, *S. mansoni* and *S. haematobium* were 18–35 °C, 16–35 °C and 18–32 °C, respectively [16,25,26]. The AGDD for each grid was calculated by summing up the difference between the mean monthly temperature (T_{ij}) at location *i* and month *j* and the efficient temperature range for parasite development:

$$AGDD_i = \sum_{j=1}^{12} (T_{ij} - T_{low}) \times day_j \times 1(T_{low} < T_{ij} < T_{high}), \quad (1)$$

where day_j indicates the number of days in month *j*, $1(\ldots)$ is the indicator function, giving the value of 1 if the condition within the parenthesis is true, otherwise 0.

The PTI_i was calculated for each pixel grid *i* in the periods 1961–1990, 2021–2050 and 2071–2100, according to Equation (2). Only *PTI* values above 1 were considered to be of relevance (i.e., areas where schistosomiasis transmission could potentially occur).

$$PTI_i = (AGDD_i/GDD_s) \times 1(AGDD_i/GDD_s > 1), \quad (2)$$

Oncomelania, the intermediate snail host of *S. japonicum*, can only survive if the January mean temperature is higher than 0 °C [17,18], while the most common *S. mansoni* snail host exists in areas where the yearly $T_{\max}$ is between 20–33 °C [27]. The corresponding optimal temperature range of the intermediate snail host for *S. haematobium* is 15.5–31 °C [28]. The vector survival threshold masks were overlapped on the PTI maps for the three different *Schistosoma* species investigated.

2.4. Geographical Information System (GIS) and Risk Assessment

We created a GIS database using ArcGIS, version 10.5 (ESRI; Redlands, CA, USA) for the investigation of baseline and change of transmission regions.

2.4.1. Baseline, Predicted Transmission Region and PTI

The PTI of the three main different schistosomiasis species for the periods 1961–1990, 2021–2050 and 2071–2100 were imported and presented as map overlays. On top of the PTI layer, we overlapped the thresholds for the intermediate hosts for the three species: 0 °C of the January T_{mean} for *Oncomelania* (*S. japonicum*), yearly $T_{\max}$ between 20 °C and 33 °C for the *Biomphalaria* snail species (*S. mansoni*) and a $T_{\max}$ between 15.5 °C and 31 °C for the *Bulinus* species (*S. haematobium*).

2.4.2. Change of Transmission Region, PTI due to Predicted Climate Change

We compared the spatial extent of the sensitive potential transmission region at two time periods: 2021–2050 vs. baseline 1961–1990 and 2071–2100 vs. baseline. We highlighted the change of PTI between the two time periods to present the transmission intensity difference due to the predicted climate change.

2.5. Model Validation by Ground Truth Data

S. japonicum was selected to evaluate the model prediction. All prediction results by pixel grids were compared with the same format data derived from the historic schistosomiasis transmission data provided by National Institute of Parasitic Diseases (NIPD), China Centers for Disease Control (CDC).

The model sensitivity and specificity of the prediction results were evaluated by the following three equations:

$$SE = \frac{Pe}{Pte}, \quad (3)$$

$$SP = \frac{Pn}{Ptn}, \quad (4)$$

$$TM = \frac{Pen}{Pa}, \quad (5)$$

where *SE* is sensitivity, *SP* is specificity, *TM* is the total agreement rate, *Pe* is the correctly predicted endemic pixels, *Pte* is all endemic pixels, *Pn* is the correctly predicted endemic pixels, *Ptn* is all non-endemic pixels, *Pen* is correctly predicted endemic and non-endemic pixels and *Pa* are all pixels.

3. Results

3.1. Change of Transmission Region and PTI for Schistosomiasis due to Climate Change

The average temperatures predicted by the IPCC for the two time periods 2021–2050 and 2071–2100, based on the average of the five GCM results, seemed increasingly likely in the event that efforts to curb the GHG emissions were not stepped up more than they were so far. Figures 2–4 use IPCC'S predicted temperatures for the two future time periods 2021–2050 and 2071–2100 but rather than comparing with a preindustrial average, we used the 1961–1990 period for which we had available PTI data as a baseline. The blue color shown in the figures designated the ocean, while the background of each plot was based on the PTI baseline.

For *S. japonicum*, we only applied the low temperature constraints. The global warming displayed heterogeneous patterns with respect to snail survival. For example, the current areas endemic for *S. japonicum* in the Sichuan Province were predicted to become unsuitable for snail habitats. On the other hand, the downstream regions between the Sichuan and Hunan/Hubei provinces corresponding to the area above the Three Gorges Dam, which is currently non-endemic, might well present a potential endemic risk in the future. The predicted potential transmission areas of *S. japonicum* moving northward was not so obvious in 2021–2050 as it might have become in the 2071–2100 period.

For *S. mansoni* and *S. haematobium*, in both timeframes forecast, the potential transmission areas could retreat from the Saharan areas as the desert might encroach on this part of the continent due to diminishing or discontinued rainfall. The future transmission areas of *S. mansoni* might shrink more than those of *S. haematobium*, while schistosomiasis in Ethiopia and other highlands in Africa could reach higher with warmer temperatures.

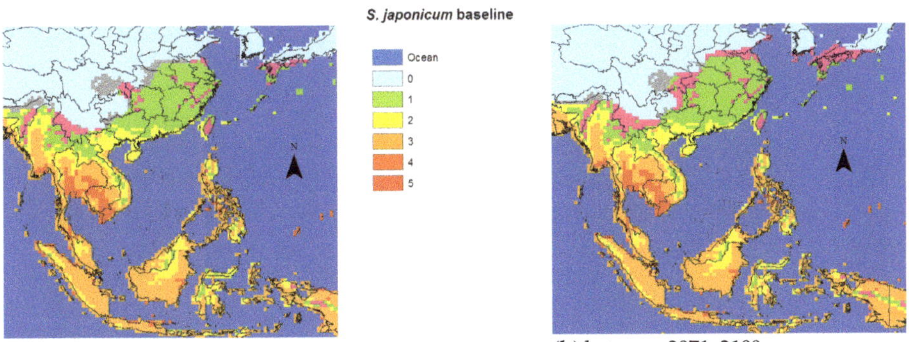

(**a**) between 2021–2050 (**b**) between 2071–2100

Figure 2. Change of risk area for *S. japonicum* vs. the baseline. (**a**) 2021–2050 vs. the baseline, (**b**) 2071–2050 vs. the baseline.

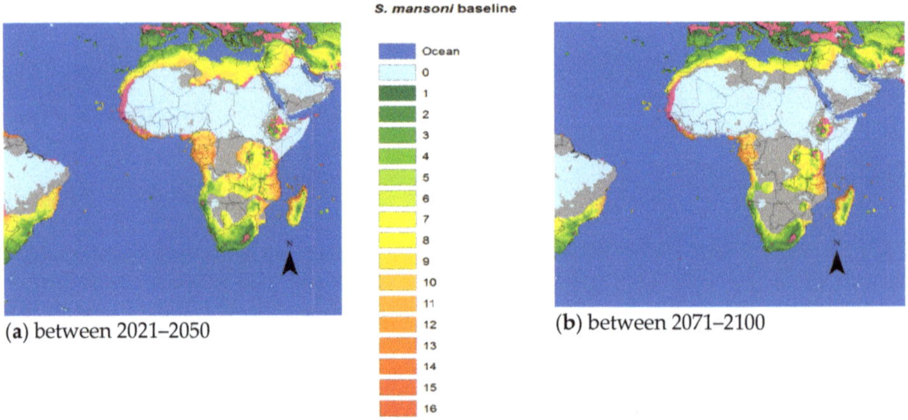

Figure 3. Change of risk area for *S. mansoni* vs. the baseline. (**a**) 2021–2050 vs. the baseline, (**b**) 2071–2050 vs. the baseline.

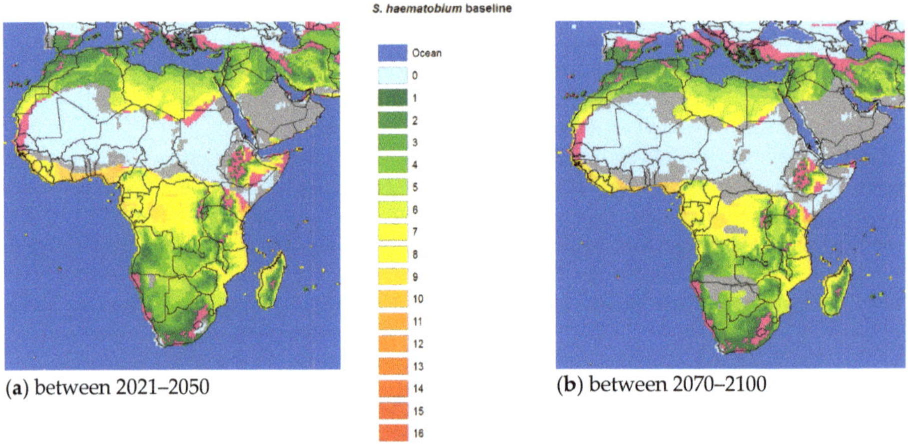

Figure 4. Change of risk area for *S. haematobium* vs. the baseline. (**a**) 2021–2050 vs. the baseline, (**b**) 2071–2050 vs. the baseline.

Suitability varies from 0 over the spectrum to the most likely (red). Grey areas signify areas that might potentially shrink as the temperature would become less suited to the specific snails for the different schistosomal species.

3.2. Model Validation by Ground Truth Data

The model prediction results were validated by the ground truth data in China. The sensitivity and specificity of model prediction were 0.78 and 0.89, respectively. The total prediction match rate was 0.88.

4. Discussion

Three schistosome species pose the main infection risk for humans. *S. japonicum* is the single schistosome species in China, the Philippines and three closely situated small foci in Celebes, Indonesia. It is transmitted by *Oncomelania* snails, whose latitudinal movements over land during most of the last million years may have been prevented by the development of the Himalaya plateau serving as a barrier. The endemic areas for *S. mansoni* and *S. haematobium* overlap to a great extent on the

African continent and in the Middle East, but not everywhere. The former, the most abundant of the schistosome species, has also found an exclusive niche in the Northeast part of South America and on some of the Caribbean islands but are now disappearing from the latter, however this is not due to climate change [29]. Its distribution is supported by the broad geographic range of *Biomphalaria* spp. snails that serve as obligatory hosts for its larval stages. Recently, however, *Bi. straminea* has been identified in the Hong Kong Special Administrative Region and Shenzhen City in the Guangdong Province of China and has remained there since the 1970s [30], a fact that could eventually result in transmission of *S. mansoni* in parallel with *S. japonicum* in China. *S. haematobium* is confined to Africa and the Middle East due to its reliance on *Bulinus* spp. intermediate snail hosts [31]. Although this schistosome species must also have been brought from Africa to Latin America during the slave trade of the 16th and 17th century, only *S. mansoni* became established there because of the absence of *Bulinus* snails. Although this information indicates that schistosome species and their specific snails can spread into various new areas, this is not of a magnitude that requires it to be considered when discussing the risk for schistosomiasis due to temperature augmentation.

To assess the potential impact of climate change on the transmission of schistosomiasis in the world we developed a biological model using available data from the literature. Compared to *S. japonicum*, both *S. mansoni* and *S. haematobium* required less total heat energy to complete one generation [17,25,26]. Therefore, the transmission intensity of the two latter species is generally somewhat stronger than that of *S. japonicum*. However, the three different intermediate snail hosts had different temperature thresholds for survival that came into play in certain geographical areas. For example, the distribution of the *Oncomelania* snail, utilized by *S. japonicum*, was constrained by the temperature in January (when below 0 °C), which effectively limited its progress northwards, while *Biomphalaria* (*S. mansoni*) and *Bulinus* (*S. haematobium*) had thermal requirements that included an annual T_{max} of 15.5–31 °C and 20–33 °C respectively [27], which is one of the factors (so far) keeping these snails from entering Europe and other northern territories. Interestingly, *S. haematobium* appears to have a better chance of a foothold in Europe than *S. mansoni*, at least in the middle part of the century (Figure 3).

With respect to snail survival, the GDD approach in 2008 predicted an extension of 662,373 and 783,883 km^2 potentially endemic areas for schistosomiasis japonica in China in 2030 and 2050, respectively [17]. Yang et al. noted that the 0–1 °C January isotherm of 1971–2000 had already shifted from 33°15′ N to 33°41′ N compared to the 1961–1990 baseline, expanding the area by 41,335 km^2, resulting in an additional 20.7 million people at risk of schistosomiasis in China [32]. For *S. japonicum*, the predicted temperature increases based on our biological model and the average ensemble of the five GCM models would result in transmission starting to extend northward by 2050 (Figure 2a) adding a considerably larger margin by 2100 (Figure 2b). It is also conceivable that the transmission intensity will increase in areas already endemic for schistosomiasis.

It is important for the existence or absence of the parasite and vital for prediction model validation that more information is made available also for *S. mansoni* and *S. haematobium*. However, the change in the geographic transmission region for these two species due to climate change is more complex than in China. With temperatures increasing above T_{max}, the historic transmission areas surrounding the Sahara region would retreat from the equator reducing the transmission regions of both species. However, the current risk areas would extend further into the northern or southern current marginal transmission areas, including the Mediterranean countries. Indeed, schistosomiasis hematobia has recently been identified in Corsica, France [33]. Although it is questionable whether this extension into Europe is due to climate change, rather large areas of southern Europe will become habitable for the snail hosts in the future (Figures 3 and 4). Overall, however, the total transmission areas should be reduced. The changing transmission patterns in terms of region and intensity are heterogeneous and new populations at risk will probably appear. Further research is warranted to work out the geographical probabilities.

A limitation of our current modelling approach is that it emphasizes the role of temperature but does not take into account the role of rainfall and the potential interaction between temperature and rainfall. It is difficult to say whether our model is conservative or whether these additional effects might further amplify the extent of changes predicted on the basis of temperature alone. Thus, recent improvements in modelling global trends in precipitation and water availability should become an integral part of present and future predictions of climate change and variability on infectious disease dynamics, including schistosomiasis. Recent years have seen widespread massive flooding, which can lead to snail dispersal and an epidemic outbreak of schistosomiasis if occurring in or close to endemic areas. In addition, the issue of altitude, that has been neglected so far, might under-evaluate changing transmission patterns in mountainous regions, which would have major implications for parts of China and many African countries. Additionally, most climate studies, including the current one, discuss large geographical scales, i.e., national, regional and global levels. To capture localized climate changes, regional climate models are needed that can assign meteorological parameters at relatively small scales also. Such climate models can provide information with useful local detail including realistic extreme events and generate detailed projections of the future climate. Any discussion of the future distribution of schistosomiasis, presumed to be induced by climate change would be futile without exact information of the prevailing distribution of the infection, both in humans and in the intermediate snail host. It is therefore critical that the diagnostic techniques applied are sensitive enough to find even the lightest infection.

This work is based on the best possible models available today on the future climate for the rest of the century. Without a doubt, however, future increased computing power will permit more comprehensive simulations, better represented parameterized processes and more accurate projections at all levels, which might well result in slightly different projections. In addition, natural phenomena, such as cataclysmic volcanic eruptions like that which occurred in Krakatoa in 1883, major meteoric hits, etc., that would completely upend any prediction of the kind discussed here cannot be completely ruled out. Even without such events, we still expect further changes in the forthcoming 6th assessment report (AR6) scheduled for release in 2022.

Author Contributions: Conceptualization, G.Y.; Formal analysis, G.Y.; Investigation, R.B.; Writing—original draft, G.Y.; Writing—review & editing, R.B.

Funding: G.Y. acknowledges the financial support from the International Development Research Centre (IDRC), Canada (grant no. 105509–00001002-024) and the National Nature Science Foundation (grant no. 81573261).

Conflicts of Interest: The authors declare no conflicts of interest.

References

1. WHO. 2012. Available online: http://www.who.int/neglected_diseases/NTD_RoadMap_2012_Fullversion.pdf (accessed on 15 October 2018).
2. Steinmann, P.; Keiser, J.; Bos, R.; Tanner, M.; Utzinger, J. Schistosomiasis and water resources development: Systematic review, meta-analysis, and estimates of people at risk. *Lancet Infect. Dis.* **2006**, *6*, 411–425. [CrossRef]
3. Hotez, P.; Alvarado, M.; Basáñez, M.; Bolliger, I.; Bourne, R.; Boussinesq, M.; Brooker, S.; Brown, A.; Buckle, G.; Budke, C.; et al. (DALYs and HALE Collaborators). The gobal burden of disease study 2010: Interpretation and implications for the neglected tropical diseases. *PLoS Negl. Trop. Dis.* **2014**, *8*, e2865. [CrossRef] [PubMed]
4. WHO. Schistosomiasis Fact Sheet of 20 February 2018. Available online: http://www.who.int/news-room/fact-sheets/detail/schistosomiasis (accessed on 20 August 2018).
5. WHO (World Health Organization). *Prevention and Control of Schistosomiasis and Soil-Transmitted Helminthiasis: Report of a WHO Expert Committee*; World Health Organization: Geneva, Switzerland, 2002.
6. Murray, C.J.; Lopez, A.D.; Jamison, D.T. The global burden of disease in 1990: Summary results, sensitivity analysis and future directions. *Bull. World Health Organ.* **1994**, *723*, 495–509.

7. Murray, C.J.L.; Vos, T.; Lozano, R.; Naghavi, M.; Flaxman, A.D.; Michaud, C.; Ezzati, M.; Shibuya, K.; Salomon, J.A.; Abdalla, S.; et al. Disability-adjusted life years (DALYs) for 291 diseases and injuries in 21 regions, 1990–2010: A systematic analysis for the Global Burden of Disease Study 2010. *Lancet* **2012**, *380*, 2197–2223. [CrossRef]
8. Hay, S.I.; Abajobir, A.A.; Abate, K.H.; Abbafati, C.; Abbas, K.M.; Abd-Allah, F.; Abdulkader, R.S.; Abdulle, A.M.; Abebo, T.A.; Abera, S.F.; et al. Global, regional, and national disability-adjusted life-years (DALYs) for 333 diseases and injuries and healthy life expectancy (HALE) for 195 countries and territories, 1990–2016: A systematic analysis for the Global Burden of Disease Study 2016. *Lancet* **2017**, *39010100*, 1260–1344. [CrossRef]
9. King, C.H. Health metrics for helminth infections. *Acta Trop.* **2015**, *141 Pt B*, 150–160. [CrossRef]
10. King, C.H. It's Time to Dispel the Myth of "Asymptomatic" Schistosomiasis. *PLoS Negl. Trop. Dis.* **2015**, *92*, e0003504. [CrossRef] [PubMed]
11. King, C.H.; Galvani, A.P. Underestimation of the global burden of schistosomiasis. *Lancet* **2018**, *39110118*, 307–308. [CrossRef]
12. Bergquist, R.; van Dam, G.J.; Xu, J. Diagnostic tests for schistosomiasis. In *Schistosoma: Biology, Pathology and Control*; Jamieson, B.G.M., Ed.; CRC Press: Boca Raton, FL, USA, 2016; pp. 401–439.
13. IPCC. Principles Governing IPCC Work, Approved 1–3 October 1998, Last Amended 14–18 October 2013. Available online: https://ipcc.ch/pdf/ipcc-principles/ipcc-principles.pdf (accessed on 5 september 2018).
14. Bonhomme, R. Bases and limits to using 'degree.day' units. *Eur. J. Agron.* **2000**, *13*, 1–10. [CrossRef]
15. Bernal, J.; Gonzalez, D. Experimental assessment of a degree-day model for predicting the development of parasites in the field. *J. Appl. Entiron.* **1993**, *116*, 459–466. [CrossRef]
16. Yang, G.J.; Utzinger, J.; Sun, L.P.; Hong, Q.B.; Vounatsou, P.; Tanner, M.; Zhou, X.N. Effect of temperature on the development of *Schistosoma japonicum* within *Oncomelania hupensis*, and hibernation of *O. hupensis*. *Parasitol. Res.* **2007**, *100*, 695–700. [CrossRef] [PubMed]
17. Zhou, X.N.; Yang, G.J.; Yang, K.; Wang, X.H.; Hong, Q.B.; Sun, L.P.; Malone, J.B.; Kristensen, T.K.; Bergquist, N.R.; Utzinger, J. Potential Impact of Climate Change on Schistosomiasis Transmission in China. *Am. J. Trop. Med. Hyg.* **2008**, *78*, 188–194. [CrossRef] [PubMed]
18. Yang, G.J.; Vounatsou, P.; Zhou, X.N.; Tanner, M.; Utzinger, J.E. Electrophoretic detection of genetic variability among Schistosoma japonicum isolates by sequence-related amplified polymorphism. *Parasitologia* **2005**, *47*, 127–134.
19. Zhu, G.; Fan, J.; Peterson, A. Schistosoma japonicum transmission risk maps at present and under climate change in mainland China. *PLoS Negl. Trop. Dis.* **2017**, *1110*, e0006021. [CrossRef] [PubMed]
20. McCreesh, N.; Nikulin, G.; Booth, M. Predicting the effects of climate change on *Schistosoma mansoni* transmission in eastern Africa. *Parasit. Vectors* **2015**, *8*, 4. [CrossRef] [PubMed]
21. Stensgaard, A.S.; Booth, M.; Nikulin, G.; McCreesh, N. Combining process-based and correlative models improves predictions of climate change effects on *Schistosoma mansoni* transmission in eastern Africa. *Geosp. Health* **2016**, *11* (Suppl. 1), 406. [CrossRef] [PubMed]
22. Moss, R.; Babiker, M.; Brinkman, S.; Calvo, E.; Carter, T.; Edmonds, J.; Elgizouli, I.; Emori, S.; Erda, L.; Hibbard, K.; et al. *Towards New Scenarios for Analysis of Emissions: Climate Change, Impacts and Response Strategies*; Intergovernmental Panel on Climate Change: Geneva, Switzerland, 2008; Volume 132.
23. IPPC Working Group I. The Scientific Basis. Available online: https://www.ipcc.ch/ipccreports/tar/wg1/029.htm (accessed on 5 September 2018).
24. Hijmans, R.J.; Cameron, S.E.; Parra, J.L.; Jones, P.G.; Jarvis, A. Very high resolution interpolated climate surfaces for global land areas. *Int. J. Clim.* **2005**, *25*, 1965–1978. [CrossRef]
25. Pflüger, W. Experimental epidemiology of schistosomiasis. I. The prepatent period and cercarial production of *Schistosoma mansoni* in *Biomphalaria* snails at various constant temperatures. *Parasitol. Res.* **1980**, *63*, 159–169.
26. Pflüger, W.; Roushdy, M.Z.; El-Emam, M. Prepatency of *Schistosoma haematobium* in snails at different constant temperatures. *J. Egypt. Soc. Parasitol.* **1983**, *13*, 513–519. [PubMed]
27. Malone, J.B.; Yilma, J.M.; McCarroll, J.C.; Erko, B.; Mukaratirwa, S.; Zhou, X. Satellite climatology and the environmental risk of Schistosoma mansoni in Ethiopia and east Africa. *Acta Trop.* **2001**, *79*, 59–72. [CrossRef]
28. Kalinda, C.; Chimbari, M.J.; Mukaratirwa, S. Schistosomiasis in Zambia: A systematic review of past and present experiences. *Infect. Dis. Poverty* **2018**, *71*, 41. [CrossRef] [PubMed]

29. Hewitt, R.; Willingham, A.L. Elimination of Schistosomiasis in the Caribbean. *TropicalMed* **2018**, in press.
30. Habib, M.R.; Guo, Y.H.; Lv, S.; Gu, W.B.; Li, X.H.; Zhou, X.N. Predicting the spatial distribution of *Biomphalaria straminea*; a potential intermediate host for *Schistosoma mansoni* in China. *Geosp. Health* **2016**, *113*, 453. [CrossRef] [PubMed]
31. Mandahl-Barth, G. The species of the genus Bulinus: Intermediate hosts of Schistosoma. *Bull. World Health Organ.* **1965**, *331*, 33–44.
32. Yang, G.; Vounatsou, P.; Zhou, X.N.; Tanner, M.; Utzinger, J. A potential impact of climate change and water resource development on the transmission of *Schistosoma japonicum* in China. *Parassitologia* **2005**, *47*, 127–134. [PubMed]
33. Berry, A.; Moné, H.; Iriart, X.; Mouahid, G.; Aboo, O.; Boissier, J.; Fillaux, J.; Cassaing, S.; Debuisson, C.; Valentin, A.; et al. *Schistosomiasis haematobium*, Corsica, France. *Emerg. Infect. Dis.* **2014**, *209*, 1595–1597. [CrossRef] [PubMed]

Tropical Medicine and Infectious Disease

MDPI

Review

Current Status of the Sm14/GLA-SE Schistosomiasis Vaccine: Overcoming Barriers and Paradigms towards the First Anti-Parasitic Human(itarian) Vaccine

Miriam Tendler *, Marília S. Almeida, Monica M. Vilar, Patrícia M. Pinto and Gabriel Limaverde-Sousa

FIOCRUZ—Instituto Oswaldo Cruz, Laboratório de Esquistossomose Experimental, Av. Brasil, 4365, Manguinhos, Rio de Janeiro 21045-900, Brazil; sirianni@ioc.fiocruz.br (M.S.A.); mvilar@ioc.fiocruz.br (M.M.V.); pmpinto@ioc.fiocruz.br (P.M.P.); gabriel.sousa@ioc.fiocruz.br (G.L.-S.)

* Correspondence: tendlermiriam@gmail.com; Tel.: +55-21-2562-1320

Received: 15 October 2018; Accepted: 12 November 2018; Published: 21 November 2018

Abstract: Schistosomiasis, a disease historically associated with poverty, lack of sanitation and social inequality, is a chronic, debilitating parasitic infection, affecting hundreds of millions of people in endemic countries. Although chemotherapy is capable of reducing morbidity in humans, rapid re-infection demonstrates that the impact of drug treatment on transmission control or disease elimination is marginal. In addition, despite more than two decades of well-executed control activities based on large-scale chemotherapy, the disease is expanding in many areas including Brazil. The development of the Sm14/GLA-SE schistosomiasis vaccine is an emblematic, open knowledge innovation that has successfully completed phase I and phase IIa clinical trials, with Phase II/III trials underway in the African continent, to be followed by further trials in Brazil. The discovery and experimental phases of the development of this vaccine gathered a robust collection of data that strongly supports the ongoing clinical phase. This paper reviews the development of the Sm14 vaccine, formulated with glucopyranosyl lipid A (GLA-SE), from the initial experimental developments to clinical trials including the current status of phase II studies.

Keywords: schistosomiasis; vaccine; Sm14; FABP

1. Introduction

Schistosomiasis is the second-most socioeconomically devastating parasitic disease after malaria. The disease is both chronic and debilitating with an estimated 200 million people infected, most of whom (85%) live in Africa. Of those infected, 120 million are symptomatic and 20 million present severe disease symptoms [1]. These estimates may err on the low side since meta-analysis has found the number of people at risk to be closer to 800 million [2]. Globally, the impact of schistosomiasis remains high and the estimated number of disability-adjusted life years (DALYs) has increased with the inclusion of previously under-recognized morbidities not previously included in the DALY index (for example, stunted growth and anemia associated with retarded intellectual development) in infants, toddlers and school age children, whose physical health and intellectual capacity are fundamental to nation development and sustainability [3,4]. In addition, high-definition circulating antigen tests, such as the POC-CCA assay, indicate that the current number of infections may be at least 10 times higher than that shown by egg detection [5]. In Brazil, the largest endemic country for schistosomiasis, 6 million individuals are estimated to be infected and 25 million are at risk of contracting the disease [6,7].

Mass chemotherapy has been the strategy of choice for the control schistosomiasis with the support of international health funding agencies. Estimates show that at least 206.5 million people were treated in 2016 [8]. However, the strategy of large-scale chemotherapeutic treatment, also equivocally called 'prophylactic treatment', over a period of 30 years has failed to control schistosome transmission. Approximately 300 million US dollars are being spent annually on treatments applied to the same populations year after year with no prospect of preventing reinfection or the need for repeat treatments [9]. 'Deworming' initiatives, originally applied to animal species only, were proposed as a tool for schistosomiasis control programs focused on school children in endemic countries [10,11].

In the veterinary field, under One Health policies for the control of helminth infections such as *Fasciola hepatica*, the major parasitic infection of livestock worldwide, there is a strong demand for the replacement of anti-helminthic drugs with vaccines. This would significantly reduce the amount of chemical residues in meat, milk and added-value products. Indeed, vaccines are considered to be the most environmentally- and human health-friendly method of control of fascioliasis in livestock [12].

The potential introduction of vaccines into schistosomiasis control programs brings hope to the poor living in endemic areas. The Brazilian Sm14 vaccine project was launched in the 1990s and strongly pushed in the context of a formal WHO program aimed at the development of an anti-schistosomiasis vaccine. The main outcome of this initiative was the selection of six priority antigen candidates of which only Sm14, continues to be developed (Table 1, adapted from [13]).

With strategic support from WHO, the Sm14 vaccine, which is based on a recombinant protein, is moving forward in an endemic country towards final development. It is being developed utilizing sophisticated and modern technological platforms and professionally conducted within a network of outstanding companies and collaborators. It is the result of long-term scientific developments carried under the coordination of FIOCRUZ, a public institution linked to the Brazilian Ministry of Health and is protected by strong patents, owned by FIOCRUZ, in all countries of interest worldwide.

Recently, the Consultative Expert Working Group on Research and Development: Financing and Coordination (CEWG/WHO) selected the Sm14 vaccine as one of six demonstration projects, globally, following an extensive review process. It was recognized as being fully in accordance with the principles of CEWG, such as clear mechanisms of de-linkage of costs from investments in research and development (R&D) from costs of final product, accessibility, affordability, viability and open knowledge innovation. The CEWG recognized that the Sm14 vaccine may become a key tool for the implementation of effective infection reduction and transmission control programs for schistosomiasis that would not rely only on chemotherapy [14].

Over recent years it has been possible to complete important milestones in the development of the vaccine including scaling up production process from laboratory bench to a clinical trial scale as well as the successful conclusion of two phase I human trials in healthy adults (male and female) living in a Brazilian non-endemic area (2011–2014) [15] together with a first phase II trial in 30 male adults living in highly endemic area for both *Schistosoma mansoni* and *S. haematobium* at the Senegal River Basin (2015–2017). In the latter, safety was extensively confirmed and strong and long-lasting immunogenicity was also demonstrated (manuscript in preparation). Master cell bank generation has recently been completed and production in good manufacturing practices (GMP) of a second Sm14 lot is currently ongoing, under the coordination of the Infectious Disease Research Institute (IDRI, Seattle, US). This article is an overview of the development of the Sm14 schistosomiasis vaccine development from antigen discovery to the current human studies (Figure 1). The need to overcome barriers for the establishment of a truly humanitarian vaccine—addressing the needs of the developing world—will be discussed.

Table 1. Schistosomiasis priority antigens selected by the WHO for independent testing (adapted from [13]).

Antigen	Size (kDa)	Stage Expressed	Description	Protection (%)	Place of Development
Glutathione S-transferase (P28/GST)	28	Adult/somula/egg	Enzyme	30–60	Institut Pasteur, Lille, France
Paramyosin (Sm97)	97	Adult/somula	Muscle protein	30	Case Western Reserve University/National Institute of Health/Cornell University, USA
IrV-5	62	Adult/somula/egg	Muscle protein	50–70	Johns Hopkins School of Medicine, Baltimore, USA
Triose phosphate isomerase (TPI)	28	Adult/somula/egg	Enzyme	30–60	Harvard School of Public Health, Boston, USA
Sm23	23	Adult/somula/egg	Integrated membrane protein	40–50	Johns Hopkins School of Medicine/Harvard School of Public Health, USA
Sm14	14	Adult/somula	Fatty acid-binding protein	65	Instituto Oswaldo Cruz, Rio de Janeiro, Brazil

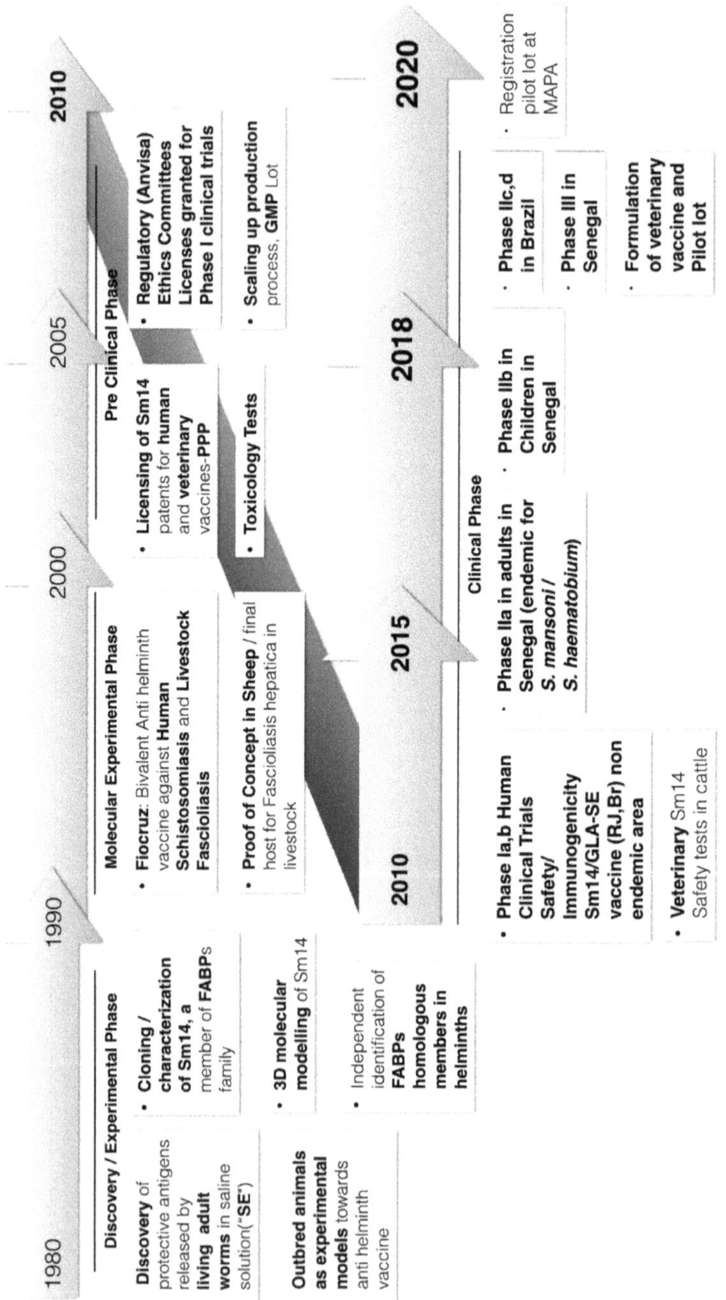

Figure 1. Timeline: Sm14/GLA-SE anti-schistosomiasis vaccine - from discovery phase to final product. MAPA: Brazilian Ministry of Agriculture.

2. Innovative Strategies Adopted for Antigen Discovery and Early Development Phases

Biotechnological advances in various areas of vaccine research have contributed to the development of safer and more effective formulations. Efforts to develop anti-helminth vaccines have been ongoing for many years and are continuing to progress in the identification of candidate antigens. These efforts have recently been boosted by the generation of a number of helminth genome sequences [16]. The development of a vaccine against schistosomiasis would represent an important step in the context of research and development in public health for poor populations infected and exposed to schistosomes. There have been initiatives to develop a vaccine against schistosomiasis from research groups in different countries. The Brazilian Sm14-based anti-schistosomiasis vaccine is the only one of these initiatives that is currently undergoing clinical trials [17].

In contrast to the current 'OMICS' strategies, in which high-throughput screening of potential target antigens are processed in parallel by automated 'discovery protocols and platforms', the Sm14 project was initiated by gathering observations from animal models of infection together with logical progression based on experimental evidence.

The first original approach was in the methodology for generating a worm extract that was subsequently used to assess protective immunity. Rather than lyophilized parasites, generally used by other research groups, a saline extract containing secreted/excreted antigens derived from living adult schistosomes was utilized for initial immunizations. The restricted number of potential protective antigens released in this saline extract allowed an accelerated identification of strong antigen candidates for molecular analysis and gene cloning [18–22]. Innovative methods were also adopted for the assessment of immunity, where the use of outbred models, in contrast to the commonly-employed inbred animals, allowed a better representation of the ultimate target population and provided a unique opportunity to develop an alternative strategy for the assessment of protective immunity. The analyses were stratified based on the measurement of frequencies of worm burdens within vaccinated animal populations as compared with non-vaccinated infected controls, as opposed to evaluation of mean values of parasite loads, as usually adopted. A solid base of pre-clinical data was generated establishing the immunization protocols that would be adopted during the following steps of the development [23–31].

As molecular biology tools evolved and gene-cloning techniques became available, several antigens released in the saline culture medium of live schistosomes, were cloned and sequenced. Serum from rabbits immunized with the 'saline extract' was used to screen an adult *S. mansoni* cDNA library and the most promising antigen was identified as a member of the fatty acid binding protein (FABP) family, termed Sm14 [32]. Molecular modeling studies from our group predicted the beta-barrel structure of the Sm14 [33] that was later experimentally confirmed by crystallography [34] and nuclear magnetic resonance [35]. These analyses allowed the engineering of a stabilizing mutation that conferred a remarkable long-term stability, while maintaining the function and immunogenicity of the antigen [36].

Sm14 was shown to be particularly important to helminths, which are not capable of synthetizing fatty acids but rely on these being provided by the host species. Lipids, apart from being constituents of membranes, have important roles in development of different lifecycle stages and the evasion of immune responses both by adult worms and larvae [37]. In addition to the publication describing the a FABP family member in *Schistosoma mansoni* [32], different groups published the identification of homologous FABP protein members from FABP family in many helminths of human and veterinary importance. Of particular importance was the identification of the *F. hepatica* FABP [38]. *F. hepatica* is the main parasite of livestock worldwide. We have managed to successfully test Sm14 vaccination against *F. hepatica* in mice, followed by two independent experiments in sheep, one of the definitive host species for fascioliasis [39]. These experiments that demonstrated that Sm14 is also protective against *F. hepatica* infection has led to Sm14 being developed in parallel as the molecular basis for a veterinary vaccine by FIOCRUZ, in collaboration with the private Brazilian company Ourofino Animal Health.

3. Clinical Studies

The licensing of the Sm14 patents for veterinary use gave birth to a public–private partnership (PPP) model of product development that rendered significant visibility to the Sm14 vaccine project. Such a gain in momentum was followed by strong support for human vaccine development by the Brazilian government project financing agency (FINEP) that allowed the use of contract research organizations (CROs) for antigen production, quality control and fill-finish in world-class academic GMP facilities based in the United States of America in collaboration with the Ludwig Institute for Cancer Research, Cornell University and the Infectious Disease Research Institute (IDRI, Seattle, USA).

In order to have a consistent, stable and defined final product for clinical human use, the Sm14 antigen was formulated with the synthetic adjuvant glucopyranosyl lipid A (GLA-SE), an adjuvant successfully tested in clinical trials with different human vaccine candidates.

In December of 2010, the Brazilian Health Regulatory Agency (ANVISA) approved a phase Ia clinical trial in 20 healthy male volunteers from a non-endemic area (Rio de Janeiro, Brazil) to evaluate the safety of the investigational product. The study was conducted by the Brazilian National Institute of Infectious Diseases (INI/FIOCRUZ). The results of this first trial demonstrated the safety of the vaccine in the studied population, showing no systemic reactogenicity. No serious adverse events were associated to the investigational product [15]. A phase Ib clinical study, to evaluate the safety and immunogenicity of the vaccine preparation in 10 healthy women volunteers, was also then successfully concluded in 2012 (manuscript in preparation).

In 2015–2016, within the scope of a CEWG Demonstration Project, a phase IIa trial was developed in 30 male adults living in a highly endemic area for both *S. mansoni* and *S. haematobium* in the Senegal River Basin. The trial was conducted by a specialized team from Espoir Pour La Santé (EPLS), linked to the Pasteur Institute of Lille (IPL, France), headed by Dr. Gilles Riveau (IPL) in conjunction with the FIOCRUZ group and the Brazilian biotechnology company Orygen Biotecnologia the license holder of Sm14 for human use (ClinicalTrials.gov Identifier: NCT03041766) [40]. The main objectives of the trial were safety and immunogenicity of the Sm14/GLA-SE vaccine. These objectives were fully achieved. The investigational product rSm14 (50 μg) formulated with GLA-SE in two dosages (2.5 μg and 5 μg/dose, denominated groups 1 and 2, respectively) and administered intramuscular (IM), was shown to be safe with no observed serious adverse events in either group. The most common reactions were local pain and heaviness of the vaccinated arm. These reactions were transitory and mild. Seroconversion of 92% of individuals after the second dose were observed, similar to the pattern observed in the phase I trials [15]. Immunogenicity based on additional cellular responses, memory cells and T cell activation markers were analyzed at IDRI in an extensive panel focusing on the identification of a vaccine-related immune response.

After the completion of the phase IIa trial and based on the observed induction of a strong and long-lasting immune response, an extension study to assess the possible persistence and profile of this response beyond the initial schedule of the trial was duly authorized by Senegalese Ministry of Health (MoH). This was carried out between August and December 2017 with the inclusion of two additional time points, 9 and 12 months, after the first vaccine injection. ELISA tests performed at Centre de Recherche Biomédicale/Espoir Pour La Santé (EPLS) showed the persistence of significant specific antibody titers up to 12 months after the first vaccination dose with Sm14/GLA-SE (manuscript in preparation).

A phase IIb trial design and protocol were defined in January 2018, based on the results of the phase IIa trial in adults. The phase IIb trial will involve 95 school children from 7–11 years of age living in the same endemic area for both *S. mansoni* and *S. hamatobium* of the Senegal River Basin region. Ethical committee approval and regulatory approval from the Senegalese MoH have been obtained. EPLS has already initiated the trial in the same region as the original phase IIa trial in adults, using the same lot of GMP Sm14 under a regimen of three IM doses of 50 μg/dose formulated with 2.5 μg of GLA-SE, 30 days apart. The phase IIa and b trials are largely funded by Orygen Biotecnologia in conjunction with FIOCRUZ and with support of CEWG-WHO platform and financial fund.

4. Sm14 +GLA-SE: A Humanitarian Anti-Schistosomiasis Vaccine

During the process of analysis by WHO member state representatives, within a regional structure, and extensive subsequent analysis by technical experts and ad hoc committees, the Sm14 schistosomiasis vaccine, was selected by the WHO Executive Board as one of the current list of six demonstration projects. A stakeholders meeting organized by WHO at its Geneva headquarters was held in June 2015 prior to the release of the first installment of funding. During the process of selection and shortlisting of the candidate demonstration projects presented projects, discussions on the scientific merits, state of the art of the project and requirement for full adherence to CEWG principles, much was learned concerning the mandatory need to assure the accessibility and affordability of this vaccine to the poor endemic countries in which it will ultimately be used [14].

From its inception, the Sm14 schistosomiasis vaccine has been designed to be both effective and low-cost. To achieve this goal, several innovations for vaccine development were implemented and a strong effort was made to choose intellectual property-free components [36]. This has led to the successful development of a very low-cost, stable product involving a large-scale production process.

De-linkage of final product price from the costs of the long R&D phases has been achieved by Sm14 being initially developed at a governmental scientific foundation (FIOCRUZ) with support from funds from public Brazilian financial institutions (FINEP and FAPERJ).

After 2005, licensing of FIOCRUZ patent rights for human use to a private Brazilian company was through contracts designed to protect the accessibility, affordability and supply strategies for the lower- and middle-income countries (LMIC) that are the target areas to receive the anti-schistosomiasis vaccine. The presently licensee company, Orygen Biotecnologia, is a startup company wholly owned by two of the largest Brazilian pharmaceutical companies. Its involvement in the final development of the Sm14 human vaccine is crucial. The company has agreed to a cost plus pricing strategy, as adopted by WHO for vaccine pricing [41].

In parallel, the veterinary anti-fasciola vaccine is being developed in keeping with current European guidelines to reduce the presence of anti-helminthic drug chemical residues in milk and meat of livestock. It is aimed at rich countries and markets and designed to contribute/support future potential large-scale delivery programs.

We are no longer at a stage when an anti-schistosomiasis vaccine is to be discussed, attacked or delayed, as it was for decades along with all anti-parasite vaccines. Our knowledge concerning vaccines has improved enormously, as have the technical resources available. Vaccines represent the intervention strategy with the best cost–benefit ratio thus far applied in public health. Moreover, transmission control of infectious/transmissible diseases has only been achieved through vaccination. Sanitation, chemotherapy and health education are not sufficient to eliminate parasitic diseases that disproportionally affect people living in poor countries. Immunization with a safe and effective vaccine can contribute to a long-term reduction of schistosome egg excretion from the host, thus truly controlling transmission. So far, there are no vaccines against the parasites that afflict countries fighting to emerge from poverty and reach better conditions of health and overall development.

The Sm14 vaccine against schistosomiasis is being developed as a humanitarian vaccine to be included in effective schistosomiasis transmission control programs that will hopefully invert the paradigm for a north-to-south route for technology generation and contribute to the broad use of the most safe, effective and environmentally and human-friendly health-promoting strategy, prophylactic vaccination.

Funding: This study was funded by FINEP (Financiadora de Estudos e Projetos), grant number 01.06.105800; FAPERJ (Fundação Carlos Chagas Filho de Amparo à Pesquisa do Estado do Rio de Janeiro), grant number E-26/010.001533/2014; IOC/FIOCRUZ (Instituto Oswaldo Cruz/Fundação Oswaldo Cruz, Ministério da Saúde) and Orygen Biotecnologia S.A.is supporting phase II/III clinical trials, process development for large scale production and steps forward to final product.

Acknowledgments: The authors would like to thank Steven Reed, Rhea Coler, Tracey Day, Anna Marie Beckman and IDRI team for immunogenicity tests and stability tests on Sm14 GMP lot; Orygen Biotechnologia technical team; Marcia Ciol, statistician from WA University; Gilles Riveau and Anne-Marie Schacht from EPLS/IPL; Tatiane dos Santos, FIOCRUZ—Instituto Oswaldo Cruz, Laboratório de Esquistossomose Experimental, for part of immunology tests.

Conflicts of Interest: The authors declare no conflict of interest.

References

1. Chitsulo, L.; Engels, D.; Montresor, A.; Savioli, L. The global status of schistosomiasis and its control. *Acta Trop.* **2000**, *77*, 41–51. [CrossRef]
2. Steinmann, P.; Keiser, J.; Bos, R.; Tanner, M.; Utzinger, J. Schistosomiasis and water resources development: Systematic review, meta-analysis, and estimates of people at risk. *Lancet Infect. Dis.* **2006**, *6*, 411–425. [CrossRef]
3. Osakunor, D.N.M.; Woolhouse, M.E.J.; Mutapi, F. Paediatric schistosomiasis: What we know and what we need to know. *PLoS Negl. Trop. Dis.* **2018**, *12*, e0006144. [CrossRef] [PubMed]
4. Poole, H.; Terlouw, D.J.; Naunje, A.; Mzembe, K.; Stanton, M.; Betson, M.; Lalloo, D.G.; Stothard, J.R. Schistosomiasis in pre-school-age children and their mothers in Chikhwawa district, Malawi with notes on characterization of schistosomes and snails. *Parasit. Vectors* **2014**, *7*, 153. [CrossRef] [PubMed]
5. Bergquist, R.; van Dam, G.J.; Xu, J. Diagnostic tests for schistosomiasis. In *Schistosoma: Biology, Pathology and Control*, 1st ed.; Jamieson, B.G.M., Ed.; CRC Press: Boca Raton, FL, USA, 2016; pp. 401–439.
6. Coura, J.R.; Amaral, R.S. Epidemiological and control aspects of schistosomiasis in Brazilian endemic areas. *Mem. Inst. Oswaldo Cruz* **2004**, *99*, 13–19. [CrossRef] [PubMed]
7. Barbosa, C.S.; Araújo, K.C.; Antunes, L.; Favre, T.; Pieri, O.S. Spatial distribution of schistosomiasis foci on Itamaracá Island, Pernambuco, Brazil. *Mem. Inst. Oswaldo Cruz* **2004**, *99*, 79–83. [CrossRef] [PubMed]
8. Schistosomiasis. Available online: http://www.who.int/news-room/fact-sheets/detail/schistosomiasis (accessed on 14 September 2018).
9. Ahuja, A.; Baird, S.; Hicks, J.H.; Kremer, M.; Miguel, E. Economics of Mass Deworming Programs. In *Child and Adolescent Health and Development*; Bundy, D.A.P., de Silva, N., Horton, S., Jamison, D.T., Patton, G.C., Eds.; The International Bank for Reconstruction and Development/The World Bank: Washington, DC, USA, 2017; ISBN 978-1-4648-0423-6.
10. Guidelines for School-Based Deworming Programs. Available online: https://www.globalpartnership.org/content/guidelines-school-based-deworming-programs (accessed on 5 September 2018).
11. WHO School Deworming at a Glance. Available online: http://www.who.int/intestinal_worms/resources/joint_statement_WHO_World_Bank/en/ (accessed on 25 September 2018).
12. Molina-Hernández, V.; Mulcahy, G.; Pérez, J.; Martínez-Moreno, Á.; Donnelly, S.; O'Neill, S.M.; Dalton, J.P.; Cwiklinski, K. *Fasciola hepatica* vaccine: We may not be there yet but we're on the right road. *Vet. Parasitol.* **2015**, *208*, 101–111. [CrossRef] [PubMed]
13. Bergquist, N.R.; Colley, D.G. Schistosomiasis vaccine: Research to development. *Parasitol. Today* **1998**, *14*, 99–104. [CrossRef]
14. WHO CEWG Demonstration Projects: Background and Process. Available online: http://www.who.int/phi/implementation/cewg_background_process/en/ (accessed on 25 September 2018).
15. Santini-Oliveira, M.; Coler, R.N.; Parra, J.; Veloso, V.; Jayashankar, L.; Pinto, P.M.; Ciol, M.A.; Bergquist, R.; Reed, S.G.; Tendler, M. Schistosomiasis vaccine candidate Sm14/GLA-SE: Phase 1 safety and immunogenicity clinical trial in healthy, male adults. *Vaccine* **2016**, *34*, 586–594. [CrossRef] [PubMed]
16. Lustigman, S.; Geldhof, P.; Grant, W.N.; Osei-Atweneboana, M.Y.; Sripa, B.; Basáñez, M.-G. A research agenda for helminth diseases of humans: Basic research and enabling technologies to support control and elimination of helminthiases. *PLoS Negl. Trop. Dis.* **2012**, *6*, e1445. [CrossRef] [PubMed]
17. Tendler, M.; Almeida, M.; Simpson, A. Development of the Brazilian anti-schistosomiasis vaccine based on the recombinant fatty acid binding protein Sm14 plus GLA-SE adjuvant. *Front. Immunol.* **2015**, *6*. [CrossRef] [PubMed]
18. Scapin, M.; Tendler, M. Immunoprecipitins in human schistosomiasis detected with adult worm antigens released by 3M KC1. *J. Helminthol.* **1977**, *51*, 71–72. [CrossRef] [PubMed]

19. Tendler, M.; Scapin, M. The presence of *Schistosoma mansoni* antigens in solutions used for storing adult worms. *Rev. Inst. Med. Trop. Sao Paulo* **1979**, *21*, 293–296. [PubMed]
20. Scarpin, M.; Tendler, M.; Messineo, L.; Katz, N. Preliminary studies with a *Schistosoma mansoni* saline extract inducing protection in rabbits against the challenge infection. *Rev. Inst. Med. Trop. Sao Paulo* **1980**, *22*, 164–172. [PubMed]
21. Tendler, M.; Scapin, M.; Tendler, M.; Scapin, M. *Schistosoma mansoni* antigenic extracts obtained by different extraction procedures. *Mem. Inst. Oswaldo Cruz* **1981**, *76*, 103–109. [CrossRef] [PubMed]
22. Tendler, M.; Lima, A.O.; Pinto, R.M.; Cruz, M.Q.; Brascher, H.M.; Katz, N.; Tendler, M.; Lima, A.O.; Pinto, R.M.; Cruz, M.Q.; et al. Immunogenetic and protective activity of an extract of *Schistosoma mansoni*. *Mem. Inst. Oswaldo Cruz* **1982**, *77*, 275–283. [CrossRef] [PubMed]
23. Tendler, M.; Pinto, R.M.; Bambirra, E.A.; Cruz, M.Q.; Lima, A.O.; Tendler, M.; Pinto, R.M.; Bambirra, E.A.; Cruz, M.Q.; Lima, A.O. Acquired resistance of mice against *S. mansoni* and lung granulomatous reaction induced by BCG. *Mem. Inst. Oswaldo Cruz* **1983**, *78*, 147–151. [CrossRef] [PubMed]
24. Tendler, M.; Magalhães Pinto, R.; Côrtes, M.; Gebara, G. *Schistosoma mansoni*: Comparative evaluation of different routes of experimental infection. *Rev. Inst. Med. Trop. São Paulo* **1985**, *27*, 111–114. [CrossRef] [PubMed]
25. Tendler, M.; Pinto, R.M.; Lima, A.O.; Gebara, G.; Katz, N. *Schistosoma mansoni*: Vaccination with adult worm antigens. *Int. J. Parasitol.* **1986**, *16*, 347–352. [CrossRef]
26. Tendler, M. *Schistosoma mansoni*: Protective antigens. *Mem. Inst. Oswaldo Cruz* **1987**, *82*, 125–128. [CrossRef] [PubMed]
27. Almeida, M.S.S.; Pinto, R.M.; Noronha, D.; Tendler, M.; Katz, N.; Almeida, M.S.S.; Pinto, R.M.; Noronha, D.; Tendler, M.; Katz, N. *Schistosoma mansoni*—NZ rabbit-model: Resistance due to infection and active immunization with adult worm antigen. *Mem. Inst. Oswaldo Cruz* **1987**, *82*, 233. [CrossRef] [PubMed]
28. Almeida, M.S.; Pinto, R.M.; Noronha, D.; Katz, N.; Tendler, M. Curative and protective activity in rabbits after reinfection with *Schistosoma mansoni*: A new model of immunity? *J. Parasitol.* **1989**, *75*, 308–310. [CrossRef] [PubMed]
29. Tendler, M.; Almeida, M.S.; Pinto, R.M.; Noronha, D.; Katz, N. *Schistosoma mansoni*-New Zealand rabbit model: Resistance induced by infection followed by active immunization with protective antigens. *J. Parasitol.* **1991**, *77*, 138–141. [CrossRef] [PubMed]
30. Tendler, M.; Pinto, R.M.; de Oliveira Lima, A.; Savino, W.; Katz, N. Vaccination in murine schistosomiasis with adult worm-derived antigens: Variables influencing protection in outbred mice. *Int. J. Parasitol.* **1991**, *21*, 299–306. [CrossRef]
31. Tendler, M.; Pinto, R.M.; de Oliveira Lima, A.; Savino, W.; Katz, N. Vaccination in murine schistosomiasis with adult worm derived antigens—II. Protective and immune response in inbred mice. *Mem. Inst. Oswaldo Cruz* **1992**, *87*, 281–286. [CrossRef] [PubMed]
32. Moser, D.; Tendler, M.; Griffiths, G.; Klinkert, M.Q. A 14-kDa *Schistosoma mansoni* polypeptide is homologous to a gene family of fatty acid binding proteins. *J. Biol. Chem.* **1991**, *266*, 8447–8454. [PubMed]
33. Tendler, M.; Brito, C.A.; Vilar, M.M.; Serra-Freire, N.; Diogo, C.M.; Almeida, M.S.; Delbem, A.C.; Silva, J.F.D.; Savino, W.; Garratt, R.C.; et al. A *Schistosoma mansoni* fatty acid-binding protein, Sm14, is the potential basis of a dual-purpose anti-helminth vaccine. *Proc. Natl. Acad. Sci. USA* **1996**, *93*, 269–273. [CrossRef] [PubMed]
34. Angelucci, F.; Johnson, K.A.; Baiocco, P.; Miele, A.E.; Brunori, M.; Valle, C.; Vigorosi, F.; Troiani, A.R.; Liberti, P.; Cioli, D.; et al. *Schistosoma mansoni* fatty acid binding protein: Specificity and functional control as revealed by crystallographic structure. *Biochemistry* **2004**, *43*, 13000–13011. [CrossRef] [PubMed]
35. Pertinhez, T.A.; Sforça, M.L.; Alves, A.C.; Ramos, C.R.R.; Ho, P.L.; Tendler, M.; Zanchin, N.I.T.; Spisni, A. Letter to the Editor: 1H, 15N and 13C resonance assignments of the apo Sm14-M20(C62V) protein, a mutant of *Schistosoma mansoni* Sm14. *J. Biomol. NMR* **2004**, *29*, 553–554. [CrossRef] [PubMed]
36. Ramos, C.R.R.; Spisni, A.; Oyama, S.; Sforça, M.L.; Ramos, H.R.; Vilar, M.M.; Alves, A.C.; Figueredo, R.C.R.; Tendler, M.; Zanchin, N.I.T.; et al. Stability improvement of the fatty acid binding protein Sm14 from *S. mansoni* by Cys replacement: Structural and functional characterization of a vaccine candidate. *Biochim. Biophys. Acta BBA-Proteins Proteom.* **2009**, *1794*, 655–662. [CrossRef] [PubMed]
37. Giera, M.; Kaisar, M.M.M.; Derks, R.J.E.; Steenvoorden, E.; Kruize, Y.C.M.; Hokke, C.H.; Yazdanbakhsh, M.; Everts, B. The *Schistosoma mansoni* lipidome: Leads for immunomodulation. *Anal. Chim. Acta* **2018**, *1037*, 107–118. [CrossRef] [PubMed]

38. Rodríguez-Pérez, J.; Rodríguez-Medina, J.R.; García-Blanco, M.A.; Hillyer, G.V. *Fasciola hepatica*: Molecular cloning, nucleotide sequence, and expression of a gene encoding a polypeptide homologous to a *Schistosoma mansoni* fatty acid-binding protein. *Exp. Parasitol.* **1992**, *74*, 400–407. [CrossRef]
39. Almeida, M.S.; Torloni, H.; Lee-Ho, P.; Vilar, M.M.; Thaumaturgo, N.; Simpson, A.J.G.; Tendler, M. Vaccination against *Fasciola hepatica* infection using a *Schistosoma mansoni* defined recombinant antigen, Sm14. *Parasite Immunol.* **2003**, *25*, 135–137. [CrossRef] [PubMed]
40. Study of Safety and Immune Response of the Sm14 Vaccine in Adults of Endemic Regions. Available online: https://clinicaltrials.gov/ct2/show/NCT03041766 (accessed on 17 September 2018).
41. *WHO Guideline on Country Pharmaceutical Pricing Policies*; WHO Guidelines Approved by the Guidelines Review Committee; World Health Organization: Geneva, Switzerland, 2013.

Tropical Medicine and Infectious Disease

MDPI

Correction

Correction: Tendler, M., et al. Current Status of the Sm14/GLA-SE Schistosomiasis Vaccine: Overcoming Barriers and Paradigms towards the First Anti-Parasitic Human(itarian) Vaccine. *Trop. Med. Infect. Dis.* 2018, *3*, 121

Miriam Tendler *, Marília S. Almeida, Monica M. Vilar, Patrícia M. Pinto and Gabriel Limaverde-Sousa

FIOCRUZ—Instituto Oswaldo Cruz, Laboratório de Esquistossomose Experimental, Av. Brasil, 4365, Manguinhos, Rio de Janeiro 21045-900, Brazil; sirianni@ioc.fiocruz.br (M.S.A.); mvilar@ioc.fiocruz.br (M.M.V.); pmpinto@ioc.fiocruz.br (P.M.P.); gabriel.sousa@ioc.fiocruz.br (G.L.-S.)

* Correspondence: tendlermiriam@gmail.com; Tel.: +55-21-2562-1320

Received: 16 January 2019; Accepted: 18 January 2019; Published: 19 January 2019

The authors wish to make the following correction to this paper [1]:

Where it reads:

"In order to have a consistent, stable and defined final product for clinical human use, the Sm14 antigen was formulated with the synthetic adjuvant glucopyranosyl lipid A (GLA-SE), clinically-approved molecule already used in a number of commercially-available human vaccines."

It should read:

"In order to have a consistent, stable and defined final product for clinical human use, the Sm14 antigen was formulated with the synthetic adjuvant glucopyranosyl lipid A (GLA-SE), an adjuvant successfully tested in clinical trials with different human vaccine candidates."

The authors would like to apologize for any inconvenience caused to the readers by this change.

Reference

1. Tendler, M.; Almeida, M.S.; Vilar, M.M.; Pinto, P.M.; Limaverde-Sousa, G. Current Status of the Sm14/GLA-SE Schistosomiasis Vaccine: Overcoming Barriers and Paradigms towards the First Anti-Parasitic Human(itarian) Vaccine. *Trop. Med. Infect. Dis.* **2018**, *3*, 121. [CrossRef] [PubMed]

Tropical Medicine and Infectious Disease

MDPI

Review

Schistosome Vaccines for Domestic Animals

Hong You, Pengfei Cai, Biniam Mathewos Tebeje, Yuesheng Li and Donald P. McManus *

Molecular Parasitology Laboratory, QIMR Berghofer Medical Research Institute, Brisbane, QLD 4006, Australia; Hong.You@qimrberghofer.edu.au (H.Y.); Pengfei.Cai@qimrberghofer.edu.au (P.C.); Biniam.Tebeje@qimrberghofer.edu.au (B.M.T.); Yuesheng.Li@qimrberghofer.edu.au (Y.L.)

* Correspondence: Don.McManus@qimrberghofer.edu.au; Tel.: +61-7-33620401

Received: 18 May 2018; Accepted: 14 June 2018; Published: 19 June 2018

Abstract: Schistosomiasis is recognized as a tropical disease of considerable public health importance, but domestic livestock infections due to *Schistosoma japonicum*, *S. bovis*, *S. mattheei* and *S. curassoni* are often overlooked causes of significant animal morbidity and mortality in Asia and Africa. In addition, whereas schistosomiasis japonica is recognized as an important zoonosis in China and the Philippines, reports of viable schistosome hybrids between animal livestock species and *S. haematobium* point to an underappreciated zoonotic component of transmission in Africa as well. Anti-schistosome vaccines for animal use have long been advocated as part of the solution to schistosomiasis control, benefitting humans and animals and improving the local economy, features aligning with the One Health concept synergizing human and animal health. We review the history of animal vaccines for schistosomiasis from the early days of irradiated larvae and then consider the recombinant DNA technology revolution and its impact in developing schistosome vaccines that followed. We evaluate the major candidates tested in livestock, including the glutathione S-transferases, paramyosin and triose-phosphate isomerase, and summarize some of the future challenges that need to be overcome to design and deliver effective anti-schistosome vaccines that will complement current control options to achieve and sustain future elimination goals.

Keywords: schistosomiasis; *Schistosoma*; vaccine; zoonosis; Asia; Africa; domestic animals; buffalo; cattle; sheep; goats

---

1. Introduction

As well as being a disease of great public health importance, schistosomiasis can also be a chronic debilitating infection of animals and a problem of considerable economic significance in Asia and many parts of Africa. It has been estimated, for example, that 165 million cattle are infected with schistosomiasis worldwide [1]. Schistosome infections of livestock are very important, if often underappreciated, and they are often causes of serious animal mortality and morbidity with several species incriminated. In South and South-East Asia, schistosomiasis is caused by the highly zoonotic *Schistosoma japonicum* and/or *S. mekongi*. *S. mattheei* and/or *S. curassoni* infect cattle, sheep and goats in southern and Central Africa, whereas *S. bovis* is a major veterinary problem in many Mediterranean and African countries, causing high levels of morbidity among susceptible ruminants (cattle, goats, sheep, horses, camels and pigs), resulting in considerably reduced economic output due to liver condemnation, reduced productivity, poor subsequent reproductive performance, increased susceptibility to other infectious agents, and death [1,2].

It has been shown also that uninfected animals grow and gain weight faster and are overall healthier than schistosome-infected animals. *S. bovis* has recently come into the spotlight as an emerging clinical health threat as well following the isolation of *S. haematobium*-*S. bovis* hybrids from children in Senegal [3] and after a recent schistosomiasis outbreak in France [4]. There are also reports of eggs indicative of potential *S. haematobium*-*S. mattheei* hybrids in Zimbabwe and in southern

African ruminants [5]. The hybridization between human and ruminant schistosomes is of particular importance as inter-species hybridization may have a considerable impact on parasite evolution, disease dynamics, transmission rates and control interventions. Laboratory hybrids acquire enhanced characteristics, including infectivity, growth rates, maturation and egg production and, in cattle, it has been reported that introgressive *Schistosoma* hybrids may affect the success of drug treatment and can cause severe disease outbreaks [6]. The zoonotic component of transmission in sub-Saharan Africa does appear to be more significant than previously assumed, and may thereby affect the recently revised WHO vision to eliminate schistosomiasis as a public health problem by 2025. Moreover, animal schistosomiasis is likely to be a significant cost to affected communities due to its direct and indirect impacts on livelihoods. These findings underscore the need for improved disease control in animals, to reduce the zoonotic transmission of *S. japonicum* and *S. mekongi*, and to prevent the spread of hybrid schistosomes to humans from animal reservoirs.

The deployment of suitable anti-schistosome vaccines for use in animals has long been advocated as part of the solution to control and eliminate schistosomiasis. Indeed, a vaccine-directed control program that reduces prevalence, intensity and transmission of the disease in animals can directly benefit both humans and animals in endemic sites and improve the local economy, features that are in clear alignment with the One Health concept synergizing human and animal health. Furthermore, genuine change of the disease spectrum in endemic areas demands lasting results and the development and positioning of an effective vaccine represents an option for long-term protection. An entirely vaccine-based approach targeting humans and animals for schistosomiasis control is unrealistic, but acceptable protection could be achieved by chemotherapy treatment followed by vaccination aimed at reducing, or markedly delaying, the development of pathology and morbidity and limiting the impact of re-infection [7,8]. Thus, the issue is not drugs competing with vaccines, but how to graft a vaccine approach onto current schistosomiasis control programs [7,8]. Mathematical modelling of schistosome transmission supports this concept, predicting that a schistosome vaccine capable of reducing the faecal egg output in bovines by 45% in conjunction with praziquantel treatment would lead to a significant reduction in the transmission of schistosomiasis japonica almost to the point of elimination [9,10]. Domesticated animals represent significant reservoirs of *S. japonicum*, and their vaccination offers an approach to control schistosomiasis by interrupting its zoonotic transmission. Pertinent to this are studies undertaken in China [11] and the Philippines [12], which showed that bovines, in particular, are major animal reservoir hosts for *S. japonicum*, responsible for up to 90% of environmental egg contamination.

2. The Early Days—Irradiated Larval Vaccines

The immunological control of animal schistosomiasis was first advanced as an option in the 1970s as in many endemic areas, particularly in Africa, the use of molluscicides or chemotherapy as interventions was either too expensive or impractical [13]. Further, cattle had been shown to develop partial immunity to reinfection with *S. bovis* and *S. mattheei*, and sheep had been shown to develop some resistance to reinfection with *S. mattheei* [13]. As well, results of experiments in calves, cattle and sheep with harmless heterologous schistosome species suggested that the presence of adult egg-producing worms was not necessary for the development of acquired immunity to reinfection; these observations suggested the possibility of developing a vaccine incorporating either non-pathogenic heterologous larvae or, alternatively, larvae of the homologous species attenuated by irradiation to prevent them reaching full maturity [13]. Cercariae and schistosomula, attenuated with gamma rays, X-rays, or ultraviolet (UV) irradiation, were subsequently reported to elicit protective immunity against schistosomiasis. Indeed, the radiation attenuated vaccine approach provided protective efficacy against *Schistosoma* species in many different host species, including mice, rats, chimpanzees and baboons. The radiation attenuated vaccine also proved to be highly effective in livestock (cattle, buffaloes, sheep and pigs), thereby establishing the potential of developing irradiated live schistosome veterinary vaccines in the laboratory and their extended application to the field.

In a pioneering study in 1976, Taylor et al. [13] demonstrated that sheep could be partially protected against *S. mattheei* by prior immunisation with live cercariae or schistosomula of *S. mattheei* irradiated at 6 krad by a [^{60}Co] source; and the study showed that effective immunisation was not dependent on the presence of a mature worm infection or on cercarial penetration of the skin by the immunising infection, as artificially transformed schistosomula were as immunogenic when injected into sheep as cercariae that penetrated the skin. The results opened up the possibility of making a live vaccine against ovine schistosomiasis, with the caveats that the problem of live parasite storage needed to be overcome and that a more efficient immunising schedule was needed. Other reports described highly effective immunisation of sheep with irradiated *S. bovis* cercariae [14] and irradiated schistosomula [15].

The first attempts at immunising cattle (zebu calves) were against *S. bovis* in Sudan and involved vaccination with 3 krad-irradiated homologous larval parasites first under experimental laboratory challenge using irradiated schistosomula or cercariae [16], and then in the field, under natural challenge when the calves (50% immunised with irradiated schistosomula) were allowed to graze in a *S. bovis*-endemic area for 10 months [17]. In both trials, vaccination was safe and, compared with control animals, the vaccinated animals had higher growth rates and significantly fewer adult worms and tissue and faecal eggs, indicating that zebu cattle could be protected effectively against *S. bovis* by vaccination with irradiated parasites.

An inherent problem in the production of a potential live radiation-attenuated vaccine at this time was the limited shelf-life of the attenuated parasites but new techniques to successfully cryopreserve schistosomula, including vitrification (solidifying a liquid without crystal formation) [18], were developed by Eric James and his team, which enabled their indefinite storage. In 1985, a cryopreserved homologous radiation-attenuated schistosomula vaccine evoked a good level of protection in sheep against *S. bovis* challenge [19].

At about the same time, effective irradiated vaccines were also being developed in China against *S. japonicum* infections, first in mice, and then in domestic pigs, sheep, cattle and buffaloes. These livestock animals, particularly water buffalo (*Bubalus bubalis*), represent important reservoirs of *S. japonicum*, so their vaccination provides a highly suitable approach to control schistosomiasis by zoonotic transmission interruption. The initial experiments were undertaken by Hsü and his team and were reported in 1983 [20] and 1984 [21]. The first study [20] used experimental infections with cattle calves receiving a vaccine of approximately 10,000 irradiated schistosomula followed by a challenge with 500 normal cercariae; the best results, in terms of reduced worm counts, involved three injections (partly given intramuscularly and partly intradermal) of larvae irradiated with 36 krad. The second study [21] was essentially a repeat with calves being perfused later (54–57 days as opposed to one month in the earlier experiment), thereby allowing the infection to mature to egg production, although the reduction in worm numbers was similar. The efficacy of this irradiated vaccine was field tested in vaccinated yearling cattle that were naturally challenged in an area in China highly endemic for schistosomiasis [21]; at perfusion, significant reductions in worm burden and liver eggs were recorded in the vaccinees compared with controls.

Although the work was undertaken in 1979 and 1980, Xu et al. [22] reported in 1993 on trials in bovines of vaccinations with single or double doses of 10,000 or 20,000 cryopreserved irradiated (CI) (20 krad) *S. japonicum* schistosomula together with 1 mL bacille Calmett-Guérin (BCG); worm numbers were reduced by 55–65% in vaccinated water buffalo (*Bubalus bubalis*) and cattle calves after being challenged with 500–1000 cercariae. A field test of the vaccine (10,000 CI schistosomula) resulted in a worm reduction of 53% in vaccinated water buffalo (*Bubalus bubalis*) calves [22]. Intradermal vaccination with 30,000 freeze-thaw (FT) schistosomula and BCG by the same group provided 57% protection in cattle. Similar levels of protection were obtained in sheep immunised with CI and FT schistosomula following challenge with 500 cercariae [23].

Cercariae have also been used as the irradiated vaccine source. Shi et al., in a report published in 1990 [24], vaccinated water buffaloes three times with 10,000 *S. japonicum* cercariae irradiated with a cheap, simple and portable UV light source at a dose of 400 μW min/cm^2. A challenge infection of 1000 untreated cercariae was given to vaccinated and naive control animals; the experiment was terminated six weeks post-challenge and, compared with controls, the vaccinated animals developed 89% resistance to infection with *S. japonicum*. Using a similar vaccination regimen, the same group undertook a study in pigs with a challenge infection of 1000 untreated cercariae given 2.5 or 6 months after the last immunization, with age-matched naïve pigs challenged as controls; immunized animals developed 90% resistance against the challenge [25].

The use of live schistosomula or cercariae vaccines attenuated by ionizing radiation or by biochemical means [26] potentially provides a method to protect domestic livestock against infection with schistosomes, but they have generally not found favour as a practical means of vaccinating domestic animals in the field (or humans) and they have never been used on a large scale. The reasons for this include: (1) the high production costs and labour-intensive efforts necessary to obtain the large numbers of cercariae required from infected snails; (2) the difficulties in standardizing the dose of ionizing radiation in order to induce larval attenuation and to ensure irradiated parasites do not retain some level of infectivity, thereby causing a breakthrough infection if insufficiently irradiated; (3) the requirement for cryo-preservation in order to store and then transport attenuated parasites over long distances; and (4) the safety issues associated with potential toxicity of administering a live vaccine and local inflammatory responses at the site of vaccination.

Thus, although in general the initial successes with irradiated schistosome vaccines were encouraging, with the research benefitting from substantial funding support during the 1970–1990s, progress stalled thereafter. This was mainly due to a change in research emphasis when the new advances in recombinant DNA technology were applied for the development of schistosome vaccines. Consequently, limited work has been undertaken on livestock animals with live attenuated schistosome vaccines in the past 25 years. In one approach protocols were established to compare the level of protection induced by recombinant and naked plasmid DNA formulations with the gold standard gamma or UV-irradiated cercarial vaccines in pigs [27,28]. Another avenue involved systematically investigating cellular and humoral immune responses generated by the protective UV-attenuated *S. japonicum* cercarial vaccine in pigs in order to identify key molecules involved in the process leading to resistance, thereby providing a paradigm for the development of an optimal vaccine formulation for both veterinary and clinical application [25,29–33].

3. The Impact of Recombinant DNA Technology on the Development of Animal Vaccines for Schistosomiasis

As indicated, in efforts to circumvent the perceived problems of using live, attenuated *S. japonicum* schistosomula or cercariae as vaccines to prevent infection in domestic livestock, and with the new techniques in genetic manipulation fast making ground, the research focus changed. Many groups attempted to reproduce or even improve on the protection afforded by substituting native antigens or chemically-defined schistosomal antigens genetically engineered in bacteria or yeast as recombinant proteins, or as plasmid DNA vaccines. The three most tested molecules tested in livestock have been glutathione S-transferases, paramyosin and triose-phosphate isomerase, details for which now follow.

3.1. The Glutathione S-Transferases

Two of the first schistosome molecules to be cloned and expressed (first in *E. coli* and then yeast) were the 28 kDa glutathione-S-transferase from *S. mansoni* (28 GST, P28 or Sm28) [34] and the 26 kDa GST homologue (termed Sj26) from *S. japonicum* [35]. The molecular cloning of the genes encoding the 28 GSTs of *S. bovis*, *S. japonicum* and *S. haematobium* soon followed [36]. The GSTs are enzyme isoforms that catalyse the detoxification of lipophilic molecules by thiol-conjugation. They were considered attractive vaccine candidates in ruminants and other mammals because it was hypothesised that antibody-mediated neutralization of this detoxification function could render the schistosome vulnerable to toxic products generated by immune attack at the tegument or in the gut [37]. Accordingly, it was shown that native GST and GP38, which shares protective epitopes with keyhole limpet haemocyanin (KLH), exhibited vaccine potential against *S. mansoni* in small animal experiments [34]. Subsequently, native forms of *S. bovis* GST and KLH were tested for vaccine efficacy against *S. bovis* in Zebu cattle, and this resulted in specific antibodies being generated against both molecules and, depending on the vaccination schedule, significant reductions in faecal and tissue eggs also resulted; notably, however, vaccination did not reduce adult worm numbers [38]. In contrast, whereas vaccination of goats [39] and sheep [40] with recombinant *S. bovis*-derived 28GST (recombinant *S. bovis* 28GST), followed by experimental challenge with *S. bovis* cercariae, resulted in reduced worm burden, there was no impairment of fecundity. In a further report, immunization of calves with recombinant *S. bovis* 28GST induced significant reductions in female worm numbers, faecal eggs counts, and the number of viable eggs (determined by miracidial counts), in animals exposed to natural *S. mattheei* infection in the field [41]. In contrast, the same immunization schedule generated no protective effect against a massive (10,000 cercariae) single experimental challenge with *S. mattheei*. Being highly susceptible to *S. mattheei* infection, calves produce high parasite recovery rates, and the effect of vaccination and the generated immune response may have been insufficient to protect the animals, raising questions of the biological relevance of massive experimental challenges in the evaluation of protective immunity to schistosomiasis [41,42].

Subsequently, although considerable work on the schistosome GST vaccines focused on *S. mansoni* and then *S. haematobium*, it was clear that the very significant inhibition of female worm fecundity and egg viability was the most evident host protective effect generated against the GSTs of all schistosome species, including *S. japonicum*, by homologous vaccination [43]. The exact mechanism whereby anti-GST antibodies affected egg production and viability remained unanswered, but the phenomenon appeared to be associated with their inhibition of the enzymatic activity of GST, the consequent impairment in prostaglandin biosynthesis (prostaglandin D2 orchestrates various stages of the host immune response), and the resultant effect on schistosome biology, including a reduction in female worm fecundity [44].

Following on from the work with *S. mansoni* GSTs, partial protection was recorded in Chinese sheep and bovines vaccinated with *S. japonicum* 28 kDa GST (Sj28GST), either as a recombinant protein or plasmid DNA vaccine [45–47], but most reports were of the vaccine potential of the 26 kDa GST isoform (Sj26GST) in different mammalian hosts [48,49] (Table 1). Recombinant (r) Sj26GST induced a prominent anti-fecundity effect, as well as a significant, albeit moderate, level of protection in terms of reduced worm burdens in sheep, cattle and pigs, following challenge infection with *S. japonicum* [48–52]. Similar levels of vaccine efficacy were obtained in water buffaloes vaccinated with purified rSj26GST [50,52]. Anti-Sj26GST antibodies were generated in the immunized water buffaloes and, following challenge with *S. japonicum*, the typical anti-fecundity effect was observed with decreased numbers (circa 50%) of faecal eggs and eggs deposited in host livers and intestines [52]. As well, the rSjc26GST vaccine reduced the egg-hatching capacity of *S. japonicum* eggs into viable miracidia by nearly 40% [52]. Encouragingly, field trials demonstrated that the protective effect of rSj26GST against *S. japonicum* could be maintained in cattle and water buffaloes for at least 12 months post-vaccination [53,54], but whereas research to improve efficacy has continued using the murine model of schistosomiasis japonica (e.g., [55]), it is disappointing that there have been no further trials of the vaccine in livestock animals. The picture is somewhat brighter in regards to paramyosin, with some of the early work and recent progress on this vaccine candidate now being described.

Table 1. *S. japonicum* vaccines tested in domestic livestock.

Host	Antigen	Method of Immunization Regimen	Vaccine Efficacy: Worm Burden Reduction %	Vaccine Efficacy: Liver Egg Burden Reduction %	Vaccine Efficacy: Fecal Egg Reduction %	Ref
Pig	UV-attenuated cercariae	Single/three immunizations	59–78	89	86–99.7	[31]
	Irradiated cercariae		>95	>95	>95	[28]
	SjC23-pcDNA3.1 DNA	Conjunction with/without IL-12	29–58	48–56		[56]
	SjTPI-pcDNA3.1 DNA	Conjunction with/without IL-12	46–48	49–66		[57]
	Paramyosin	Conjugated with alum or TiterMax	32–34			[27]
Water buffalo	Paramyosin	Montanide ISA 206	52–58			[58]
	SjCTPI DNA	Fused to bovine heat shock protein 70	41–51	42–62	33–52 (miracidial hatching)	[10]
	SjC23DNA	(Hsp70) and boosted with a plasmid DNA encoding IL-12	45–51	43–54	47–52 (miracidial hatching)	
	Sjc26GST (field study)	Twenty months after vaccination, the infection rate in buffaloes was reduced by 60–68%				[53]
	Sjc26GST		22	50	50	[52]
	Sj28GST (field study)	Injected with Freund's adjuvants	37	33	62 (miracidial hatching)	[46]
	Cryopreserved-irradiated and freeze-thaw schistosomula	Single/twice intradermal vaccination	62–65			[22]
	Cercariae UV irradiated	Six immunizations	89			[24]
Goat	Sj31 and Sj32	DNA priming-protein boosting	21–32	47–52	48–54 (miracidial hatching)	[59]
Cattle	Sj26GST		30	60		[54]
	Sj28GST-DNA	Three immunizations	44	19	77	[47]
	Sj23-DNA		33	34	66	
	Sj28GST + Sj23-DNA		38	48	68	
Sheep	Sj26GST	Injected with Freund's adjuvants	54–62	42–55	11–38	[45,46]
	Sj28GST		61–69	59–69	43–60	
	Sj23		58–66	56–66	40–58	
	Native Paramyosin			68	43	
	Paramyosin			56	16	

3.2. Paramyosin

Paramyosin is a large (97 kDa) coiled-coil myofibrillar protein restricted to invertebrates. In schistosomes it is found on the tegumental surface of lung stage schistosomula, in the cercarial secretory glands, and in the muscles of adult worms and larvae [60]. This molecule first generated interest as a vaccine candidate based on results of experiments in mice targeting *S. mansoni* [60]. Trials in sheep with native and an expressed and purified recombinant fragment of Chinese strain *S. japonicum* paramyosin (Sj-97) resulted in significant partial protection being obtained [45]. Subsequently, vaccine experiments in pigs [27] and water buffaloes [61], using full length Chinese *S. japonicum* paramyosin, yielded further encouraging protective efficacy against challenge infection, although the protection was again only partial. At this time (the early 2000s) the limitations to wide-spread use of recombinant (r) Sj-97 as a vaccine were the size of the protein, the inadequate expression levels obtained, resulting in low yields of the recombinant protein, its insolubility in yeast and bacterial expression systems, the inevitable costs of its up-scaled production and purification, and the funds required for large-scale buffalo vaccine trials in the field; this resulted in a halting in its progression as a priority vaccine candidate.

In 2008, however, Jiz et al. [62] published a new robust method for the pilot-scale expression and purification of rSj-97 by its extraction from *E. coli* inclusion bodies and purification with sequential anion-exchange, hydroxyapatite, and size exclusion chromatography. The purified protein was greater than 95% pure, free of significant endotoxin contamination, adopted an alpha-helical coiled-coil tertiary structure, bound immunoglobulin and collagen, and represented a significant step forward towards preclinical evaluation of paramyosin as a vaccine for schistosomiasis [63]. The same team showed that the rSj-97 vaccine, adjuvanted with Montanide ISA 206, was safe, well tolerated and robustly immunogenic among water buffaloes resident in four villages in Leyte, the Philippines, an area highly endemic for schistosomiasis japonica [64]. They conducted three vaccine trials (in 2008, in 2013 and in 2016) to assess the level of protection generated in water buffaloes with the rSj-97 vaccine; animals received and tolerated well three doses (250 µg/dose or 500 µg/dose) of rSj97 plus Montanide ISA 206 at 4 weekly intervals before a challenge infection with 1000 *S. japonicum* cercariae [58]. The 3×250 µg/dose of rSj97 (2008 and 2013 trials) did not result in a significant reduction in worm burden in vaccinated animals compared with controls injected with ISA 206 emulsified with lyophilisation buffer, but the increased dosage (3×500 µg/dose of rSj97) in the 2013 and 2016 trials resulted in a significantly lower worm burden (by 57.8% in both trials) in vaccinated water buffaloes compared with controls [58]. The trialled rSj97/ISA206 vaccine resulted in a mixed immune response with induction of both IgG1 and IgG2 anti-paramyosin antibodies, but no conclusive correlation was found between isotype distribution and protection [58]. The group also reported undertaking a trial in buffaloes with the rSj97-ISA206 vaccine followed by six months of community-based field exposure after vaccination [58], but the results have not yet been released.

3.3. Triose-Phosphate Isomerase (TPI)

Another leading anti-schistosome vaccine candidate is triose-phosphate isomerase (TPI). Following its uptake in schistosomes, glucose is metabolised via glycolysis to provide critical energy in the form of ATP to ensure parasite survival; TPI is a highly efficient enzyme and pivotal in this process, converting glyceraldehyde-3-phosphate to dihydroxyacetone phosphate. It is located in most cells of the adult schistosome and on the surface membranes of newly transformed schistosomula, the stage in the mammalian host that is considered the most likely target of an anti-schistosome vaccine [50]; a plasmid DNA vaccine encoding *S. japonicum* Chinese strain TPI (SjCTPI) was shown to reduce worm burdens in mice and pigs [57,65]. Subsequently, the efficacy of SjCTPI and the 23 kDa integral membrane protein tetraspanin (SjC23), independently, and as fusions with bovine heat-shock protein 70 (Hsp70), co-administered with an interleukin-12-expressing plasmid as adjuvant, were assessed as DNA vaccines in China in water buffaloes against experimental *S. japonicum* challenge [10]. The most encouraging vaccine was the SjCTPI-Hsp70 construct, which reduced worm burdens by

51.2%, reduced liver eggs by 61.5%, reduced faecal eggs by 52.1% and resulted in a 52.1% reduction in hatching of faecal miracidia [10]. The SjCTPI-Hsp70 vaccine has subsequently undergone field testing in bovines against natural *S. japonicum* challenge in China. The trial comprised a four-year double-blind cluster randomised intervention in 12 administrative villages around the schistosomiasis-endemic Dongting Lake in Hunan Province, designed to assess the impact of a multi-component integrated control strategy, including bovine vaccination using a heterologous 'prime-boost' delivery of the SjCTPI vaccine, on schistosome transmission. The study design and baseline results have been published [66]. In brief, the integrated control strategies included: (a) Combined human mass chemotherapy and the bovine SjCTPI vaccine or placebo vaccine; (b) Combined mollusciciding of snails and bovine SjCTPI vaccine or placebo vaccine; (c) No other intervention (treatment of infected individuals only) and bovine SjCTPI vaccine or placebo vaccine. The primary end-point for the study is human infection rate, with secondary endpoints including bovine infection rate, snail infection prevalence and the density of infected snails.

4. Challenges and Opportunities for the Future

In summary, many of the *S. japonicum* vaccines tested in domestic livestock include enzymes, muscle components and membrane proteins (Table 1) [67,68]. DNA vaccines have found particular appeal as they generate both T-cell and B-cell (or antibody-mediated) immune responses, their preparation and production are convenient and cost-effective, and they can even be used in the field without a cold chain. Another advantage of applying DNA vaccines compared with other approaches is the possibility of targeting the in vivo expressed recombinant antigen to different cell compartments. Furthermore, methods such as prime-boost regimens and the use of adjuvants (such as IL-12) in combination with a DNA vaccine can enhance its protective efficacy.

Other than some proteomic analyses of *S. bovis* and the *S. bovis*-host interface, aimed at identifying potential new vaccine and drug targets [69], it is surprising that no recent research has been reported in the development and testing of different vaccines targeting schistosomiasis infections caused by *S. bovis* and *S. mattheei* in livestock, despite the early encouraging successes. This may be somewhat short-sighted as it has been recently argued that animal schistosomiasis likely causes a considerable drain, both directly and indirectly, on the local economy of many poor communities in sub-Saharan Africa [70]. Further, the zoonotic component of schistosomiasis transmission in Africa appears to be far more significant and important than previously thought [6], and this may impact on the current WHO vision to eliminate schistosomiasis as a public health issue by 2025. Consequently, it has been considered that extending treatment to include animal hosts in a One Health approach, as has been successfully undertaken in China, would be both of economic and public health benefit. The positioning of an animal-based transmission blocking vaccine as part of an integrated control package fits well into this scenario, as was recognised as an outcome of two workshops co-sponsored by the Bill and Melinda Gates Foundation and the National Institute of Allergy and Infectious Diseases on schistosomiasis elimination strategies and the potential role of a vaccine [71,72]. Some proposed Preferred Product Characteristics for a clinical versus a veterinary vaccine against schistosomiasis were formulated at one of these workshops, indicating that the safety profile of the latter is more straightforward and less rigorous [71]. Whereas this characteristic could potentially reduce the costs of deploying a schistosomiasis vaccine for use in livestock as opposed to one for human application, an evaluation of the economics and benefits of applying the two different types of vaccine needs to be undertaken.

One significant challenge impacting on the future development of veterinary-targeted vaccines to aid in the control of schistosomiasis continues to be our rather scanty knowledge of the immunology of schistosome infections in natural livestock hosts, especially bovines, compared with experimental model animals, such as mice. This is due, in part, to the high cost of purchasing and maintaining large animals for immunobiological studies and the scarcity and high price of immunological reagents for studying the relevant immune responses. Nevertheless, some recent research has provided new insights on immunity against schistosomiasis japonica in field-exposed natural hosts such as cattle and water buffalo, particularly the immune response generated against migrating schistosome larvae, the likely targets of an anti-schistosome vaccine. In an important study, McWilliam et al. [73] investigated the immune response evoked in the lungs and skin, the major sites of larval migration, in previously *S. japonicum*-exposed and re-challenged water buffaloes. A powerful allergic-type response was generated in the skin with IL-5 transcript levels being elevated, with IL-10 levels decreased. In addition, a Th1 type immune profile was demonstrated in stimulated cells from the lung-draining lymph node, whereas a predominant Th2 type immune response was apparent in stimulated cells from the skin-draining lymph node; these immune responses reflected the timing of parasite migration and occurred consecutively. The intense Th2 type profile generated at the cercarial penetration site differs markedly from that evident in mice, suggesting a possible mechanism of immunity. Furthermore, the study suggested that a reduced/delayed immune response occurred in buffaloes challenged with high numbers of cercariae compared with lower numbers, particularly in the skin.

In tandem with studies comparing immune responses in buffalo (in which age-related resistance likely occurs) and yellow cattle (in which it does not) against schistosomiasis [74,75], and further immunological exploration of the self-cure effect in older buffalo and other livestock hosts such as pigs against schistosomes [76], the investigation by McWilliam et al. [73] provides a unique, in-depth appreciation of the immunobiology of schistosomiasis in a natural host. Such studies can aid in the design and delivery of more effective anti-schistosome vaccines that will complement current control options so as to achieve and sustain future elimination goals.

Author Contributions: D.P.M. conducted the literature review, and drafted and revised the manuscript. H.Y., B.M.T., L.Y. and P.C. revised the manuscript and provided intellectual content. All authors read and approved the final manuscript.

Funding: This research was funded by the National Health and Medical Research Council of Australia (NHMRC) grant number APP1132975.

Acknowledgments: The authors would like to thank the National Health and Medical Research Council of Australia (NHMRC) for providing financial support for their research on schistosomiasis through Project (APP1002245, APP1098244) and Program (APP1037304, APP1132975) grants. DPM is a NHMRC Senior Principal Research Fellow (APP1102926).

Conflicts of Interest: The authors declare no conflict of interest. Ethical clearance was not required for the review.

References

1. De Bont, J.; Vercruysse, J. Schistosomiasis in cattle. *Adv. Parasitol.* **1998**, *41*, 285–364. [PubMed]
2. Charlier, J.; van der Voort, M.; Kenyon, F.; Skuce, P.; Vercruysse, J. Chasing helminths and their economic impact on farmed ruminants. *Trends Parasitol.* **2014**, *30*, 361–367. [CrossRef] [PubMed]
3. Webster, B.L.; Diaw, O.T.; Seye, M.M.; Webster, J.P.; Rollinson, D. Introgressive hybridization of *Schistosoma haematobium* group species in Senegal: Species barrier break down between ruminant and human schistosomes. *PLoS Negl. Trop. Dis.* **2013**, *7*, e2110. [CrossRef] [PubMed]
4. Boissier, J.; Grech-Angelini, S.; Webster, B.L.; Allienne, J.F.; Huyse, T.; Mas-Coma, S.; Toulza, E.; Barre-Cardi, H.; Rollinson, D.; Kincaid-Smith, J.; et al. Outbreak of urogenital schistosomiasis in Corsica (France): An epidemiological case study. *Lancet Infect. Dis.* **2016**, *16*, 971–979. [CrossRef]
5. King, K.C.; Stelkens, R.B.; Webster, J.P.; Smith, D.F.; Brockhurst, M.A. Hybridization in parasites: Consequences for adaptive evolution, pathogenesis, and public health in a changing world. *PLoS Pathog.* **2015**, *11*, e1005098. [CrossRef] [PubMed]
6. Leger, E.; Webster, J.P. Hybridizations within the genus *Schistosoma*: Implications for evolution, epidemiology and control. *Parasitology* **2017**, *144*, 65–80. [CrossRef] [PubMed]
7. Bergquist, R.; Utzinger, J.; McManus, D.P. Trick or treat: The role of vaccines in integrated schistosomiasis control. *PLoS Negl. Trop. Dis.* **2008**, *2*, e244. [CrossRef] [PubMed]
8. Bergquist, R.M.; Donald, M. Schistosomiasis vaccine development: The missing link. In *Schistosoma Biology, Pathology, Control*; Jamieson, B.G.M., Ed.; CRC Press: Boca Raton, FL, USA, 2017; pp. 462–478.

9. Williams, G.M.; Sleigh, A.C.; Li, Y.; Feng, Z.; Davis, G.M.; Chen, H.; Ross, A.G.; Bergquist, R.; McManus, D.P. Mathematical modelling of schistosomiasis japonica: Comparison of control strategies in the People's Republic of China. *Acta Trop.* **2002**, *82*, 253–262. [CrossRef]
10. Da'dara, A.A.; Li, Y.S.; Xiong, T.; Zhou, J.; Williams, G.M.; McManus, D.P.; Feng, Z.; Yu, X.L.; Gray, D.J.; Harn, D.A. DNA-based vaccines protect against zoonotic schistosomiasis in water buffalo. *Vaccine* **2008**, *26*, 3617–3625. [CrossRef] [PubMed]
11. Gray, D.J.; Williams, G.M.; Li, Y.; Chen, H.; Li, R.S.; Forsyth, S.J.; Barnett, A.G.; Guo, J.; Feng, Z.; McManus, D.P. A cluster-randomized bovine intervention trial against *Schistosoma japonicum* in the People's Republic of China: Design and baseline results. *Am. J. Trop. Med. Hyg.* **2007**, *77*, 866–874. [PubMed]
12. Gordon, C.A.; Acosta, L.P.; Gray, D.J.; Olveda, R.M.; Jarilla, B.; Gobert, G.N.; Ross, A.G.; McManus, D.P. High prevalence of *Schistosoma japonicum* infection in Carabao from Samar Province, the Philippines: Implications for transmission and control. *PLoS Negl. Trop. Dis.* **2012**, *6*, e1778. [CrossRef] [PubMed]
13. Taylor, M.G.; James, E.R.; Nelson, G.S.; Bickle, Q.; Dunne, D.W.; Webbe, G. Immunisation of sheep against *Schistosoma mattheei* using either irradiated cercariae or irradiated schistosomula. *J. Helminthol.* **1976**, *50*, 1–9. [CrossRef] [PubMed]
14. Hussein, M.F.; Bushara, H.O. Investigations on the development of an irradiated vaccine for animal schistosomiasis. In *Nuclear Techniques in Animal Production and Health*; International Atomic Energy Agency: Vienna, Austria, 1976; pp. 421–431.
15. Taylor, M.G.; James, E.R.; Bickle, Q.; Hussein, M.F.; Andrews, B.J.; Dobinson, A.R.; Nelson, G.S. Immunization of sheep against *Schistosoma bovis* using an irradiated schistosomular vaccine. *J. Helminthol.* **1979**, *53*, 1–5. [CrossRef] [PubMed]
16. Bushara, H.O.; Hussein, M.F.; Saad, A.M.; Taylor, M.G.; Dargie, J.D.; Marshall, T.F.; Nelson, G.S. Immunization of calves against *Schistosoma bovis* using irradiated cercariae of schistosomula of *S. bovis*. *Parasitology* **1978**, *77*, 303–311. [CrossRef] [PubMed]
17. Majid, A.A.; Bushara, H.O.; Saad, A.M.; Hussein, M.F.; Taylor, M.G.; Dargie, J.D.; Marshall, T.F.; Nelson, G.S. Observations on cattle schistosomiasis in the Sudan, a study in comparative medicine. III. Field testing of an irradiated *Schistosoma bovis* vaccine. *Am. J. Trop. Med. Hyg.* **1980**, *29*, 452–455. [CrossRef] [PubMed]
18. James, E.R. Cryopreservation of helminths. *Parasitol. Today* **1985**, *1*, 134–139. [CrossRef]
19. James, E.R.; Dobinson, A.R.; Lucas, S.B.; Andrews, B.J.; Bickle, Q.D.; Taylor, M.G.; Ham, P.J. Protection of sheep against *Schistosoma bovis* using cryopreserved radiation-attenuated schistosomula. *J. Helminthol.* **1985**, *59*, 51–55. [CrossRef] [PubMed]
20. Hsu, S.Y.; Hsu, H.F.; Xu, S.T.; Shi, F.H.; He, Y.X.; Clarke, W.R.; Johnson, S.C. Vaccination against bovine schistosomiasis japonica with highly X-irradiated schistosomula. *Am. J. Trop. Med. Hyg.* **1983**, *32*, 367–370. [CrossRef] [PubMed]
21. Hsu, S.Y.; Xu, S.T.; He, Y.X.; Shi, F.H.; Shen, W.; Hsu, H.F.; Osborne, J.W.; Clarke, W.R. Vaccination of bovines against schistosomiasis japonica with highly irradiated schistosomula in China. *Am. J. Trop. Med. Hyg.* **1984**, *33*, 891–898. [CrossRef] [PubMed]
22. Xu, S.; Shi, F.; Shen, W.; Lin, J.; Wang, Y.; Lin, B.; Qian, C.; Ye, P.; Fu, L.; Shi, Y.; et al. Vaccination of bovines against schistosomiasis japonica with cryopreserved-irradiated and freeze-thaw schistosomula. *Vet. Parasitol.* **1993**, *47*, 37–50. [PubMed]
23. Xu, S.; Wu, H.; Fu, L.; Tzian, T.; Lin, B.; Tzian, T.; Chu, H. Tests to immunize sheep by freezing *Schistosoma japonicum* larva vaccines. *China J. Vet. Sci. Technol.* **1990**, *2*, 19–20.
24. Shi, Y.E.; Jiang, C.F.; Han, J.J.; Li, Y.L.; Ruppel, A. *Schistosoma japonicum*: An ultraviolet-attenuated cercarial vaccine applicable in the field for water buffaloes. *Exp. Parasitol.* **1990**, *71*, 100–106. [CrossRef]
25. Shi, Y.E.; Jiang, C.F.; Han, J.J.; Li, Y.L.; Ruppel, A. Immunization of pigs against infection with *Schistosoma japonicum* using ultraviolet-attenuated cercariae. *Parasitology* **1993**, *106*, 459–462. [CrossRef] [PubMed]
26. Chi, L.W.; Andreus, J.; Yates, R.A.; Kiley, L.A.; Liu, S.X. Worm burden and lymphocyte response in mice immunized with *N*-methyl-*N*′-nitro-*N*-nitrosoguanidine attenuated cercariae of *Schistosoma japonicum*. *Chin. Med. J.* **1988**, *101*, 181–186. [PubMed]
27. Chen, H.; Nara, T.; Zeng, X.; Satoh, M.; Wu, G.; Jiang, W.; Yi, F.; Kojima, S.; Zhang, S.; Hirayama, K. Vaccination of domestic pig with recombinant paramyosin against *Schistosoma japonicum* in China. *Vaccine* **2000**, *18*, 2142–2146. [CrossRef]

28. Bickle, Q.D.; Bogh, H.O.; Johansen, M.V.; Zhang, Y. Comparison of the vaccine efficacy of gamma-irradiated *Schistosoma japonicum* cercariae with the defined antigen Sj62(IrV-5) in pigs. *Vet. Parasitol.* **2001**, *100*, 51–62. [CrossRef]
29. Abdel-Hafeez, E.H.; Kikuchi, M.; Watanabe, K.; Ito, T.; Yu, C.; Chen, H.; Nara, T.; Arakawa, T.; Aoki, Y.; Hirayama, K. Proteome approach for identification of schistosomiasis japonica vaccine candidate antigen. *Parasitol. Int.* **2009**, *58*, 36–44. [CrossRef] [PubMed]
30. Tian, F.; Lin, D.; Wu, J.; Gao, Y.; Zhang, D.; Ji, M.; Wu, G. Immune events associated with high level protection against *Schistosoma japonicum* infection in pigs immunized with UV-attenuated cercariae. *PLoS ONE* **2010**, *5*, e13408. [CrossRef] [PubMed]
31. Lin, D.; Tian, F.; Wu, H.; Gao, Y.; Wu, J.; Zhang, D.; Ji, M.; McManus, D.P.; Driguez, P.; Wu, G. Multiple vaccinations with UV-attenuated cercariae in pig enhance protective immunity against *Schistosoma japonicum* infection as compared to single vaccination. *Parasites Vectors* **2011**, *4*. [CrossRef] [PubMed]
32. Tian, F.; Hou, M.; Chen, L.; Gao, Y.; Zhang, X.; Ji, M.; Wu, G. Proteomic analysis of schistosomiasis japonica vaccine candidate antigens recognized by UV-attenuated cercariae-immunized porcine serum IgG2. *Parasitol. Res.* **2013**, *112*, 2791–2803. [CrossRef] [PubMed]
33. Abdel-Hafeez, E.H.; Watanabe, K.; Kamei, K.; Kikuchi, M.; Chen, H.; Daniel, B.; Yu, C.; Hirayama, K. Pilot study on interferon-gamma-producing T cell subsets after the protective vaccination with radiation-attenuated cercaria of *Schistosoma japonicum* in the miniature pig model. *Trop. Med. Health* **2014**, *42*, 155–162. [CrossRef] [PubMed]
34. Balloul, J.M.; Sondermeyer, P.; Dreyer, D.; Capron, M.; Grzych, J.M.; Pierce, R.J.; Carvallo, D.; Lecocq, J.P.; Capron, A. Molecular cloning of a protective antigen of schistosomes. *Nature* **1987**, *326*, 149–153. [CrossRef] [PubMed]
35. Saint, R.B.; Beall, J.A.; Grumont, R.J.; Mitchell, G.F.; Garcia, E.G. Expression of *Schistosoma japonicum* antigens in *Escherichia coli*. *Mol. Biochem. Parasitol.* **1986**, *18*, 333–342. [CrossRef]
36. Trottein, F.; Godin, C.; Pierce, R.J.; Sellin, B.; Taylor, M.G.; Gorillot, I.; Silva, M.S.; Lecocq, J.P.; Capron, A. Inter-species variation of schistosome 28-kDa glutathione S-transferases. *Mol. Biochem. Parasitol.* **1992**, *54*, 63–72. [CrossRef]
37. Mitchell, G.F. Glutathione *S*-transferases—Potential components of anti-schistosome vaccines? *Parasitol. Today* **1989**, *5*, 34–37. [CrossRef]
38. Bushara, H.O.; Bashir, M.E.; Malik, K.H.; Mukhtar, M.M.; Trottein, F.; Capron, A.; Taylor, M.G. Suppression of *Schistosoma bovis* egg production in cattle by vaccination with either glutathione S-transferase or keyhole limpet haemocyanin. *Parasite Immunol.* **1993**, *15*, 383–390. [CrossRef] [PubMed]
39. Boulanger, D.; Trottein, F.; Mauny, F.; Bremond, P.; Couret, D.; Pierce, R.J.; Kadri, S.; Godin, C.; Sellin, E.; Lecocq, J.P.; et al. Vaccination of goats against the trematode *Schistosoma bovis* with a recombinant homologous schistosome-derived glutathione S-transferase. *Parasite Immunol.* **1994**, *16*, 399–406. [CrossRef] [PubMed]
40. Boulanger, D.; Schneider, D.; Chippaux, J.P.; Sellin, B.; Capron, A. *Schistosoma bovis*: Vaccine effects of a recombinant homologous glutathione S-transferase in sheep. *Int. J. Parasitol.* **1999**, *29*, 415–418. [CrossRef]
41. De Bont, J.; Vercruysse, J.; Grzych, J.M.; Meeus, P.F.; Capron, A. Potential of a recombinant *Schistosoma bovis*-derived glutathione S-transferase to protect cattle against experimental and natural *S. mattheei* infection. *Parasitology* **1997**, *115*, 249–255. [CrossRef] [PubMed]
42. Grzych, J.M.; De Bont, J.; Liu, J.; Neyrinck, J.L.; Fontaine, J.; Vercruysse, J.; Capron, A. Relationship of impairment of schistosome 28-kilodalton glutathione S-transferase (GST) activity to expression of immunity to *Schistosoma mattheei* in calves vaccinated with recombinant *Schistosoma bovis* 28-kilodalton GST. *Infect. Immun.* **1998**, *66*, 1142–1148. [PubMed]
43. Capron, A. Schistosomiasis: Forty years' war on the worm. *Parasitol. Today* **1998**, *14*, 379–384. [CrossRef]
44. Herve, M.; Angeli, V.; Pinzar, E.; Wintjens, R.; Faveeuw, C.; Narumiya, S.; Capron, A.; Urade, Y.; Capron, M.; Riveau, G.; et al. Pivotal roles of the parasite PGD2 synthase and of the host D prostanoid receptor 1 in schistosome immune evasion. *Eur. J. Immunol.* **2003**, *33*, 2764–2772. [CrossRef] [PubMed]
45. Taylor, M.G.; Huggins, M.C.; Shi, F.; Lin, J.; Tian, E.; Ye, P.; Shen, W.; Qian, C.G.; Lin, B.F.; Bickle, Q.D. Production and testing of *Schistosoma japonicum* candidate vaccine antigens in the natural ovine host. *Vaccine* **1998**, *16*, 1290–1298. [CrossRef]

46. Shi, F.; Zhang, Y.; Ye, P.; Lin, J.; Cai, Y.; Shen, W.; Bickle, Q.D.; Taylor, M.G. Laboratory and field evaluation of *Schistosoma japonicum* DNA vaccines in sheep and water buffalo in China. *Vaccine* **2001**, *20*, 462–467. [CrossRef]
47. Shi, F.; Zhang, Y.; Lin, J.; Zuo, X.; Shen, W.; Cai, Y.; Ye, P.; Bickle, Q.D.; Taylor, M.G. Field testing of *Schistosoma japonicum* DNA vaccines in cattle in China. *Vaccine* **2002**, *20*, 3629–3631. [CrossRef]
48. McManus, D.P. Prospects for development of a transmission blocking vaccine against *Schistosoma japonicum*. *Parasite Immunol.* **2005**, *27*, 297–308. [CrossRef] [PubMed]
49. Wu, Z.D.; Lu, Z.Y.; Yu, X.B. Development of a vaccine against *Schistosoma japonicum* in China: A review. *Acta Trop.* **2005**, *96*, 106–116. [CrossRef] [PubMed]
50. McManus, D.P.; Loukas, A. Current status of vaccines for schistosomiasis. *Clin. Microbiol. Rev.* **2008**, *21*, 225–242. [CrossRef] [PubMed]
51. Liu, S.X.; Song, G.C.; Xu, Y.X.; Yang, W.; McManus, D.P. Anti-fecundity immunity induced in pigs vaccinated with recombinant *Schistosoma japonicum* 26 kDa glutathione-*S*-transferase. *Parasite Immunol.* **1995**, *17*, 335–340. [CrossRef] [PubMed]
52. Shuxian, L.; Yongkang, H.; Guangchen, S.; Xing-song, L.; Yuxin, X.; McManus, D.P. Anti-fecundity immunity to *Schistosoma japonicum* induced in Chinese water buffaloes (*Bos buffelus*) after vaccination with recombinant 26 kDa glutathione-S-transferase (reSjc26GST). *Vet. Parasitol.* **1997**, *69*, 39–47. [CrossRef]
53. He, Y.K.; Liu, S.X.; Zhang, X.Y.; Chen, G.C.; Luo, X.S.; Li, Y.S.; Xu, Y.X.; Yu, X.L.; Yang, R.Q.; Chen, Y.; et al. Field assessment of recombinant *Schistosoma japonicum* 26 kDa glutathione S-transferase in Chinese water buffaloes. *Southeast Asian J. Trop. Med. Hyg.* **2003**, *34*, 473–479.
54. Wu, Z.; Liu, S.; Zhang, S.; Tong, H.; Gao, Z.; Liu, Y.; Lin, D.; Liu, Z.; Wu, G.; Yi, H.; et al. Persistence of the protective immunity to *Schistosoma japonicum* in Chinese yellow cattle induced by recombinant 26 kDa glutathione-S-transferase (reSjc26GST). *Vet. Parasitol.* **2004**, *123*, 167–177. [CrossRef] [PubMed]
55. Cheng, P.C.; Lin, C.N.; Peng, S.Y.; Kang, T.F.; Lee, K.M. Combined IL-12 Plasmid and recombinant SjGST enhance the protective and anti-pathology effect of SjGST DNA vaccine against *Schistosoma japonicum*. *PLoS Negl. Trop. Dis.* **2016**, *10*. [CrossRef] [PubMed]
56. Zhu, Y.; Ren, J.; Da'dara, A.; Harn, D.; Xu, M.; Si, J.; Yu, C.; Liang, Y.; Ye, P.; Yin, X.; et al. The protective effect of a *Schistosoma japonicum* Chinese strain 23 kDa plasmid DNA vaccine in pigs is enhanced with IL-12. *Vaccine* **2004**, *23*, 78–83. [CrossRef] [PubMed]
57. Zhu, Y.; Si, J.; Harn, D.A.; Xu, M.; Ren, J.; Yu, C.; Liang, Y.; Yin, X.; He, W.; Cao, G. *Schistosoma japonicum* triose-phosphate isomerase plasmid DNA vaccine protects pigs against challenge infection. *Parasitology* **2006**, *132*, 67–71. [CrossRef] [PubMed]
58. Wu, H.W.; Fu, Z.Q.; Lu, K.; Pond-Tor, S.; Meng, R.; Hong, Y.; Chu, K.; Li, H.; Jiz, M.; Liu, J.M.; et al. Vaccination with recombinant paramyosin in Montanide ISA206 protects against *Schistosoma japonicum* infection in water buffalo. *Vaccine* **2017**, *35*, 3409–3415. [CrossRef] [PubMed]
59. Tang, L.; Zhou, Z.; Chen, Y.; Luo, Y.; Wang, L.; Chen, L.; Huang, F.; Zeng, X.; Yi, X. Vaccination of goats with 31 kDa and 32 kDa *Schistosoma japonicum* antigens by DNA priming and protein boosting. *Cell. Mol. Immunol.* **2007**, *4*, 153–156. [PubMed]
60. Gobert, G.N.; Stenzel, D.J.; Jones, M.K.; Allen, D.E.; McManus, D.P. *Schistosoma japonicum*: Immunolocalization of paramyosin during development. *Parasitology* **1997**, *114*, 45–52. [CrossRef] [PubMed]
61. McManus, D.P.; Wong, J.Y.; Zhou, J.; Cai, C.; Zeng, Q.; Smyth, D.; Li, Y.; Kalinna, B.H.; Duke, M.J.; Yi, X. Recombinant paramyosin (rec-Sj-97) tested for immunogenicity and vaccine efficacy against *Schistosoma japonicum* in mice and water buffaloes. *Vaccine* **2001**, *20*, 870–878. [CrossRef]
62. Jiz, M.; Wu, H.W.; Meng, R.; Pond-Tor, S.; Reynolds, M.; Friedman, J.F.; Olveda, R.; Acosta, L.; Kurtis, J.D. Pilot-scale production and characterization of paramyosin, a vaccine candidate for schistosomiasis japonica. *Infect. Immun.* **2008**, *76*, 3164–3169. [CrossRef] [PubMed]
63. Jiz, M.A.; Wu, H.; Olveda, R.; Jarilla, B.; Kurtis, J.D. Development of paramyosin as a vaccine candidate for schistosomiasis. *Front. Immunol.* **2015**, *6*. [CrossRef] [PubMed]
64. Jiz, I.M.; Mingala, C.N.; Lopez, I.F.M.; Chua, M.; Gabonada, F.G., Jr.; Acosta, L.P.; Wu, H.; Kurtis, J.D. A field trial of recombinant *Schistosoma japonicum* paramyosin as a potential vaccine in naturally-infected water buffaloes. *Ann. Parasitol.* **2016**, *62*, 295–299.

65. Zhu, Y.; Si, J.; Ham, D.A.; Yu, C.; He, W.; Hua, W.; Yin, X.; Liang, Y.; Xu, M.; Xu, R. The protective immunity produced in infected C57BL/6 mice of a DNA vaccine encoding *Schistosoma japonicum* Chinese strain triose-phosphate isomerase. *Southeast Asian J. Trop. Med. Public Health* **2002**, *33*, 207–213. [PubMed]
66. Gray, D.J.; Li, Y.S.; Williams, G.M.; Zhao, Z.Y.; Harn, D.A.; Li, S.M.; Ren, M.Y.; Feng, Z.; Guo, F.Y.; Guo, J.G.; et al. A multi-component integrated approach for the elimination of schistosomiasis in the People's Republic of China: Design and baseline results of a 4-year cluster-randomised intervention trial. *Int. J. Parasitol.* **2014**, *44*, 659–668. [CrossRef] [PubMed]
67. Tebeje, B.M.; Harvie, M.; You, H.; Loukas, A.; McManus, D.P. Schistosomiasis vaccines: Where do we stand? *Parasites Vectors* **2016**, *9*. [CrossRef] [PubMed]
68. You, H.; McManus, D.P. Vaccines and diagnostics for zoonotic schistosomiasis japonica. *Parasitology* **2015**, *142*, 271–289. [CrossRef] [PubMed]
69. De la Torre-Escudero, E.; Perez-Sanchez, R.; Manzano-Roman, R.; Oleaga, A. *Schistosoma bovis*-host interplay: Proteomics for knowing and acting. *Mol. Biochem. Parasitol.* **2017**, *215*, 30–39. [CrossRef] [PubMed]
70. Gower, C.M.; Vince, L.; Webster, J.P. Should we be treating animal schistosomiasis in Africa? The need for a One Health economic evaluation of schistosomiasis control in people and their livestock. *Trans. R. Soc. Trop. Med. Hyg.* **2017**, *111*, 244–247. [CrossRef] [PubMed]
71. Mo, A.X.; Colley, D.G. Workshop report: Schistosomiasis vaccine clinical development and product characteristics. *Vaccine* **2016**, *34*, 995–1001. [CrossRef] [PubMed]
72. Mo, A.X.; Agosti, J.M.; Walson, J.L.; Hall, B.F.; Gordon, L. Schistosomiasis elimination strategies and potential role of a vaccine in achieving global health goals. *Am. J. Trop. Med. Hyg.* **2014**, *90*, 54–60. [CrossRef] [PubMed]
73. McWilliam, H.E.; Piedrafita, D.; Li, Y.; Zheng, M.; He, Y.; Yu, X.; McManus, D.P.; Meeusen, E.N. Local immune responses of the Chinese water buffalo, *Bubalus bubalis*, against *Schistosoma japonicum* larvae: Crucial insights for vaccine design. *PLoS Negl. Trop. Dis.* **2013**, *7*, e2460. [CrossRef] [PubMed]
74. Wang, T.; Zhang, S.; Wu, W.; Zhang, G.; Lu, D.; Ornbjerg, N.; Johansen, M.V. Treatment and reinfection of water buffaloes and cattle infected with *Schistosoma japonicum* in Yangtze River Valley, Anhui province, China. *J. Parasitol.* **2006**, *92*, 1088–1091. [CrossRef] [PubMed]
75. Yang, J.; Fu, Z.; Feng, X.; Shi, Y.; Yuan, C.; Liu, J.; Hong, Y.; Li, H.; Lu, K.; Lin, J. Comparison of worm development and host immune responses in natural hosts of *Schistosoma japonicum*, yellow cattle and water buffalo. *BMC Vet. Res.* **2012**, *8*. [CrossRef] [PubMed]
76. Li, Y.S.; McManus, D.P.; Lin, D.D.; Williams, G.M.; Harn, D.A.; Ross, A.G.; Feng, Z.; Gray, D.J. The *Schistosoma japonicum* self-cure phenomenon in water buffaloes: Potential impact on the control and elimination of schistosomiasis in China. *Int. J. Parasitol.* **2014**, *44*, 167–171. [CrossRef] [PubMed]

Tropical Medicine and Infectious Disease

MDPI

Review

Use of Geospatial Surveillance and Response Systems for Vector-Borne Diseases in the Elimination Phase

John B. Malone [1,*], Robert Bergquist [2], Moara Martins [1] and Jeffrey C. Luvall [3]

1 Pathobiological Sciences, School of Veterinary Medicine, Louisiana State University, Baton Rouge, LA 70803, USA; moaramartins@gmail.com
2 Ingerod, SE-454 94 Brastad, Sweden; robert.bergquist@outlook.com
3 National Aeronautics Space Administration (NASA), MSFC ST11, NSSTC, 320 Sparkman Drive, Huntsville, AL 35805, USA; jluvall@nasa.gov
* Correspondence: vtmalon@lsu.edu; Tel.: +225-614-6103

Received: 28 December 2018; Accepted: 15 January 2019; Published: 18 January 2019

Abstract: The distribution of diseases caused by vector-borne viruses and parasites are restricted by the environmental requirements of their vectors, but also by the ambient temperature inside the host as it influences the speed of maturation of the infectious agent transferred. The launch of the Soil Moisture Active Passive (SMAP) satellite in 2015, and the new ECOSTRESS instrument onboard the International Space Station (ISS) in 2018, established the leadership of the National Aeronautics Space Administration (NASA) in ecology and climate research by allowing the structural and functional classification of ecosystems that govern vector sustainability. These advances, and the availability of sub-meter resolution data from commercial satellites, contribute to seamless mapping and modelling of diseases, not only at continental scales (1 km^2) and local community or agricultural field scales (15–30 m^2), but for the first time, also at the habitat–household scale (<1 m^2). This communication presents current capabilities that are related to data collection by Earth-observing satellites, and draws attention to the usefulness of geographical information systems (GIS) and modelling for the study of important parasitic diseases.

Keywords: GIS; remote-sensing; satellite; international space station; ECOSTRESS; worldview; spatio-temporal epidemiology; climate change; parasite; schistosomiasis, leishmaniasis

1. Introduction

Disease and location were already linked by Hippocrates in the fourth century before the Christian era, and Snow famously traced a cholera outbreak to a particular water pump in London in the mid-1800s. Interestingly, this was before anybody had any idea about bacteria and viruses, even though van Leeuwenhoek probably saw the former in his rudimentary microscope, 170 years before Snow's findings. However, some decades later, communicable diseases and their propagation were already quite well understood, but what was now missing was the technology needed to translate the data collected over large areas into reliable risk maps. Remote sensing (RS), first from airplanes, since the 1970s from satellites, and very recently also from drones, changed all that. RS became the impetus to the merger of Earth sciences, computer technology, and advanced statistics eventually granting access to an array of advanced tools that are highly suitable for epidemiological investigation [1–4]. Such techniques are particularly useful for the study of those parasitic infections that rely on intermediate hosts (vectors) to complete their life cycles, since these vectors (commonly insects but also molluscs) are highly sensitive to a range of environmental variables. In addition, temperature also limits the maturation of the parasite's intermediate stage(s) inside the vector which, together with other variables, makes it possible to estimate disease distributions with a good level of accuracy. Indeed, the number of publications promoting the use of remotely sensed variables, such as land use, temperature, rainfall, humidity, vegetation etc., to effectively decide the distributions of infectious microorganisms, is increasing exponentially, as exemplified by Rogers and Randolph [5], Foley [6], Bergquist [7], Lord et al. [8], Misslin et al. [9], and a multitude of other authors. Temperature plays a major role for vector presence, and climate change has by now made it possible for diseases to start expanding their endemic areas, or can be expected to do so. For example, several tick-borne infections around the world [10], dirofilariasis in northern Europe [11], and schistosomiasis in northern China [12,13] are currently on the move. Pollution, and resistance to pesticides and drugs, as well as the general fall-out from globalization, are other factors driving such changes [14]. Previously locally confined infections that have lately become wide-spread are becoming more numerous on a monthly basis, e.g., the parasite *Babesia*, the spirochete *Borrelia*, and viruses such as chikungunya, Rift Valley virus (RFV), West Nile virus (WNV), and the Zika virus, to mention the most well-known [15].

2. Data Collection

Advanced laptop computers and widespread access to the Internet have created a broad accessibility of RS data from Earth-observing satellites. While this has made epidemiology more dependent on satellite-generated data, the discipline has also undergone a paradigmatic change, thanks to geographical information systems (GIS) that facilitate the management and processing of epidemiological data. The stronger potential to match the suitability of various environments to parasite life cycles and transmission dynamics provides a new way to address the nidality concept introduced by Pavlovskii as far back as 1945 [16]. Based on his ideas, geography and environmental variables associated with health data have led to the concept of disease ecology, where RS provides useful insights on the different factors related to transmission levels and disease distributions, while mapping and modelling facilitates interpretation, synthesis, and recognition of outbreak frequencies [17].

The GIS approach supports overlay and network analysis by documenting neighborhoods, buffers and spatial parameters, and today's epidemiologists have access to a multitude of ecological and climatic data that were never before available in such amounts and with such ease. The visualization of epidemiological datasets in a geographical context, e.g., linking spatial data from virtual globes with GIS software packages supports prediction and risk profiling [18], while sharing epidemiological data in real-time, is helpful, not only for individual researchers, but also for decision-makers. The growth of the Internet has distributed GIS widely, connecting with other platforms, such as web map servers, libraries, spatial database management systems, and software development frameworks. The field has thus become multi-participatory, such as allowing the advantage of cloud computing opportunities that facilitate GIS access for anyone, anywhere. However, while the development of near real-time surveillance systems, based on GIS, global positioning systems (GPS) and RS, facilitate the establishment of accurate, up-to-date early-warning systems (EWS), it is important to understand that GIS neither makes the actual field collection of parasites and vector easier, nor does it assure the quality of the information gained [19,20].

In the published literature on health applications of the geospatial sciences since the 1980s, malaria and schistosomiasis are the focus of the first and second most numerous articles, respectively. It is likely that schistosomiasis will continue to be a barometer of progress in geospatial health sciences, when the attention of researchers is drawn to emerging issues, such as the efficiencies of integrated control of malaria, and the neglected tropical diseases (NTDs), which include schistosomiasis. The spatial, temporal, and spectral resolution of the satellite-based sensors, and the capabilities of computer-based models has led to an improved understanding of geographical areas, and how they can support the transmission of various infections. In addition, improved surveillance, risk-mapping, and access to large databases promise stronger possibilities for understanding the complex relationship between the environment and infection with regard to infections. For example, like so many other parasitic diseases, the interaction between the human definitive host and the intermediate snail host in schistosomiasis, depends strongly on ambient environmental variables, above all temperature. While the latter and accessibility to water, humidity, vegetation, and shade limit the snail distribution, the ambient temperature in the snail governs the speed of maturation of the infectious agent inside [21].

3. GEOHealth: Part of the Global Earth Observation System of Systems (GEOSS)

Major scientific groups are interested in public health applications of the geospatial sciences, e.g., the Earth Science area of the National Aeronautics Space Administration (NASA) (http://www.nasa.gov/) has moved towards a strategic goal that includes the study of climate and environmental change and the potential impact on public health issues, such as infectious diseases, emergency preparedness and response (https://www.earthobservations.org/documents/cop/he_henv/2011032). NASA's Public Health Program, chronicled by Luvall [22], is a growing part of the organization. In addition, the Group on Earth Observations (GEO) (https://www.earthobservations.org/geoss.php), an international agency with support from over 100 governmental departments, non-governmental organizations (NGOs), and scientific organizations has an interest in health, and so has the International Society for Photogrammetry and Remote Sensing (ISPRS) (http://www.isprs.org/). Yet another group, the International Medical Geology Association (MEDGEO) (http://rock.geosociety.org) has similar goals in its stated mission focused on the science dealing with the relationships between geological factors and health.

The growing availability of digital data for geospatial studies made possible by RS and resources from national space agencies, such as NASA in the USA, the French National Centre for space studies (Centre National d'Études Spatiales (CNES) [23], the European Space Agency (ESA) and the Japan Aerospace Exploration Agency (JAXA) [24] has led to the establishment of scientific teams that are interested in exploiting geospatial health applications for specific pursuits, e.g., public health research. Several dedicated journals have emerged, e.g., Geospatial Health (http://www.geospatialhealth.net) [25], the International Journal of Health Geographics (http://www.ij-healthgeographics.com) and Spatial and Spatio-Temporal Epidemiology (http://www.journals.elsevier.com/spatial-and-spatiotemporal-epidemiology/). The net result is that geospatial mapping and multidisciplinary modelling are becoming mainstream science in the health community at large. It is therefore of great potential value to cross-fertilize and reinforce linkages of diverse interest groups on health applications of the geospatial sciences. NASA programs promote linkages with the Group on Earth Observations (GEO) mission to build and utilize GEOSS (https://www.earthobservations.org/geoss.php) under the public health societal benefit area in which health scientists working on very different health issues can collaborate in the use of a standardized, interoperable, open-source global resource data portal. It would be expedient if the Earth observations health network (GEOHealth) within the GEOSS framework would gain stronger traction along the lines in the Box 1 below.

Box 1. The GEOHealth Mandate.

GEOHealth collaborates on activities relating to the GEO societal benefit area on Public Health and GEOSS, enabling the collaboration of governmental, inter-governmental, and non-governmental organizations to organize and improve mapping and predictive modelling of the distribution of infectious, vector-borne, and non-contagious diseases globally and make these data, information, and forecasts more accessible to policy and decision-makers, managers, experts, and other users. Such a network would progress from a Community of Practice to an Initiative and then a Flagship in the GEO work plan. This voluntary partnership would be guided by a steering committee comprising the key stakeholders, initially the ISPRS VIII/2 Working Group (http://www2.isprs.org/commissions/comm8/wg2.html) and the International Society of Geospatial Health (GnosisGIS) (www.gnosisgis.org) actively recruiting other organizations to join. GEOHealth draws on GEO's data-sharing principles to promote full and open exchange of data, and on the GEOSS common infrastructure, to enable interoperability through the adoption of consistent standards. To assist both holders and users of health information to engage with GEOHealth, an active website would need to be established, containing links to information resources, activities, GEOHealth documents, meetings, and other resources that are relevant to the this mandate, including GnosisGIS, ISPRS VIII/2, the American Society of Tropical Medicine and Hygiene (ASTMH), and other groups interested in this endeavor to commit to the global vision of GEOHealth [26].

Is it possible to develop a dynamical 3-dimensional (3D) or even 4D (adding the temporal dimension) models of disease, such as bi-weekly global reports on the major endemic diseases? We are close to succeeding in this endeavor, facilitated by new satellite systems, big data, climatology advances, and novel sensors, such as the global precipitation model (GPM), the soil moisture active passive (SMAP), the Operational Land Imager (OLI), and the Thermal Infrared Sensor (TIRS), which replaces the Thematic Mapper Plus (ETM+) onboard the Landsat 8 satellite (summarized in Table 1). In addition, ESA's Copernicus Sentinel mission includes a range of satellites carrying radar and multi-spectral imaging instruments for land, ocean, and atmospheric monitoring. Perhaps most importantly, the sub-meter resolution data now available from the image-focused Worldview 2, 3, and 4 satellites (https://www.digitalglobe.com/about/our-constellation) can provide community risk assessments. Adding to this, the elective value-added potential of the low-altitude sensors on drone airborne vehicles as a source of very high-resolution data collection within a user-set agenda [27,28].

Future NASA satellite missions, such as the Hyperspectral Infrared Imager or HyspIRI (http://hyspiri.jpl.nasa.gov/), will provide further enhanced capability to map vector-borne and other environmentally sensitive diseases, based on global hyperspectral visible and multispectral thermal data products (5-day, 60 m^2 thermal and 19-day, 30 m^2 hyperspectral repeat intervals) that will enable structural and functional classification of ecosystems, and the measurement of key environmental parameters, such as temperature and soil moisture. A new generation of sensors offer new capabilities, e.g., the ECOSTRESS instrument added to the International Space Station (ISS) on 29 June, 2018 (http://www.nasa.gov/jpl/nasas-ecostress) has started to monitor plant health using surface temperature measurements (and derived evapotranspiration values) with a 3-day to 5-day diurnal pair coverage, 38×57 m spatial resolution at varying times during the day due to the ISS orbit precession [22]. Timely adoption of these data resources in health surveillance and response systems will require close cooperation between NASA and public health scientists. In addition, very high-resolution satellite data collected by GeoEye-1, Worldview1-4, Quickbird-2 are available for both historical and current time periods from Digital Globe (https://www.digitalglobe.com/), a company recently acquired by Maxar Technologies (https://www.maxar.com/). These advances finally allow seamless mapping and modelling of diseases, not only at continental scales (1 km^2) and local community-agricultural field scales (15–30 m^2), but for the first time, also at the habitat-household scale (<1 m^2) within individual communities.

A geospatial surveillance and response system resource for vector-borne disease in the Americas is currently being constructed using NASA satellite data, GIS, and ecological niche modelling to characterize the environmental and socioeconomic suitability, and the potential for the spread of selected endemic and epizootic vector-borne diseases in the Americas. The initial focus will be on developing prototype geospatial models on visceral leishmaniasis, an expanding endemic disease in Latin America, and models for dengue and other emerging *Aedes aegypti*-borne viruses (dengue, Zika, chikungunya) that have potential for epizootic spread from Latin America and the Caribbean to North America. We are planning to use the same resource data and modelling methods for surveillance and response systems for other vector-borne diseases, including schistosomiasis in the elimination phase. The GEOHealth concept would be a convenient way for incorporating the results into the interoperable, open-access standards of the GEOSS. Dissemination and training programs can then be implemented to promote geospatial mapping and modelling of vector-borne diseases, as envisioned in GEOSS. Implementation of GEOHealth requires, however, an initial effort to compile, design, and construct interoperable data structures that are anticipated to be useful for vector-borne disease surveillance and response systems based on the project investigators' experience, literature reports and availability. In this way, all data will be resampled and projected in geographic formats compatible with other GEOHealth project data parameters, and available in ASCII form needed, e.g., for use in Maxent (https://www.gbif.org/tool/81279/maxent) [29] or Bayesian (OpenBUGS) mapping and modelling software. Data portal construction methods would be similar to that reported for a prior Pan American Health Organization (PAHO) project on mapping and modelling six neglected tropical diseases in

Latin America and the Caribbean region [30]. To economize on the size of data storage requirements, data available for multiple years, e.g., the United States Geologic Survey (USGS) Landsat Legacy data would be acquired and archived in the data portal archive at 5-year intervals (2005, 2010, and 2015) with a step-by-step tutorial on how investigators can download additional data in the same format. Investigators would be able to examine data to evaluate usefulness using limited example data, with instructions on how to obtain similar additional complete data on specific time frames and scales, as needed from open-source archives linked to specified internet sites, e.g., the USGS Earth Resources Observation Systems (EROS) Data Center (https://eros.usgs.gov) which was established to study land change and to produce land change data products used by researchers, resource managers, and policy makers around the world.

Data from the GEOHealth common resource data portal could then be used to demonstrate the feasibility of improved disease risk assessment models in prototype surveillance and response system models, as compared to previously reported models for vector-borne diseases that have a fundamentally different epidemiology, including schistosomiasis. We aim to develop geospatial development rate models that can simulate and display temporal progression (e.g., as 8-day snapshots) of vector–parasite life cycles and geospatial risk, based on comprehensive daily climate re-analysis data, night and day land surface temperatures (LST_{night}, LST_{day}), the normalized difference vegetation index (NDVI), the normalized difference moisture index (NDMI), and the normalized difference wetness index (NDWI) available from the Moderate Resolution Imaging Spectroradiometer (MODIS) on board the Terra and Aqua satellites The Visible-Infrared Imaging Radiometer Suite (VIIRS) will extend the MODIS program in the future. These data should used in the context of topography, land use, and population patterns. A major gap in the past has been environmental moisture data, which can now be addressed using newly available sensor systems data from SMAP, GPM, GOES-16, and ECOSTRESS (Table 1).

Table 1. Recently launched Earth-observing satellite resources for mapping and modelling GeoHealth applications.

Satellite Platform	Frequency	Swath	Sensor	Spatial Resolution	Applications/Comments
GPM [a] Launched Feb. 2014	Integrated multi-satellite retrievals (IMERGE) 0.5 hours	Dual-frequency Precipitation Radar (DPR) 125–245 km; Global Microwave Imager (GMI) 885 km	Core Observatory radar/radiometer system	1 km	Measures precipitation using a reference standard to unify measurements from a constellation of related research and operational satellites. Extends Tropical Rainfall Measuring Mission (TRMM) records
GOES [b] 16 Launched Nov. 2014	5–15 min	Full disk image of the Earth consisting of 22 swaths	Advanced Baseline Imager (ABI) with 16 bands	0.5–1 km–2 km	Meteorology; Geostationary orbit over the western hemisphere
Suomi-NPP [c] Launched Oct. 2011	Daily	3000 km	Visible-Infrared Imaging Radiometer Suite (VIIRS)	1 km	8-day Land Surface Temperature (LST) measurements for day and night. Extends MODIS [d], AVHRR [e]
Soil Moisture Active Passive (SMAP)	3 h		L band Radar and Microwave Imager	3–10 km	Measures water content in the top 5 cm of the soil
Landsat 8 Launched Jan. 2013	16 days	185 km	Operational Land Imager (OLI), Thermal Infrared Sensor (TIRS)	OLI: Panchrom. = 15 m VIS-NIR-SWIR [f] = 30 m TIRS: thermal bands = 100 m	OLI and TIRS replace the Thematic Mapper (TM) and the enhanced Thematic Mapper Plus (ETM+) on previous Landsat satellites (Landsat legacy data has a continuous record since 1972
Sentinel 1 (A&B) A launched 2014 B launched 2015 Sentinel 2 A launched 2015 B launched 2016 Sentinel 3 A launched 2015 B launched 2016	12 days 10 days 27 days	250 km 290 km 1270 km	C-band Synthetic Aperture Radar (C-SAR) Multi-spectral instrument (MSI) with 13 channels in VIS-NIR-SWIR [f] Radar altimeter, micro wave radiometer, sea and land surface temperature radiometer	5 and 20 m 10, 20 and 60 m 300 m	EU contribution to GEOSS with applications related to land, coastal water with respect to natural disasters, resources, environment, weather, seasonal forecasting and climate. Monitors plant growth and forests, changes in land cover marine and ecosystems through leaf chlorophyll and water content indexes
Worldview 3 Aug. 2013 Worldview 4 Nov. 2016	<1 day	13.1 km	Pan, 8 Multi-spectral, 8 SWIR	Panchromatic = 31 cm Multispectral = 1.24 m	Optical data collection at the habitat-household level
International Space Station (ISS)	3 days	385–415 km	ECOSTRESS [g] Launched July 2018	38 × 57 m	Measures plant evapotranspiration (ET)

[a] Global Precipitation Measurement (mission); [b] Geostationary Operational Environmental Satellites; [c] National Polar-Orbiting Partnership; [d] Moderate Resolution Imaging Spectroradiometer (MODIS); [e] Advanced Very High Resolution Radiometer; [f] Visual, Near Infrared and Short-Wave Infrared; [g] ECOsystem Spaceborne Thermal Radiometer Experiment on International Space Station. Table sources: https://earthdata.nasa.gov/user-resources/remote-sensors. Additional info pm Sentinel: https://directory.eoportal.org/web/eoportal/satellite-missions/c-missions/copernicus-sentinel-1.

4. Mapping and Modelling NTDs in the Americas

Disease and vector occurrence data that are available at the national, state-wide and local community scale from earlier NTD studies in Brazil [30,31] funded by PAHO served as input for mapping disease and vector data using climate- and satellite-derived environmental data at the regional scale (1 km^2 spatial resolution), the state-wide scale (15–30–60 m^2 spatial resolution) and individual community scales (sub-meter spatial resolution). High-frequency climate and satellite sensor data can be made available in near real-time by access to Internet linkages to active program data. The selection of relevant environmental parameters to include in geospatial models, e.g., for visceral leishmaniasis, was based on results of regression analysis of disease and vector occurrence data, with variance inflation factor analysis to eliminate autocorrelation bias, according to the method of Mischler et al. [30]. Significantly associated Bioclim risk factors were included in Maxent as variables, and run with known vector and disease occurrence point data to develop probability risk surface maps that can be generated and incorporated as data layers in ArcGIS 10.6 mapping and modelling software. The relative contribution of each environmental variable to geospatial risk maps was evaluated by jackknife statistics, a part of the Maxent software package, to evaluate seasonality and relative risk as seen in Figure 1, Figure 2, and Figure 3 (from the doctoral thesis by Moara de Santana Martins [31]).

High resolution, biology-based geospatial mapping, and modelling methods can be developed and implemented by government agencies as the key to more rational, targeted control in surveillance and response systems for schistosomiasis that can interrupt and reverse the expansion to new endemic areas. Schistosomiasis in the elimination phase will require more sensitive case-finding diagnostic methods and satellite surveillance at the habitat–household resolution to pick up diminishing numbers of cases as control program success progresses. Sustained continuing surveillance programs are then required to prevent re-emergence.

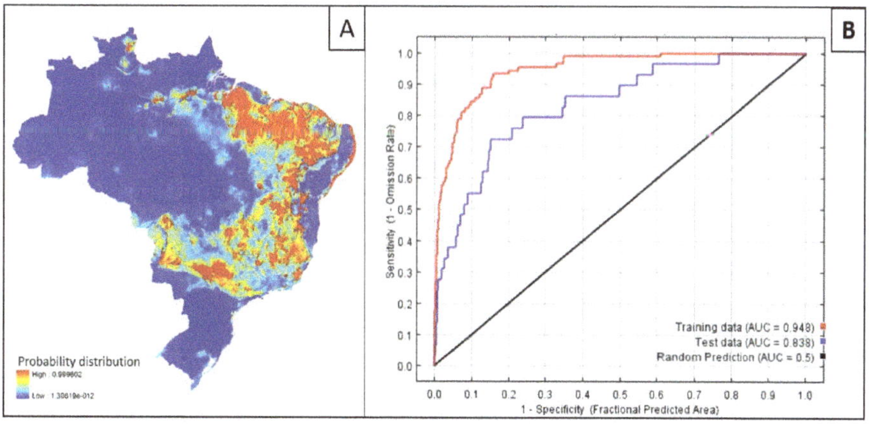

Figure 1. (**A**) Maxent-generated ecological niche model for predicting suitability for visceral leishmaniasis in Brazil based on the national surveillance program incidence data and Bioclim variables. (**B**) The accuracy of the model (0.838) was evaluated using Maxent by the area under the curve (AUC) of the receiver operating characteristic (ROC).

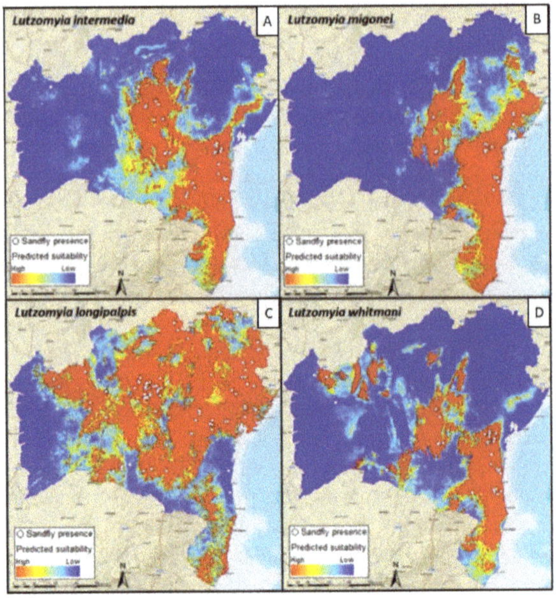

Figure 2. Maxent-predicted suitability for sand fly species of medical importance collected in Bahia state, Brazil. The output maps for the distribution of species incriminated as vectors of parasites that cause cutaneous leishmaniasis (**A**,**B**,**D**) and visceral leishmaniasis (**C**) were based on MODIS vegetation indices and Bioclim variables. Red areas indicate a higher suitability for vector occurrence.

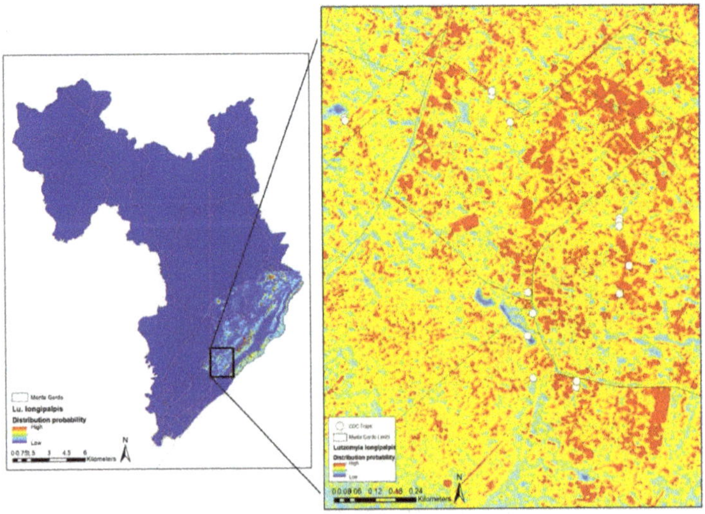

Figure 3. Maxent predicted the suitability for *Lutzomyia longipalpis* in Monte Gordo community-based on CDC trap data points and sub-meter spatial resolution WorldView2 imagery. The administrative boundaries of the municipality and districts (red lines) of Camacari, Bahia, Brazil are shown in the left panel. The predicted suitability of *Lutzomyia longipalpis* in Monte Gordo district is shown in the right panel based on CDC trap data and three vegetation indices derived from WorldView2 imagery, normalized difference vegetation index (NDVI), normalized difference soil index (NDSI), and normalized difference water index (NDWI). The inset box shows the model output and CDC trap locations. Highly suitable areas for the vector are shown in red.

5. Schistosomiasis

Of all the vector-borne diseases, schistosomiasis was the topic of pioneer GIS studies done by Cross et al. [32], using the Landsat MSS (https://lta.cr.usgs.gov/MSS) satellite data and rainfall–temperature weather variables for geospatial risk assessment in the Philippines. Other early work was done as part of the Schistosomiasis Research Project (SRP) in Egypt, funded by the United States Agency for International Development (USAID), which showed that the Advanced very-high-resolution radiometer (AVHRR) temperature difference (dT) imagery could be used to map the risk of schistosomiasis in the Nile Delta [33], and that this was associated with the effect of the local hydrologic regime and shallow water table on the snail host–schistosome development cycle [34]. This work showed how well the GIS could address the classic concept of the 'landscape epidemiology', and Pavlovskii's 'essential nidality of disease' concept [16] by virtue of its potential to match the relative suitability of various environments to the parasite life cycle and the transmission dynamics of host–parasite systems [35]. A more modern aspect is the attempt to predict the potential for future areas becoming endemic for schistosomiasis, due to the spread of the intermediate snail host, due to climate change [36].

5.1. Africa

With the African continent carrying the main burden off schistosomiasis by far, key countries in sub-Saharan Africa were selected for implementation of the 'Schistosomiasis Control Initiative' (SCI) (http://wwwsci-ntds.org), now the major control program in Africa. Basically a programme for the distribution of praziquantel, SCI, which applied GIS and RS to collect and record the cross-sectional national surveys on the distribution and intensity of schistosomiasis at the regional scale that were eventually used to guide optimal treatment strategies [37]. In this way, geospatial technology became linked to spatial information on climate, elevation, proximity to streams and water bodies activating innovative Bayesian geostatistical prediction models. Another activity was the Contrast project—a multi-disciplinary, 4-year alliance to optimize schistosomiasis control and transmission surveillance—that complemented the CSI by introducing an interactive agenda operating simultaneously at the molecular, biological, spatial, and social levels to identify risk factors governing the frequency and transmission dynamics of schistosomiasis [38]. The overall approach emphasized detailed knowledge of the distribution and abundance of snail hosts, bringing together existing information into a single database in an open-source Google Earth platform with Internet connection [39].

The accumulated experience on the transmission control of the Contrast program, facilitated by geospatial methods, contributed to the shift from an exclusive focus on morbidity control, to the adoption of the schistosomiasis elimination agenda in low-transmission countries [40]. In May 2012, the World Health Assembly passed a resolution calling upon member states to intensify schistosomiasis control and to initiate interventions towards local elimination [41]. This resulted in a focus on what was to be called the NTDs, and marked the start of a new era in the ambitious goal of elimination of schistosomiasis as a public health problem. The emergence of GIS, and access to Earth-observing satellite data as major tools in schistosomiasis research, and their integration into control strategies, has been excellently reviewed from the African scene by Mayangadze [42].

5.2. China and Southeast Asia

The International Symposium on Schistosomiasis, held in Shanghai, China [43] marked the beginning of geospatial tools for schistosomiasis control there. Using the NDVI, Land Surface Temperature (LST) and the Digital Elevation Model (DEM) extracted from MODIS and the Advanced Spaceborne Thermal Emission and Reflection Radiometer (ASTER) sensors onboard the Terra satellite, Zhu et al. [44] found that an ecological niche model integrated with NDVI, LST, elevation, slope, and distance from every village to its nearest stream could adequately predict snail habitats in the mountainous regions.

Even if snails can survive dry periods, water is the guarantee for their long-term survival and reproduction. The focus on snail habitats made GIS and RS necessary tools for the identification of land use, water bodies, vegetation, temperature, humidity LST, and vegetation and water indices [45]. These tools, including spatial statistics, are exceptionally useful for extracting and handling environmental data [46–49], and emphasized the importance of detailed updated information with wide geographical coverage. They further highlighted the advantages of RS technology over manual snail documentation, while Wang et al. [49] reported that a simple combination of the two indexes, normalized difference wetness index (NDWI) and normalized difference vegetation index (NDVI), made it possible to directly estimate the snail habitats quantitatively. This type of information should be useful for areas endemic for schistosomiasis japonica outside China, such as The Philippines and strongly limited endemic areas, such as those in the Sulawesi Island of Indonesia, where the exact borders of endemicity are difficult to settle. This could also be of value in the areas endemic for *S. mekongi* in Cambodia and Laos.

Schistosomiasis has a long history in The Philippines, with the disease ensconced in more than half of the country's 78 provinces. Apart from the paper by Cross et al. [32], referred to above, relatively few papers on geospatial technology have appeared in the Philippines. Malone et al. [50], focusing on the implementation of a geospatial health infrastructure in Southeast Asia for the control of schistosomiasis, pointed out that health workers have not rapidly taken advantage of the widely available, low-cost spatial data resources for epidemiological modelling. Although the situation has since improved in China, the use of geospatial tools in The Philippines is still at the build-up stage [51,52].

5.3. Latin America

Adoption of geospatial approaches to schistosomiasis control in Latin America emerged in a similar timeframe as that in Africa and Asia. Analysis of the role of environmental factors for prevalence in representative Brazilian municipalities in a GIS shows that the population density and the duration of the annual dry period are the most significant determinants [53]. A follow-up study has given additional data on the temperature difference, and NDVI collected by the satellite-borne AVHRR sensor that was used for a GIS environmental risk assessment model for schistosomiasis in Brazil [54]. Joining the consensus in Brazil on the potential value of geospatial methods, Gazzinelli and Kloos [55] promoted use of spatial tools, while Guimarães et al. [56,57] reported the successful use of social, meteorological, and RS-derived digital elevation and NDVI data to delimit the risk for schistosomiasis at the municipality level in the state of Minas Gerais.

A special issue of *Geospatial Health*, published in 2012, was devoted to geospatial applications for NTDs, including schistosomiasis, in South America and the Caribbean [58]. Of particular interest for the Brazilian distribution of schistosomiasis is the presence of two compatible snail host species: *Biomphalaria glabrata*, and *B. straminea* and that competitive selection makes *B. glabrata* dominate in irrigation systems, while *B. straminea* is more common in natural water sources [38,59]. Given the importance of socioeconomic and environmental risk factors in the persistence of transmission of NTDs, geospatial mapping and modelling was recognized early on, to be useful for the prediction of the distribution, and the prevalence of these diseases, and to identify areas where hotspots or disease overlap occurs. Significantly, the potential influence of climate change was often considered [16,35,60].

6. Healthy Futures

Concerns about the potential effects of impending climate change on vector-borne diseases was the focus of a major project funded in 2010–2014 by the European Commission's 7th Framework (FP7)—Healthy Futures. The aim of his project was to contribute to reducing the future burden of three, water-related high-impact vector-borne diseases (VBD) in Africa—malaria, schistosomiasis, and rift valley fever (RVF). The project consortium comprised an inter-disciplinary group of climatologists, disease modellers, and experts in the environmental, health, and socio-economic sciences, together with staff in government health ministries in the East African Community (EAC).

A total of 15 institutions made up the consortium, located in 10 different countries, five African (Rwanda, Kenya, Uganda, Tanzania, South Africa) and five European (Ireland, Sweden, Austria, Italy, UK). VBD's were expected to be sensitive to changes in environmental conditions, such as increased ambient temperature or changes in the timing and levels of rainfall associated with climate change. Dynamical simulation models were developed for each of the three targeted diseases based on data generated by the MODIS and the Tropical Rainfall Measuring Mission (TRMM) sensors. The climate surrogate data gathered covered the EAC at 1-km resolution at Earth surface. Model output risk maps were produced using ArcGIS software (http://www.esri.com/software/arcgis) based on current climate data and long-term climate change projections, as proposed by the Intergovernmental Panel on Climate Change (IPCC) in 2013. Predicted changes in the distribution and transmission patterns for malaria [61,62] schistosomiasis [63]), and RVF [64] were represented as maps covering the EAC, and decision support frameworks were developed for use by the scientific community and stakeholders in the EAC.

Notably, an integrated, open-source Atlas based on the key results of the Healthy Futures project was produced [65]. This online resource provides information on past, present, and future conditions of the risk for malaria, schistosomiasis, and RVF and allows the exploration and visualization of results through web-based interactive tools. The Atlas embodies a guided access to information on climate change, the potentiality of disease occurrence, and population vulnerability, with respect to these three diseases in the EAC region through direct access to downloadable datasets and metadata integrated in the Healthy *Futures* Metadata Portal. Current available information can be directly accessed through the Healthy Futures website (http://www.healthyfutures.eu).

Information can be queried based on three prime selection criteria: (i) the infectious diseases targeted; (ii) time, allowing for comparisons of current conditions with a range of future projections, while allowing access to information on historic outbreaks; and (iii) different components of risk. Future climate change projections based on two representative concentration pathways (RCPs) emission scenarios RCP4.5 (mid-level change) and RCP8.5 (high-level change) for each decade to 2100 throughout the EAC study area can thus be made available. Relative values of social vulnerability are mapped based on a range of indicators, such as susceptibility to disease (e.g., immunity, malnutrition, poverty, conflict, remoteness) and lack of resilience (e.g., education level, access to health facilities, number of dependents), while social and susceptibility indicators are weighted and combined in the form of a composite map indicator of geospatial risk [66]. The original Metadata Portal is hosted by the International Livestock Research Institute in Nairobi (ILRI). The metadata platform software used is freely available from ESRI (http://www.esri.com/software/arcgis/geoportal). The Portal uses the CSW (Catalogue Service for the Web) standard of the Open Geospatial Consortium (OGC) (http://www.opengeospatial.org), which makes it interoperable with other metadata portals and programs.

If successfully adopted and further developed, the Atlas will be among the first of its kind in geospatial health research to offer public health practitioners, scientists, and stakeholders a tool to enable the identification of likely VBD hotspots under different climate change scenarios at policy-relevant time-intervals over the coming century. Twelve articles emanating from the Healthy Futures 'Remote Sensing of Environment project' were published in a special issue of Geospatial Health (http://www.geospatialhealth.net) in 2016. The emergence of GIS and Earth-observing satellite data as a major tool in schistosomiasis research, and their integration into real-world control strategies has been acknowledged by a large number of research teams.

7. Future Potential

The NASA GEOSS program is currently divided geographically into an AfriGEOSS and AmeriGEOSS data resource effort, with the potential to add other defined regions, and it is these continental databases that will be used to develop GEOHealth applications, consistent with the NASA societal benefit area of public health. The members of the GEOHealth CoP (www.geohealthcop.org/) aim to both use and contribute GEOSS interoperable resource databases.

The results of the Healthy Futures project provide an excellent candidate for developing public health applications within the AfriGEOSS program. The current NASA project 'GeoHealth: A Surveillance and Response System Resource for Vector Borne Disease in the Americas' aims to contribute interoperable resource data and methods that are essential for vector-borne disease mapping and modelling in the Western Hemisphere, as part of the AmeriGEOSS program. Other data from Health and Air Quality Applications of the Applied Sciences program offer broader potential geospatial resources [66]. Global health databases, e.g., on schistosomiasis [38] and on sand flies [6] are emerging, that can be accessed for relevant health data to develop mapping and modelling applications, along with the addition of data from the existing literature, and results of new research projects in the future.

The virtual globe concept is not new, but the essential idea is now coming into its own. Many and various efforts in this direction have been made over the last 10–15 years. However, the field did not take off until user-friendly applications started to appear [67]. Intuitive technologies, such as Google Earth, enable scientists around the world to share data in a readily understandable fashion without the need for much technical assistance. In 2008, Elvidge and Tuttle felt that three-dimensional software modelling of the Earth leading to virtual globes would revolutionize Earth observation, data access, and integration [68]. Stensgaard et al. [38] and Yang et al. [18] used Google Earth for the management and control of vector-borne diseases, including schistosomiasis. The authors of this paper believe that the use of this approach can lead to a better understanding of the epidemiology and ecology of the neglected tropical diseases, including schistosomiasis, and other environmentally sensitive infectious diseases in the multidimensional environments in which they occur.

8. Conclusions

Currently available global geospatial data are underutilized by medical researchers. This may be due to the lack of the ability to bridge barriers to awareness, prioritization, or training deficits, which are needed for the interdisciplinary interaction of medical scientists with environmental scientists. The development of a GEOHealth platform would facilitate and encourage research to utilize and implement currently available geospatial analysis tools and new global data systems in surveillance and response systems for vector-borne diseases.

Recently launched earth-observing satellite systems provide new opportunities to improve existing geospatial risk models that have already been effectively used to guide control programs for both filariasis [69] and soil transmitted helminths (STH) [70]. In particular, higher-resolution environmental analysis and the ability to evaluate life cycle drivers, as well as limiting moisture factors by new sensors such as SMAP and ECOSTRESS, are very promising tools for ecological niche modeling.

What is needed is an open-source, inter-operable platform that is freely accessible by the global health community to link public health workers with the most current potential earth observation resources from the geospatial sciences community. We propose that geospatial data resources from NASA and other national space agencies *can* be organized through a GEOSS virtual globe to make this possible. The vision, organization, and structure of the GEOHealth network is offered as a framework for initial effort as a vehicle for translational research, dissemination, and implementation in national public health systems in collaboration with GEO.

Given the strong progress on schistosomiasis elimination in several countries, China in particular, and the strong follow-up of the pioneer RS and GIS studies centered on this disease, it might well be used as model for the development and application of the new generation of space-based tools for NTD elimination.

Author Contributions: Conceptualization, J.B.M. and R.B.; methodology, J.B.M. and J.C.L.; software, M.M.; validation, J.B.M., R.B. and J.C.L.; formal analysis, J.B.M. and R.B.; investigation, M.M. and J.B.M..; resources, J.C.L.; data curation, J.B.M.; writing—original draft preparation, J.B.M. and R.B.; writing—review and editing, J.B.M. and R.B..; visualization, M.M.; supervision, J.B.M.; project administration, J.B.M.; funding acquisition, J.B.M. and J.C.L.

Funding: This research was funded by the National Aeronautics and Space Administration (NASA) grant number 80NSSC18K0517.

Conflicts of Interest: The authors declare no conflict of interest. The funders had no role in the design of the study; in the collection, analyses, or interpretation of data; in the writing of the manuscript, or in the decision to publish the results.

References

1. Bergquist, R. New tools for epidemiology: A space odyssey. *Mem. Inst. Oswaldo Cruz* **2011**, *106*, 892–900. [CrossRef] [PubMed]
2. Bergquist, R.; Tanner, M. Visual approaches for strengthening research, science communication and public health impact. *Geospat. Health* **2012**, *6*, 155–156. [CrossRef] [PubMed]
3. Malone, J.B.; Tourre, Y.M.; Faruque, F.; Luvall, J.C.; Bergquist, R. Towards establishment of GeoHealth, an open-data portal for health mapping and modelling based on Earth observations by remote sensing. *Geospat. Health* **2014**, *8*, 599–602. [CrossRef] [PubMed]
4. Bergquist, R.; Rinaldi, L. Health research based on geospatial tools: A timely approach in a changing environment. *J. Helminthol.* **2010**, *84*, 1–11. [CrossRef] [PubMed]
5. Rogers, D.J.; Randolph, S.E. Climate change and vector-borne diseases. *Adv. Parasitol.* **2006**, *62*, 345–381. [PubMed]
6. Foley, D.H.; Wilkerson, R.C.; Dornak, L.L.; Pecor, D.B.; Nyari, A.S.; Rueda, L.M.; Long, L.S.; Richardson, J.H. SandflyMap: Leveraging spatial data on sand fly vector distribution for disease risk assessments. *Geospat. Health* **2012**, *6*, 25–30. [CrossRef] [PubMed]
7. Bergquist, R. Climate and the distribution of vector-borne diseases: What's in store? *Geospat. Health* **2017**, *12*, 549. [CrossRef] [PubMed]
8. Lord, J.S.; Torr, S.J.; Auty, H.K.; Brock, P.M.; Byamungu, M.; Hargrove, J.W.; Morrison, L.J.; Mramba, F.; Vale, G.A.; Stanton, MC. Geostatistical models using remotely-sensed data predict savanna tsetse decline across the interface between protected and unprotected areas in Serengeti, Tanzania. *J. Appl. Ecol.* **2018**, *4*, 1997–2007. [CrossRef]
9. Misslin, R.; Vaguet, Y.; Vaguet, A.; Daudé, É. Estimating air temperature using MODIS surface temperature images for assessing *Aedes aegypti* thermal niche in Bangkok, Thailand. *Environ. Monit. Assess.* **2018**, *190*, 537. [CrossRef]
10. Randolph, S.E.; Rogers, D.J. Tick-borne disease systems: Mapping geographic and phylogenetic space. *Adv. Parasitol.* **2006**, *62*, 263–291.
11. Genchi, C.; Mortarino, M.; Rinaldi, L.; Cringoli, G.; Traldi, G.; Genchi, M. Changing climate and changing vector-borne disease distribution: The example of *Dirofilaria* in Europe. *Vet. Parasitol.* **2011**, *176*, 295–299. [CrossRef] [PubMed]
12. Yang, G.J.; Vounatsou, P.; Zhou, X.N.; Tanner, M.; Utzinger, J. A potential impact of climate change and water resource development on the transmission of *Schistosoma japonicum* in China. *Parassitologia* **2005**, *47*, 127–134. [PubMed]
13. Zhou, X.N.; Yang, G.J.; Yang, K.; Wang, X.H.; Hong, Q.B.; Sun, L.P.; Malone, J.B.; Kristensen, T.K.; Bergquist, N.R.; Utzinger, J. Potential impact of climate change on schistosomiasis transmission in China. *Am. J. Trop. Med. Hyg.* **2008**, *78*, 188–194. [CrossRef] [PubMed]
14. Harrus, S.; Baneth, G. Drivers for the emergence and re-emergence of vector-borne protozoal and bacterial diseases. *Int. J. Parasitol.* **2005**, *35*, 1309–1318. [CrossRef] [PubMed]
15. Bergquist, R.; Stensgaard, A.S.; Rinaldi, L. Vector-borne diseases in a warmer world: Will they stay or will they go? *Geospat. Health* **2018**, *13*, 699. [CrossRef] [PubMed]
16. Pavlovskii, E.N. The ecological parasitology. *J. Gen. Biol.* **1945**, *6*, 65–92.
17. Rinaldi, L.; Hendrickx, G.; Cringoli, G.; Biggeri, A.; Ducheyne, E.; Catelan, D.; Morgan, E.; Williams, D.; Charlier, J.; von Samson-Himmelstjerna, G.; et al. Mapping and modelling helminth infections in ruminants in Europe: Experience from GLOWORM. *Geospat. Health* **2015**, *19*, 257–259. [CrossRef] [PubMed]
18. Yang, K.; Sun, LP.; Huang, Y.X.; Yang, G.J.; Wu, F.; Hang, D.R.; Li, W.; Zhang, J.F.; Liang, Y.S.; Zhou, X.N. A real-time platform for monitoring schistosomiasis transmission supported by Google Earth and a web-based geographical information system. *Geospat. Health* **2012**, *6*, 195–203. [CrossRef]

19. Rinaldi, L.; Musella, V.; Biggeri, A.; Cringoli, G. New insights into the application of geographical information systems and remote sensing in veterinary parasitology. *Geospat. Health* **2006**, *1*, 33–47. [CrossRef]
20. Kistemann, T.; Dangendorf, F.; Schweikart, J. New perspectives on the use of Geographical Information Systems (GIS) in environmental health sciences. *Int. J. Hyg. Environ. Health* **2002**, *205*, 169–181. [CrossRef] [PubMed]
21. Malone, J.B. Biology-based mapping of vector-borne parasites by geographic information systems and remote sensing. *Parassitologia* **2005**, *47*, 27–50. [PubMed]
22. Luvall, J.C. The power of the pixel—A thermodynamic paradigm for studying disease vector's habitats & life cycles using NASA's Remote sensing data. Presented at the 8th International Symposium on Geospatial Health, New Orleans, LA, USA, 1–2 November 2014.
23. Marechal, F.; Ribeiro, N.; Lafaye, M.; Guell, A. Satellite imaging and vector-borne diseases: The approach of the French National Space Agency (CNES). *Geospat. Health* **2008**, *3*, 1–5. [CrossRef] [PubMed]
24. Igarashi, T.; Kuze, A.; Sobue, S.; Yamamoto, A.; Yamamoto, K.; Oyoshi, K.; Imaoka, K.; Fukuda, T. Japan's efforts to promote global health using satellite remote sensing data from the Japanese aerospace exploration agency (JAXA) for prediction of infectious diseases and air quality. *Geospat. Health* **2014**, *8*, S603–S610. [CrossRef] [PubMed]
25. Utzinger, J.; Rinaldi, L.; Malone, J.B.; Krauth, S.J.; Kristensen, T.K.; Cringoli, G.; Bergquist, R. Geospatial health: The first five years. *Geospat. Health* **2011**, *6*, 137–154. [CrossRef] [PubMed]
26. De Roeck, E.; Van Coillie, F.; De Wulf, R.; Soenen, K.; Charlier, J.; Vercruysse, J.; Hantson, W.; Ducheyne, E.; Hendrickx, G. Fine-scale mapping of vector habitats using very high resolution satellite imagery: A case-study on liver fluke. *Geospat. Health* **2014**, *8*, S671–S683. [CrossRef] [PubMed]
27. Capolupo, A.; Pindozzi, S.; Okello, C.; Boccia, L. Indirect technology for detecting areas object of illegal spills, harmful to human health, by applying drones, photogrammetry and hydrological models. *Geospat. Health* **2014**, *8*, S699–S707. [CrossRef] [PubMed]
28. Phillips, S.J.; Anderson, R.P.; Schapire, R. Maximum entropy modeling of species geographic distributions. *Ecol. Model.* **2006**, *190*, 231–259. [CrossRef]
29. Mischler, P.; Kearney, M.; McCarroll, J.C.; Scholte, R.G.; Vounatsou, P.; Malone, J.B. Environmental and socio-economic risk modelling for Chagas disease in Bolivia. *Geospat. Health* **2012**, *6*, S59–S66. [CrossRef]
30. Martins, M. The Use of Geographic Information Systems and Ecological Niche Modeling to Map Transmission Risk for Visceral Leishmaniasis in Salvador, Bahia, Brazil. Ph.D. Thesis, Louisiana State University, Baton Rouge, LA, USA, 2015.
31. Cross, E.R.; Perrine, R.; Sheffield, C. Predicting areas endemic for schistosomiasis using weather variables and a Landsat database. *Mil. Med.* **1984**, *149*, 542–544. [CrossRef]
32. Malone, J.B.; Huh, O.K.; Fehler, D.P.; Wilson, P.A.; Wilensky, D.E.; Holmes, R.A.; Elmagdoub, A.I. Temperature data from satellite imagery and the distribution of schistosomiasis in Egypt. *Am. J. Trop. Med. Hyg.* **1994**, *50*, 714–722. [CrossRef]
33. Abdel Rahman, M.S.; El Bahy, M.M.; El Bahy, N.M.; Malone, J.B. Development and validation of a satellite based Geographic information system (GIS) model for epidemiology of *Schistosoma* risk assessment at snail level in Kafr El Sheikh governorate. *J. Egypt. Soc. Parasitol.* **1997**, *27*, 299–316. [PubMed]
34. *Geospatial Surveillance and Response Systems for Schistosomiasis*; Malone, J.B.; Bergquist, R.; Rinaldi, L., Eds.; CRC Press: Boca Raton, FL, USA, 2016; Chapter 28; p. 523.
35. Yang, G.J.; Bergquist, R. Potential Impact of Climate Change on Schistosomiasis: A Global Assessment Attempt. *Trop. Med. Infect. Dis.* **2018**, *3*, 117. [CrossRef]
36. Clements, A.C.; Deville, MA.; Ndayishimiye, O.; Brooker, S.; Fenwick, A. Spatial co-distribution of neglected tropical diseases in the East African Great Lakes region: Revisiting the justification for integrated control. *Trop. Med. Int. Health* **2010**, *15*, 198–207. [CrossRef]
37. Bergquist, R. Closing in on 'perhaps the most dreadful of the remaining plagues': An independent view of the multidisciplinary alliance to optimize schistosomiasis control in Africa. *Acta Trop.* **2013**, *128*, 179–181. [CrossRef] [PubMed]
38. Stensgaard, A.S.; Saarnak, C.F.L.; Utzinger, J.; Vounatsou, P.; Simoonga, C.; Mushinge, G.; Rahbek, C.; Møhlenberg, F.; Kristensen, T.K. Virtual globes and geospatial health: The potential of new tools in the management and control of vector-borne diseases. *Geospat. Health* **2009**, *3*, 127–141. [CrossRef] [PubMed]

39. Rollinson, D.; Knopp, S.; Levitz, S.; Stothard, J.R.; Tchuente, L.A.; Garba, A.; Mohammed, K.A.; Schur, N.; Person, B.; Colley, D.G.; et al. Time to set the agenda for schistosomiasis elimination. *Acta Trop.* **2013**, *128*, 423–440. [CrossRef]
40. WHO. Accelerating Work to Overcome the Global Impact of Neglected Tropical Diseases: A Roadmap for Implementation. 2012. Available online: http://www.who.int/neglected_diseases/NTD_RoadMap_2012_Fullversion.pdf (accessed on 17 January 2012).
41. Mayangadze, T.; Chimbari, M.J.; Gebreslasie, M.; Mukaratirwa, S. Application of geo-spatial technology in schistosomiasis modeling in Africa: A review. *Geospat. Health* **2015**, *10*, 326. [CrossRef]
42. Zhou, X.N.; Chen, M.G.; McManus, D.; Bergquist, R. Schistosomiasis control in the 21st century. Proceedings of the International Symposium on Schistosomiasis, Shanghai, 4–6 July 2001. *Acta Trop.* **2001**, *82*, 95–114.
43. Zhu, H.R.; Liu, L.; Zhou, X.N.; Yang, G.J. Ecological Model to Predict Potential Habitats of Oncomelania hupensis, the Intermediate Host of Schistosoma japonicum in the Mountainous Regions, China. *PLoS Negl. Trop. Dis.* **2015**, *9*, e0004028. [CrossRef]
44. Wang, Y.; Zhuang, D.A. Rapid Monitoring and Evaluation Method of Schistosomiasis Based on Spatial Information Technology. *Int. J. Environ. Res. Publ. Health* **2015**, *12*, 15843–15859. [CrossRef]
45. Yang, G.J.; Vounatsou, P.; Zhou, X.N.; Tanner, M.; Utzinger, J.A. Bayesian-based approach for spatio-temporal modeling of county level prevalence of *Schistosoma japonicum* infection in Jiangsu province. *China Int. J. Parasitol.* **2005**, *35*, 155–162. [CrossRef] [PubMed]
46. Yang, G.J.; Vounatsou, P.; Tanner, M.; Zhou, X.N.; Utzinger, J. Remote sensing for predicting potential habitats of *Oncomelania hupensis* in Hongze, Baima and Gaoyou lakes in Jiangsu province, China. *Geospat. Health* **2006**, *1*, 85–92. [CrossRef] [PubMed]
47. Guo, J.G.; Vounatsou, P.; Cao, C.L.; Utzinger, J.; Zhu, H.Q.; Anderegg, D.; Zhu, R.; He, Z.Y.; Li, D.; Hu, F. A geographic information and remote sensing based model for prediction of *Oncomelania hupensis* habitats in the Poyang Lake area, China. *Acta Trop.* **2005**, *96*, 213–222. [CrossRef] [PubMed]
48. Wang, Z.L.; Zhu, R.; Zhang, Z.J.; Yao, B.D.; Zhang, L.J.; Gao, J.; Jiang, Q.W. Identification of snail habitats in the Poyang Lake region, based on the application of indices on joint normalized difference vegetation and water. *Zhonghua Liu Xing Bing Xue Za Zhi* **2012**, *33*, 823–827. (In Chinese)
49. Malone, J.B.; Yang, G.J.; Leonardo, L.; Zhou, X.N. Implementing a geospatial health data infrastructure for control of Asian schistosomiasis in the People's Republic of China and the Philippines. *Adv. Parasitol.* **2010**, *73*, 1–100. [CrossRef]
50. Leonardo, L.R.; Crisostomo, B.A.; Solon, J.A.; Rivera, P.T.; Marcelo, A.B.; Villasper, J.M. Geographical information systems in health research and services delivery in the Philippines. *Geospat. Health* **2007**, *1*, 147–155. [CrossRef]
51. Leonardo, L.R.; Rivera, P.T.; Crisostomo, B.A.; Sarol, J.N.; Bantayan, N.C.; Tiu, W.U.; Bergquist, N.R. A study of the environmental determinants of malaria and schistosomiasis in the Philippines using Remote Sensing and Geographic Information Systems. *Parassitologia* **2005**, *47*, 105–114.
52. Bavia, M.E.; Hale, L.T.; Malone, J.B.; Braud, D.H.; Shane, S. Geographic information systems and the environmental risk of schistosomiasis in Bahia, Brazil. *Am. J. Trop. Med. Hyg.* **1999**, *60*, 566–572. [CrossRef]
53. Bavia, M.E.; Malone, J.B.; Hale, L.; Dantes, A.; Marroni, L.; Reis, R. Use of thermal and vegetation index data from earth observing satellites to evaluate the risk of schistosomiasis in Bahia, Brazil. *Acta Trop.* **2001**, *79*, 79–85. [CrossRef]
54. Gazzinelli, A.; Kloos, H. The use of spatial tools in the study of *Schistosoma mansoni* and its intermediate host snails in Brazil: A brief review. *Geospat. Health* **2007**, *2*, 51–58. [CrossRef]
55. Guimarães, R.J.; Freitas, C.C.; Dutra, L.V.; Moura, A.C.; Amaral, R.S.; Drummond, S.C.; Scholte, R.G.; Carvalho, O.S. Schistosomiasis risk estimation in Minas Gerais State, Brazil, using environmental data and GIS techniques. *Acta Trop.* **2008**, *108*, 234–241. [CrossRef] [PubMed]
56. Guimarães, R.J.; Freitas, C.C.; Dutra, L.V.; Scholte, R.G.; Martins-Bedé, F.T.; Fonseca, F.R.; Amaral, R.S.; Drummond, S.C.; Felgueiras, C.A.; Oliveira, G.C.; et al. A geoprocessing approach for studying and controlling schistosomiasis in the state of Minas Gerais, Brazil. *Mem. Inst. Oswaldo Cruz* **2010**, *105*, 524–531. [CrossRef] [PubMed]
57. Malone, J.B.; Bergquist, N.R. Mapping and modelling neglected tropical diseases and poverty in Latin America and the Caribbean. *Geospat. Health* **2012**, *6*, S1–S5. [CrossRef] [PubMed]

58. Barboza, D.M.; Zhang, C.; Santos, N.C.; Silva, M.M.; Rollemberg, C.V.; de Amorim, F.J.; Ueta, M.T.; de Melo, C.M.; de Almeida, J.A.; Jeraldo, V.; et al. Biomphalaria species distribution and its effect on human Schistosoma mansoni infection in an irrigated area used for rice cultivation in northeast Brazil. *Geospat. Health* **2012**, *6*, S103–S109. [CrossRef] [PubMed]
59. Scholte, R.G.C.; Carvlho, O.S.; Malone, J.B.; Utzinger, J.; Vounatsou, P. Spatial distribution of *Biomphalaria* spp., the intermediate host snails of *Schistosoma mansoni*, in Brazil. *Geospat. Health* **2012**, *6*, S95–S101. [CrossRef] [PubMed]
60. Stensgaard, A.S.; Utzinger, J.; Vounatsou, P.; Hürlimann, E.; Saarnak, C.F.L.; Mubita, P.; Simoonga, C.; Kabatereine, N.B.; Tchuem Tchuenté, L.A.; Simoonga, C.; et al. Large-scale determinants of intestinal schistosomiasis and intermediate host snail distribution across Africa: Does climate matter? *Acta Trop.* **2013**, *128*, 378–390. [CrossRef] [PubMed]
61. Tompkins, A.; Caporaso, L. Assessment of malaria transmission changes in Africa, due to the climate impact of land use change using Coupled Model Intercomparison Project Phase 5 earth system models. *Geospat. Health* **2016**, *11*. [CrossRef] [PubMed]
62. Bizimana, J.P.; Kienberger, S.; Hagenlocher, M.; Twarabamenye, E. Modelling homogeneous regions of social vulnerability to malaria in Rwanda. *Geospat. Health* **2016**, *11*. [CrossRef] [PubMed]
63. McCreech, N.; Nikulin, G.; Booth, M. Predicting the effects of climate change on *Schistosoma mansoni* transmission in eastern Africa. *Parasites Vectors* **2015**, *8*, 4. [CrossRef]
64. Taylor, D.; Hagenlocher, M.; Jones, A.; Kienberger, S.; Leedale, J.; Morse, A. Environmental change and Rift Valley fever in eastern Africa: Projecting beyond Healthy futures. *Geospat. Health* **2016**, *11*. [CrossRef]
65. Hagenlocher, M.; Castro, M.C. Mapping malaria risk and vulnerability in the United Republic of Tanzania: A spatial explicit model. *Popul. Health Metr.* **2015**, *13*, 2. [CrossRef] [PubMed]
66. Chapman, H. NASA Health and Air Quality (HAQ) Newsletter, Volume 16, June–September 2018. Available online: https://appliedsciences.nasa.gov/system/files/sites/default/files/HAQ%20Newsletter%20Jun-Sept18.pdf (accessed on 11 October 2018).
67. Boulos, M.N. Web GIS in practice III: Creating a simple interactive map of England's Strategic Health Authorities using Google Maps API, Google Earth KML, and MSN Virtual Earth Map Control. *Int. J. Health Geogr.* **2005**, *21*, 22. [CrossRef] [PubMed]
68. Elvidge, C.D.; Tuttle, B.T. How virtual globes are revolutionizing Earth observation data access and integration. *Int. Arch. Photogram. Rem. Sens. Spat. Inf. Sci.* **2008**, *37*, 137–139.
69. Sabeson, S.; Raju, K.; Subramanian, S.; Srivastava, P.; Jambulingam, P. Lymphatic filariasis transmission risk map of India based on a geo-environmental risk model. *Vector Borne Zoonotic Dis.* **2013**, *13*, 657–665. [CrossRef] [PubMed]
70. Yaro, C.A.; Kogi, E.; Luka, S.A. Spatial distribution and modeling of soil transmitted helminthes infection in Nigeria. *Research J. Parasitol.* **2018**, *13*, 19–35. [CrossRef]

Tropical Medicine and Infectious Disease

MDPI

Review

Artemether and Praziquantel: Origin, Mode of Action, Impact, and Suggested Application for Effective Control of Human Schistosomiasis

Robert Bergquist [1] and Hala Elmorshedy [2,3,*]

1 Ingerod, SE-454 94 Brastad, Sweden; robert.bergquist@outlook.com
2 College of Medicine, Princess Nourah bint Abdulrahman University, Riyadh 11671, Saudi Arabia
3 Department of Tropical Health, High Institute of Public Health, Alexandria University, Alexandria 21561, Egypt
* Correspondence: elmorshedyh@hotmail.com

Received: 19 November 2018; Accepted: 11 December 2018; Published: 19 December 2018

Abstract: The stumbling block for the continued, single-drug use of praziquantel (PZQ) against schistosomiasis is less justified by the risk of drug resistance than by the fact that this drug is inactive against juvenile parasites, which will mature and start egg production after chemotherapy. Artemisinin derivatives, currently used against malaria in the form of artemisinin-based combination therapy (ACT), provide an opportunity as these drugs are not only active against malaria plasmodia, but surprisingly also against juvenile schistosomes. An artemisinin/PZQ combination would be complementary, and potentially additive, as it would kill two schistosome life cycle stages and thus confer a transmission-blocking modality to current chemotherapy. We focus here on single versus combined regimens in endemic settings. Although the risk of artemisinin resistance, already emerging with respect to malaria therapy in Southeast Asia, prevents use in countries where ACT is needed for malaria care, an artemisinin-enforced praziquantel treatment (APT) should be acceptable in regions of North Africa (including Egypt), the Middle East, China, and Brazil that are not endemic for malaria. Thanks to recent progress with respect to high-resolution diagnostics, based on circulating schistosome antigens in humans and molecular approaches for snail surveys, it should be possible to keep areas scheduled for schistosomiasis elimination under surveillance, bringing rapid response to bear on problems arising. The next steps would be to investigate where and for how long APT should be applied to make a lasting impact. A large-scale field trial in an area with modest transmission should tell how apt this approach is.

Keywords: schistosomiasis; elimination; praziquantel; artemether; combination therapy

1. Background

The World Health Organization (WHO) includes schistosomiasis among the neglected tropical diseases (NTDs) and has selected it for elimination [1]; this may be premature as there is still a large discrepancy between the number of people requiring preventive chemotherapy (PCT) and those presently receiving it [2]. The disease is caused by trematode parasites with a predilection for abdominal capillary veins in the mammalian definitive host. Various freshwater snails act as intermediate hosts for the six different species capable of infecting humans. Out of these, *Schistosoma mansoni*, *S. haematobium*, and *S. japonicum* together cause almost all cases of schistosomiasis, which amounts to about 240 million infected and 700 million at risk worldwide [3]. The prevalence is often focal with high transmission in some spots and none in others and the lesions caused, intestinal or urogenital depending on the species of the parasite, tend to be chronic rather than acute. The attributes of infection include poor sanitation, proximity to water bodies, type and extent of water contact, snail population density, as well as age and gender of the human population in the endemic areas. For example, the prevalence and intensity of infection are significantly higher in males and in school-age children [2,4,5]. Theoretically, successful schistosomiasis control should be possible through a multidisciplinary approach focusing on chemotherapy, snail control, provision of water, sanitation, and hygiene (WASH) as well as behavioural change [6,7]. Nevertheless, elimination will be difficult to achieve in practice, and very few endemic countries have been entirely successful in controlling the disease. Interestingly, Japan managed to eradicate the infection (in 1977), mainly thanks to snail control based on environmental management, as described by Tanaka and Tsuji [2,4,5].

The cornerstone strategy for schistosomiasis control was for a long time directed at its snail intermediate host using broad-spectrum molluscicides. However, when praziquantel (PZQ) was introduced [8] and soon afterwards used for mass drug administration (MDA), it not only replaced other drugs thanks to safety, high efficacy and easy administration [9–11] but effectively became the only approach. This modality also changed the focus from snail control and infection prevention to morbidity reduction, reflected in a declining disability-adjusted life years (DALY) metric for schistosomiasis [12,13].

In China, Chairman Mao Zedong, not only instigated the National Schistosomiasis Control Programme [14] but also took an interest in malaria. The launch of the malaria research programme (under code name 523) in 1967 focused on herbs used in traditional Chinese medicine. Working in this programme, Youyou Tu, soon identified the ingredient artemisinin (qinghaosu) in extracts from wormwood (*Artemisia annua*) as a powerful antimalarial [15,16]. Qinghaosu has been used in China for more than 2,000 years for the treatment of fevers, and the story of how it was discovered has eloquently been told by Faurant [17] and Miller [18]. Already in 1971, Chinese chemists isolated the active lactone with its peroxide grouping [19]. However, this knowledge did not reach the West until the late 1970s when it was mentioned in a Welcome News Supplement [20]. Youyou Tu's own remarks [15] at the Fourth Meeting of the WHO Scientific Working Group on the Chemotherapy of Malaria, held in Beijing 1981, provided further details of the new drug. The landmark work carried out under her direction [21] constituted a break-through for malaria therapy and led to the development of artemisinin-based combination therapy (ACT) that has since revolutionized the care of malaria patients [22] eventually leading to Youyou Tu being awarded the Nobel prize in Medicine for 2015, together with Campbell and Ōmura for ivermectin [23,24]. However, the story does not end there since, amazingly, it was found that the artemisinin do not only affect the malaria parasites, but are also active against juvenile schistosomes, which was first shown by Chen et al. [25] at the end of the golden decade of antiparasitic drug discovery in the 1970s. In fact, this discovery predates that of scholarly articles on qinghaosu's use against malaria, which remains its main application.

2. Pharmacological Aspects

Single-celled malaria plasmodia and schistosome worms are phylogenetically very distant from each other, and one might think that the damage caused by the artemisinins to both these organisms would be due to different principles. However, there are reasons to believe otherwise, considering that both parasites feed by the digestion of haemoglobin in host erythrocytes, leading to a surplus of haeme (protoporphyrin-IX with a ferric ion at its centre) or haemin (ferriprotoporphyrin-IX characterized by an extra chloride ion bound to the ferric ion), both of which produce destructive hydroxyl radicals capable of provoking the alkylation of parasite proteins [26]. Faced with this threat, both parasites detoxify these compounds by crystallizing them into the inert polymer haemozoin (ferriprotoporphyrin-IX) that is found in quantity, both in *Plasmodium* [27] and adult schistosomes [28]. It seems that haeme and haemin are implicated in the destruction of *Plasmodium* and *Schistosoma* due to interference with the formation of hemozoin. Various drugs besides artemisinins (e.g., trioxalanes [29–31], trioxaquines [32], and ozonides [33,34]) are also capable to form alkylates with free haeme and haemin and use them for further alkylation, this time between parasite proteins.

Indeed, this seems to be an example of independent parallel evolution making chemical pathways available when needed, thus appearing de novo without connection to previous genetic information.

2.1. The Artemisinins

The active principle in qinghaosu is a lactol endoperoxide, which was used to produce artemether (ART) and artesunate, two semisynthetic artemisinin derivatives which become active after being metabolised in the blood into dihydro-artemisinin [35]. The current working hypothesis is that this drug acts through haeme-dependent reduction to sequentially generate free radicals: the haeme iron first attacks and breaks the endoperoxide linkage to artemisinin, producing an oxygen-free radical, which is then rearranged to produce a carbon-free radical that causes lethal damage through the alkylation of parasite proteins [36]. Work by Xiao et al. [31,37–39] and Chaturvedi et al. [36], further developed and summarized by Xiao and Sun [26], indicates that the same pathway is followed with respect to *Schistosoma*. Antioxidant enzymes systems available in adult worms, but not common in immature ones, can prevent this effect. However, to be effective, the drug needs to be ingested by the parasite, enabling the interaction with haemin or haeme causing damage to the worm gut by generating one or many substances toxic to these worms in amounts overwhelming the pathway leading to the hemozoin. The fact that the gut suffers particularly severe damage after ART treatment supports this chain of events [37]. A disadvantage of the artemisinin derivatives is their short in vivo half-life, typically ~2 h in humans [40].

2.2. Praziquantel

In spite of being used for 40 years, and most of that time in the form of MDA, the exact molecular mechanism of PZQ remains unknown. However, the drug has no effect on the enzymes discussed above but relies on a rapid influx of Ca^{2+} into the worm (interestingly, immature forms are refractory), leading to intense muscular paralysis together with damage to the tegument [41,42]. How this disruption is linked to the original binding of the drug is still unknown, but it is thought that the exposure of parasite surface antigens leads to recognition and parasite clearance through immunological means, something which may indirectly account for the difference in sensitivity between juvenile and mature stages [43]. Although the receptor is not known, it has been shown that PZQ disrupts ion transport and recent experimental evidence indicates that transient potential (TRP) channels are targeted by the drug; this could result in the increased permeability of adult schistosome cell membranes towards calcium ions [44].

2.3. Combination Treatment

With artemisinins active against immature schistosome worms [25,45,46] and PZQ primarily targeting adults [47,48], the combination of PZQ and ART presents a chemotherapeutic perfect storm against this parasite as shown in Figure 1, where the y-axle shows the cidal effect expressed as percentage of killed parasites in the experimental animals used. Although small susceptibility variations with respect to parasite age can be seen between the species, there is also a short period coinciding with a larval age between 4 and 5 weeks when all three species are partially refractory against both ART and PZQ. However, the main difference between the two drugs is that the former is predominantly active against juvenile stages and the latter against adult stages. In addition, although PZQ shows a similar activity against *S. haematobium* and *S. japonicum* worms, there is quite a different picture when given to *S. mansoni*, as it obviously also has some activity against juvenile stages.

S. mansoni reactions to ART according to experiments by Xiao et al. [46] and to PZQ by Gönnert and Andrews [48], were confirmed by Sabah et al. [47]; *S. japonicum* to ART by Xiao et al. [39] and to PZQ by Xiao et al. [49], were confirmed by Wu et al. [50]; and *S. haematobium* to PZQ by Botros et al. [51]. Note that *S. haematobium* reactions to ART represent indirect information on parasite susceptibility based on tegumental damage [52,53] and cannot therefore be directly compared with other measurements presented in this figure.

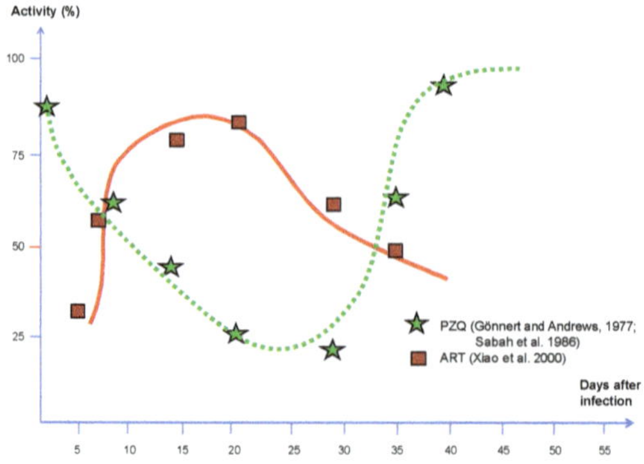

S. mansoni

(**A**)

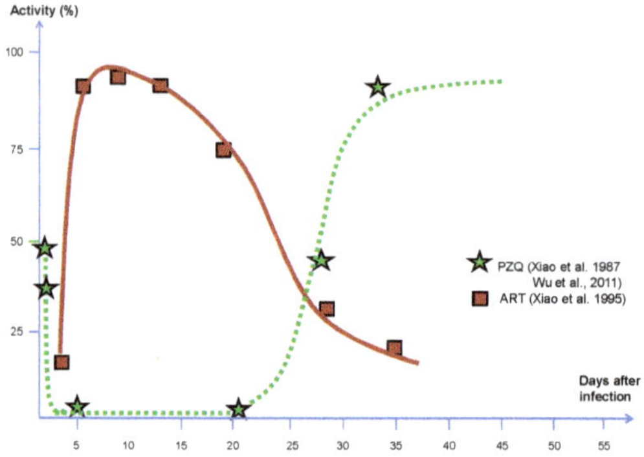

S. japonicum

(**B**)

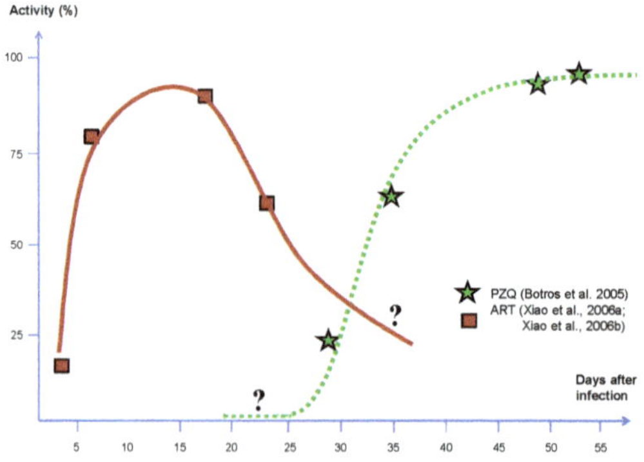

S. haematobium

(**C**)

Figure 1. Activity of artemether and praziquantel in relation to different stages of maturity in all three main schistosome species. (**A**) *S. mansoni*; (**B**) *S. japonicum*; (**C**) *S. haematobium*.

3. Drug Resistance

3.1. *Artemether*

Resistance to artemisinins in malaria parasites, defined as a slower rate of parasite clearance in patients under treatment, has emerged in Southeast Asia's Mekong region [54]. The parasites are thought to mount a defensive stress response, and recent evidence suggests that this response in certain mutants is enhanced, thus promoting parasite survival leading to drug resistance [55]. These authors have shown that the enhanced cellular defence response that underlies resistance development enables very early ring stages to withstand drug exposure for longer. However, in this case, the intrinsic sensitivity to artemisinin is retained [55], which is an encouraging sign that might also play a role in schistosomiasis therapy in due course, although there is as of yet no knowledge about this. On the other hand, drug resistance may still appear in the longer perspective, and might well do so if the drug were to be incorporated in widespread control schemes. It should also be said that the determination of whether or not resistance has developed is not straightforward when the drugs are used against schistosomiasis as the parasites are localized in abdominal veins, that is, in areas where they cannot be directly observed.

A major problem preventing the use of ART for schistosomiasis control is the increased risk for the spread of drug resistance against malaria. This is very clearly a big risk, and the use of the drug against schistosomiasis should be restricted to areas outside those where there is any trace of malaria transmission. As can be seen in Figure 2, there are such areas—in China, Brazil, Mediterranean Africa including Egypt, and the Middle East—where a combination treatment would be particularly useful at the elimination stage.

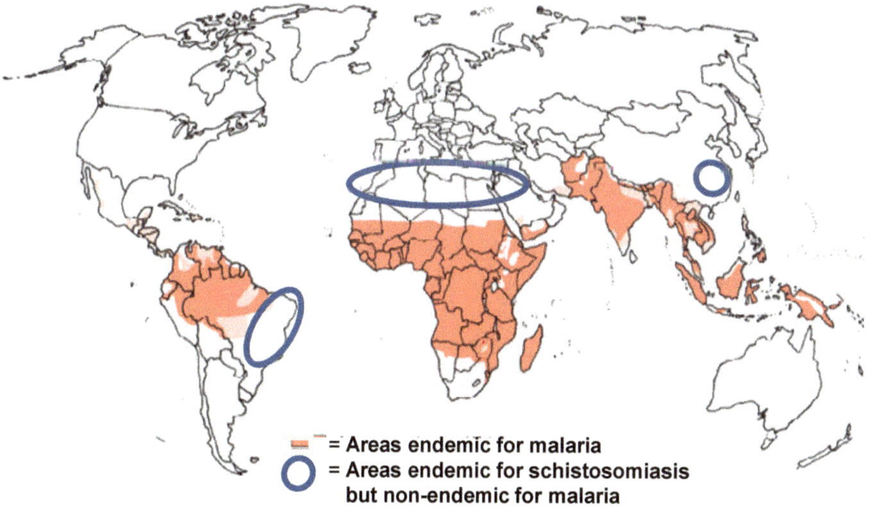

Figure 2. Areas where artemisinin derivates can be used for transmission interruption of schistosomiasis.

3.2. *Praziquantel*

Drug resistance, to be expected after long-term use of repeated, extensive application, is a clear risk, but evidence with respect to PZQ remains scant. However, if it were to emerge, current efforts to eliminate schistosomiasis would be severely challenged requiring alternative and/or complementary drugs [56,57]. Ominously, drug resistance against PZQ has been generated in the laboratory following treatments of *S. mansoni* strains with subcurative drug doses [58–61], proving that it cannot be ruled out. Furthermore, resistant *S. mansoni* isolates have been reported from various African sites (Egypt and Kenya in particular [62–64]), while several cases of failed parasite clearance following a standard treatment for *S. haematobium* infections in Africa have also been shown [65–67]. In China, the emergence of drug resistance has also been experimentally produced [68,69], including reports of resistant *S. japonicum* isolates [70]. Based on the evidence referred to above, it can be concluded that drug resistance in the field is a clear possibility and it is just a question of how fast it will spread once established.

Even if the influx of calcium ions into the worm after exposure to PZQ is regularly observed, the molecular mechanism of PZQ's mode of action is not fully unravelled. The lack of widespread resistance after long-term use may be due to the presence of multiple pharmacologically relevant targets, and Thomas and Timson [71] suggest that PZQ may act, at least in part, on a protein–protein interaction and that altered drug metabolism or enhanced drug efflux are the most likely ways resistance may arise. Additionally, laboratory tests to identify resistance to PZQ have demonstrated a specific region in the parasite genome which might be responsible for reduced drug susceptibility [72].

4. Trials and Community-based Studies

Although annual or biennial MDA with PZQ controls schistosomiasis morbidity well, even in high-transmission areas, it does not generally achieve any significant reduction in transmission [73]. ART, on the other hand, has been shown to do so in several randomized control studies [74–78], at least during the limited time covered by the studies. With regard to single-drug trials using artemether, Utzinger et al. [79] investigated the use of ART for prevention of *S. mansoni* infection using a randomized, double-blind, placebo-controlled trial in Côte d'Ivoire, demonstrating that ART resulted in a significantly lower incidence of infection (24% versus 48.6%, relative risk: 0.50 [95% CI 0.35–0.71], $p = 0.00006$), translating into a 50% risk reduction. A follow-up study on the application of ART against *S. haematobium* in the same country found similar results, although the protective efficacy was considerably lower [78]. A few studies more similar to interventions have been carried out. In Nigeria, for example, PZQ combined with artesunate was used for the treatment of urinary schistosomiasis in 312 randomly selected schoolchildren, reaching a cure rate of 89%, something statistically significant. Two groups, given either monotherapy with PZQ and artesunate to compare, showed a 73% and 71% cure, respectively, demonstrating that the use of combination treatment is both safe and more effective than treatment with either drug alone [76].

Results of a systematic reviews and meta-analysis of a large number of clinical trials have demonstrated the superior performance of the combined drug regimens versus single-drug application, as shown by Wu et al. [45], Liu et al. [35] and Perez del Villar et al. [80]. The first two reviews concerned *S. japonicum* infections only, out of which the former reports ten randomized controlled trials with participants ranging from 318 to 5098; four were multi-centre studies, and six were carried out at single centres. Artemisinin compounds (artesunate or ART) had few side effects and were found to be effective at 7-day and 15-day intervals (preferentially when used at 15-day intervals) for preventing infection during short-term exposures, such as during flooding relief work [45]. Liu et al. [35] state that protection was considerably higher when using combination therapy (84–97%), while it was only 52% with monotherapy (PZQ at 40 mg/Kg), while increasing the dosage to 60 or 100 mg/Kg resulted in a protection rate up to 91%. Interestingly, the protection rate of artemisinin derivates alone exceeded that of PZQ alone with protection rates reaching 97%, the highest rates achieved when the number of doses (3–8) were increased and the interval between them shortened from 1 month to 1 week. Confirming these results, not only for *S. japonicum* but also for *S. haematobium* and *S. mansoni*, Perez del Villar et al. [80] also reported better results with combination therapy than that achieved using either drug alone. In addition, the reviews convey the impression that ART, rather than artesunate, is the preferable choice when combined with PZQ.

In Egypt, good PZQ coverage has resulted in a substantial drop of infection intensities in most endemic settings [81–83]. However, despite a regular distribution of PZQ since almost 20 years, transmission continues at an appreciable and unacceptable level in many foci, especially in the Nile Delta. The experience in Kafer El-Sheikh Governorate, located close to the end of the Rosetta branch of the Nile River in the northern part of the Delta, is one of the hotspot areas with regard to transmission that clearly reflects the failure of controlling schistosomiasis with PZQ alone. As shown by Barakat et al. [81,82] and Haggag et al. [84], the prevalence and intensity of infection in children newly enrolled in primary schools remain almost unaffected [75]. In addition, premature interruption of MDA programmes due to the insensitivity of routinely used diagnostic tests often result in the re-emergence of infection in the span of a few years with concern that the prevalence and intensity of infection might again bounce back to higher levels.

Our own field experience in Kafer El-Sheikh Governorate have clearly demonstrated the remarkably positive effect of giving ART and PZQ in combination [74]. We conducted a double-blind, randomized controlled trial with 913 children, in which two groups (experimental and controls) received 40 mg/kg body weight of PZQ twice, four weeks apart at baseline. Afterwards, the experimental group received 6 mg/kg body weight of ART every 3 weeks in 5 cycles during the transmission season, and the control group received a placebo. At the end of the study, prevalence of infection in the group receiving ART was approximately half that of the placebo group: 6.7% versus 11.6%, and incidence of new infection for the ART group was 2.7% versus 6.5% for the placebo group, i.e., a clearly significant risk reduction. What was unique about this study is that we treated the patent infection with two doses of PZQ 4 weeks apart, 40 mg/Kg each to maximize the cure rate, thereby achieving the aim to evaluate the prophylactic effect of ART alone. It should be added that five annual rounds of PZQ treatment with a coverage rate above 90% in the same area was shown to have reduced the incidence from 29% to 12 %, while the incidence dropped from approximately 19% in 2000 to 12% in 2001 [85]. Another study including 2382 individuals of both sexes and all ages in five high-risk Nile Delta villages in Kafer El-Sheikh showed an overall prevalence of schistosomiasis of 29% with a generally low intensity of infection. Although this result was deemed positive compared to the situation before MDA using PZQ was implemented, the outcome was tempered by the insight that transmission remained largely uninterrupted after long-term uninterrupted control activities [75]. To ensure better cure rates in this area, prevent rapid re-infection, and avoid the potential development of drug resistance, the use of ART/PZQ combinations should be instituted.

5. Discussion

Treatment failure can be due to drug resistance against PZQ, but it can also be due to a lack of therapeutic efficacy of the drug with respect to juvenile trematode flukes as shown by Doenhoff et al. [86]. In this connection, it should also be considered that PZQ, though it has a strong curative effect, never reaches 100% efficacy. These facts together reveal that this drug is not transmission-blocking, making the goal of elimination of schistosomiasis illusory if not combined with other drugs or tools, such as snail control, health education, water, sanitation, and hygiene (WASH). Overall, complementing PZQ with ART would not only target all stages of the parasite, from its penetration into the host (when PZQ has an ultra-short activity to the organism covering only a few hours) over its first weeks of growth to the adult stage. Importantly, by targeting the stages before egg production has started, the artemisinin derivates are truly a transmission-blocking drugs. In addition, its already high efficacy can be raised to almost 100% by using several doses provided on a weekly basis [46]; however, this approach would not be realistic in practise. This is of course only acceptable for short periods, when prevention is needed for which it has successfully been applied in flooding interventions in China [35,45]. Prolonged treatment periods have not been tried.

The successful outcome of 40 years of schistosomiasis chemotherapy using PZQ, most of this time in the form of MDA is of a magnitude relieving morbidity and suffering of millions of people. This accomplishment has led to thoughts of worldwide elimination of the disease in the next decade, though others feel that it might take longer [87]. The stumbling block is that PZQ does not block transmission. This can, however, be achieved by conferring a transmission-blocking modality to current chemotherapy through the addition of artemisinin derivatives that act before the infection results in adult worms capable of producing eggs. However, due to the risk of drug resistance, which is already emerging in Southeast Asia, APT cannot be recommended in areas where ACT is needed for malaria care. On the other hand, China, Mediterranean Africa, and also large areas elsewhere where schistosomiasis and malaria do not overlap are also locations where the elimination of schistosomiasis would have the best chance of rapid success. As side effects of an ART treatment are mild or non-existent, we propose a precision treatment approach, involving repeated ART treatments (monthly or bimonthly) backed up with PZQ biannually until elimination has been achieved. However, the elimination of schistosomiasis from sub-Saharan Africa cannot depend on artemisinin derivates, due to the need to reserve these drugs for malaria treatment; it will therefore require more complicated, long-term schemes, preferably including a vaccine. It is encouraging that, thanks to high-resolution diagnostics, both for humans [88] and snails [89], it should be possible to keep areas scheduled for elimination under surveillance so that rapid response can be raised whenever needed [90].

Thanks to donors supporting purchase and distribution of PZQ (e.g., the Schistosomiasis Control Initiative working in Africa (http://www.imperial.ac.uk/schistosomiasis-control-initiative), the drug been made available free of charge in all large endemic areas. However, as pointed above, there is still a shortfall with respect to PZQ [2]. The addition of ART would raise the cost further but before requesting the extra funds, more convincing data is required. Although the field trials mentioned here support combination therapy, testing in conjunction with more sensitive and quantitative diagnostic tools will be needed to take us closer to the goal of applying ART/PZQ therapy for schistosomiasis elimination in non-malarious areas. Indeed, such diagnostic assays [91–93] have already shown that the extent of schistosome infection has been greatly underestimated, due to the diagnostic deficit of stool examination and urine filtration which are still commonly used in the endemic areas [94].

6. Conclusions

The obvious problem with PZQ is that it does not block transmission. Snail control has been tried with questionable results since the snails hosts of *S. mansoni* and *S. haematobium* are non-amphibious and can survive long dry periods. The outcome in China has been better, although not completely successful there either, since the intermediate snail host of *S. japonicum* is amphibious and therefore slightly easier to control. Other underlying factors favouring transmission are ecological conditions, poor sanitation, and the high intensity of unprotected water contact. Under such circumstances, additional control measures need to be adopted. One of these measures would be to change the current MDA strategy to include a combination of PZQ and ART in certain areas based on the rationale that it would confer a transmission-blocking modality to current chemotherapy. thereby ensuring higher cure rates, reducing (possibly even preventing) transmission and rapid re-infection, and avoiding a potential development of resistance to either drug.

The spatiotemporal risk for reinfection dominates in endemic areas, which in principle would require keeping people on constant chemotherapy, at least for a period of time. Although this is not a realistic approach, a strategy consisting of PZQ provided at 6-month intervals together with a monthly ART treatment might be the recipe for not only achieving elimination, but in fact also making local eradication possible. It remains to be investigated how long APT regimens should last and how realistic this approach would be.

Author Contributions: Both authors produced the main body of text together. R.B. conceived the draft, focusing on drug origin and mode of action studies. H.M. contributed field use of combined treatment and clinical trials.

Funding: This research received no external funding.

Conflicts of Interest: The authors declare no conflict of interest.

References

1. WHO. Accelerating Work to Overcome the Global Impact of Neglected Tropical Diseases. Available online: http://www.who.int/neglected_diseases/NTD_RoadMap_2012_Fullversion.pdf (accessed on 3 December 2018).
2. WHO. Schistosomiasis Fact Sheet of 20 February 2018. Available online: http://www.who.int/news-room/fact-sheets/detail/schistosomiasis (accessed on 20 August 2018).
3. Hotez, P.J.; Asojo, O.A.; Adesina, A.M. Nigeria: "Ground Zero" for the high prevalence neglected tropical diseases. *PLoS Negl. Trop. Dis.* **2012**, *6*, e1600. [CrossRef]
4. Barakat, R.; El Morshedy, H. Efficacy of two praziquantel treatments among primary school children in an area of high *Schistosoma mansoni* endemicity, Nile Delta, Egypt. *Parasitology* **2011**, *138*, 440–446. [CrossRef]
5. El-Khoby, T.; Galal, N.; Fenwick, A.; Barakat, R.; El-Hawey, A.; Nooman, Z.; Habib, M.; Abdel-Wahab, F.; Gabr, N.S.; Hammam, H.M.; et al. The epidemiology of schistosomiasis in Egypt: Summary findings in nine governorates. *Am. J. Trop. Med. Hyg.* **2000**, *62*, 88–99. [CrossRef]
6. Gryseels, B. Schistosomiasis. *Infect. Dis. Clin. N. Am.* **2012**, *26*, 383–397. [CrossRef]
7. Sow, S.; de Vlas, S.J.; Stelma, F.; Vereecken, K.; Gryseels, B.; Polman, K. The contribution of water contact behavior to the high *Schistosoma mansoni* Infection rates observed in the Senegal River Basin. *BMC Infect. Dis.* **2011**, *11*, 198. [CrossRef]
8. Davis, A.; Wegner, D.H. Multicentre trials of praziquantel in human schistosomiasis: Design and techniques. *Bull. World Health Organ.* **1979**, *57*, 767–771.
9. Colley, D.G.; Bustinduy, A.L.; Secor, W.E.; King, C.H. Human schistosomiasis. *Lancet* **2014**, *383*, 2253–2264. [CrossRef]
10. Zhou, X.N.; Bergquist, R.; Leonardo, L.; Yang, G.J.; Yang, K.; Sudomo, M.; Olveda, R. Schistosomiasis japonica control and research needs. *Adv. Parasitol.* **2010**, *72*, 145–178. [CrossRef]
11. King, C.H. Parasites and poverty: The case of schistosomiasis. *Acta Trop.* **2010**, *113*, 95–104. [CrossRef]
12. Hay, S.I.; Abajobir, A.A.; Abate, K.H.; Abbafati, C.; Abbas, K.M.; Abd-Allah, F.; Abdulkader, R.S.; Abdulle, A.M.; Abebo, T.A.; Abera, S.F.; et al. Global, regional, and national disability-adjusted life-years (DALYs) for 333 diseases and injuries and healthy life expectancy (HALE) for 195 countries and territories, 1990–2016: A systematic analysis for the Global Burden of Disease Study 2016. *Lancet* **2017**, *390*, 1260–1344. [CrossRef]
13. Murray, C.J.; Vos, T.; Lozano, R.; Naghavi, M.; Flaxman, A.D.; Michaud, C.; Ezzati, M.; Shibuya, K.; Salomon, J.A.; Abdalla, S.; et al. Disability-adjusted life years (DALYs) for 291 diseases and injuries in 21 regions, 1990–2010: A systematic analysis for the Global Burden of Disease Study 2010. *Lancet* **2012**, *380*, 2197–2223. [CrossRef]
14. Chen, J.; Xu, J.; Bergquist, R.; Li, S.Z.; Zhou, X.N. "Farewell to the God of Plague": The Importance of Political Commitment Towards the Elimination of Schistosomiasis. *Trop. Med. Infect. Dis.* **2018**, *3*, 108. [CrossRef]
15. Tu, Y. The discovery of artemisinin (qinghaosu) and gifts from Chinese medicine. *Nat. Med.* **2011**, *17*, 1217–1220. [CrossRef]
16. Tu, Y. The development of the antimalarial drugs with new type of chemical structure–qinghaosu and dihydroqinghaosu. *Southeast Asian J. Trop. Med. Publ. Health* **2004**, *35*, 250–251.
17. Faurant, C. From bark to weed: The history of artemisinin. *Parasite* **2011**, *18*, 215–218. [CrossRef]
18. Miller, L.H.; Su, X. Artemisinin: Discovery from the Chinese herbal garden. *Cell* **2011**, *146*, 855–858. [CrossRef]
19. Klayman, D.L. Qinghaosu (artemisinin): An antimalarial drug from China. *Science* **1985**, *228*, 1049–1055. [CrossRef]
20. Gardner, B. A present from Chairman Mao. Welcome News Supplement 6: Research Directions in Malaria. *Wellcome Trust* **2002**, *25* Suppl. 6.
21. Li, Y.; Wu, Y.L. How Chinese scientists discovered qinghaosu (artemisinin) and developed its derivatives? What are the future perspectives? *Med. Trop. Rev. Corps Sante Colonial* **1998**, *58*, 9–12.
22. Ansari, M.T.; Saify, Z.S.; Sultana, N.; Ahmad, I.; Saeed-Ul-Hassan, S.; Tariq, I.; Khanum, M. Malaria and artemisinin derivatives: An updated review. *Mini Rev. Med. Chem.* **2013**, *13*, 1879–1902. [CrossRef]
23. Tu, Y. Artemisinin-A Gift from Traditional Chinese Medicine to the World (Nobel Lecture). *Angew. Chem.* **2016**, *55*, 10210–10226. [CrossRef] [PubMed]

24. Tambo, E.; Khater, E.I.; Chen, J.H.; Bergquist, R.; Zhou, X.N. Nobel prize for the artemisinin and ivermectin discoveries: A great boost towards elimination of the global infectious diseases of poverty. *Infec. Dis. Poverty* **2015**, *4*, 58. [CrossRef] [PubMed]
25. Chen, D.J.; Fu, L.F.; Shao, P.P.; Wu, F.Z.; Fan, C.Z.; Shu, H.; Ren, C.X.; Sheng, X.L. Experimental studies on antischistosomal activity of qinghaosu. *Chin. Med. J.* **1980**, *60*, 422–425.
26. Xiao, S.H.; Sun, J. *Schistosoma* hemozoin and its possible roles. *Int. J. Parasitol.* **2017**, *47*, 171–183. [CrossRef] [PubMed]
27. Pagola, S.; Stephens, P.W.; Bohle, D.S.; Kosar, A.D.; Madsen, S.K. The structure of malaria pigment beta-haematin. *Nature* **2000**, *404*, 307–310. [CrossRef] [PubMed]
28. Homewood, C.A.; Jewsbury, J.M. Comparison of malarial and schistosome pigment. *Trans. R. Soc. Trop. Med. Hyg.* **1972**, *66*, 1–2. [CrossRef]
29. Meunier, B.; Robert, A. Heme as trigger and target for trioxane-containing antimalarial drugs. *Acc. Chem. Res.* **2010**, *43*, 1444–1451. [CrossRef] [PubMed]
30. Creek, D.J.; Charman, W.N.; Chiu, F.C.; Prankerd, R.J.; Dong, Y.; Vennerstrom, J.L.; Charman, S.A. Relationship between antimalarial activity and heme alkylation for spiro- and dispiro-1,2,4-trioxolane antimalarials. *Antimicrob. Agents Chemother.* **2008**, *52*, 1291–1296. [CrossRef]
31. Xiao, S.H.; Keiser, J.; Chollet, J.; Utzinger, J.; Dong, Y.; Endriss, Y.; Vennerstrom, J.L.; Tanner, M. In vitro and in vivo activities of synthetic trioxolanes against major human schistosome species. *Antimicrob. Agents Chemother.* **2007**, *51*, 1440–1445. [CrossRef]
32. Pradines, V.; Portela, J.; Boissier, J.; Cosledan, F.; Meunier, B.; Robert, A. Trioxaquine PA1259 alkylates heme in the blood-feeding parasite *Schistosoma mansoni*. *Antimicrob. Agents Chemother.* **2011**, *55*, 2403–2405. [CrossRef]
33. Dong, Y.; Wang, X.; Kamaraj, S.; Bulbule, V.J.; Chiu, F.C.; Chollet, J.; Dhanasekaran, M.; Hein, C.D.; Papastogiannidis, P.; Morizzi, J.; et al. Structure-Activity Relationship of the Antimalarial Ozonide Artefenomel (OZ439). *J. Med. Chem.* **2017**, *60*, 2654–2668. [CrossRef] [PubMed]
34. Xue, J.; Wang, X.; Dong, Y.; Vennerstrom, J.L.; Xiao, S.H. Effect of ozonide OZ418 against *Schistosoma japonicum* harbored in mice. *Parasitol. Res.* **2014**, *113*, 3259–3266. [CrossRef]
35. Liu, R.; Dong, H.F.; Guo, Y.; Zhao, Q.P.; Jiang, M.S. Efficacy of praziquantel and artemisinin derivatives for the treatment and prevention of human schistosomiasis: A systematic review and meta-analysis. *Parasites Vectors* **2011**, *4*, 201. [CrossRef] [PubMed]
36. Chaturvedi, D.; Goswami, A.; Saikia, P.P.; Barua, N.C.; Rao, P.G. Artemisinin and its derivatives: A novel class of anti-malarial and anti-cancer agents. *Chem. Soc. Rev.* **2010**, *39*, 435–454. [CrossRef] [PubMed]
37. Xiao, S.H.; Mei, J.Y.; Jiao, P.Y. *Schistosoma japonicum*-infected hamsters (Mesocricetus auratus) used as a model in experimental chemotherapy with praziquantel, artemether, and OZ compounds. *Parasitol. Res.* **2011**, *108*, 431–437. [CrossRef] [PubMed]
38. Xiao, S.; Chollet, J.; Utzinger, J.; Matile, H.; Mei, J.; Tanner, M. Artemether administered together with haemin damages schistosomes in vitro. *Trans. R. Soc. Trop. Med. Hyg.* **2001**, *95*, 67–71. [PubMed]
39. Xiao, S.H.; You, J.Q.; Yang, Y.Q.; Wang, C.Z. Experimental studies on early treatment of schistosomal infection with artemether. *Southeast Asian J. Trop. Med. Publ. Health* **1995**, *26*, 306–318.
40. Djimde, A.; Lefevre, G. Understanding the pharmacokinetics of Coartem. *Malar. J.* **2009**, *8* (Suppl. 1), S4. [CrossRef]
41. Chan, J.D.; Zarowiecki, M.; Marchant, J.S. Ca^{2+} channels and praziquantel: A view from the free world. *Parasitol. Int.* **2013**, *62*, 619–628. [CrossRef] [PubMed]
42. Xiao, S.; Binggui, S.; Chollet, J.; Tanner, M. Tegumental changes in 21-day-old *Schistosoma mansoni* harboured in mice treated with artemether. *Acta Trop.* **2000**, *75*, 341–348. [CrossRef]
43. Cupit, P.M.; Cunningham, C. What is the mechanism of action of praziquantel and how might resistance strike? *Future Med. Chem.* **2015**, *7*, 701–705. [CrossRef] [PubMed]
44. Bais, S.; Greenberg, R.M. TRP channels as potential targets for antischistosomals. *Int. J. Parasitol. Drugs Drug Resist.* **2018**, *8*, 511–517. [CrossRef] [PubMed]
45. Wu, T.X.; Liu, G.J.; Zhang, M.M.; Wang, Q.; Ni, J.; Wei, J.F.; Zhou, L.K.; Duan, X.; Chen, X.Y.; Zheng, J.; et al. Systematic review of benefits and harms of artemisinin-type compounds for preventing schistosomiasis. *Zhonghua Yi Xue Za Zhi* **2003**, *83*, 1219–1224. [PubMed]

46. Shuhua, X.; Chollet, J.; Weiss, N.A.; Bergquist, R.N.; Tanner, M. Preventive effect of artemether in experimental animals infected with *Schistosoma mansoni*. *Parasitol. Int.* **2000**, *49*, 19–24. [CrossRef]
47. Sabah, A.A.; Fletcher, C.; Webbe, G.; Doenhoff, M.J. *Schistosoma mansoni*: Chemotherapy of infections of different ages. *Exp. Parasitol.* **1986**, *61*, 294–303. [CrossRef]
48. Gonnert, R.; Andrews, P. Praziquantel, a new board-spectrum antischistosomal agent. *Zeitschrift fur Parasitenkunde* **1977**, *52*, 129–150. [CrossRef] [PubMed]
49. Xiao, S.H.; Yue, W.J.; Yang, Y.Q.; You, J.Q. Susceptibility of *Schistosoma japonicum* to different developmental stages to praziquantel. *Chin. Med. J.* **1987**, *100*, 759–768.
50. Wu, W.; Wang, W.; Huang, Y.X. New insight into praziquantel against various developmental stages of schistosomes. *Parasitol. Res.* **2011**, *109*, 1501–1507. [CrossRef]
51. Botros, S.; Pica-Mattoccia, L.; William, S.; El-Lakkani, N.; Cioli, D. Effect of praziquantel on the immature stages of *Schistosoma haematobium*. *Int. J. Parasitol.* **2005**, *35*, 1453–1457. [CrossRef]
52. Xiao, S.U.; Utzinger, J.; Shen, B.G.; Tanner, M.; Chollet, J. Ultrastructural alterations of adult *Schistosoma haematobium* harbored in mice following artemether administration. *Zhongguo Ji Sheng Chong Xue Yu Ji Sheng Chong Bing Za Zhi* **2006**, *24*, 321–328.
53. Shu-Hua, X.; Utzinger, J.; Chollet, J.; Tanner, M. Effect of artemether administered alone or in combination with praziquantel to mice infected with Plasmodium berghei or *Schistosoma mansoni* or both. *Int. J. Parasitol.* **2006**, *36*, 957–964. [CrossRef] [PubMed]
54. WHO. Q&A on artemisinin resistance. 2018. Available online: https://www.who.int/malaria/media/artemisinin_resistance_qa/en/ (accessed on 11 November 2018).
55. Tilley, L.; Straimer, J.; Gnadig, N.F.; Ralph, S.A.; Fidock, D.A. Artemisinin Action and Resistance in *Plasmodium falciparum*. *Trends Parasitol.* **2016**, *32*, 682–696. [CrossRef] [PubMed]
56. Bergquist, R.; Utzinger, J.; Keiser, J. Controlling schistosomiasis with praziquantel: How much longer without a viable alternative? *Infect. Dis. Poverty* **2017**, *6*, 74. [CrossRef] [PubMed]
57. Cioli, D.; Valle, C.; Angelucci, F.; Miele, A.E. Will new antischistosomal drugs finally emerge? *Trends Parasitol.* **2008**, *24*, 379–382. [CrossRef] [PubMed]
58. Lotfy, W.M.; Hishmat, M.G.; El Nashar, A.S.; Abu El Einin, H.M. Evaluation of a method for induction of praziquantel resistance in *Schistosoma mansoni*. *Pharm. Biol.* **2015**, *53*, 1214–1219. [CrossRef] [PubMed]
59. Couto, F.F.; Coelho, P.M.; Araujo, N.; Kusel, J.R.; Katz, N.; Jannotti-Passos, L.K.; Mattos, A.C. *Schistosoma mansoni*: A method for inducing resistance to praziquantel using infected Biomphalaria glabrata snails. *Mem. Inst. Oswaldo Cruz* **2011**, *106*, 153–157. [CrossRef] [PubMed]
60. Ismail, M.; Metwally, A.; Farghaly, A.; Bruce, J.; Tao, L.F.; Bennett, J.L. Characterization of isolates of *Schistosoma mansoni* from Egyptian villagers that tolerate high doses of praziquantel. *Am. J. Trop. Med. Hyg.* **1996**, *55*, 214–218. [CrossRef] [PubMed]
61. Fallon, P.G.; Doenhoff, M.J. Drug-resistant schistosomiasis: Resistance to praziquantel and oxamniquine induced in *Schistosoma mansoni* in mice is drug specific. *Am. J. Trop. Med. Hug.* **1994**, *51*, 83–88. [CrossRef]
62. Mwangi, I.N.; Sanchez, M.C.; Mkoji, G.M.; Agola, L.E.; Runo, S.M.; Cupit, P.M.; Cunningham, C. Praziquantel sensitivity of Kenyan *Schistosoma mansoni* isolates and the generation of a laboratory strain with reduced susceptibility to the drug. *Int. J. Parasitol. Drugs Drug Resist.* **2014**, *4*, 296–300. [CrossRef]
63. Melman, S.D.; Steinauer, M.L.; Cunningham, C.; Kubatko, L.S.; Mwangi, I.N.; Wynn, N.B.; Mutuku, M.W.; Karanja, D.M.; Colley, D.G.; Black, C.L.; et al. Reduced susceptibility to praziquantel among naturally occurring Kenyan isolates of *Schistosoma mansoni*. *PLoS Negl. Trop. Dis.* **2009**, *3*, e504. [CrossRef]
64. Ismail, M.; Botros, S.; Metwally, A.; William, S.; Farghally, A.; Tao, L.F.; Day, T.A.; Bennett, J.L. Resistance to praziquantel: Direct evidence from *Schistosoma mansoni* isolated from Egyptian villagers. *Am. J. Trop. Med. Hyg.* **1999**, *60*, 932–935. [CrossRef]
65. Alonso, D.; Munoz, J.; Gascon, J.; Valls, M.E.; Corachan, M. Failure of standard treatment with praziquantel in two returned travelers with *Schistosoma haematobium* infection. *Am. J. Trop. Med. Hyg.* **2006**, *74*, 342–344. [CrossRef] [PubMed]
66. Silva, I.M.; Thiengo, R.; Conceicao, M.J.; Rey, L.; Lenzi, H.L.; Pereira Filho, E.; Ribeiro, P.C. Therapeutic failure of praziquantel in the treatment of *Schistosoma haematobium* infection in Brazilians returning from Africa. *Mem. Inst. Oswaldo Cruz* **2005**, *100*, 445–449. [CrossRef] [PubMed]

67. Silva, I.M.; Pereira Filho, E.; Thiengo, R.; Ribeiro, P.C.; Conceicao, M.J.; Panasco, M.; Lenzi, H.L. Schistosomiasis haematobia: Histopathological course determined by cystoscopy in a patient in whom praziquantel treatment failed. *Rev. Inst. Med. Trop. São Paulo* **2008**, *50*, 343–346. [CrossRef] [PubMed]
68. Liang, Y.S.; Li, H.J.; Dai, J.R.; Wang, W.; Qu, G.L.; Tao, Y.H.; Xing, Y.T.; Li, Y.Z.; Qian, K.; Wei, J.Y. Studies on resistance of *Schistosoma* to praziquantel XIII resistance of *Schistosoma japonicum* to praziquantel is experimentally induced in laboratory. *Chin. J. Schistosomiasis Control* **2011**, *23*, 605–610.
69. Li, H.J.; Liang, Y.S.; Dai, J.R.; Wang, W.; Qu, G.L.; Li, Y.Z.; Xing, Y.T.; Tao, Y.H.; Qian, K.; Jia, Y.; et al. Studies on resistance of Schistosoma to praziquantel XIV experimental comparison of susceptibility to praziquantel between PZQ-resistant isolates and PZQ-susceptible isolates of *Schistosoma japonicum* in stages of adult worms, miracidia and cercariae. *Chin. J. Schistosomiasis Control* **2011**, *23*, 611–619.
70. Ke, Q.; You-Sheng, L.; Wei, W.; Guo-Li, Q.; Hong-Jun, L.; Zhen-Kun, Y.; Zheng-Yang, Z.; Yuntian, X.; Jian-Rong, D. Studies on resistance of *Schistosoma* to praziquantel XVII Biological characteristics of praziquantel-resistant isolates of Schistosoma japonicum in mice. *Chin. J. Schistosomiasis Control* **2017**, *29*, 683–688. [CrossRef]
71. Thomas, C.M.; Timson, D.J. The mechanism of action of praziquantel: Six hypotheses. *Curr. Top. Med. Chem.* **2018**. [CrossRef]
72. World Health Organization. Seventh Meeting of the Working Group on Monitoring of Neglected Tropical Diseases Drug Effi Cacy. Geneva, 26–27 February 2018. Available online: http://apps.who.int/iris/bitstream/handle/10665/273620/WHO-CDS-NTD-PCT-2018.06-eng.pdf?ua=1 (accessed on 3 November 2018).
73. King, C.H. The evolving schistosomiasis agenda 2007-2017-Why we are moving beyond morbidity control toward elimination of transmission. *PLoS Negl. Trop. Dis.* **2017**, *11*, e0005517. [CrossRef]
74. Elmorshedy, H.; Tanner, M.; Bergquist, R.N.; Sharaf, S.; Barakat, R. Prophylactic effect of artemether on human schistosomiasis mansoni among Egyptian children: A randomized controlled trial. *Acta Trop.* **2016**, *158*, 52–58. [CrossRef]
75. Elmorshedy, H.; Bergquist, R.; El-Ela, N.E.; Eassa, S.M.; Elsakka, E.E.; Barakat, R. Can human schistosomiasis mansoni control be sustained in high-risk transmission foci in Egypt? *Parasites Vectors* **2015**, *8*, 372. [CrossRef] [PubMed]
76. Inyang-Etoh, P.C.; Ejezie, G.C.; Useh, M.F.; Inyang-Etoh, E.C. Efficacy of a combination of praziquantel and artesunate in the treatment of urinary schistosomiasis in Nigeria. *Trans. R. Soc. Trop. Med. Hyg.* **2009**, *103*, 38–44. [CrossRef] [PubMed]
77. Hou, X.Y.; McManus, D.P.; Gray, D.J.; Balen, J.; Luo, X.S.; He, Y.K.; Ellis, M.; Williams, G.M.; Li, Y.S. A randomized, double-blind, placebo-controlled trial of safety and efficacy of combined praziquantel and artemether treatment for acute schistosomiasis japonica in China. *Bull. World Health Organ.* **2008**, *86*, 788–795. [CrossRef] [PubMed]
78. N'Goran, E.K.; Utzinger, J.; Gnaka, H.N.; Yapi, A.; N'Guessan, N.A.; Kigbafori, S.D.; Lengeler, C.; Chollet, J.; Shuhua, X.; Tanner, M. Randomized, double-blind, placebo-controlled trial of oral artemether for the prevention of patent *Schistosoma haematobium* infections. *Am. J. Trop. Med. Hyg.* **2003**, *68*, 24–32. [CrossRef] [PubMed]
79. Utzinger, J.; N'Goran, E.K.; N'Dri, A.; Lengeler, C.; Xiao, S.; Tanner, M. Oral artemether for prevention of *Schistosoma mansoni* infection: Randomised controlled trial. *Lancet* **2000**, *355*, 1320–1325. [CrossRef]
80. Perez del Villar, L.; Burguillo, F.J.; Lopez-Aban, J.; Muro, A. Systematic review and meta-analysis of artemisinin based therapies for the treatment and prevention of schistosomiasis. *PLoS ONE* **2012**, *7*, e45867. [CrossRef] [PubMed]
81. Barakat, R.; El Morshedy, H.; Farghaly, A. *Neglected Tropical Diseases—Middle East and North Africa*; McDowell, M.A., Rafati, S., Eds.; Springer: New York, NY, USA, 2014.
82. Barakat, R.M. Epidemiology of Schistosomiasis in Egypt: Travel through Time: Review. *J. Adv. Res.* **2013**, *4*, 425–432. [CrossRef]
83. Barakat, R.; Farghaly, A.; El Morshedy, H.; Hassan, M.; Miller de, W. Impact of National Schistosomiasis Control Program in Kafr El-Sheikh governorate, Nile Delta, Egypt: An independent evaluation. *J. Egypt. Public Health Assoc.* **1998**, *73*, 737–753.
84. Haggag, A.A.; Rabiee, A.; Abd Elaziz, K.M.; Gabrielli, A.F.; Abdel Hay, R.; Ramzy, R.M.R. Mapping of *Schistosoma mansoni* in the Nile Delta, Egypt: Assessment of the prevalence by the circulating cathodic antigen urine assay. *Acta Trop.* **2017**, *167*, 9–17. [CrossRef]

85. Barakat, R.; Elmorshedy, H. Annual report of the project entitled: "Establishment and monitoring of cohort school children in Kafer El-Sheikh Governorate, Egypt, in preparation for schistosomiasis vaccine candidate testing when appropriate". Vaccine Development Project (SVDP); Funded by USAID& Egyptian Ministry of Health and Population (EMHP), 1996-2001. Unpublished work.
86. Doenhoff, M.J.; Cioli, D.; Utzinger, J. Praziquantel: Mechanisms of action, resistance and new derivatives for schistosomiasis. *Curr. Opin. Infect. Dis.* **2008**, *21*, 659–667. [CrossRef]
87. Fenwick, A.; Jourdan, P. Schistosomiasis elimination by 2020 or 2030? *Int. J. Parasitol.* **2016**, *46*, 385–388. [CrossRef] [PubMed]
88. Coulibaly, J.T.; N'Gbesso, Y.K.; Knopp, S.; N'Guessan, N.A.; Silue, K.D.; van Dam, G.J.; N'Goran, E.K.; Utzinger, J. Accuracy of urine circulating cathodic antigen test for the diagnosis of *Schistosoma mansoni* in preschool-aged children before and after treatment. *PLoS Negl. Trop. Dis.* **2013**, *7*, e2109. [CrossRef]
89. Qin, Z.Q.; Jing, X.; Feng, T.; Lv, S.; Qian, Y.; Zhang, L.; Li, Y.L.; Chao, L.V.; Bergquist, R.; Li, S.Z.; Zhou, X.N. Field evaluation of a loop-mediated isothermal amplification (LAMP) platform for the detection of *Schistosoma japonicum* infection in Oncomelania hupensis snails. *Trop. Med. Infect. Dis.* **2018**. [CrossRef]
90. Bergquist, R.; Yang, G.J.; Knopp, S.; Utzinger, J.; Tanner, M. Surveillance and response: Tools and approaches for the elimination stage of neglected tropical diseases. *Acta Trop.* **2015**, *141*, 229–234. [CrossRef] [PubMed]
91. Ogongo, P.; Kariuki, T.M.; Wilson, R.A. Diagnosis of schistosomiasis mansoni: An evaluation of existing methods and research towards single worm pair detection. *Parasitology* **2018**, *145*, 1355–1366. [CrossRef] [PubMed]
92. Corstjens, P.L.; De Dood, C.J.; Kornelis, D.; Fat, E.M.; Wilson, R.A.; Kariuki, T.M.; Nyakundi, R.K.; Loverde, P.T.; Abrams, W.R.; Tanke, H.J.; et al. Tools for diagnosis, monitoring and screening of *Schistosoma* infections utilizing lateral-flow based assays and upconverting phosphor labels. *Parasitology* **2014**, *141*, 1841–1855. [CrossRef]
93. Bergquist, R. Good things are worth waiting for. *Am. J. Trop. Med. Hyg.* **2013**, *88*, 409–410. [CrossRef] [PubMed]
94. Colley, D.G.; Andros, T.S.; Campbell, C.H., Jr. Schistosomiasis is more prevalent than previously thought: What does it mean for public health goals, policies, strategies, guidelines and intervention programs? *Infect. Dis. Poverty* **2017**, *6*, 63. [CrossRef] [PubMed]

MDPI
St. Alban-Anlage 66
4052 Basel
Switzerland
Tel. +41 61 683 77 34
Fax +41 61 302 89 18
www.mdpi.com

Tropical Medicine and Infectious Disease Editorial Office
E-mail: tropicalmed@mdpi.com
www.mdpi.com/journal/tropicalmed

www.ingramcontent.com/pod-product-compliance
Lightning Source LLC
LaVergne TN
LVHW071938080526
838202LV00064B/6631